Statistics for Veterinary and
Animal Science

Statistics for Veterinary and Animal Science

Third Edition

Aviva Petrie, BSc, MSc, CStat, CSci, FHEA
Senior Lecturer in Statistics and Head of the Biostatistics Unit
UCL Eastman Dental Institute
University College London

Honorary Lecturer in Medical Statistics
London School of Hygiene and Tropical Medicine
University of London
London
UK

Paul Watson, BSc, BVetMed, PhD, DSc, FRCVS
Emeritus Professor of Reproductive Cryobiology
The Royal Veterinary College
University of London
London
UK

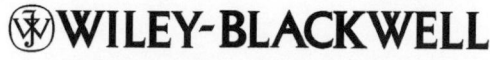
A John Wiley & Sons, Ltd., Publication

This edition first published 2013 © 2013 by John Wiley & Sons, Ltd

Wiley-Blackwell is an imprint of John Wiley & Sons, formed by the merger of Wiley's global Scientific, Technical and Medical business with Blackwell Publishing.

Registered office: John Wiley & Sons, Ltd, The Atrium, Southern Gate, Chichester, West Sussex, PO19 8SQ, UK

Editorial offices: 9600 Garsington Road, Oxford, OX4 2DQ, UK
The Atrium, Southern Gate, Chichester, West Sussex, PO19 8SQ, UK
111 River Street, Hoboken, NJ 07030-5774, USA

For details of our global editorial offices, for customer services and for information about how to apply for permission to reuse the copyright material in this book please see our website at www.wiley.com/wiley-blackwell.

Library of Congress Cataloging-in-Publication Data is available for this title.

A catalogue record for this book is available from the British Library.

Wiley also publishes its books in a variety of electronic formats. Some content that appears in print may not be available in electronic books.

Cover image: Horse illustration: all-silhouettes.com
Pig and dog illustration: Neubau Welt
Cover design by www.hisandhersdesign.co.uk

Set in 10/12 pt Times Ten by Toppan Best-set Premedia Limited

C9780470670750_221123

Contents

Colour plate section can be found facing page 240

Preface to third edition

The continuing interest in our textbook together with the ongoing development of statistical applications in veterinary and animal science has encouraged us to prepare this third edition of *Statistics for Veterinary and Animal Science*. We have introduced some new material but we want to reassure all readers that our original intention of this being an introductory text still stands. Again, you will find everything that you need to begin to understand statistics and its application to your scientific and clinical endeavours; it remains an introduction for the novice with emphasis on understanding the application, rather than exhibiting mathematical competence in the calculations. Readily available statistical software packages, which provide the mechanics of the calculations, have become more extensive in the range of procedures they offer. Accordingly, we have augmented our text, within the bounds of an introductory exposition, to match their development.

As in previous editions, we use two commonly employed statistical software packages, SPSS and Stata, to analyse the data in our examples. We believe that by presenting you with different forms of computer output, you will have the confidence and proficiency to interpret output from other statistical packages. The previous edition of the book had an accompanying CD which contained the data sets (in ASCII, Excel, SPSS and Stata) used as examples in the text. These data sets are now available at www.wiley.com/go/petrie/statisticsforvets, and will be helpful if you wish to get to grips with various statistical techniques by attempting the analyses yourselves. You will find a website icon next to the examples for which the data are available on the website.

Please note that, although we have provided details of a considerable number of websites that you may find useful, we cannot guarantee that these website addresses will remain correct over the course of time because of the mutability of the internet.

Some sections of the book are, as in previous editions, in small print and are accompanied by a jumping horse symbol. These sections contain information that relates to more advanced or obscure topics, and you may skip (jump over) them without loss of continuity. Our teaching experience has demonstrated that one of hardest tasks for the novice when analysing his or her own data set is deciding which test or procedure is most appropriate. To overcome this difficulty, we provide two flow charts (Figure E.2 for binary data and Figure E.3 for numerical data) which lead you through the various questions that need to be asked to aid that decision. Another flow chart (Figure E.1) organizes the tests and procedures into relevant groups and indicates the particular section of the book where each is located: you can find these flow charts in the Appendix as well as on the inside back/front covers for easy reference.

Many of the chapters in this third edition are similar to those in the second edition, apart from some minor modifications and additional exercises. However, Chapter 5 has been extended to include techniques for recognizing and dealing with confounding, and this chapter now provides a description of the different types of missing data that might be encountered. We have added a section on checking the assumptions underlying a logistic regression model to Chapter 11, and have included modifications of the sample size estimation process to take account of different group sizes and losses to follow-up in Chapter 13. Chapter 14 has been expanded considerably by extending the sections on diagnostic tests, measuring agreement and survival analysis as well as Bayesian analysis. Chapter 15 is entirely new, bringing together a group of specialist topics – ethical issues of animal investigation (some of which was in Chapter 5 of the second edition), spatial statistics, surveillance and its importance, and statistics in molecular and quantitative genetics. While none of these is intended as more than an introduction, you will find references to help you explore the topics more fully should you so desire. The section on evidence-based veterinary medicine (EBVM) in Chapter 16 is unchanged from that in the second edition's Chapter 15, but in the third edition this chapter no longer provides guidelines for reporting results. Instead, we have devoted the new Chapter 17 to this topic by presenting different published guidelines relevant to veterinary medicine (i.e. for reporting of livestock trials, research using laboratory animals, diagnostic accuracy studies, observational studies in epidemiology, and systematic reviews and meta-analyses) as a ready reference for those wanting to follow best practice both in planning and in writing up their research. Lastly, in Chapter 18, which is entirely new, we bring together the concepts of EBVM and the guidelines provided in Chapter 17 by proffering a template for the critical appraisal of randomized controlled trials and observational studies. We use this template to critically appraise two published papers, both of which are reproduced in full, and hope that by providing these examples, we will help you develop your own skills in what is an essential, but frequently overlooked, component of statistics.

We are indebted as always to those who, for earlier editions of this book, have offered their data to us to use for examples or exercises, have assisted with the presentation of the illustrations and tables, and have provided critical advice on the text. These colleagues are all identified in the prefaces to the first and second editions. As in earlier editions, we have occasionally taken summary data or abstracts from published papers and have used them to develop exercises or to illustrate techniques: we extend our thanks to the authors and the publishers for the use of this material. For this third edition, we are most grateful to Dr Geoff Pollott and Professor Dirk Pfeiffer (both of the Royal Veterinary College, University of London) for their critical reading and suggestions for sections of Chapter 15. We wish to record our particular thanks to Professor Garry Anderson (University of Melbourne) for his critique of much of the new text. His suggestions have drawn our attention to errors and have considerably improved the presentation. Nonetheless, we remain responsible for all contained herein, and offer it, with all its shortcomings, to our readership.

This preface would not be complete without acknowledging our marriage partners, Gerald and Rosie, and our children, Nina, Andrew and Karen, and Oliver and Anna, who have allowed us once again to engage with this task to their inevitable exclusion, and offer them our most grateful thanks.

Aviva Petrie
Paul Watson
2013

Preface to second edition

It is six years since this book was first available, and we are glad to acknowledge the positive responses we have received to the first edition and the evident uptake of the text for a number of courses around the world. In the intervening period much has happened to encourage us to update and expand our initial text. However, many of the chapters which were in the first edition of the book are changed only slightly, if at all, in this second edition. To these chapters, we have added some exercises and further explanations (for example, on equivalence studies, confounding, interactions and bias, Bayesian analysis and Cox survival analysis) to make the book more comprehensive. We have nevertheless retained our original intent of this being an introductory text starting with very basic concepts for the complete novice in statistics. You will still find sections marked for skipping unless you have a particular need to explore them, and these include the newer more complex analysis methods. This edition also contains the glossaries of notation and of terms, but we have expanded them to reflect the enhanced content of the text. For easy reference, the flow charts for choosing the correct statistical analyses in different situations are now found immediately before the index, and we hope these will serve to guide you to the appropriate procedures and text relating to their use.

Computer software to deal with increasingly sophisticated analytical tools has been developed in recent years in such a way that the associated methodology is more readily accessible to those who previously believed such techniques were out of their reach. As a consequence, we have substantially enhanced the material relating to regression analysis and created a new chapter (Chapter 11) to describe some advanced regression techniques. The latter incorporates the sections on multiple regression and an expanded section on logistic regression from Chapter 10 of the first edition, and introduces Poisson regression, different regression methods which can be used to analyse clustered data, maximum likelihood estimation and the concept of the generalized linear model. Because we have inserted this new Chapter 11, the numbering of the chapters which follow does not accord with that of the corresponding chapters in the first edition.

Chapter 15 is an entirely new chapter which is devoted in large part to introducing the concepts of evidence-based veterinary medicine (EBVM), stressing the role of statistical knowledge as a basis for its practice. The methodology of EBVM describes the processes for integrating, in a systematic way, the results of scientifically conducted studies into day-to-day clinical practice with the aim of improving clinical outcome. This requires the practitioner to develop the skills to evaluate critically the efforts of others in respect of the design of studies, and of the presentation, analysis and interpretation of results. The recognition of the value of the evidence-based approach to veterinary medicine has followed a similar emphasis in human clinical medicine, and is influencing the whole veterinary profession. Accordingly, it is also very much a part of the mainstream veterinary curriculum. Whether you are a practitioner of veterinary medicine or of one of the allied sciences, you will now more than ever need to be conversant with modern biostatistical analysis. Knowing how best to report your own results is also vital if you are to impart knowledge correctly, and so, to this end, we include in Chapter 15 a section on the CONSORT Statement, designed to standardize clinical trial reporting.

Although we refer only to two common statistical packages in the text, SPSS and Stata, sufficient information is given to interpret output from other packages, even though the layout and content may differ to some degree. We have also mentioned a number of websites containing useful information, and which were correct at the time of printing. Given the mutability of the internet, we cannot guarantee that such sites will stay available.

Also included with this edition is a CD containing the data sets used as examples in the text. You can use these data sets to consolidate the learning process. It is only when you attempt the analyses yourself that you are fully able to get to grips with the techniques. Each data set is presented in four different formats (ASCII, Excel, SPSS and Stata), so you should be able to access the data and use the software that is available to you.

We would like to acknowledge the generosity of the late Dr Penny Barber, Mark Corbett, Dr J. E. Edwards, Professor Jonathan Elliott, Professor Gary England, Dr Oliver Garden, Dr Ilke Klaas, Dr Teresa Martinez, Dr Anne Pearson, Dr P. D. Warriss, Professor Avril Waterman-Pearson and Dr Susannah Williams who shared their original data with us, and to others who have allowed us to use their published data. In places, we have taken published summary data and constructed a primary data set to suit our own purposes; if we have misrepresented our colleagues' data, we accept full responsibility. We are particularly grateful to Alex Hunte who lent us his skills in refining the illustrations in the first edition, and to Dr David Moles who assisted with the preparation of the statistical tables. We especially thank Dr Ben Armstrong, Professor Caroline Sabin and Dr Ian Martin who kindly gave us their critical advice as the text of the first edition was developed, and Professor John Smith who was instrumental in getting us to consider writing the book in the first place. In addition, we acknowledge our debt to a host of other colleagues who have helped with discussions over the telephone, with their expertise in areas we are lacking, and in their encouragement to complete what we hope will be a useful contribution to the field of veterinary and animal science. We are particularly indebted to those of our colleagues who have graciously pointed us to our errors, which we hope are now corrected.

Lastly, we again acknowledge with gratitude the patience and encouragement of our marriage partners, Gerald and Rosie, and our children, Nina, Andrew and Karen, and Oliver and Anna, who have once more graciously allowed us to become absorbed in the book and have had to suffer neglect in the process. We trust that they still appreciate the worthiness of the cause!

Aviva Petrie
Paul Watson

Preface to first edition

Although statistics is anathema to many, it is, unquestionably, an essential tool for those involved in animal health and veterinary science. It is imperative that practitioners and research workers alike keep abreast with reports on animal production, new and emerging diseases, risk factors for disease and the efficacy of the ever-increasing number of innovations in veterinary care and of developments in training methods and performance. The most cogent information is usually contained in the appropriate journals; however, the usefulness of these journals relies on the reader having a proper understanding of the statistical methodology underlying study design and data analysis. The modern animal scientist and veterinary surgeon therefore need to be able to handle numerical data confidently and properly. Often, for us, as teachers, there is little time in busy curricula to introduce the subject slowly and systematically; students find they are left bewildered and dejected because the concepts seem too difficult to grasp. While there are many excellent introductory books on medical statistics and on statistics in other disciplines such as economics, business studies and engineering, these books are unrelated to the world of animal science and health, and students soon lose heart. It is our intention to provide a guide to statistics relevant to the study of animal health and disease. In order to illustrate the principles and methods, the reader will find that the text is well endowed with real examples drawn from companion and agricultural animals. Although veterinary epidemiology is closely allied to statistics, we have concentrated only on statistical issues as we feel that this is an area which, until now, has been neglected in veterinary and animal health sciences.

Our book is an introductory text on statistics. We start from very simple concepts, assuming no previous knowledge of statistics, and endeavour to build up an understanding in such a way that progression on to advanced texts is possible. We intend the book to be useful for those without mathematical expertise but with the ability to utilize simple formulae. We recognize the influence of the computer and so we avoid the description of complex hand calculations. Instead, emphasis is placed on understanding of concepts and interpretation of results, often in the context of computer output. In addition to acquiring an ability to perform simple statistical techniques on original data, the reader will be able critically to evaluate the efforts of others in respect of the design of studies, and of the presentation, analysis and interpretation of results. The book can be used either as a self-instructional text or as a basis for courses in statistics. In addition, those who are further on in their studies will be able to use the text as a reference guide to the analysis of their data, whether they be postgraduate students, veterinary practitioners or animal scientists in various other settings. Every section contains sufficient cross referencing for the reader to find the relevant background to the topic.

We would like to acknowledge the generosity of Penny Barber, Mark Corbett, Dr J. E. Edwards, Dr Jonathan Elliott, Dr Gary England, Dr Oliver Garden, Dr Anne Pearson, Dr P. D. Warriss, Professor Avril Waterman-Pearson and Susannah Williams, who shared their original data with us. In places, we have taken published summary data and constructed a primary data set to suit our own purposes; if we have misrepresented our colleagues' data, we accept full responsibility.

We are particularly grateful to Alex Hunte who lent us his skills in preparing the illustrations, and to Dr David Moles who assisted with the preparation of the statistical tables. We especially thank Dr Ben Armstrong, Dr Caroline Sabin and Dr Ian Martin who kindly gave us their critical advice as the text was developed. Professor John Smith was instrumental in getting us to consider writing the text in the first place, and we thank him for his continual encouragement. In addition, we acknowledge our debt to a host of other colleagues who have helped with discussions over the telephone, with their expertise in areas we are lacking, and in general encouragement to complete what we hope will be a useful contribution to the field of veterinary and animal science.

Lastly, we acknowledge with gratitude the patience and encouragement of our families. Our marriage partners, Gerald and Rosie, have endured with fortitude our neglect of them while this work was in preparation. In particular, our children, Nina, Andrew and Karen, and Oliver and Anna, have had to cope with our absorption with the project and lack of involvement in their activities. We trust they will recognize that it was in a good cause.

Aviva Petrie
Paul Watson

About the companion website

This book is accompanied by a companion website:

www.wiley.com/go/petrie/statisticsforvets

The website includes:
- Data files which relate to some of the examples in the text. Each data file is provided for download in four different formats: ASCII, Excel, SPSS and Stata.
- Examples relating to the data files are indicated in the text using the following icon:

1 The whys and wherefores of statistics

1.1 Learning objectives

By the end of this chapter, you should be able to:

- State what is meant by the term 'statistics'.
- Explain the importance of a statistical understanding to the animal scientist.
- Distinguish between a qualitative/categorical and a quantitative/numerical variable.
- List the types of scales on which variables are measured.
- Explain what is meant by the term 'biological variation'.
- Define the terms 'systematic error' and 'random error', and give examples of circumstances in which they may occur.
- Distinguish between precision and accuracy.
- Define the terms 'population' and 'sample', and provide examples of real (finite) and hypothetical (infinite) populations.
- Summarize the differences between descriptive and inferential statistics.

1.2 Aims of the book

1.2.1 What will you get from this book?

All the biological sciences have moved on from simple qualitative description to concepts founded on numerical measurements and counts. The proper handling of these values, leading to a correct understanding of the phenomena, is encompassed by statistics. This book will help you appreciate how the theory of statistics can be useful to you in veterinary and animal science. Statistical techniques are an essential part of communicating information about health and disease of animals, and their agricultural productivity, or value as pets, or in the sporting or working environment. We, the authors, aim to introduce you to the subject of statistics, giving you a sound basis for managing straightforward study design and analysis. Where necessary, we recommend that you extend your knowledge by reference to more specialized texts. Occasionally, we advocate that you seek expert statistical advice to guide you through particularly tricky aspects.

You can use this book in two ways:

1. The chapter sequence is designed to develop your understanding systematically and we therefore recommend that, initially, you work through the chapters in order. You will find certain sections marked in small type with a symbol, which indicates that you can skip these, at a first read through, without subsequent loss of continuity. These marked sections contain information you will find useful as your knowledge develops. Chapters 11, 14 and 15 deal with particular types of analyses which, depending on your areas of interest, you may rarely need.
2. When you are more familiar with the concepts, you can use the book as a reference manual;

Statistics for Veterinary and Animal Science, Third Edition. Aviva Petrie and Paul Watson.
© 2013 John Wiley & Sons, Ltd. Published 2013 by John Wiley & Sons, Ltd.

you will find sufficient cross-referenced information in any section to answer specific queries.

1.2.2 What are learning objectives?

Each chapter has a set of **learning objectives** at the beginning. These set out in task-oriented terms what you should be able to 'do' when you have mastered the concepts in the chapter. You can therefore test your growing understanding; if you are able to perform the tasks in the learning objectives, you have understood the concepts.

1.2.3 Should you use a computer statistics package?

We encourage you to use available computer statistics packages, and therefore we do not dwell on the development of the equations on which the analyses are based. We do, however, present the equations (apart from when they are very complex) for completeness, but you will normally not need to become familiar with them since computer packages will provide an automatic solution. We provide computer output, produced when we analyse the data in the examples, from two statistical packages, mostly from SPSS (IBM SPSS Version 20 (www-01.ibm. com/software/analytics/spss, accessed 9 October 2012)) and occasionally from Stata (Stata 12, StataCorp, 2011, *Stata Statistical Software: Release 12*. College Station, TX: StataCorp LP (www. stata.com/products, accessed 9 October 2012)). Although the layout of the output is particular to each individual package, from our description you should be able to make sense of the output from any other major statistical package.

1.2.4 Will you be able to decide when and how to use a particular procedure?

Our main concern is with the *understanding* that underlies statistical analyses. This will prevent you falling into the pitfalls of misuse that sur-round the unwitting user of statistical packages. We present the subject in a form that we hope is accessible, using examples showing the application of the subject to veterinary and animal science. A brief set of exercises is provided at the end of each chapter, based on the ideas presented within. These exercises should be used to check your understanding of the concepts and procedures; solutions to the exercises are given at the back of the book. The two exceptions are Chapter 17, which provides reporting guidelines and Chapter 18 in which we ask you to critically appraise two published articles, preferably before looking at the 'model answers' provided in the chapter.

1.2.5 Use of the glossaries of notation and terms

Statistical nomenclature is often difficult to remember. We have gathered the most common symbols and equations used throughout this book into a Glossary of notation in Appendix C. This gives you a readily accessible reminder of the meaning of the terminology.

You will find a Glossary of terms in Appendix D. In this glossary, we define common statistical terms which are used in this book. They are also defined at the appropriate places in relevant chapters, but the glossary provides you with a ready reference if you forget the meaning of a term. Terms that are in the glossary are introduced in the text in bold type. Note, however, that there are some instances where bold is purely used for extra emphasis.

1.3 What is statistics?

The number of introductory or elementary texts on the subject of statistics indicates how important the subject has become for everyone in the biological sciences. However, the fact that there are many texts might also suggest that we have yet to discover a foolproof method of presenting what is required.

The problem confronted in biological statistics is as follows. When you make a set of numerical observations in biology, you will usually find that the values are scattered. You need to know whether the values differ because of factors you are interested in (e.g. treatments) or because they are part of a 'background' natural variation. You need to evaluate what the numbers actually mean, and to represent them in a way that readily communicates their meaning to others.

The subject of statistics embraces:

- The design of the study in order that it will reveal the most information efficiently.
- The collection of the data.
- The analysis of the data.
- The presentation of suitably summarized information, often in a graphical or tabular form.
- The interpretation of the analyses in a manner that communicates the findings accurately.

Strictly, this broad numerical approach to biology is correctly termed '**biometry**' but we shall adopt the more generally used term '**statistics**' to cover all aspects. Statistics (meaning this entire process) has become one of the essential tools in modern biology.

1.4 Statistics in veterinary and animal science

One of the common initial responses of both veterinary students and animal science students is: Why do I need to study statistics? The mathematical basis of the subject causes much uncertainty, and the analytical approach is alien. However, in professional life, there are many instances of the relevance of statistics:

- The **published scientific literature** is full of studies in which statistical procedures are employed. Look in any of the relevant scientific journals and notice the number of times reference is made to mean ± SEM (standard error of mean), to statistical significance, to P-values or to t-tests or Chi-squared analysis or analysis of variance or multiple regression analysis. The information is presented in the usual brief form and, without a working knowledge of statistics, you are left to accept the conclusions of the author, unable to examine the strength of the supporting data. Indeed, with the advent of computer-assisted data handling, many practitioners can now collect their own observations and summarize them for the advantage of their colleagues; to do this, they need the benefit of statistical insights.

- The subject of **epidemiology** (see Section 5.2) is gaining prominence in veterinary and animal science, and the concepts of **evidence-based veterinary medicine** (see Section 1.5 and Chapter 16) are being explicitly introduced into clinical practice. As never before, there is an essential need for you to understand the types of trials and investigations that are carried out and to know the meaning of the terms associated with them.

- In the animal health sciences, there are an increasing number of independent **diagnostic services** that will analyse samples for the benefit of health monitoring and maintenance. Those running such laboratory services must always be concerned about quality control and accuracy in measurements made for diagnostic purposes, and must be able to supply clear guidelines for the interpretation of results obtained in their laboratories.

- The **pharmaceutical and agrochemical industries** are required to demonstrate both the safety and the efficacy of their products in an indisputable manner. Such data invariably require a statistical approach to establish and illustrate the basis of the claim for both these aspects. Those involved in pharmaceutical product development need to understand the importance of study design and to ensure the adequacy of the numbers of animals used in treatment groups in order to perform meaningful experiments. Veterinary product licensing committees require a thorough understanding of statistical science so that they can appreciate the data presented to substantiate the claims for a novel therapeutic substance. Finally, practitioners and animal carers are faced with the blandishments of sales representatives with competing claims, and must evaluate the literature which is offered in support of specific agents, from licensed drugs to animal nutrition supplements.

- Increasingly, there is concern about the regulation of **safety and quality of food for human consumption**. Where products of animal origin are involved, the animal scientist and the veterinary profession are at the forefront. Examples are: pharmaceutical product withdrawal times before slaughter based on the pharmacokinetics and pharmacodynamics of the products, the withholding times for milk after therapeutic treatment of the animal, tissue residues of herbicides and insecticides, and the possible contamination of carcasses by antibiotic-resistant bacteria. In every case, advice and appropriate regulations are established by experimental studies and statistical evaluation. The experts need to be aware of the appropriate statistical procedures in order to play their proper roles.

In all these areas, a common basic vocabulary and understanding of biometrical concepts is assumed to enable scientists to communicate accurately with one another. It is important that you gain mastery of these concepts if you are to play a full part in your chosen profession.

1.5 Evidence-based veterinary medicine

The veterinary profession is following the medical profession in introducing a more objective basis to its practice. Under the term **evidence-based veterinary medicine** (EBVM) – by which we mean the conscientious, explicit and judicious use of current best evidence to inform clinical judgements and decision-making in veterinary care (see Cockcroft and Holmes, 2003) – we are now seeing a move towards dependence upon good scientific studies to underpin clinical decisions. In many ways, practice has implicitly been about using clinical experience to make the best decisions, but what has changed is the explicit use of the accessible information. No longer do clinicians have to depend on their own clinical experience and judgement alone; now they can benefit from other studies in a formalized manner to assist their work. The clinician has to know what information is relevant and how to access this

evidence, and be able to use rigorous methods to assess it. Generally, this requires a familiarity with the terminology used and an understanding of the principles of statistical analysis. Moreover, the wider world of animal science is finding a need to understand these ideas as the evidence-based concepts are being applied not only in the treatment of clinical disease but also in aspects of production and performance.

One of the differences between the application of EBVM in veterinary science and in human medicine is that in the latter the body of literature is now very large, and this makes finding relevant information easier. In the veterinary field, EBVM is still hampered by the relatively small amount and variable quality of the evidence available. Nevertheless, EBVM is gaining momentum, and we have devoted Chapter 16 to its concepts. One of the key requirements of EBVM is reliably reported information and, as in the human medical field, the veterinary publishing field is in the process of consolidating a set of guidelines for good reporting. We have addressed this in Chapter 17, outlining the information that is available at the time of writing. As critical appraisal of the published literature is invariably an essential component of evaluating evidence, we have devoted Chapter 18 to it. In this chapter, we provide templates for critically appraising randomized controlled trials and observational studies, and invite you to develop your skills by critically appraising two published articles.

1.6 Types of variable

A **variable** is a characteristic that can take values which *vary* from individual to individual or group to group, e.g. height, weight, litter size, blood count, enzyme activity, coat colour, percentage of the flock which are pregnant, etc. Clearly some of these are more readily quantifiable than others. For some variables, we can assign a number to a category and so create the appearance of a numerical scale, but others have a true numerical scale on which the values lie. We take **readings** of the variable which are measurements of a biological characteristic, and these become the **values** which we use for the statistical procedures. Both these terms are in general use, and both refer to the original measurements, the **raw data**.

Numerical data take various forms; a proper understanding of the nature of the data and the classification of variables is an important first step in choosing an appropriate statistical approach. The flow charts shown in Appendix E, and on the inside front and back covers, illustrate this train of thought, which culminates in a suitable choice of statistical procedure to analyse a particular data set.

We distinguish the main types of variable in a systematic manner by determining whether the variable can take 'one of two distinct values', 'one of several distinct values' or 'any value' within the given range. In particular, the variable may be one of the following:

1. **Categorical (qualitative) variable** – an individual belongs to any one of two or more distinct categories for this variable. A *binary* or dichotomous variable is a particular type of categorical variable defined by only *two* categories; for example, pregnant or non-pregnant, male or female. We customarily summarize the information for the categorical variable by determining the number and percentage (or proportion) of individuals in each category in the sample or population. Particular scales of a categorical variable are:
   - **Nominal scale** – the distinct categories that define the variable are unordered and each can be assigned a name, e.g. coat colours (piebald, roan or grey).
   - **Ordinal scale** – the categories that constitute the variable have some intrinsic order; for example, body condition scores, subjective intensity of fluorescence of cells in the fluorescence microscope, degree of vigour of motility of a semen sample. These 'scales' are often given numerical values 1 to n.
2. **Numerical (quantitative) variable** – consisting of numerical values on a well-defined scale, which may be:
   - **Discrete (discontinuous) scale**, i.e. data can take only particular integer values, typically counts, e.g. litter size, clutch size, parity (number of pregnancies within an animal).
   - **Continuous scale**, for which all values are theoretically possible (perhaps limited by an upper and/or lower boundary), e.g. height, weight, speed, concentration of a chemical constituent of the blood or urine. Theoretically, the number of values that the continuous variable can take is infinite since the scale is a continuum. In practice, continuous data are restricted by the degree of accuracy of the measurement process. By definition, the interval between two adjacent points on the scale is of the same magnitude as the interval between two other adjacent points, e.g. the interval on a temperature scale between 37°C and 38°C is the same as the interval between 39°C and 40°C.

1.7 Variations in measurements

It is well known that if we repeatedly observe and quantify a particular biological phenomenon, the measurements will rarely be identical. Part of the variability is due to an inherent variation in the biological material being measured. For example, not all cows eat the same quantity of grass per day even if differences both in body weight and water content of the feed are taken into account. We shall use the term '**biological variation**' for this phenomenon, although some people use the term 'biological error'. (Biological error is actually a misleading term since the variability is not in any sense due to a mistake.)

By the selection of individuals according to certain characteristics in advance of the collection of data, we may be able to *reduce* the range of biological variation but we cannot eliminate it. Selection is often based on animal characteristics (e.g. species, strain, age, sex, degree of maturity, body weight, show-jumpers, milking herds, hill sheep, etc.), the choice of which depends upon the particular factors under investigation. However, the result is then only valid for that *restricted population* and we are not justified in extrapolating beyond that population. For example, we should not assume that a study based on beef cattle applies to other types of cattle.

In addition to biological variation, there will most likely be differences in repeated measurements of the same subject within a very short period of time. These are **technical variations or errors**, due to a variety of instrumental causes and to human error. We may properly consider them to be errors since they represent departures from the true values.

1.7.1 Biological variation

The causes of biological variation, which makes one individual differ from the next or from one time to another, may be obvious or subtle. For example, variations in any characteristic may be attributable to:

- Genetics – e.g. greater variability in the whole cow population compared with just Friesians.
- Environment – e.g. body weight varies with diet, housing, intercurrent disease, etc.
- Gender – sexual dimorphism is common.
- Age – many biological data are influenced by age and maturity, e.g. the quantity of body fat.

In a heterogeneous population, the biological variation may be considerable and may mask the variation due to particular factors under investigation. Statistical approaches must take account of this inherent variability. The problem for the scientist, having measured a range of results of a particular feature in a group of individuals, is to distinguish between the sources of variation.

Here are two examples of problems created by biological variation:

- Two groups of growing cattle have been fed different diets. The ranges of the recorded weights at 6 months of age show an overlap in the two groups. Is there a real difference between the groups?
- You have the results of an electrolyte blood test which shows that the serum potassium level is elevated. By how much must it be elevated before you regard it as abnormal?

1.7.2 Technical errors

A technical or measurement error is defined as the difference between an observed reading and its 'true' value. Measurement errors are due to factors which are, typically, **human** (e.g. variations within and between observers) or **instrumental**, but may also be attributed to differences in conditions (e.g. different laboratories).

Technical errors may be systematic or random. A **systematic error** is one in which the observed values have a tendency to be above (or below) the true value; the result is then said to be *biased*. When the observed values are evenly distributed above and below the true value, **random errors**, due to unexplained sources, are said to be occurring. Random variation can be so great as to obscure differences between groups but this problem may be minimized by taking repeated observations.

(a) Human error

Human error can occur whenever a person is performing either an unfamiliar task or a routine or monotonous task; fatigue increases the chances of error. Errors due to these factors are usually random, and providing steps are taken to minimize them (e.g. practice to acquire a proper level of skill, avoiding long periods of monotonous labour, and checking results as measurements are made), they are generally not of great concern.

Other sorts of human error can arise because of data handling. **Rounding errors** can introduce inaccuracies if performed too early in an analysis. If you use a computer to manage your data, you need not be concerned about this, since computer algorithms generally avoid rounding errors by carrying long number strings even if these are not displayed.

Another recognized human error is called **digit preference**. Whenever there is an element of judgement involved in making readings from instruments (as in determining the last digit of a number on a scale), certain digits between 0 and 9 are more commonly chosen than others to represent the readings; such preferences differ between individuals. This may introduce either a random or a systematic error, the magnitude of which will depend on the importance of the last digit to the results.

(b) Instrumental error

Instrumental errors arise for a number of reasons (Figure 1.1). Providing we are aware of the potential problem, the causes are often correctable or reducible.

- With a *systematic offset* or *zero error*, a 'blank' sample consistently reads other than zero. It is common in colorimetry and radioisotope measurements (Figure 1.1a).
- *Non-linearity* is a systematic error, commonly seen in the performance of strain gauges, thermocouples and colorimeters (Figure 1.1b).
- *Proportional* or *scale error* is usually due to electronic gain being incorrectly adjusted or altered after calibration; it results in a systematic error (Figure 1.1c).
- *Hysteresis* is a systematic error commonly encountered in measurements involving galvanometers. It may require a standard measurement procedure, e.g. always adjusting input *down* to desired level (Figure 1.1d).
- *Instability* or *drift* – electronic gain calibration may drift with temperature and humidity giving rise to an intermittent but systematic error, resulting in an unstable baseline (Figure 1.1e).
- *Random errors* are commonly seen in attempts to measure with a sensitivity beyond the limits of resolution of an instrument (Figure 1.1f). Most instruments carry a specification of their accuracy, for example it is no use attempting to measure to the nearest gram with a balance accurate only to 10 g.

Two or more of these sources of error may occur simultaneously. Technical errors of all kinds can be minimized by careful experimentation. This is the essence of **quality control** and is of paramount importance in a diagnostic laboratory. Quality control in the laboratory is about ensuring that processes and procedures are carried out in a consistently satisfactory manner so that the results are trustworthy. We introduce some additional terms in order to understand these concepts more fully.

1.8 Terms relating to measurement quality

Two terms which are of major importance in understanding the principles of biological measurement are **precision** and **accuracy**. It is essential they are understood early in a consideration of the nature of data measurement.

- **Precision** refers to how well repeated observations agree with one another.
- **Accuracy** refers to how well the observed value agrees with the true value.

To understand these terms consider the diagrams in Figure 1.2, in which the bull's-eye represents the true value: in Figure 1.2a there is poor accuracy and poor precision, in Figure 1.2b there is poor accuracy and good precision, while in Figure 1.2c there is both good accuracy and good precision.

It is possible to have a diagnostic method (e.g. blood enzyme estimation) that gives good precision but poor accuracy (Figure 1.2b) because of systematic error. In an enzyme activity estimation, such an error might be due to variation in temperature.

Several other terms, all of which describe aspects of **reliability**, are in use and these are defined as follows:

- **Repeatability** is concerned with gauging the similarity of replicate, often duplicate, measurements of a particular technique or instrument or observer under identical conditions, e.g. measurements made by the same observer in the same laboratory. It assesses technical errors (see Section 14.4).
- **Reproducibility** (sometimes called **method agreement**) is concerned with determining how well two or more approaches to measuring the same quantity agree with one another, e.g. measurements made by the same observer but using different methods, or by different

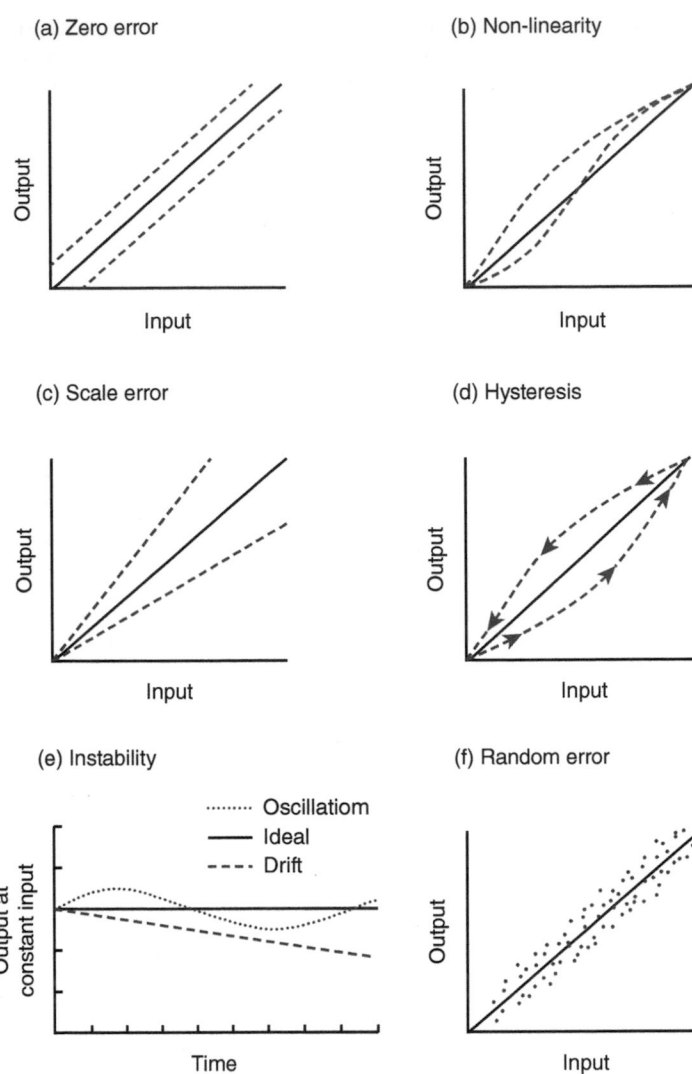

Figure 1.1 Types of instrumental error. 'Input' refers to the true value of the measurements being recorded, 'output' refers to the recorded response, and the solid line refers to the situation when the output values equal the input values. Errors in measurements are represented by dots or dashed lines.

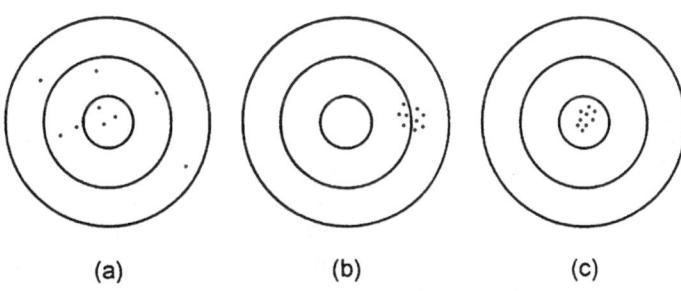

Figure 1.2 Diagram representing the concepts of accuracy and precision: (a) represents poor accuracy and precision, (b) represents poor accuracy but good precision, and (c) represents both good accuracy and precision.

observers using the same method, or by observers using the same method but in different laboratories (see Section 14.4).

- **Stability** concerns the long-term repeatability of measurement. Diagnostic laboratories will usually have reference material kept for checking stability over time.
- **Validity** is concerned with determining whether the measurement is actually measuring what it purports to be measuring. In the clinical context, the measurement is compared with a 'gold standard' (see Section 14.2).

1.9 Populations and samples

The concept of a **population** from which our measurements are a **sample** is fundamental. A population includes all representatives of a particular group, whereas a sample is a subgroup drawn from the population. We aim to choose a sufficiently large sample in such a manner that it is representative (i.e. is typical) of the population (see Sections 1.9.2, 4.2 and 13.3).

1.9.1 Types of population

In this book we usually use the word 'animal' to suggest the unit of investigation, but we also use other terms such as 'individual' or 'case'. We want you to become familiar with different terminology. A population of animals may be represented by:

- The individuals, e.g. all cattle, all beef cattle, all Herefords, all the herd.
- The measurements of a particular variable on every animal, e.g. liver weight, bone length, blood hormone or enzyme level.
- Numbers of items (in a given area, volume or time), e.g. blood cell counts or faecal egg counts, counts of radioactive particle emissions.

The population may be either a **real (or finite) group** or a **hypothetical (or infinite) group**. For example, if we are interested in the growth rate of pigs in Suffolk, then the population is all pigs in Suffolk. This is a real or finite population. If, however, we want to know the effect of an experimental diet in these pigs, we will feed the test diet to a sample of pigs which now comprises the only representatives of a hypothetical population fed on the test diet. Theoretically, at least, we could actually measure the entire population in finite cases, but infinite populations are represented *only* by the sample.

1.9.2 Random sampling and random allocation

We examine a sample with a view to making statements about the population. The sample must therefore be *representative* of the population from which it is taken if it is to give useful results applicable to the population at large. In order for the sample to be representative, strictly, there should be **random selection** from *all* possible members of the entire population, implying that the individuals should be selected using a method based on chance (see Section 13.6). However, in reality, random selection is generally not feasible (for example, in an observational study (see Section 5.2.1) or in a clinical study when the disease under investigation is rare). In that case, it is important that we try to ensure that the individuals in the sample are a true reflection of those in the population of interest, and that, if groups are to be compared, we check that the individuals in the different groups are comparable with similar baseline characteristics.

It is essential to use an objective method to achieve random sampling, and a method based on a random number sequence is the method of choice. The sequence may be obtained from a table of random numbers (see Table A.11) or be generated by a computer random number generator or, if only a small sequence, it could be generated by a mechanical method such as rolling a die, although the latter approach is not recommended.

Note that for allocating individuals into treatment groups in an experimental situation, principles of **random allocation (randomization)** should also be employed to avoid subjective influence and ensure that the groups are comparable (see Section 5.6). Again, a random number sequence is recommended to provide objective allocation of individuals or treatments so that the causes of any subsequent differences in performance between the groups can be properly identified.

1.10 Types of statistical procedures

Statistical procedures can be divided into descriptive statistics and inferential statistics.

- **Descriptive statistics**. We use these techniques to reduce a data set to manageable proportions, summarizing the trends and tendencies within it, in order to represent the results clearly. From these procedures we can produce diagrams, tables and numerical descriptors. Numerical descriptors include measures that convey where the centre of the data set lies, like the arithmetic mean or median, and measures of the scatter or dispersion of the data, such as the variance or range. These are described more fully in Chapter 2.
- **Inferential statistics**. Statistical inference is the process of generalizing from the sample to the population: it enables us to draw conclusions about certain features of the population when only a subset of it, the sample, is available for investigation. One aspect of inferential statistics is the **estimation** of population parameters using sample data. A parameter, such as the mean or proportion, describes a particular feature of the distribution of a variable in the entire population (see Section 4.3.2). Usually, estimation is followed by a procedure called **hypothesis testing**, another aspect of inferential statistics that investigates a particular theory about the data. Hypothesis tests allow conclusions relating to the population to be drawn from the information in a sample. You can only use these tests properly, and so avoid the pitfalls of misinterpretation of the data, when you have a knowledge of their inherent assumptions. Some of these techniques are simple and require little expertise to master, while others are complex and are best left to the qualified statistician. Details of these procedures can be found in Chapters 6–14; the

flow charts in Appendix E provide a quick guide to the choice of the correct test.

1.11 Conclusion

We develop the ideas presented in this chapter in subsequent chapters. As we have said, the concepts are introduced building on one another, and you will need a sound understanding of the earlier theory in order to appreciate the material presented later.

The best incentive for wrestling with statistical concepts is the need to know the meaning of a data set of your own. Remember – statistical procedures cannot enhance poor data. Providing the data have been acquired with sufficient care and in sufficient number, the statistical procedures can supply you with sound summary statements and interpretative guidelines; the interpretation is still down to you! In the chapters that follow, the emphasis is on developing your understanding of the procedures and their limitations to aid your interpretation. We hope you find the experience of getting to grips with your data rewarding, and discover that statistics can be both satisfying and fun!

Exercises

The statements in questions 1.1–1.3 are either TRUE or FALSE.

1.1 Biological variation:
(a) Is the main cause of differences between animals.
(b) Is the term given to differences between animals in a population.
(c) Is the reason why statistics is necessary in animal science.
(d) Makes it impossible to be sure of any aspect of animal science.
(e) Is the term given to the variation in ability of a technician performing a monotonous task throughout the day.

1.2 A sample is *randomly* drawn from a population:
(a) To reduce the study to a manageable size.

(b) To ensure that the full range of possibilities is included.

(c) To obtain 'normal' animals.

(d) To obtain a representative group.

(e) To avoid selector preferences.

1.3 A nominal scale of measurement is used for data that:

(a) Comprise categories which cannot be ordered.

(b) Are not qualitative.

(c) Take many possible discrete quantitative values.

(d) Are evaluated as percentages.

(e) Are ranked.

1.4 Decide whether the following errors are likely to be systematic or random (S or R):

(a) The water bath that holds samples for an enzyme assay fails during incubation.

(b) A clinician reading a clinical thermometer has a digit preference for the numbers 0 and 5.

(c) The calibration on a colorimeter was not checked before use.

(d) Scales for measuring the weight of animal feed packs are activated sometimes before the sack is put on and sometimes after, depending on the operator.

(e) A chemical balance weighing to 100 mg is used to weigh quantities of 2550 mg.

1.5 Decide whether the following are either real or hypothetical populations (R or H):

(a) Milking cows in a trial for the effectiveness of a novel mastitis treatment.

(b) Horses in livery stables in the southeast of England.

(c) Fleas on dogs in urban Liverpool.

(d) Fleas on dogs treated with an oral monthly ectoparasite treatment.

(e) Blood glucose levels in diabetic dogs.

1.6 Identify the appropriate type of variable (nominal, ordinal, discrete or continuous: N, O, D or C) for the following data:

(a) Coat colour of cats: in a colony of 35 cats there were one white, three black, seven ginger, seven agouti, 11 tortoiseshell and six of other colours.

(b) Percentages of motile spermatozoa in the ejaculates of six bulls at an artificial insemination centre collected on a single day during March: they were 73%, 81%, 64%, 76%, 69% and 84%.

(c) Spectrophotometer measurements of maximum light absorbance at a wavelength of 280 nm of solutions of egg yolk proteins: they were 0.724, 0.591 and 0.520 arbitrary units.

(d) The motility of a series of frozen and thawed samples of spermatozoa estimated on an arbitrary scale of 0–10 (0 indicating a completely immotile sample).

(e) Plasma progesterone levels (ng/ml) measured monthly in pregnant sheep throughout gestation by means of radioimmunoassay.

(f) Kittens classified 1 week post-natally as either flat-chested (abnormal) or normal.

(g) The optical density of negative micrographs of fluorescent cells calculated from measurements obtained with a densitometer: the results for groups A, B and C were 0.814, 0.986 and 1.103 units, respectively.

(h) Litter sizes of rabbits during an investigation of behavioural disturbances about the time of implantation.

(i) Body condition scores of goats.

(j) Numbers of deaths due to particular diseases in a year studied in an epidemiological investigation.

(k) Radioactivity determined by scintillation counts per minute in a β-counter.

(l) The gestation length (days) in cattle carrying twins and in those carrying singletons.

2 Descriptive statistics

2.1 Learning objectives

By the end of this chapter, you should be able to:

- Explain, with diagrams, the concepts of frequency distributions.
- Interpret diagrams of the frequency distributions of both categorical and numerical data.
- Identify frequency distributions that are skewed to the right and skewed to the left.
- Describe and conduct strategies to compare frequency distributions that have different numbers of observations.
- List the essential attributes of good tables and good diagrams.
- Interpret a pie chart, bar chart, dot diagram and histogram and state their appropriate uses.
- Interpret a stem-and-leaf diagram and a box-and-whisker plot, and state their appropriate uses.
- Interpret a scatter diagram and explain its usage.
- List different measures of location and identify their strengths and limitations.
- List different measures of dispersion and identify their strengths and limitations.
- Summarize any given data set appropriately in tabular and/or diagrammatic form to demonstrate its features.

2.2 Summarizing data

We collect data with the intention of gleaning information which, usually, we then convey to interested parties. This presents little problem when the data set comprises relatively few observations made on a small group of animals. However, as the quantity of information grows, it becomes increasingly difficult to obtain an overall 'picture' of what is happening.

The first stage in the process of obtaining this picture is to organize the data to establish how often different values occur (see frequency distributions in Section 2.3). Then it is helpful to further condense the information, reducing it to a manageable size, and so obtain a snapshot view as an aid to understanding and interpretation. There are various stratagems that we adopt; most notably, we can use:

- **Tables** to exhibit features of the data (see Section 2.4).
- **Diagrams** to illustrate patterns (see Section 2.5).
- **Numerical measures** to summarize the data (see Section 2.6).

2.3 Empirical frequency distributions

2.3.1 What is a frequency distribution?

A **frequency distribution** shows the frequencies of occurrence of the observations in a data set. Often the distribution of the observed data is

Statistics for Veterinary and Animal Science, Third Edition. Aviva Petrie and Paul Watson.
© 2013 John Wiley & Sons, Ltd. Published 2013 by John Wiley & Sons, Ltd.

called an **empirical frequency distribution**, in contrast to the **theoretical probability distribution** (see Section 3.3) determined from a mathematical model.

It is vital that you clearly understand the distinction between categorical and numerical variables (see Section 1.6) before you make any attempt to form a frequency distribution since the variable type will dictate the most appropriate form of display.

- When a variable is **categorical** or **qualitative**, then the observed frequency distribution of that variable comprises the frequency of occurrence of the observations in every class or category of the variable (see Section 2.5.1). We can display this information in a table in which each class is represented, or in a diagram such as a bar chart or a pie diagram.

  For example, if the variable represents different methods of treatment to prevent hypomagnesaemia in dairy cows, the numbers of farms observed using each method would comprise the frequency distribution. The data can be illustrated in a pie chart (see Figure 2.3).

- When the variable of interest is **numerical** or **quantitative** (either discrete or continuous), then the information is most easily assimilated by creating between five and 15 non-overlapping, preferably equal, intervals or classes that encompass the range of values of the variable. It is essential that the class intervals are *unambiguously* defined such that an observation falls into one class only. These classes are adjacent when the data are discrete, and contiguous when the data are continuous. We determine the number of observations belonging to each class (the class frequency). The complete set of class frequencies is a frequency distribution. We can present it in the form of a table or a diagram (see Section 2.5.2) such as a bar chart (discrete variable) or a histogram (continuous variable).

  For example, columns 1 and 2 of Table 2.1 show the frequency distribution of the threshold response of sheep to a mechanical stimulus applied to the forelimb; Figure 2.5 is a histogram of the data. These data reflect sensitivity

to pain sensation in the extremities of sheep at pasture, and were derived as the control data in a study of the relationship of pain threshold and the incidence of foot rot; a higher threshold was associated with a greater incidence of disease (Ley *et al.*, 1995).

2.3.2 Relative frequency distributions

Although creating a frequency distribution is a useful way of describing a set of observations, it is difficult to compare two or more frequency distributions if the total number of observations in each distribution is different. A way of overcoming this difficulty is to calculate the proportion or percentage of observations in each class or category. These are called **relative frequencies** and each is obtained by dividing the frequency for that category by the total number of observations (column 3 of Table 2.1). The sum of the relative frequencies of all the categories is unity (or 100%) apart from rounding errors.

Table 2.1 Frequency distribution of mechanical threshold of 470 sheep.

Class limits of mechanical threshold (newtons)	Frequency	Relative frequency (%)	Cumulative relative frequency (%)
1.0–1.9	9	1.9	1.9
2.0–2.9	44	9.4	11.3
3.0–3.9	88	18.7	30.0
4.0–4.9	137	29.1	59.1
5.0–5.9	69	14.7	73.8
6.0–6.9	37	7.9	81.7
7.0–7.9	21	4.5	86.2
8.0–8.9	17	3.6	89.8
9.0–9.9	19	4.0	93.8
10.0–10.9	14	3.0	96.8
11.0–11.9	4	0.9	97.7
12.0–12.9	6	1.3	98.9
13.0–13.9	2	0.4	99.4
14.0–14.9	3	0.6	100.0
Total	470	100.0	

2.3.3 Cumulative relative frequency distributions

Sometimes it is helpful to evaluate the number (the cumulative frequency) or percentage (cumulative relative frequency) of individuals that are contained in a category and in all lower categories. Generally, we find that cumulative relative frequency distributions are more useful than cumulative frequency distributions. For example, we may be interested in using the data of Table 2.1 to determine the percentage of sheep whose mechanical threshold is less than 7.01 newtons. We form a **cumulative relative frequency distribution** by adding the relative frequencies of individuals contained in each category and all lower categories, and repeating this process for each category. The cumulative relative frequencies are tabulated in column 4 of Table 2.1 and the distribution is drawn in the **cumulative relative frequency polygon** of Figure 2.1.

We can evaluate the **percentiles** (often called *centiles*) of the frequency distribution from this cumulative frequency distribution. Percentiles are the values of the variable that divide the total frequency into 100 equal parts. They are used to divide the frequency distribution into useful groups when the observations are arranged in

order of magnitude. In particular, the 50th percentile (called the **median** – see Section 2.6.1(b)) is the value of the variable that divides the distribution into two halves; 50% of the individuals have observations less than the median, and 50% of the individuals have observations greater than the median. Often the 25th and the 75th percentiles are quoted (these are called the **lower (first) quartile** and **upper (third) quartile**, respectively); 25% of the observations lie below the lower quartile and 25% of the observations lie above the upper quartile, the distance between these quartiles being the **interquartile range**. The 5th and 95th percentiles enclose the central 90% of the observations. We show how to evaluate these percentiles from the cumulative frequency distribution polygon in Figure 2.1.

2.4 Tables

A table is an orderly arrangement, usually of numbers or words in rows and columns, which exhibits a set of facts in a distinct and comprehensive way. The layout of the table will be dictated by the data, and therefore will vary for different types of data. It is useful, however, to remember the most important principles that

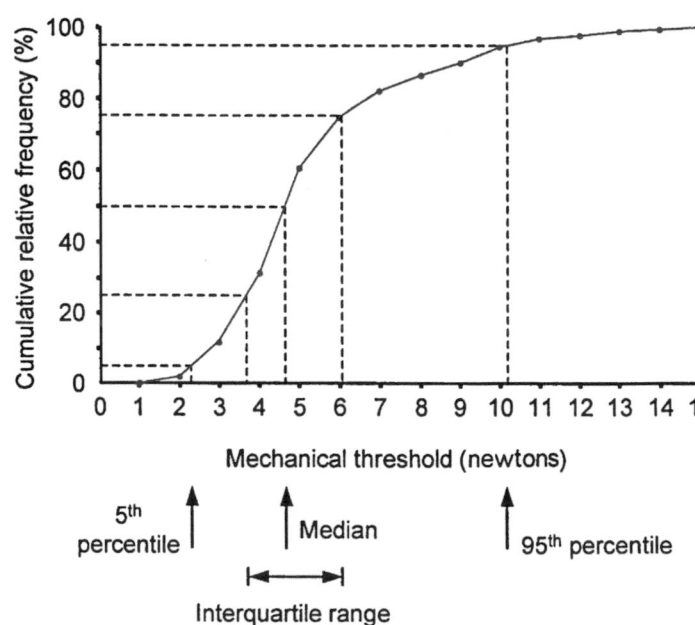

Figure 2.1 Cumulative relative frequency polygon of the mechanical threshold of sheep (data from Ley *et al.*, 1995, with permission from the authors and BMJ Publishing Group Ltd).

Box 2.1   Rules for well-constructed tables

- Include a concise, informative and unambiguously defined title.
- Give a brief heading for each row and column.
- Include the units of measurement.
- Give the number of items on which any summary measure (e.g. a percentage) is based.
- When providing a summary statistic (e.g. the mean) always include a measure of precision (e.g. a confidence interval – see Section 4.5).
- Give figures only to the degree of accuracy that is appropriate (as a guideline, one significant figure more than the raw data).
- Do not give too much information in a table.
- Remember that it is easier to scan information down columns rather than across rows.

Box 2.2   Rules for well-constructed diagrams

- Keep it simple and avoid unnecessary 'frills' (e.g. making a simple pie chart, histogram or bar chart three-dimensional).
- Include a concise, informative and unambiguously defined title.
- Label all axes, segments and bars, if necessary using a legend or key showing the meaning of the different symbols used.
- Present the units, the numbers on which summary measures are based, and measures of variability where appropriate.
- Avoid exaggerating the scale on an axis, perhaps by omitting the zero point, so as to distort the results.
- Include a break in the scale only if there is no other satisfactory way of demonstrating the extremes.
- Show coincident points in a scatter diagram.
- Ensure that the method of display conveys all the relevant information (e.g. pairing).

govern well-constructed tables; we outline them in Box 2.1.

2.5 Diagrams

A diagram is a graphic representation of data and may take several forms. It is often easier to discern important *patterns* from a diagram rather than a table, even though the latter may give more precise numerical information. Diagrams are most useful when we want to convey information quickly, and they should serve as an adjunct to more formal statistical analysis. You will find the guidelines in Box 2.2 helpful when you construct a diagram.

2.5.1 Categorical (qualitative) data

When data are categorical or qualitative, then each observation belongs to one of a number of distinct categories or classes. We can determine the number or percentage of individuals falling into each class or category and display this information in a *bar chart* or a *pie chart*.

(a) Bar chart

A **bar chart** is a diagram in which every category of the variable is represented; the length of each bar, which should be of constant width, depicts

the number or percentage of individuals belonging to that category. Figure 2.2 is an example of a bar chart. The length of the bar is proportional to the frequency or relative frequency in the relevant category, so it is essential that the scale showing the frequency or relative frequency should start at zero for each bar.

You may find in other people's work that the frequency in a category is indicated by a pictorial representation of a relevant object. Typically, this object in a veterinary study will be the animal under investigation. Such a diagram is called a **pictogram**. There is an inherent danger of misinterpretation when making crude comparisons by eye of the frequencies in different categories. Is it height or area or volume of the object which represents the frequencies? To a certain extent, this problem can be overcome by using equally sized images, so that the frequency in a category is indicated by the appropriate number of repetitions of the image. The effect is similar to a bar chart, with each 'bar' containing varying numbers of images. However, because of the potential for confusion, we do not recommend that you use pictograms to display frequencies.

(b) Pie chart

A **pie chart** is a circle divided into segments with each segment portraying a different category

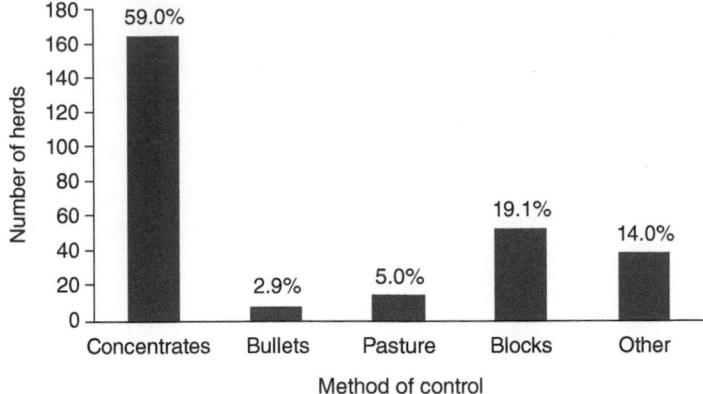

Figure 2.2   Bar chart showing the number of herds in which specific methods of control of hypomagnesaemia were used by dairy farmers in 278 dairy herds (data from McCoy *et al.*, 1996, with permission from BMJ Publishing Group Ltd).

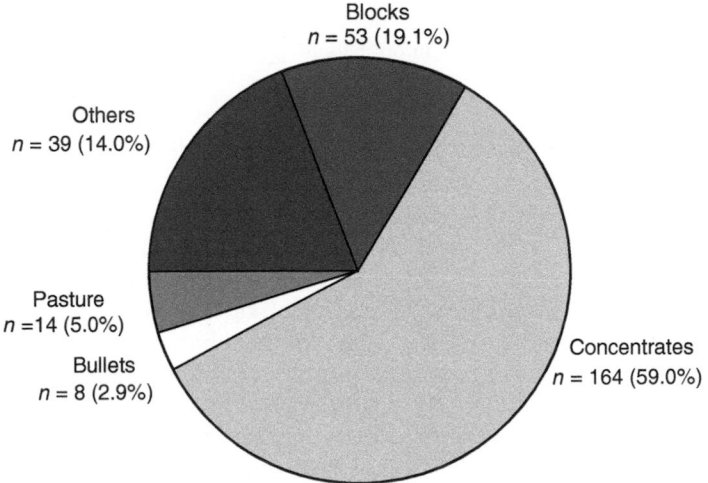

Figure 2.3   Pie chart showing the percentage of herds in which specific methods of control of hypomagnesaemia were used by dairy farmers in 278 dairy herds (redrawn from McCoy *et al.*, 1996, with permission from BMJ Publishing Group Ltd).

of the qualitative variable (Figure 2.3). The total area of the circle represents the total frequency, and the area or angle of a given sector is proportional to the percentage of individuals falling into that category. A pie chart should include a statement of the percentage or actual number of individuals in each segment. Generally, we prefer the bar chart to the pie chart as the former is easier to construct and is more useful for comparative purposes, partly because it is easier to compare lengths by eye rather than angles.

2.5.2 Numerical (quantitative) data

When the data are numerical or quantitative, we may show every data value, for example in a *dot*

diagram, or we may display only a summary of the data, for example in a *histogram*.

(a) Dot diagram

If the data set is of a manageable size, the best way of displaying it is to show every value in a **dot diagram/plot**. When we investigate a single numerical variable, we can mark each observation as a dot on a line calibrated in the units of measurement of that variable, plotted horizontally or vertically.

- If the data are in a single group, the diagram will look like Figure 2.9.
- When we are comparing the observations in two or more groups, we can draw a dot diagram

(a)

(b)

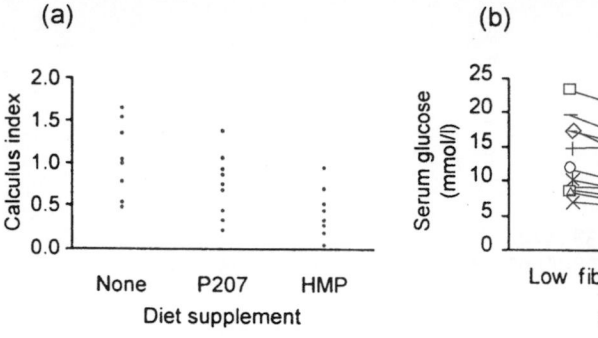

Figure 2.4 (a) Dot diagram showing the calculus index on teeth in three groups of dogs on different diets (based on summary data from Stookey *et al.*, 1995). (b) Dot diagram showing the change in serum glucose concentration in each of 11 diabetic dogs on high- and low-fibre diets (based on summary data from Nelson *et al.*, 1998).

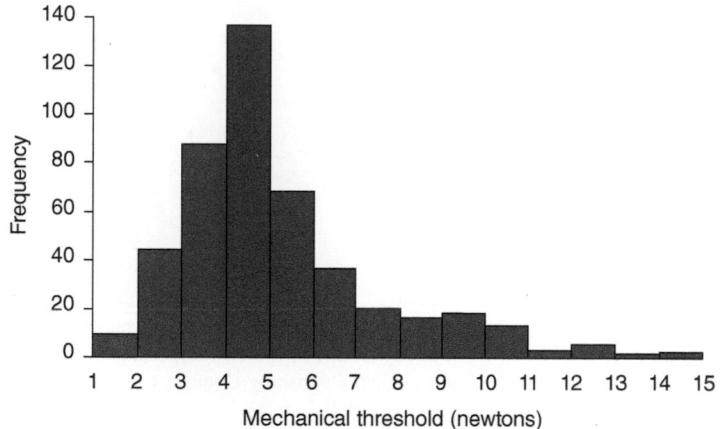

Figure 2.5 Histogram of the mechanical threshold of 470 sheep (data from Ley *et al.*, 1995, with permission from the authors and BMJ Publishing Group Ltd).

with the horizontal axis designating the groups, and the vertical axis representing the scale of measurement of the variable. Then, in a single diagram, we can show the values for each group in a vertical dot plot, facilitating the comparison of groups as well as providing a visual display of the distribution of the variable in each group (Figure 2.4a).

- When an individual reading in one group bears a direct relationship to that in another group (e.g. from two litter mates, or before and after within an individual) we can join the related dots in a pair by a straight line (Figure 2.4b). The directions of the slope of the lines may indicate a difference between the groups.

(b) Histogram

The frequency distribution of a quantitative variable (see Section 2.3.1) can be displayed as a **histogram**. This is a two-dimensional diagram in which usually the horizontal axis represents the unit of measurement of the variable of interest, with each class interval being clearly delineated. We construct rectangles above each class interval so that the *area* of the rectangle is proportional to the frequency for that class. If the intervals are of equal width, then the height of the rectangle is proportional to the frequency.

The histogram gives a good picture of the frequency distribution of the variable (Figure 2.5). The distribution is **symmetrical** if its shape to the right of a central value is a mirror image of that to the left of the central value. The **tails** of the frequency distribution represent the frequencies at the extremes of the distribution. The frequency distribution is **skewed to the right (positively skewed)** if the right-hand tail is extended, and **skewed to the left (negatively skewed)** if the left-hand tail is extended. The distribution of the data in Figure 2.5 is skewed to the right; it is

Frequency	Stem and leaf
6	1 * 04&
3	1 . &
20	2 * 111123344&
24	2 . 5566778889
40	3 * 0011111222222334444
48	3 . 555555566666777788888899
65	4 * 00011111111122222222333333334444
72	4 . 555555566666666777777788888888899999
39	5 * 000011112222334444
30	5 . 55666777889999
18	6 * 00123344
19	6 . 557788889&
9	7 * 014&
12	7 . 5689&
8	8 * 024&
9	8 . 59&
8	9 * 34&
6	9 . 56

Extremes (9.7), (9.8), (9.9), (10.0), (10.2), (10.3), (10.4)
Extremes (10.5), (10.7), (10.8), (10.9), (11.0), (11.3), (11.5)
Extremes (11.8), (12.0), (12.3), (12.4), (12.6), (12.8), (12.9)

Stem width: 1.00
Each leaf: 2 case(s)
& denotes a fractional leaf (i.e. one case)
*   indicates that there are 2 branches for that stem unit

Figure 2.6 Stem-and-leaf diagram of the mechanical threshold of sheep (data from Ley *et al.*, 1995, with permission from the authors and BMJ Publishing Group Ltd).

not uncommon to find biological data which are skewed to the right.

You should note that although the histogram is similar to the bar chart, the rectangles in a histogram are contiguous because the numerical variable is continuous, whereas there are spaces between the bars in a bar chart.

(c) Stem-and-leaf diagram

We often see a mutation of the histogram, called a **stem-and-leaf diagram**, in computer outputs. Each vertical rectangle of the histogram is replaced by a row of numbers that represent the relevant observations. The stem is the core value of the observation (e.g. the unit value before the decimal place) and the leaves are represented by a sequence of ordered single digits, one for each observation, that follow the core value (e.g. the first decimal place). Plotting the data in this way provides an easily assimilated description of the distribution of the data whilst, at the same time,

showing the raw data. Figure 2.6 is a stem-and-leaf diagram for the mechanical threshold data for sheep.

(d) Box-and-whisker plot

Another diagram that we often see in computer outputs, the **box-and-whisker plot** (or **box plot**), provides a summary of the distribution of a data set. The scale of measurement of the variable is usually drawn vertically. The diagram comprises a box with horizontal limits defining the upper and lower quartiles (see Section 2.3.3) and representing the interquartile range (see Section 2.6.2(b)), enclosing the central 50% of the observations, with the median (see Section 2.6.1(b)) marked by a horizontal line within the box. The whiskers are vertical lines extending from the box as low as the 2.5th percentile and as high as the 97.5th percentile (sometimes the percentiles are replaced by the minimum and maximum values of the set of observations). Figure 2.7 is a

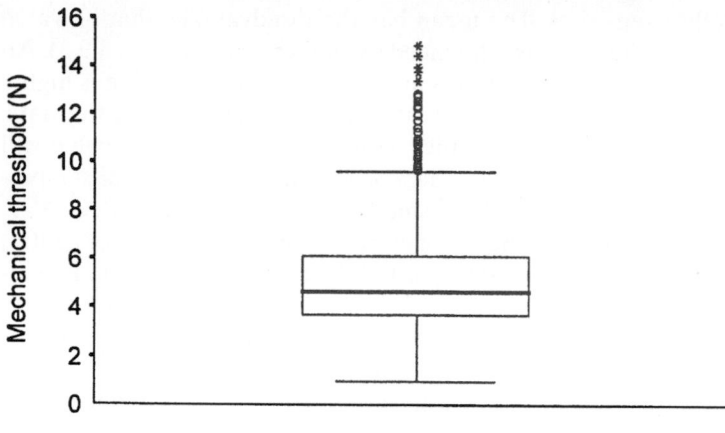
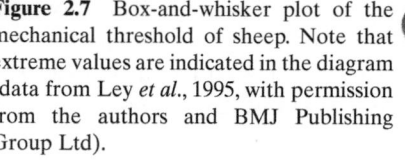

Figure 2.7 Box-and-whisker plot of the mechanical threshold of sheep. Note that extreme values are indicated in the diagram (data from Ley *et al.*, 1995, with permission from the authors and BMJ Publishing Group Ltd).

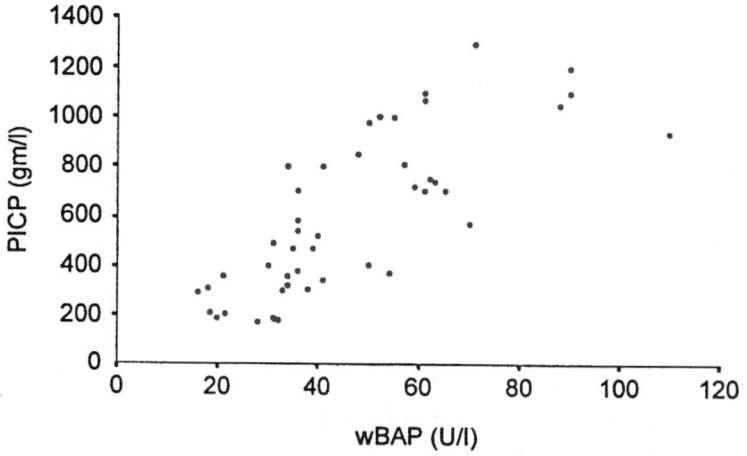

Figure 2.8 Scatter diagram showing the relationship between two measures of bone formation: bone alkaline phosphatase activity (wBAP) and Type I collagen concentration (PICP) (redrawn from Jackson *et al.*, 1996, with permission from Elsevier Ltd).

box-and-whisker plot of the mechanical threshold data for sheep. The box-and-whisker plot is particularly useful when a number of data sets are to be compared in a single diagram (see Figure 7.2).

(e) Scatter diagram

The **scatter diagram** is an effective way of presenting data when we are interested in examining the relationship between two variables which may be numerical or ordinal. The diagram is a two-dimensional plot in which each axis represents the scale of measurement of one of the two variables. Using this rectangular co-ordinate system, we relate the value for an individual on the horizontal scale (the *abscissa*) to the corresponding value for that individual on the vertical scale (the *ordinate*) by marking the relevant point with an appropriate symbol (Figure 2.8). Coincident points should be identifiable. We can discern possible relationships between the variables by observing the scatter of points, and then we may join the points to produce a line graph, or draw a line that best represents the relationship (see Chapter 10). If two or more treatment groups are represented, they can be distinguished by colour or dot symbols, such as a cross or circle.

2.6 Numerical measures

Using a visual display as a means of describing a set of data helps us get a 'feel' for the data, but our impressions are subjective. It is usually essential that we supplement the visual display with the appropriate numerical measures that summarize the data. If we are able to determine some form of average that measures the central tendency of the data set, and if we know how widely scattered the observations are in either direction from that average, then we will have a reasonable 'picture' of the data. These two characteristics of a set of observations measured on a numerical variable are known as **measures of location** and **measures of dispersion**.

Note that it is customary to distinguish between measures in the population (called *parameters*) and their sample estimates (called *statistics*) by using Greek letters for the former and Roman letters for the latter (see the Glossary of notation in Appendix C).

2.6.1 Measures of location (averages)

The term **average** refers to any one of several measures of the **central tendency** of a data set.

(a) Arithmetic mean

The most commonly used measure of central tendency is the **arithmetic mean** (usually abbreviated to the **mean**). It is obtained by adding together the observations in a data set and dividing by the number of observations in the set.

If the continuous variable of interest is denoted by x and there are n observations in the sample, then the sample mean (pronounced x bar) is

$$\bar{x} = \frac{\sum x}{n}$$

Example
The following are plasma potassium values (mmol/l) of 14 dogs:

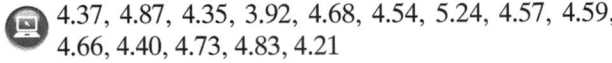 4.37, 4.87, 4.35, 3.92, 4.68, 4.54, 5.24, 4.57, 4.59, 4.66, 4.40, 4.73, 4.83, 4.21

$$\bar{x} = \frac{63.96}{14} = 4.57 \text{ mmol/l}$$

- The mean has the disadvantage that its value is influenced by outliers (see Section 5.9.3). An **outlier** is an observation whose value is highly inconsistent with the main body of the data. An outlier with an excessively large value will tend to increase the mean unduly, whilst a particularly small value will decrease it.
- The mean is an appropriate measure of central tendency if the distribution of the data is symmetrical. The mean will be 'pulled' to the right (increased in value) if the distribution is skewed to the right, and 'pulled' to the left (decreased in value) if the distribution is skewed to the left.

(b) Median

Another frequently used measure of central tendency is the **median**. The median is the central value in the set of n observations which have been arranged in **rank order**, i.e. the observations are arranged in an increasing (or decreasing) order of magnitude. The median is the middle value of the ordered set with as many observations above it as below it (Box 2.3). The median is the 50th percentile (see Section 2.3.3).

Example
The weights (grams) of 19 male Hartley guinea pigs were:

314, 991, 789, 556, 412, 499, 350, 863, 455, 297, 598, 510, 388, 642, 474, 333, 421, 685, 536

If we arrange the weights in rank order, they become:

297, 314, 333, 350, 388, 412, 421, 455, 474, **499**, 510, 536, 556, 598, 642, 685, 789, 863, 991

The median, shown in bold, is the $(19 + 1)/2 = $ 10th weight in the ordered set; this is 499 g.

Box 2.3   Calculating the median

- *If n is odd*, then the median is found by starting with the smallest observation in the ordered set and then counting until the $(n + 1)/2$th observation is reached. This observation is the median.
- *If n is even*, then the median lies midway between the central two observations.

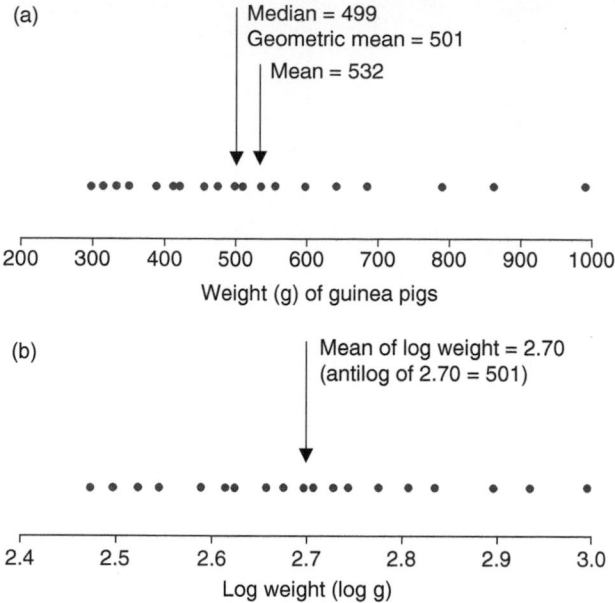

Figure 2.9 Dot plots for (a) the weights, and (b) the $\log_{10}$ weights of 19 guinea pigs.

- The arithmetic mean and the median are close or equal in value if the distribution is symmetrical.
- The advantage of the median is that it is not affected by outliers or if the distribution of the data is skewed. Thus the median will be less than the mean if the data are skewed to the right, and greater than the mean if the data are skewed to the left.
- A disadvantage of the median is that it does not incorporate all the observations in its calculations, and it is difficult to handle mathematically.

(c) Geometric mean

If we take the logarithm (generally to base 10 or to base e) of each value of a data set which is skewed to the right, we usually find that the distribution of the log-transformed data becomes more symmetrical. In this case, the arithmetic mean of the log-transformed values is a useful measure of location. However, it has the disadvantage that it is measured on a log scale. We therefore convert it back to the original scale by taking its antilogarithm; this is the **geometric**

mean. The distribution of biological data, if not symmetrical, is frequently skewed to the right; we could then calculate the geometric mean to represent an average value.

For example, Figure 2.9 shows the distribution of the guinea pig weights given in the example in Section 2.6.1(b) illustrated in a dot plot, first as the untransformed data (Figure 2.9a) and then as the log-transformed data (Figure 2.9b). You can see that the transformation improves symmetry, and the geometric mean is smaller than the arithmetic mean and closer to the median. It is important to realize that we apply the transformation to each value of the raw data and *not* to the class limits of grouped data, even when the data are presented as a frequency distribution. Figure 2.10b shows the effect of this log transformation on the distribution of the mechanical threshold data summarized in Table 2.1 and displayed in Figure 2.10a. The mean of the log mechanical threshold data is 0.6778 log newtons; the antilog of this mean, the geometric mean, is 4.76 newtons. Note that the arithmetic mean is 5.25 newtons and the median is 4.65 newtons. You can see that the distribution is more symmetrical, and the geometric mean represents the central tendency of the transformed data much

(a) Histogram of raw data

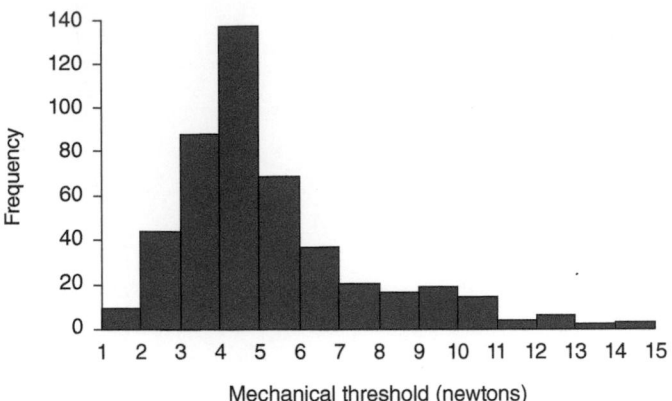

(b) Histogram of log₁₀ data

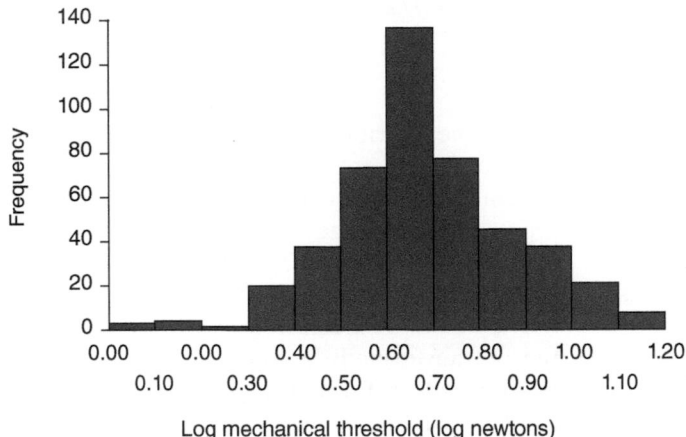

Figure 2.10 Histograms of the mechanical threshold of sheep showing (a) the raw data, and (b) the log₁₀-transformed data (data from Ley *et al.*, 1995, with permission from the authors and BMJ Publishing Group Ltd).

better than the arithmetic mean of the untransformed data.

- The geometric mean is always less than the arithmetic mean if the data are skewed to the right.
- The geometric mean is usually approximately equal to the median if the data are skewed to the right. We often prefer to use the geometric mean rather than the median for right-skewed data because the properties of the distribution of the mean (from which the geometric mean is calculated using the log data) are more useful than those of the median.

(d) Mode

A well-known but infrequently used measure of central tendency is the **mode**. It is the most commonly occurring observation in a set of observations. The mode often has a different value from both the arithmetic mean and the median. The **modal group** or **modal class** is the group or class into which most observations fall in a histogram.

In the mechanical threshold data of Table 2.1 and Figure 2.5, the modal group represents values from 4.0 to 4.9 newtons. In another context, we might use the mode to indicate the most common litter size in a breed of dogs, e.g. the most common litter size of bearded collie dogs is seven.

For the following reasons, statisticians tend not to favour the mode as a tool for summarizing data:

- The mode is determined by disregarding most of the observations.
- The mode depends on the accuracy with which the data are measured.
- Some distributions do not have a mode, whilst other distributions may have more than one mode. A distribution that has a single mode or modal group is called **unimodal**; a distribution that has two humps (i.e. modes or modal groups) separated by a trough is called **bimodal** even if the frequency of occurrence of the observations in the two modes or modal classes is not equal.

2.6.2 Measures of dispersion (spread)

There are a number of measures of the spread of the data, each of which has different attributes.

(a) Range

The **range** is defined as the difference between the largest and smallest observations. In the mechanical threshold data from Table 2.1, the range is 13.9 newtons, being the difference between the maximum value of 14.9 newtons and the minimum value of 1.0 newton.

- The range is an easily determined measure of dispersion of the observations of a numerical variable.
- It gives undue weight to extreme values and will, therefore, overestimate the dispersion of most of the observations if outliers are present.
- The range tends to increase in value as the number of observations in the sample increases.

(b) Interquartile range

The **interquartile range** is the range of values that encloses the central 50% of the observations

if the observations are arranged in order of magnitude. It is defined as the difference between the first and third quartiles (see Section 2.3.3). In the mechanical threshold data, the interquartile range is from 3.68 to 6.10 newtons (see Figure 2.1).

- The interquartile range is influenced neither by the presence of outliers nor by the sample size.
- It suffers from the disadvantage, in common with the range, of ignoring most of the observations as it is calculated from just two of them.

(c) Variance

The **variance** is determined by calculating the *deviation* of each observation from the mean. This deviation will be large if the observation is far from the mean, and it will be small if the observation is close to the mean. Some sort of average of these deviations therefore provides a useful measure of spread. However, some of the deviations are positive and some are negative, depending on whether the observation is greater or less than the mean, and their arithmetic mean is zero. The effect of the sign of the deviation can be annulled by squaring every deviation, since the square of both positive and negative numbers is always positive. The arithmetic mean of these squared deviations is called the variance.

In fact, when we select a sample of n observations from our population, we divide the sum of the squared deviations in the sample by $n-1$ instead of n. It can be shown that this produces a better estimate (i.e. *unbiased*, see Sections 4.4.3 and 4.4.4) of the population variance. Thus, the sample variance, s^2, which estimates the population variance, σ^2, is given by

$$s^2 = \frac{\sum(x-\bar{x})^2}{n-1}$$

We rarely calculate the variance from first principles in this age of hand-held calculators and computers, and so we make no attempt here to show the mechanics of the calculation.

Example

The plasma potassium data of 14 dogs, for which the mean was calculated as 4.57 mmol/l (see Section 2.6.1(a)), gives a sample variance of

$$s^2 = \frac{1.32297}{13} = 0.10177 \,(\text{mmol/l})^2$$

If you were reporting the variance, you would probably correct it to one decimal place more than the original data. This variance would therefore be reported as 0.102 $(\text{mmol/l})^2$.

- The variance uses every available observation.
- Although the variance is a sensible measure of spread, it is not intuitively appealing as its dimensionality is different from that of the original measurements.

(d) Standard deviation

The **standard deviation** (often abbreviated to **SD**) is equal to the square root of the variance. The standard deviation may be regarded as a kind of average of the deviations of the observations from the arithmetic mean. It is often denoted by s in the sample, estimating σ in the population, and is given by

$$s = \sqrt{\text{Variance}} = \sqrt{\frac{\sum (x - \bar{x})^2}{n-1}}$$

We can calculate the standard deviation on a calculator rather than by substituting the actual observations into the above formula. (Note: most calculators have two SD function keys, one for the population SD and one for its estimate from the sample. These may be marked as σ (for the population) and s (for the sample). On some calculators, you may find them marked as σ_n (for the population) and s_{n-1} or σ_{n-1} (for the sample). The use of σ_{n-1} is confusing because it is contrary to the generally accepted convention of nomenclature.)

Example

In the plasma potassium data of 14 dogs used as the example for the calculations of the mean and the variance

$$s = \sqrt{0.10177} = 0.319 \,\text{mmol/l}$$

- The SD uses all the observations in the data set.
- The SD is a measure of spread whose dimensionality is the same as that of the original observations, i.e. it is measured in the same units as the observations.
- The SD is of greatest use in relation to a symmetrically distributed data set that follows the Gaussian or Normal distribution (see Section 3.5.3). In this case, it can be shown that the interval defined by the (mean ± 2 SD) encompasses the central 95% (approximately) of the observations in the population. In the example above, the interval is 4.57 ± 2(0.319), i.e. from 3.93 to 5.21 mmol/l.
- For data that are Normally distributed, four times the standard deviation gives us an indication of the *range* of the majority of the values in the population. In the plasma potassium example, this is 4 × 0.319 = 1.28 mmol/l.

Sometimes the standard deviation is expressed as a percentage of the mean; we call this measure the **coefficient of variation** (**CV**). It is a dimensionless quantity that can be used for comparing relative amounts of variation. However, these comparisons are entirely subjective because its theoretical properties are complex, so we do not recommend its use.

2.7 Reference interval

Sometimes we are interested in describing the range of values of a variable that defines the healthy population; we call this the **reference interval** or the **reference range**. Because of the problem caused by outliers, we calculate the reference range as the interval that encompasses, say, the central 90%, 95% or 99% of the observations obtained from a large representative sample of the population. We usually calculate the values encompassing 95% of the observations; the reference range is then defined by the mean ± 1.96 SD (the 1.96 is often approximated by 2) provided the data have an approximately Normal distribution (see Section 3.5.3). If the data are not Normally distributed, we can still calculate the reference range as the interval defined by the 2.5th and 97.5th percentiles of the empirical distribution of the observations. More information about the calculation of the reference interval may be found in, for example, Geffré *et al.* (2011).

We can use the reference interval to determine whether an individual animal may be classified as belonging to the population of healthy animals. If the animal under consideration has a value for this variable which lies outside the specified range for the healthy population, we may conclude that the animal is unlikely to belong to the normal population and is a diseased animal. For example, plasma creatinine values above the reference interval of 40–180 mmol/l were used to diagnose renal failure in cats in a study by Barber and Elliott (1998).

Note that the reference interval or range is sometimes called the normal range. The latter term is best avoided because of the confusion between 'normal' implying healthy and 'Normal' in the statistical sense describing a particular theoretical distribution. In this book we distinguish the two by small and capital letters but they may still be misconstrued.

Exercises

The statements in questions 2.1–2.4 are either TRUE or FALSE.

2.1 An appropriate diagram to show the frequency distribution of a continuous variable is:
(a) A histogram.
(b) A pie chart.
(c) A stem-and-leaf plot.
(d) A bar chart.
(e) A box-and-whisker plot.

2.2 An appropriate measure of central tendency for continuous data that are skewed to the right is:
(a) The arithmetic mean.
(b) The geometric mean.
(c) The antilog of the arithmetic mean of the log-transformed data.
(d) The median.
(e) The 50th percentile.

2.3 The standard deviation:
(a) Is a measure of dispersion.
(b) Is the difference between the 5th and 95th percentiles.
(c) Is greater than the range of the observations.
(d) Measures the average deviation of the observations from the mean.
(e) Is the square of the variance.

2.4 The reference range (containing 95% of the observations) for a particular variable:
(a) Cannot be calculated if the data are skewed.
(b) May be used to determine whether or not an animal is likely to be diseased if its value for the variable is known.
(c) Can be evaluated from a small sample of data.
(d) Is equal to the mean ± SD if the data are Normally distributed.
(e) Is equal to the difference between the largest and smallest observations in the data set.

2.5 The following data show the resting pulmonary ventilation in 25 adult sheep (l/min):

8.3	8.0	9.9	6.1	5.5
10.3	6.5	7.6	7.6	7.6
6.9	10.3	7.8	7.3	8.9
10.1	7.6	9.1	8.3	4.8
10.2	6.5	9.1	7.0	11.9

Draw histograms of the data with:
(a) Class interval 1.0 l/min, lowest class 4.25–5.24 l/min.
(b) Class interval 0.2 l/min, lowest class 4.80–4.99 l/min.
(c) Class interval 5.0 l/min, lowest class 4.50–9.49 l/min.

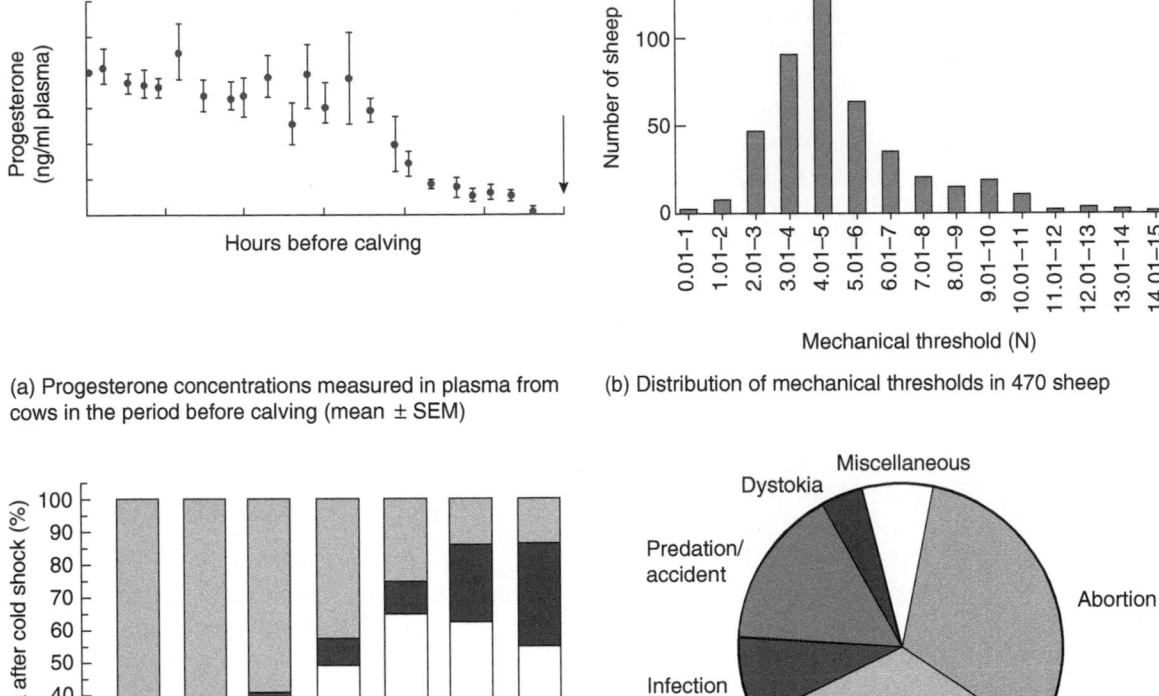

(a) Progesterone concentrations measured in plasma from cows in the period before calving (mean ± SEM)

(b) Distribution of mechanical thresholds in 470 sheep

(c) Categorization of boar spermatozoa into ☐live acrosome-intact, ■ live acrosome-damaged, and ▨ dead subgroups after cold shock at various times after ejaculation

(d) Relative importance of different causes of lamb deaths

Figure 2.11   Illustrations taken from the literature: (a) Parker *et al.* (1988), reproduced from the *Veterinary Record* with permission from BMJ Publishing Group Ltd; (b) Ley *et al.* (1995), reproduced with permission from the authors and BMJ Publishing Group Ltd; (c) Tamuli and Watson (1994), reproduced from the *Veterinary Record* with permission from BMJ Publishing Group Ltd; and (d) Merrell (1998), redrawn with permission from the author.

All the histograms should appear on the same sheet of graph paper and should not be superimposed. Use the same scales for all of them. Which is the most appropriate histogram for demonstrating the distribution of the data? Explain your answer.

2.6 The diagrams in Figure 2.11 have errors in their presentation. Identify the incorrect features and suggest what is required to rectify the errors.

2.7 The following data, 44.4, 67.6, 76.2, 64.7, 80.0, 64.2, 75.0, 34.2, 29.2, represent the infection of goats with the viral condition *peste des petits ruminants*, expressed as the percentage morbidity in Indian villages (Kulkarni *et al.*, 1996, reproduced from the *Veterinary Record* with permission from BMJ Publishing Group Ltd). Calculate the median.

2.8 Calculate the mean and the median of the following data set. What evidence is there for concluding that the data are or are not symmetrically distributed?

Body weights of 16 weanling female mice in grams:

54.1	49.8	24.0	46.0	44.1	34.0	52.6	54.4
56.1	52.0	51.9	54.0	58.0	39.0	32.7	58.5

2.9 Use a calculator with statistical functions to calculate the range, the variance and the standard deviation of the sample data which follows (Gunning & Walters, 1994, reproduced from the *Veterinary Record* with permission from BMJ Publishing Group Ltd).

Vitamin E concentration (mmol/l) in 12 heifers showing clinical signs of an unusual myopathy:

4.2	3.3	7.0	6.9	5.1	3.4	2.5	8.6	3.5
2.9	4.9	5.4						

2.10 Explain the meaning of the following terms, indicating how each is determined:
(a) Percentile.
(b) Median.
(c) Interquartile range.
(d) Reference range.

3

Probability and probability distributions

3.1 Learning objectives

By the end of this chapter, you should be able to:

- Calculate the mathematical probability of the occurrence of particular outcomes in simple events, such as dice-throwing and coin-tossing.
- Elaborate the simple rules of probability – the addition rule and the multiplication rule for independent and dependent events – and illustrate each with a simple example.
- Explain what is meant by a probability density function.
- List the properties of the Normal distribution.
- Describe the Standardized Normal Deviate.
- Explain how you might verify approximate Normality in a data set.
- List situations when a Lognormal distribution might apply.
- Define conditions under which measurements follow the Binomial distribution, and give an example.
- State when the Binomial distribution is approximated by the Normal distribution.
- Define conditions under which measurements follow the Poisson distribution, and give an example.
- State when the Poisson distribution is approximated by the Normal distribution.

3.2 Probability

3.2.1 Relevance of probability to statistics

So far, we have discussed the processes involved in summarizing and displaying the results obtained from a group of animals. The approaches, collectively known as **descriptive statistics**, are an important first step to any analysis. However, usually we want to generalize the results from a representative sample to the larger population from which they came; that is, we want to make *inferences* about the population using the sample data.

For example, suppose the mean and standard deviation of serum iron concentration in a random sample of 59 Simmental cows are 27.64μmol/l and 6.36μmol/l, respectively. It is unlikely that the results obtained in this sample are identical to those that would be observed in the population of Simmental cows. However, we want to use this information to infer something about this population. There is invariably some doubt associated with the inferences drawn about the population; this doubt is quantified by a **probability** which is fundamental to statistical inference as it provides the link between the sample and the population. We discuss the concepts of **inferential statistics** in Chapter 4 when

Statistics for Veterinary and Animal Science, Third Edition. Aviva Petrie and Paul Watson.
© 2013 John Wiley & Sons, Ltd. Published 2013 by John Wiley & Sons, Ltd.

the notion of sampling and sampling distributions is introduced, and develop the theory in subsequent chapters. Here we introduce the concepts of probability.

3.2.2 Definitions of probability

There are several approaches to defining a probability:

- We can take the **subjective** or personal view of probability, which is to regard it as a measure of the strength of belief an individual has that a particular event will occur. For example, 'That cow has a 60% chance of calving tonight'. This subjective or personal view of probability is often called Bayesian probability (see Section 14.3.4) when it represents the extent to which it is supported by the available evidence. Whilst this approach to defining a probability has the advantage that it is possible to assign a probability to any event, this is more than offset by the fact that different people are likely to assign different probabilities to the same event, often influenced by irrelevant considerations.
- A second approach to defining a probability relies on having an understanding of the theoretical **model** defining the set of all possible outcomes of a trial; we evaluate the probability solely on the basis of this model, without recourse to performing the experiment at all. It is often called an *a priori* probability. So, for example, we know that there are two equally likely outcomes when an unbiased coin is tossed: either a head or a tail. This is the model from which we can deduce that the probability of a defined event, obtaining a head, say, is 1/2 = 0.5.
- The third approach to defining a probability, and the one commonly used in statistical inference, is to regard a probability as the proportion of times a particular outcome (the event) will occur in a very large number of 'trials' or 'experiments' performed under similar conditions. The result of any one trial should be independent of the result of any other trial, so whether or not the event occurs in any one

trial should not affect whether or not the event occurs in any other trial. As an example, if we are interested in estimating the probability of a litter size greater than three in a colony of guinea pigs, we would have to count the number of such litters over a lengthy period, say a year, and divide it by the total number of litters. This is the **frequency** definition of probability because it relies on counting the frequency of occurrence of the event in a large number of repetitions of similar trials. The probability defined in this way is thus the *relative frequency* of the event in repeated trials under similar conditions. See also Section 14.3.3 for the distinction between the frequentist understanding of probability and significance testing propounded by Ronald Fisher, Jerzy Neyman and Egon Pearson and the more abstract interpretation of probability put forward by Bayesians.

It is interesting to note that the various definitions of probability are not entirely distinct. The proportion of times that an event would be observed if an experiment were to be repeated a large number of times approaches the *a priori* probability. So, if a coin were tossed five times, we would not be very surprised to observe four heads; however if the coin were tossed 1000 times, we would be more likely to observe approximately 500 heads. Thus, the values for the probability defined using both the *a priori* approach and the frequency approach coincide when the experiment is repeated many times. Similarly, the subjective view of probability cannot be divorced from the frequency view, as the former is usually based on experience, which in turn relies on previous occurrences of similar events. For example, the likely incidence of liver fluke infestation can be forecast on the basis of the previous year's rainfall, and is founded on a large database of rainfall/fluke incidence relationships.

3.2.3 Properties of a probability

It is clear that, since a probability can be defined as a relative frequency or a proportion, its numerical value must be equal to or lie between 0 and 1.

- A probability of 0 means that the event *cannot* occur.
- A probability of 1 (unity) means that the event *must* occur.

We often convert probabilities into percentages (with a range 0–100%) or express them as ratios (e.g. a one-in-three chance of an event occurring).

Sometimes we focus our interest not on a particular event occurring but on that event *not* occurring, i.e. on the *complementary event*. It follows from the properties of a probability that the probability of the event not occurring is 1 minus the probability of the event occurring. So, if the probability of a kitten contracting feline viral rhinotracheitis after vaccination at 9 and 13 weeks of age is 0.04 (in a particular location and time), then the probability of being adequately protected is 0.96.

3.2.4 Rules of probability

Two simple rules governing probabilities are the addition and multiplication rules. For simplicity, we define them for only two events, A and B, but they can be extended to multiple events.

- **Addition rule**. When two events are *mutually exclusive*, implying that the two events cannot occur at the same time, then the probability of *either* of the two events occurring is the *sum* of the probability of each event. Thus,

$$Pr(A \text{ or } B) = Pr(A) + Pr(B)$$

  For example, assuming that we have a carton of 50 dog biscuits, with 10 of each of five different shapes, the probability of picking either a diamond shape or a round shape from the carton is the sum of the probability of a diamond (10/50 = 1/5) and the probability of a round (10/50 = 1/5) which is 2/5 or 0.4.
- **Multiplication rule**. When two events are *independent*, so that the occurrence or non-

occurrence of one event does not affect the occurrence or non-occurrence of the other event, then the probability of *both* events occurring is the *product* of the individual probabilities. Thus,

$$Pr(A \text{ or } B) = Pr(A) \times Pr(B)$$

For example, if we have two cartons of dog biscuits, as in the addition rule example, the probability of picking a diamond shape from both cartons is 1/5 × 1/5, equal to 1/25 or 0.04.

When two events are *not independent*, we have to adopt a different rule, which relies on an understanding of **conditional probability**. The probability of an event B occurring when we know that A has already occurred is called the conditional probability of B, and is written as $Pr(B \text{ given } A)$ or $Pr(B|A)$. Thus the event B is dependent on A. If we have two such dependent events, the probability of both events occurring is equal to the probability of one of them occurring times the conditional probability of the other occurring. So,

$$Pr(A \text{ or } B) = Pr(A) \times Pr(B \text{ given } A)$$

For example, if we have a carton of dog biscuits as in the addition rule example, the probability of picking a second diamond shape after we have already picked one diamond shape (and given it to Max to eat!) is equal to the probability of picking the first diamond shape (10/50 = 1/5) times the probability of picking the second diamond shape out of the remaining 49 biscuits (9/49), i.e. it is 0.037.

3.3 Probability distributions

3.3.1 Introduction

We introduced **empirical frequency distributions** in Section 2.3; these allow us to assimilate a large amount of *observed* data and condense them into a form, typically a table or a diagram, from which we can interpret their salient features. Another type of distribution is a **probability distribution**; this is a *theoretical* model that we use to calculate the probability of an event occurring. The probability distribution shows how the set of all possible mutually exclusive events is distributed, and can be presented as an *equation*, a *chart* or a *table*. We may regard a probability distribution as the theoretical equivalent of an empirical relative frequency distribution, with its own mean and variance.

A variable which can take different values with given probabilities is called a **random variable**. A probability distribution comprises all the values that the random variable can take, with their associated probabilities. There are numerous probability distributions which may be distinguished by whether the random variable is **discrete**, taking only a finite set of possible values, or **continuous**, taking an infinite set of possible values in a range of values (see Section 1.6). A discrete random variable with only two possible values is called a **binary variable**, e.g. pregnant or not pregnant, diseased or healthy.

3.3.2 Avoiding the theory!

We discuss some of the more common distributions in this chapter although, for simplicity, we omit the mathematical equations that define the distributions. You do not need to know the equations for the procedures we describe in this text, since the required probabilities are tabulated.

We are aware that much of the theory associated with probability distributions presents difficulties to the novice statistician. Moreover, it is possible to perform analyses on a variable without this knowledge. We have therefore chosen not to present more details of these distributions than we believe are absolutely necessary for you to proceed. Advanced statistics texts and many elementary texts cover this in more detail.

3.4 Discrete probability distributions

3.4.1 Definition

Box 3.1 defines a discrete probability distribution. An example of a *discrete* random variable

Box 3.1 Definition of a discrete probability distribution

> A discrete probability distribution attaches a probability to every possible mutually exclusive event defined by a discrete random variable; the sum of these probabilities is 1 (unity).

is seen in simple Mendelian inheritance. Consider the situation where we have a pair of alleles represented by T, the dominant allele, and t, the recessive allele. In Manx cats the dominant mutant, T, is associated with the tailless condition but the homozygous combination, TT, is lethal and these embryos do not develop. The heterozygous condition, Tt or tT, results in the tailless Manx cat, and the homozygous tt condition is the normal cat with a tail. When two Manx cats (heterozygous) are mated, there are four equally likely genotypic outcomes: TT, Tt, tT and tt (Figure 3.1a).

Figure 3.1b is a chart of the discrete probability distribution of the dominant allele, T. The probability distribution for this random variable is the complete statement of the three possible phenotypic outcomes with their associated probabilities. In the chart, the horizontal axis describes the set of the three possible outcomes defining the random variable, and the vertical axis measures the probability of each outcome. Each probability is quantified by the length of a bar; the sum of the three probabilities attached to the possible outcomes is unity (i.e. $0.25 + 0.50 + 0.25 = 1$). As can be seen in Figure 3.1b, in this case there are only three viable genotypes (tt, Tt, tT), giving rise to a ratio of phenotypically Manx cats to normal cats of 2:1. It is easy to see that the diagrammatic representation of a probability distribution bears a strong resemblance to the empirical bar chart in which the vertical axis represents relative frequency, as in Figure 2.2.

There are many different discrete probability distributions. The two distributions which are particularly relevant to biological science are the **Binomial** and **Poisson** distributions. As we explain in Section 3.6.1, these two discrete distributions are often approximated by a continuous distribution.

(a)

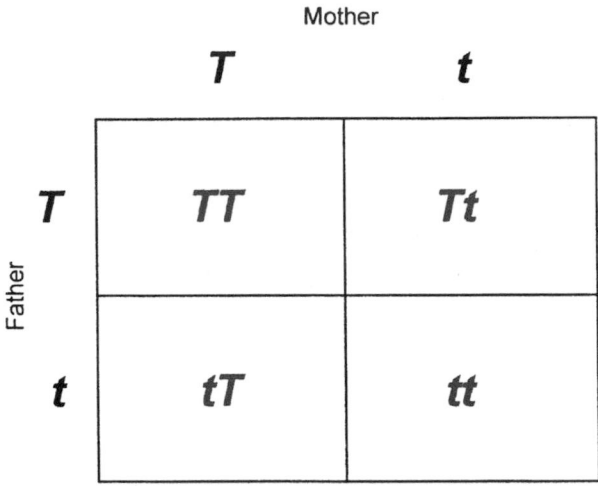

(b)

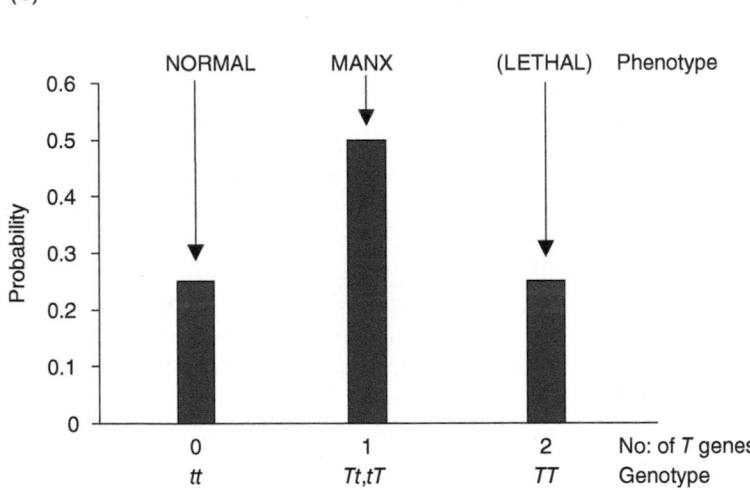

Figure 3.1 Genetic characteristics of cats whose parents are each of Manx genotype *Tt*. (a) The four possible genotypic outcomes. (b) The probability distribution of the number of *T* genes, the random variable that determines the phenotype of the cat.

3.4.2 Binomial distribution

The **Binomial distribution** is relevant in the situation in which we are investigating a *binary* response. There are only two possible outcomes to what we shall term a 'trial': either the animal is pregnant or it is not; either the animal shows clinical signs of infectious disease or it does not. It is common in statistical theory to use the terminology 'success' in a trial to represent the situation when the individual possesses the char-

acteristic (e.g. disease) or the event occurs (e.g. pregnancy). Likewise, 'failure' is used to represent the complementary event, i.e. the situation when the individual does not possess the characteristic (e.g. is disease-free) or the event does not occur (e.g. not pregnant). We define the Binomial distribution in Box 3.2.

So for example, suppose we take blood samples from six cattle randomly selected from the population. Each animal in the population is either seropositive for *Leptospira* (success)

Box 3.2   The Binomial distribution

> The random variable in the Binomial distribution represents the number of successes in a series of *n* independent trials in which each trial can result in either a success (with probability, π) or a failure (with probability, $1 - \pi$). In theory, there are $n + 1$ possible outcomes in this situation as it is possible to observe either 0 successes or 1 or 2 or 3 or . . . up to *n* successes in the *n* trials. The Binomial distribution attaches a probability to each outcome. The mean and variance of the distribution are $n\pi$ and $n\pi(1 - \pi)$, respectively.

Box 3.3   The Poisson distribution

> The random variable of a Poisson distribution represents the *count* of the number of events occurring randomly and independently in time or space at a constant rate, μ, on average. The mean and variance of the distribution are equal to μ.

or not (failure), i.e. we have a binary response variable. We know that the prevalence (see Box 5.1) of *Leptospira* in the cattle population is approximately 30% (this is π). We can use this information and our knowledge of the Binomial distribution to attach a probability to each of the possible outcomes – the probability that none is positive for *Leptospira*, or alternatively, that 1, 2, 3, . . . , up to 6 are positive. These probabilities are, respectively, 0.1176, 0.3025, 0.3241, 0.1852, 0.0595, 0.0102 and 0.0007, which, when added, sum to 1 (apart from rounding errors).

(a) Importance of the Binomial distribution

The Binomial distribution is particularly important in statistics because of its role in analysing *proportions*. A proportion is derived from a binary response variable, e.g. the proportion of animals with disease if each animal either has or does not have the disease. We can use our knowledge of the Binomial distribution (usually its Normal approximation, see Section 3.6.1) to make inferences about proportions (see Sections 4.7 and 9.3.1). As an example, Little *et al.* (1980) used the differences in the proportions of leptospiral-positive antisera in groups of aborting and normal animals to investigate the role of leptospiral infection in abortion in cows. It was shown that the aborting cows had a significantly higher proportion of *Leptospira*-positive antibody levels than the normal animals.

3.4.3 Poisson distribution

Another discrete probability distribution which occurs in veterinary and animal science is the

Poisson distribution. We define the Poisson distribution in Box 3.3.

For example, using the Poisson distribution, we can attach probabilities to a particular count – the number (say, 5550) of scintillation events caused by a radioactive sample in a scintillation counter per unit time, or the number (say, 35) of blood cells per unit volume of a diluted sample, or the number (say, 60) of parasitic eggs per unit volume or weight of faecal sample, or the number (say, 2) of poisonous plants per quadrat across a field. Usually, for convenience, we employ the Normal approximation to the Poisson distribution for analysing these data (see Section 3.6.1).

3.5 Continuous probability distributions

3.5.1 Relationship between discrete and continuous probability distributions

In order to understand the relationship between discrete and continuous probability distributions:

- Refer to Figure 3.2a, an example of a very simple discrete probability distribution. All possible events are represented on the horizontal axis. The vertical length of each line represents the probability of the event. Since all events are represented, and the total probability must equal unity, the sum of the lengths of all the lines also equals 1.
- Refer to Figure 3.2b, an illustration of a discrete probability distribution in which there are a large, but still finite, number of possible discontinuous values of the random variable. Again, the sum of the lengths of all the lines equals unity.

(a) Categorical random variable taking only three values

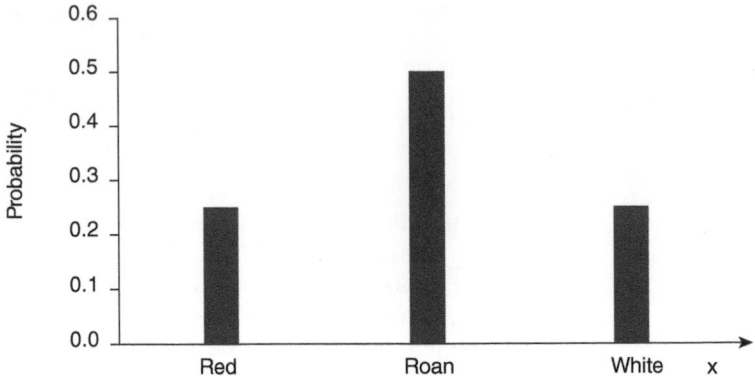

(b) Discrete random variable taking 15 values

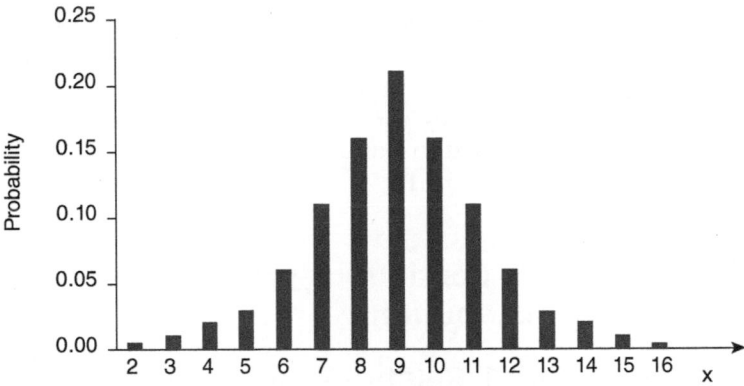

(c) Probability density function of a continuous random variable

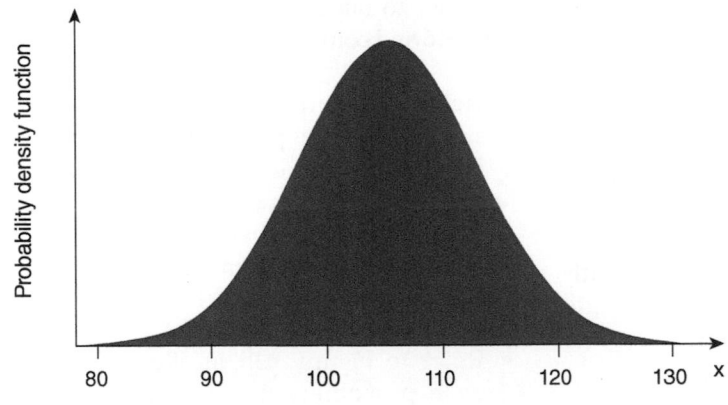

Figure 3.2 Example showing the probability distributions of categorical and numerical random variables: (a) x = coat colour of Shorthorn cattle, (b) x = raccoon litter size, and (c) x = height of donkeys (cm).

Box 3.4 Properties of a continuous probability distribution

> - A continuous probability distribution is defined by a probability density function.
> - The total area under the probability density function is 1 (unity).
> - The probability that the continuous random variable lies between certain limits is equal to the area under the probability density function between these limits.

- Now refer to Figure 3.2c. This figure represents the probability distribution of a continuous random variable. In contrast to a discrete probability distribution, here the variable can take an infinite number of values so it is impossible to draw separate lines. The shaded *area* now represents the total probability of unity. The curve that defines the area is called a **probability density function** which is described by an equation. Box 3.4 summarizes the properties of a continuous probability distribution.

3.5.2 Calculating probabilities from the probability density function

If the variable of interest is continuous, then the probability that its value lies in a particular interval is given by the relevant area under the curve of the probability density function (Figure 3.3). We can determine the area under the curve for a range of values of the random variable by a mathematical process (called integration) applied to the equation. Rather than having to do this, there are special tables that relate areas under the curve to probabilities for the well-known continuous distributions, such as the **Normal**, **Student's** *t*-, **Chi-squared** and *F*-distributions, each defined by its own equation.

3.5.3 Normal (or Gaussian) distribution

(a) Empirical distributions and Normality

The **Normal** or **Gaussian distribution**, named after C. F. Gauss, an 18th century German math-

ematician, is the most important of the continuous distributions because of its role in sampling theory, which we consider in Chapter 4. The term 'Normal' is not meant to imply that the probability distribution of the random variable is typical, even though it is a good approximation to the distribution of many naturally occurring variables, or that it represents a 'non-diseased' group of individuals. To distinguish the Normal distribution from any other interpretation of normal, we use an upper case N in the former instance throughout this book.

The Normal distribution is a theoretical distribution. We often find that observations made on a variable in a group of individuals have an empirical frequency distribution which is similar to a Normal distribution. We then make the assumption that the distribution of that variable in the population is Normal. If this is a reasonable assumption, we can use the properties of the Normal distribution to evaluate required probabilities. For example, the 6-furlong finish times for Thoroughbreds on Louisiana racetracks have an empirical distribution which is approximately Normal (Martin *et al.*, 1996). We show, in Section 3.5.3(c), how we can use the 6-furlong finish time to calculate the probability that a racehorse has a finish time faster than 72 seconds.

(b) Description

As well as possessing the property, in common with other continuous distributions, that the area under the curve defined by its probability density function is unity, the Normal distribution has several useful properties. These are listed in Box 3.5 and demonstrated in Figure 3.4.

(c) Areas under the curve and the Standard Normal distribution

In order to calculate the probability that a value of the variable, x, is greater than x_1 (see Figure 3.3c), you can use Appendix Table A.1. We will take you through a four-step process:

1. Recognize that the probability that x has a value greater than x_1 is equal to the area under the Normal distribution curve to the right of x_1.

(a)

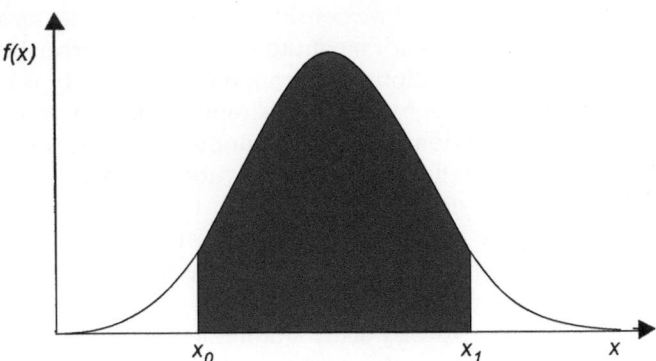

(b)

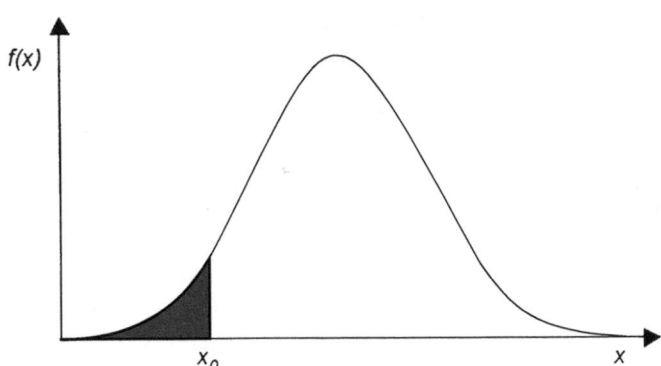

(c)

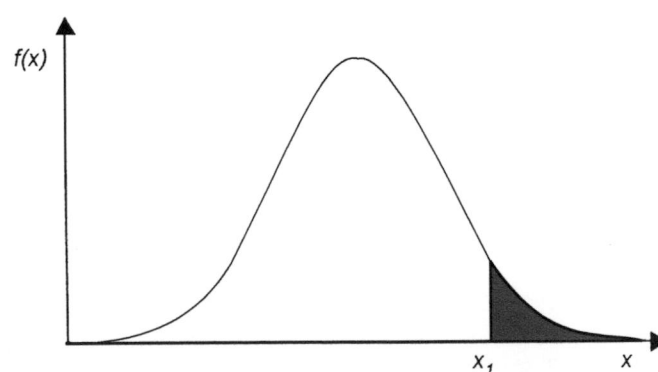

Figure 3.3 Relationship between the area under the probability density function, $y = f(x)$, for the random variable, x, and probability. The total area under $f(x)$ is 1; the shaded area in (a) represents Prob $\{x_0 < x < x_1\}$, in (b) Prob $\{x < x_0\}$, and in (c) Prob $\{x > x_1\}$.

Box 3.5   Properties of the Normal distribution

- The Normal distribution is completely described by two parameters: the mean and the standard deviation. These are usually denoted by the Greek letters μ and σ, respectively. The mathematical formula for the probability density function is omitted for simplicity.
- It is unimodal.
- It is symmetrical about its mean. This implies that the curve to the right of the mean is a mirror image of the curve to the left of the mean. It is often described as 'bell-shaped'.
- Its mean, median and mode are all equal.
- If the standard deviation remains unchanged, increasing the value of the mean shifts the curve horizontally to the right. Conversely, decreasing the value of the mean shifts the curve horizontally to the left (Figure 3.4a).
- A decrease in the standard deviation of the curve makes the curve thinner, taller and more peaked. Conversely, an increase in the standard deviation makes the curve fatter, shorter and flatter (Figure 3.4b).
- The limits $(\mu - \sigma)$ and $(\mu + \sigma)$ contain 68.3% of the distribution (Figure 3.5a).
- The limits $(\mu - 1.96\sigma)$ and $(\mu + 1.96\sigma)$ contain 95% of the distribution (see Figure 3.5a). This fact is often used in the calculation of a reference range (see Section 2.7).
- The limits $(\mu - 2.58\sigma)$ and $(\mu + 2.58\sigma)$ contain 99% of the distribution (Figure 3.5a).

- The Standard Normal distribution is symmetrical around its mean of 0. Thus the tail area to the right of a value z_1 is the same as the tail area to the left of $-z_1$; equivalently, the probability that $z > z_1$ is equal to the probability that $z < -z_1$. Table A.1 provides the sum of these two tail area probabilities for various values of z. The values of z are sometimes called **critical values** or **percentage points**, as each defines a percentage of the total area under the probability density function.
- To obtain the area to the right of z_1 from Table A.1, we have to divide the probability obtained from the table by 2. This is because the probabilities in the table relate to both tails of the Standard Normal distribution, whereas here we are interested only in the right tail.
- You should be aware that the Standard Normal distribution is not always tabulated in the same way as in Table A.1. For example, you might find that only the right tail or the left tail area is tabulated. However, you can always determine the probability that is required for your problem by subtraction and/or multiplying or dividing by 2, as long as you remember that the Standard Normal distribution is symmetrical and that the total area under the curve is 1.

2. Define the mean and the standard deviation of your Normal distribution. In general terms, we call these μ and σ, respectively.
3. Convert this Normal distribution into a **Standard Normal distribution** (see Figure 3.5b) which has a mean of 0 and a standard deviation of 1 (unity). This is the distribution of a new variable, z, which is called a **Standardized Normal Deviate (SND)**. In general terms

$$z = \frac{x - \mu}{\sigma}$$

And, in this particular example, the value of the SND which corresponds to x_1 is

$$z_1 = \frac{x_1 - \mu}{\sigma}$$

4. Use Table A.1 to determine the specified area. Instructions for the procedure are given with the table, which has an accompanying illustrative diagram. It is important to realize that:

Suppose we want to apply this theory to a practical example. We know that the six-furlong finish time for Thoroughbreds on Louisiana racetracks is approximately Normally distributed in the population with a mean of 75.2 seconds (s) and a standard deviation of 2.2 s (Martin *et al.*, 1996). We want to determine the probability of a racehorse having a finish time of less than, say, 72.0 s. The value of z corresponding to $x_1 = 72.0$ is $z_1 = (72.0 - 75.2)/(2.2) = -1.45$ (which is -1.4545 corrected to two decimal places). Since we are only interested in the probability in the lower tail of the distribution, and the Standard Normal distribution is symmetrical about zero so that the area to the left of a SND of -1.45 is equal to that to the right of a SND of $+1.45$, the required probability is half the tabulated two-tailed probability corresponding to a SND of 1.45. Thus, from Table

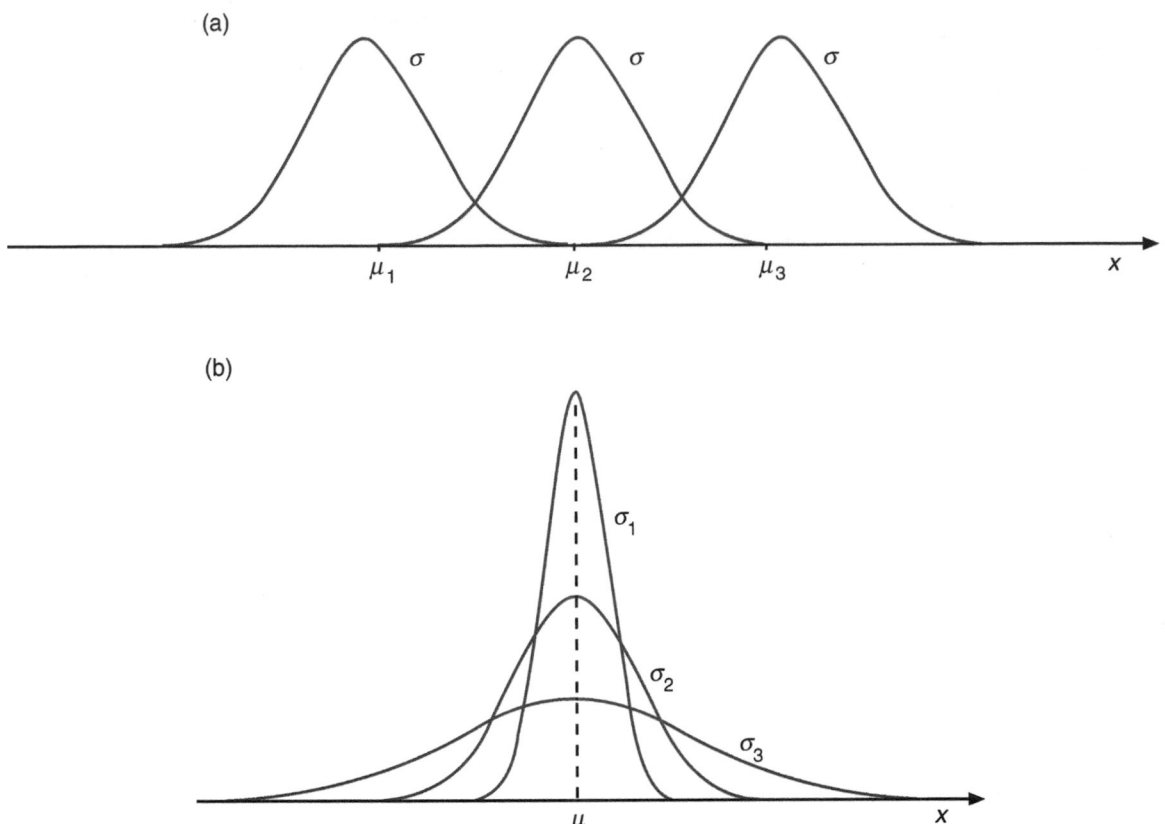

Figure 3.4   The effect on the Normal distribution of changing the parameters μ and σ: (a) with different means, $\mu_1 < \mu_2 < \mu_3$, and the same standard deviation, σ, and (b) with different standard deviations, $\sigma_1 < \sigma_2 < \sigma_3$, and the same mean, μ.

A.1 we find that the probability is $0.5 \times 0.1471 = 0.0736$; we would expect about 7% of the racehorses to have finish times quicker than 72.0 s.

(d) Determining the Standardized Normal Deviate from a defined probability

It may be that we are interested not in evaluating a probability (area under the curve) from a particular value of the SND, z, but in the reverse procedure, i.e. in determining the value of z from a specified probability. Naturally, it is possible to do this from Table A.1 but, for simplicity and convenience, we give the z-values for some common probabilities in Appendix Table A.2. We show z-values both for the situation in which the

probability of interest corresponds to the sum of the right- and left-hand tail areas (a **two-tailed probability**), and for the situation in which all the probability of interest corresponds only to the right-hand tail area (a **one-tailed probability**). Two-tailed probabilities are more often relevant than one-tailed probabilities; we discuss this in Section 6.3 in relation to one- and two-sided tests of hypotheses. Note that we may also require a z-value in order to calculate a confidence interval (see Sections 4.5.2 and 4.7).

Suppose we want to know the two values of z that encompass the central 95% of the distribution; this leaves 2.5% of the distribution in each tail, i.e. 5% of the entire distribution is in the two tails. Thus, we enter Table A.2 and note that the value of z which corresponds to a two-tailed

(a)

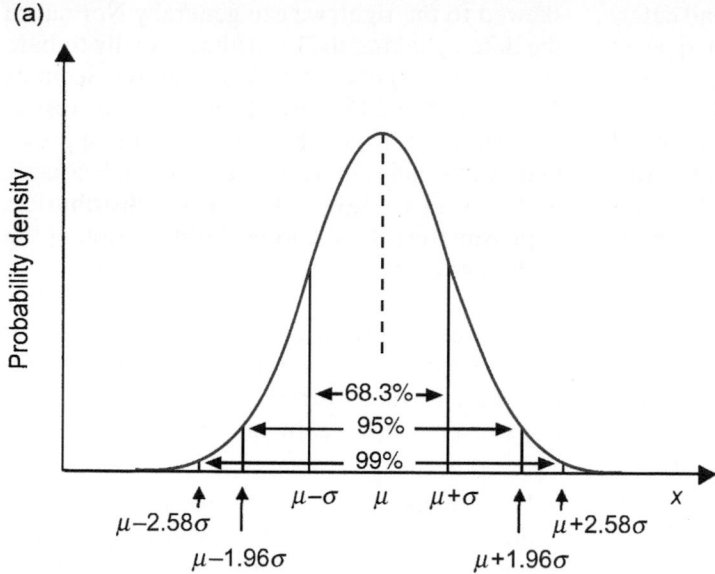

(b)

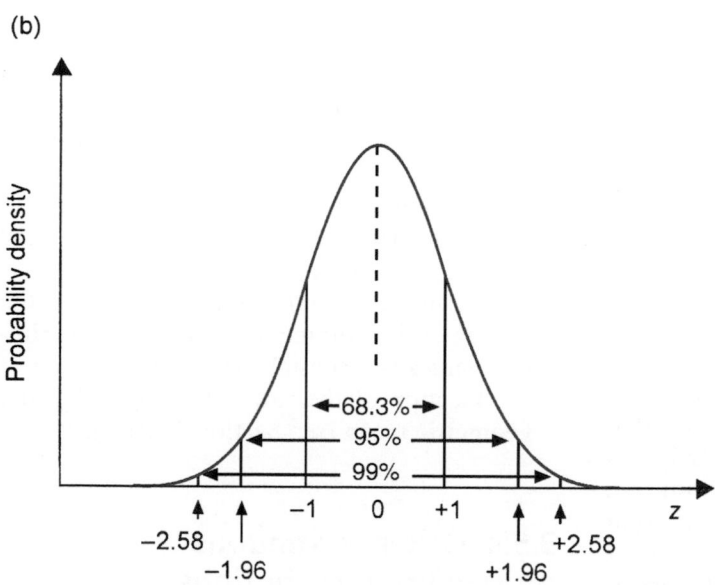

Figure 3.5 Areas under (a) the Normal curve; the random variable, x, has mean = μ and standard deviation = σ; and (b) the Standard Normal curve; the random variable, $z = (x - \mu)/\sigma$, has mean = 0 and standard deviation = 1.

probability of 0.05 is 1.96. You can now see how the value given in the penultimate bullet point of Box 3.5 is derived.

(e) Establishing Normality

The assumption of Normality is important if we wish to use the properties of the Normal distribu-

tion to calculate relevant probabilities. We stress, however, that although the assumption of Normality is inherent in many statistical procedures, the procedures are often valid providing the data are *approximately* Normally distributed.

- The easiest approach to establishing approximate Normality is to produce a histogram of the empirical frequency distribution and determine, by eye, whether the distribution appears unimodal, bell-shaped and symmetrical. Alternatively, a box-and-whisker plot will indicate whether or not the distribution is symmetrical and approximately Normal. This subjective approach is often adequate but it does not work well when the number of observations is small, say, less than 20.

- We can use more formal ways of establishing whether data approximate a Normal distribution. One such method is to produce a graph called a **Normal plot** in which the horizontal axis represents the ordered numerical values of the variable, and the vertical axis represents the corresponding Standardized Normal Deviates. If the data are Normally distributed, then the plot points will conform to a straight line; if the data are not Normally distributed, then the points will deviate from the straight line so that a curve is produced. Often, we find it easier to judge whether the data follow a straight line than whether the histogram of the raw data is symmetrical. Hence, although this technique is also subjective, the Normal plot is commonly produced, usually on a computer, in an attempt to verify the assumption of Normality. We show an example in Figure 3.6 in which the distribution of the sheep mechanical threshold data is not Normal (Figure 3.6a) but that of the log-transformed data is more nearly Normal (Figure 3.6b).
- Occasionally, an objective test for Normality is required. The **Shapiro–Wilk W test** is available in many computer packages, as is the Lilliefors modification of the **Kolmogorov–Smirnov test**, both of which are extremely tedious to perform by hand. We can also derive measures of **skewness** (describing symmetry) and **kurtosis** (describing peakedness) for the observed data set and determine how these measures deviate from what would be expected if the data were Normally distributed.

(f) Lognormal distribution

Many biological variables, such as, for example, parasite infestation data, display a distribution with a long tail to the right. When data are skewed to the right, we can generally Normalize the data by taking the logarithm (usually to base 10 or to base e) of each observation (see Sections 2.6.1(c) and 13.2.1). The distribution of the resulting transformed variable will often be approximately Normal (Figure 3.6). The original variable is then said to have a **Lognormal distribution**, approximating the theoretical distribution of the same name.

The advantage of transforming data in this way so as to produce a transformed variable which is Normally distributed is that the properties of the Normal distribution are relevant to the transformed variable. In particular:

- We can use the probabilities (areas) of the Standard Normal curve to evaluate particular population limits. So, 95% of the distribution of the logarithmic values lie in the interval defined by their mean ± 1.96 times their standard deviation. For example, for the sheep mechanical threshold data in Figure 2.10, 95% of the log-transformed threshold values would be expected to fall between $0.6778 \pm 1.96 \times 0.1927$, i.e. between 0.3001 and 1.0555 log newtons. Hence, by finding the antilogs of these values, we would expect 95% of the threshold values in the population to lie between 1.20 and 11.36 newtons.
- Furthermore, it is interesting to note that the antilog of the arithmetic mean of the logarithmic values is a sensible summary measure of the location of the raw data; it is called the **geometric mean** (see Section 2.6.1(c)).

3.5.4 Other continuous probability distributions

There are numerous continuous probability distributions apart from the Normal distribution. Three particularly well known and useful distributions are the t-, Chi-squared (χ^2) and F-distributions. You may find the discussions of these distributions too theoretical and laborious for comfort. You could skip them at this stage and refer to them only when (or if!) the need arises.

(a)

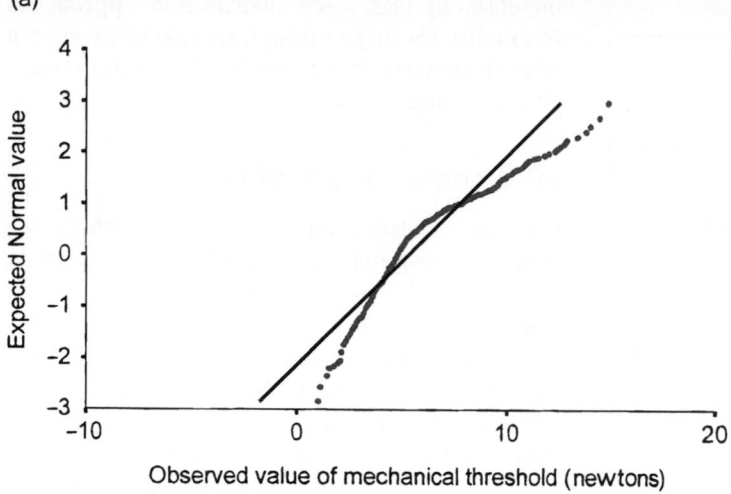

(b)

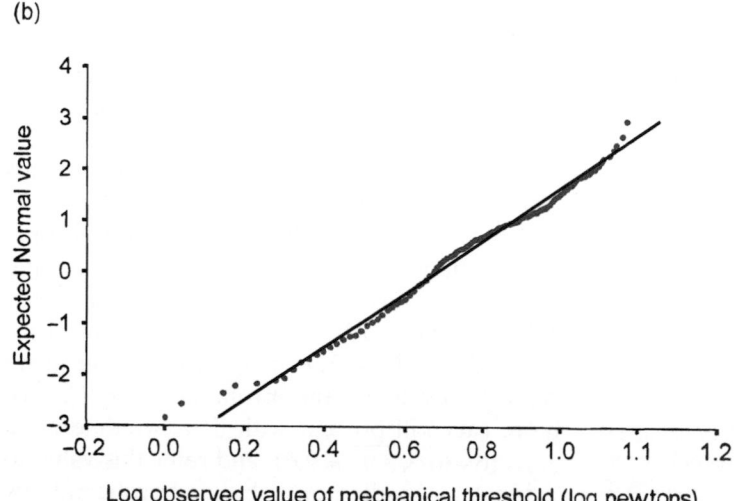

Figure 3.6 Normal plots of the data shown in Figure 2.10. (a) Normal plot of mechanical threshold. (b) Normal plot of log mechanical threshold.

(a) Student's *t*-distribution

'Student', a pseudonym for W. S. Gosset, described the *t*-distribution in 1908 although it was perfected by R. A. Fisher in 1926. This distribution has revolutionized the statistical analysis of small samples. We give the percentage points of the *t*-distribution in Appendix Table A.3, and summarize its properties in Box 3.6.

As we explain in Chapter 7, we use the *t*-distribution when we wish to test a hypothesis about a mean or a difference between two means.

(b) Chi-squared distribution

We give the percentage points of the **Chi-squared (χ^2) distribution** in Appendix Table A.4, and summarize its properties in Box 3.7. We use the Chi-squared distribution when we analyse categorical data (see Chapter 9).

Box 3.6 Properties of the *t*-distribution

- The *t*-distribution is symmetrical about the mean and is bell-shaped.
- It is completely characterized by what are called the degrees of freedom (*df*) so that knowledge of the degrees of freedom allows the probabilities of the *t*-distribution to be computed. We consider the degrees of freedom more fully in Section 6.3.6. For the moment, it is sufficient to note that they have a close affinity to sample size.
- The *t*-distribution is indistinguishable from the Standard Normal distribution when the degrees of freedom are large; as the degrees of freedom decrease, the *t*-distribution becomes more and more spread out compared with the Standard Normal distribution.

Box 3.7 Properties of the Chi-squared distribution

- The Chi-squared distribution can only take positive values and is highly skewed (see diagram attached to Table A.4).
- The degrees of freedom characterize this distribution, so that knowledge of them allows us to determine the relevant probabilities under the curve.
- As the degrees of freedom increase, the distribution becomes more and more symmetrical and eventually approaches Normality.

Box 3.8 Properties of the *F*-distribution and use of Table A.5

- The *F*-distribution is the distribution of a ratio (see Section 3.6.2).
- It is characterized by two separate degrees of freedom: those attached to the numerator and those attached to the denominator of the ratio that defines it.
- Although the ratio could be either greater or less than 1, the tabulated probabilities of the *F*-distribution relate to a ratio that is always greater than or equal to 1, i.e. the numerator is greater than or equal to the denominator. Thus the tabulated values refer only to the upper tail of the distribution. Extra care has to be taken in evaluating the appropriate probabilities from Table A.5 (see Sections 8.3.1 and 8.3.3).

(c) *F*-distribution

We give the percentage points of the **F-distribution** in Appendix Table A.5, and summarize its properties in Box 3.8. We may use the *F*-distribution to compare two variances if each is calculated from Normally distributed data (see Section 8.3). The main use of the *F*-distribution, however, is in a technique called the analysis of variance, which we discuss in Section 8.5. □

3.6 Relationships between distributions

3.6.1 Normal approximations of the Binomial and Poisson distributions

The Binomial and Poisson distributions are skewed when sample sizes are small, although they become more symmetrical as sample sizes increase. In fact, each distribution approaches Normality for large enough sample sizes when a smooth curve is drawn joining the discrete probability values.

(a) Binomial distribution

Consider a Binomial situation in which we observe a proportion, p, of successes in n trials. It is reasonable to use the Normal approximation of the Binomial distribution if both np and $n(1 - p)$ are greater than 5. The mean and variance of this Normal distribution are estimated by np and $np(1 - p)$, respectively. This approximation is particularly useful in statistical inference, for testing hypotheses about and calculating confidence intervals for proportions (see Chapter 9).

Example

Suppose that on a typical day, 18 cats are presented to a veterinary clinic, and six are seen to have fleas. The observed proportion (an estimate of the true proportion) of infested cats is 6/18 = 0.33. Hence, $np = 18 \times 0.33 = 6$, and $n(1 - p) = 18 \times 0.67 = 12$, and a Normal approximation is appropriate. The mean and variance of this Normal distribution are estimated by $np = 18 \times 0.33 = 6$ and $np(1 - p) = 18 \times 0.33 \times 0.67 = 3.98$, respectively. Thus, if we want to evaluate the probability that 10 or more cats will present with fleas, we determine $z_1 = (10 - 6)/\sqrt{3.98} = 2.01$, and refer this value to Table A.1. Dividing the tabulated probability by 2 because we are only interested in the upper tail of the distribution, we find that the required probability is approximately 0.02 (this is 0.0222 corrected to two decimal places). In fact, we should have applied the continuity correction (see Section 3.6.1(c)).

(b) Poisson distribution

The Normal approximation of a Poisson distribution is acceptable if the average rate of occurrence of the event of interest, μ, is not too small (it should be greater than, say, 5). You will then find that the sample mean and variance are approximately equal to μ. This follows from the property of the Poisson distribution that the variance equals the mean. For example, we could analyse worm burden data using the Normal approximation to the Poisson distribution, providing that the average faecal egg counts per gram of wet weight faeces does not fall below 5. □

(c) Continuity correction

These two Normal approximations are useful because we can use tables of the Standard Normal distribution to evaluate probabilities for random variables that follow the Binomial or Poisson distributions. However, note the following:

- The Poisson and Binomial distributions both relate to discrete random variables.
- The Normal distribution relates to continuous random variables.

Therefore, if we use tables of the Normal distribution to provide approximations of the Binomial and Poisson distributions, we should apply a **continuity correction** to adjust for this discrepancy. We subtract 0.5 from the absolute value (i.e. ignoring the sign) of the difference between x and μ in the numerator of the Standardized Normal Deviate, so our adjusted value is

$$z' = \frac{|x - \mu| - 0.5}{\sigma}$$

So, strictly, in the flea-infested cats example described in Section 3.6.1(a), we should have applied the continuity correction to the determination of the probability that 10 or more cats will present with fleas, i.e. $z_1 = \{|10 - 6| - 0.5\}/\sqrt{3.98} = 1.75$. Referring to Table A.1, we find that the required probability is $(0.0801)/2 = 0.04$. We can see that, for small numbers, the continuity correction makes a substantial difference.

3.6.2 Mathematical interrelationships

You may find these theoretical concepts difficult, immaterial or boring, in which case you should skip this section! Otherwise, you may find it interesting to note the following:

- The t-, Chi-squared (χ^2) and F-distributions each represent a specific function, expressed mathematically, of a Normally distributed variable.
- The Chi-squared distribution with k degrees of freedom is defined as the distribution of the sum of the squares of

k independent variables, each of which has a Standard Normal distribution.
- If the degrees of freedom are 1, then the Chi-squared distribution is the square of the Standard Normal distribution.
- The distribution of a mean of a Normally distributed variable divided by its estimated standard error follows a t-distribution.
- The variance estimated from a sample of observations of a Normally distributed variable follows a Chi-squared distribution multiplied by σ^2, where σ^2 is the true variance of the variable in the population.
- The F-distribution is the distribution of the ratio of two independent variables, each with a Chi-squared distribution and each divided by its degrees of freedom.
- The ratio of two variances estimated from independent samples of observations of a Normally distributed variable follows the F-distribution.
- The F-distribution is related to both the t- and Chi-squared distributions. When the degrees of freedom of the numerator of the F-ratio are 1, the tabulated values of the F-distribution correspond to those of the t-distribution on the same number of degrees of freedom as those in the denominator of the F-ratio. When the degrees of freedom of the denominator are extremely large, tending to infinity, then the tabulated values of the F-distribution are the same as those of the Chi-squared distribution when the latter are divided by the degrees of freedom of the numerator of the F-ratio. □

Exercises

The statements in questions 3.1–3.3 are either TRUE or FALSE.

3.1 The random variable, x, is Normally distributed. This implies that:
(a) Its distribution is skewed to the right.
(b) The mean and the median of its distribution are equal.
(c) The limits defined by the mean ± SD contain approximately 95% of the distribution.
(d) The distribution has a mean of 0 and a standard deviation of 1.
(e) All the animals on which this variable is measured are healthy.

3.2 The random variable, z, has a Standard Normal distribution. This implies that:
(a) z is a discrete random variable.
(b) The mean and standard deviation of its distribution are equal.
(c) The total area under its probability density function is 1.

(d) If $z = (x - \mu)/\sigma$, where x is a Normally distributed random variable, then z has a mean equal to μ and a standard deviation equal to σ.

(e) Approximately 68% of the distribution lies between the limits $z = -1$ and $z = +1$.

3.3 Indicate whether the following statements are true or false:

(a) A random variable that follows the Binomial distribution can take more than two values.

(b) The Binomial distribution is the most widely used theoretical distribution in biological statistics.

(c) If sample data approximate a Normal distribution, then the data have been selected from a healthy population.

(d) The mean and variance of the Standard Normal distribution depend on the data set.

(e) The Lognormal distribution is obtained after we take logs of data that follow the Normal distribution.

3.4 A family is trying to decide whether to purchase a puppy bitch or a dog. Dad wants to have a bitch. Because they cannot agree on the pros and cons, Dad suggests that they roll dice to make the decision:

(a) He suggests that his youngest daughter has a go at rolling the two dice once; if she succeeds in getting a 'double' (i.e. two sixes, two fives, ... , or two ones), then they will opt for a bitch, but if not they will have a dog. As she is about to roll, he does his calculations in his head of the probabilities involved and he has second thoughts.

(b) Instead, he proposes that his daughter rolls just one die, but three times. If she fails to get a 'six' in the three tries, then they will purchase a bitch. He believes that now he has the odds with him. Is he right?

Calculate the probability of getting a bitch in (a) and (b). Show how these dice rollings illustrate both the addition and the multiplication rules of probability. What type of probability approach is this (subjective, model, frequency)?

3.5 Do you think the data sets in (a) and (b) which follow are Normally distributed? If you conclude that either is not approximately Normal,

would a log transformation achieve approximate Normality?

(a) The following data (based on the summary data in Coyne *et al.*, 1996) are oxytetracycline measurements from muscle samples from Atlantic salmon (*Salmo salar*). The antibiotic was added to the water over a 10-day period for therapeutic purposes; measurements were taken of muscle concentrations ($\mu g/g$ of muscle tissue) at the 8th day to check effective levels after dosing.

1.3	1.6	1.5	0.5	1.8
1.9	2.5	1.4	0.0	2.1
2.1	0.4	0.3	0.7	0.8
1.2	0.1	1.2	0.8	1.9
0.6	1.7	2.5	2.5	2.4

(b) The following are alkaline phosphatase levels in the serum of 12 normal adult dogs (IU/l).

5.4	7.3	20.3	17.5	35.9	16.8
28.6	54.3	10.0	14.0	11.7	24.3

3.6 The cell counts of erythrocytes in horse blood per small square of the counting chamber are determined. What theoretical distribution would these counts be expected to follow most closely? How can you check whether the counts follow this distribution?

3.7 The mean packed cell volume (PCV) of healthy cats approximates a Normal distribution with mean of 0.37 l/l and a standard deviation of 0.066 l/l.

(a) What percentage of cats have values above 0.40 l/l?

(b) What percentage of cats have values below 0.30 l/l?

(c) What percentage of cats have values between 0.30 and 0.40 l/l?

(d) What is the range containing the central 90% of PCV values?

3.8 (a) What is the area of the Standard Normal curve:
   (i) Above 2.00?
   (ii) Below -1.00?

(b) What is the percentage point (i.e. *z*-value) of the Standard Normal curves for which there is:
  (i) 5% of the total area in the upper tail?
  (ii) 2.5% of the total area in the lower tail?

3.9 A Friesian cow is inseminated on a particular day and sustains the pregnancy to term. The gestation period has an assumed Normal distribution with a mean of 278 days. What is the probability of the cow calving later than 278 days from insemination? If two Friesian cows are inseminated on the same day (and both sustain their pregnancies to term), what is the probability of both of them calving before 278 days later?

3.10 Mollie is very excited as her guinea pigs have just produced four pups (two male and two female) and she is giving her friends, Stephen and Stephanie, one each as a present. She thinks it would be fun to give Stephen a male pup and Stephanie a female pup; she does not want to demonstrate bias in her selection so she decides she will choose them randomly from the litter. Each pup is of approximately the same weight and is equally active. She closes her eyes and reaches for a pup to give to Stephen. She finds that it is male. So far so good! She closes her eyes again and reaches for a second pup out of those remaining. What is the probability that the second guinea pig that she chooses, and which she will give to Stephanie, is female? What, then, is the probability that she can achieve her aim of giving a male pup to Stephen and a female pup to Stephanie after random selection?

4 Sampling and sampling distributions

4.1 Learning objectives

By the end of this chapter, you should be able to:

- Explain the need to distinguish between a sample and the population.
- Explain the concept of a sampling distribution.
- Give the formula for the standard error of the mean.
- Calculate the standard error of the mean.
- Distinguish between the standard deviation and the standard error of the mean.
- Give applications of the standard deviation and the standard error of the mean.
- Explain why a confidence interval is useful.
- Calculate a confidence interval for the mean when the population standard deviation is unknown.
- Interpret the confidence interval for the mean.
- Explain how the standard error of the proportion is calculated and interpret it.
- Calculate a confidence interval for the proportion.

4.2 Distinction between the sample and the population

It is a rare situation, indeed, when we are able to study a whole population of individuals. There may be constraints imposed by time and economic or practical considerations that preclude examination of the whole population. It would be most unusual, for example, to be able to investigate all the Thoroughbred mares in Great Britain. In this situation, we would be most likely to take what we would hope to be a representative sample of animals from the Thoroughbred population (we discuss, in Section 13.6, the principles of **sampling** and the methods by which we can select our sample). We then have to generalize the results from our sample to the population from which it was taken.

The price that we pay for sampling is that we cannot make statements of absolute certainty about the population. Instead, we are able only to surmise about what we expect in the population, and there will always be some doubt associated with the conclusions that we draw about the population. We express this doubt as a probability (see Section 3.2). The larger the sample and the more representative it is of the population, the smaller our uncertainty and the more likely it is that our conclusions are correct.

4.3 Statistical inference

4.3.1 Introduction

This process of generalizing to the population from the sample is called **statistical inference**. Statistical inference enables us to draw conclusions about certain features of a population when only a subgroup of that population, the sample, is available for investigation. It is very important

Statistics for Veterinary and Animal Science, Third Edition. Aviva Petrie and Paul Watson.
© 2013 John Wiley & Sons, Ltd. Published 2013 by John Wiley & Sons, Ltd.

that we are aware of the distinction between the sample and the population from which it is taken, as a major component of statistical theory is statistical inference.

There are two aspects of statistical inference that play an important role in statistical analysis: these are **estimation** and **hypothesis testing**. We discuss estimation in this chapter. Hypothesis testing is concerned with deciding whether the results we obtain from our sample enable us to discredit a particular hypothesis about the population or whether they lend support to it. We introduce the concepts of hypothesis testing in Chapter 6.

4.3.2 Estimation of population parameters by sample statistics

The purpose of sampling is to learn something about the population. Usually, we want to know about various features, termed **parameters**, which characterize the distribution of a variable in the population. We can describe the distribution if we know their values. The parameters that characterize the better-known discrete and continuous probability distributions are discussed in Sections 3.4 and 3.5. In particular, the parameters that characterize the Normal distribution are the arithmetic mean and the standard deviation.

It is impossible to determine the population mean exactly when we have selected only a sample of observations from that population. For example, we do not know the precise value for the mean number of races that Thoroughbred mares have run when we only have the results of a selected sample. The best we can do is *estimate* its value from the sample, i.e. we have to calculate the *sample* **statistic** whose value is as close as possible to the true value of the parameter in the population. The population parameter and its sample statistic are usually calculated using the same formula, but the former uses population values and the latter uses sample values. For example, it can be shown that the sample mean is the best estimate of the population mean. The sample mean is the sum of all the observations *in the sample* divided by the number of observations *in the sample*; the population mean is the sum of all the observations *in the population* divided by the number of observations *in the population*. However, one noteworthy exception is that the population variance and its sample estimate are not calculated using exactly the same formula (see Section 2.6.2(c)).

4.3.3 Notation for population parameters and sample statistics

As it is important to maintain a distinction between the population parameters and the sample statistics that estimate them, it is helpful to use different notation for each. It is customary to use Greek letters for the population parameters and Roman letters for the sample statistics (see Glossary of notation in Appendix C).

4.3.4 Sampling error

It is unlikely that the value of the sample statistic is exactly equal to the value of the population parameter that it is estimating. We have to recognize that there is always likely to be error in the estimate because we have sampled the population and are not looking at it in its entirety. We call this **sampling error**. We need to establish the precision (see Section 1.8) of the sample statistic as an estimate of the population parameter. For this purpose, we calculate the **standard error of the estimate**.

Suppose we want to know the average milk yield of Holstein–Friesian dairy cows. Milk yield is a *continuous* variable so we will use this example to develop the ideas of sampling error in relation to the mean (see Section 4.4).

Furthermore, we might be interested in the proportion of cows that had been exposed to leptospirosis. Either a cow has or does not have a positive titre for *Leptospira* (Little *et al.*, 1980), so this is a *binary* variable. We will use this example to explore sampling error in relation to a proportion (see Section 4.6).

We will not discuss sampling error in relation to the variance as you are unlikely to need it in practice; you can obtain details in texts such as Armitage *et al.* (2002).

4.4 Sampling distribution of the mean

4.4.1 Sampling error in relation to the sample mean

Let us suppose that we are interested in making inferences about the population mean of a numerical variable, such as milk yield.

The first step is to take a representative sample of observations from the population. By 'representative' we mean, of course, that we have taken steps, such as random selection, to ensure that we have a sample that properly reflects the population. (Further details of sampling methods are given in Section 13.6.) We calculate the mean milk yield of this sample of observations to provide an estimate of the true mean milk yield in the population. Because of **sampling error** (see Section 4.3.4), it is unlikely that its value is exactly equal to the population mean. The extent to which a sample mean differs from the population mean depends on both the following:

- The size of the sample (the sampling error is greater for a smaller sample).
- The variability of the observations (the sampling error is greater if the observations are more diverse).

4.4.2 Concept of the distribution of the sample means

The sample mean from one sample will probably be slightly different from that obtained if we were to take another sample of the same size from the population. Expressed in another way, there is **sampling variation** resulting from the fact that the value of the sample mean varies according to the particular sample chosen.

We can get some feel for this sampling variation by considering a *hypothetical* probability distribution, i.e. the distribution of sample means that we would obtain if we were to repeat the sampling procedure and take all possible samples, each of the same size, from the population and calculate the sample mean from every sample.

We must stress that this is a hypothetical distribution because, in practice, we usually make inferences about the population mean from only a single sample from a population. However, by studying the properties of this theoretical distribution of the sample means, called the **sampling distribution of the mean**, we can evaluate the sampling error of the sample mean.

4.4.3 Properties of the sampling distribution of the mean

Figure 4.1 shows a diagrammatic representation of the distribution of the sample means. Just as with any other continuous distribution, we can look at its shape, and obtain measures of location and spread as summary measures of its important features. We list the properties of the distribution of the sample means below:

- Its **distribution** is *Normal* if the distribution of the parent population is Normal. Furthermore, the sampling distribution is approximately Normal even if the distribution of the parent population is not Normal, provided the size of the samples, assumed constant, is large enough, say greater than about 30. This is expressed mathematically in the *central limit theorem*, and is a very useful result which contributes to the importance of the Normal distribution in statistical inference. The resemblance of the sampling distribution of the mean to a Normal distribution improves as the size of the samples increases.
- The **mean** of the distribution of sample means is the mean of the parent population. We say that the sample mean is an **unbiased** (free from **bias** – see also Section 5.4) estimate of the population mean; i.e. *it is unbiased because the mean of the sampling distribution of the sample statistic coincides with the parameter that the statistic is estimating*. Furthermore, we know that the sample means are distributed symmetrically around the true mean because of the Normality property.
- The **standard deviation** of the distribution of the sample means, each from a sample of size n, is given by $\sigma/\sqrt{n}$, where σ is the standard

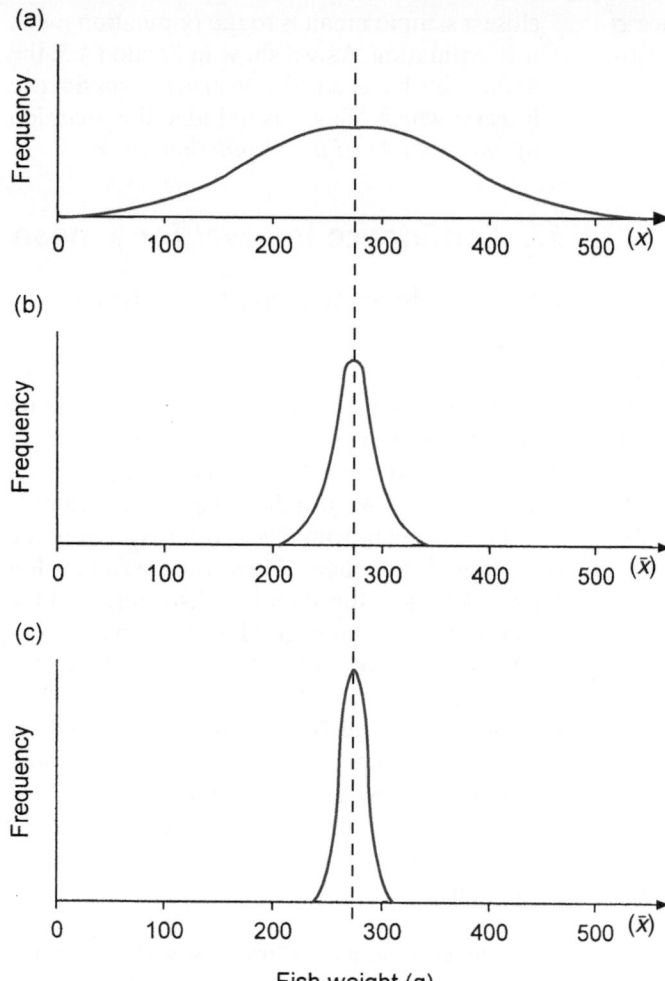

Figure 4.1 The effect of sample size on the sampling distribution of the mean. (a) Normal distribution of the population values (x) of fish weights, with mean = 272 g and SD = 96.4 g. (b) Sampling distribution of mean $(\bar{x})$ with sample size = 25. (c) Sampling distribution of mean $(\bar{x})$ with sample size = 100.

deviation of the observations in the population. The standard deviation of the sampling distribution of the mean is a measure of the dispersion of the sample means. It is known as the **standard error of the mean**. When there is no ambiguity, it may be called simply the standard error, and is often abbreviated to SE or **SEM**. So

$$SEM = \frac{\sigma}{\sqrt{n}}$$

From the formula, we can see that the standard error of the mean increases with increasing values of σ (i.e. as the variability of the parent population increases) and is smaller with larger samples. For example, for a given population with a fixed standard deviation, if we want to halve the standard error, we must quadruple the sample size. Therefore, we have a more precise estimate of the population mean if the sample size is large.

4.4.4 Estimation of the standard error using sample data

The SEM $= \sigma/\sqrt{n}$, where σ is the standard deviation of the observations in the population. If we are using our sample to estimate the population mean, it is very unlikely that we will have knowledge of σ. Hence we will have to replace σ in the formula for the SEM by its sample estimate, s. Thus, the estimate from the sample is

$$SEM = \frac{s}{\sqrt{n}}$$

where $s = \sqrt{\dfrac{\sum (x - \bar{x})^2}{n-1}}$

Example

The most recent standard lactations (305 days) of a random sample of 256 Holstein–Friesian cows, of mixed numbers of lactations, gave an estimated mean milk yield of 9414 kg with an estimated standard deviation of 2353 kg. The estimated standard error of the mean is therefore $2353/\sqrt{256} = 147$ kg.

4.4.5 Distinction between the standard deviation and the standard error of the mean

We have introduced you to the SD in Section 2.6.2(d) and the SEM in this chapter. But what are they for? They have very different applications; it is important that you have a clear understanding of the distinction between the standard deviation of the observations and the standard error of the mean. The two are frequently confused, with the consequence that the wrong measure is used to describe the variability of interest; this may lead to a misinterpretation of the data.

- The **standard deviation** is a measure of the *scatter of the observations* (see Section 2.6.2(d)). It gives an indication of how close the observations are to their mean; it may be thought of as a kind of average measure of the deviation of each observation from the mean. It may be used to construct a **reference interval** (see Section 2.7) which defines the *range of most of the observations* in a population.
- The **standard error of the mean** is a measure of the *precision of the sample mean* as an estimate of the population mean. It evaluates the sampling error by giving an indication of how

close a sample mean is to the population mean it is estimating. As we show in Section 4.5, the SEM may be used to construct a **confidence interval** which allows us to judge the *precision of our estimate of the population mean*.

4.5 Confidence interval for a mean

4.5.1 Understanding confidence intervals

We have stressed that the sampling distribution of the mean is a hypothetical distribution. In practice, we do not take repeated samples from our population; we usually take just one sample and use the mean from this sample as an estimate of the population mean. However, we can exploit the properties of the sampling distribution of the mean to indicate how 'good' our estimate is.

The best way of establishing whether the estimate is good is to calculate what is called the **confidence interval for the mean**. This interval, defined by its upper and lower limits (the **confidence limits**), is generally interpreted as the range of values within which we expect the true population mean to lie with a certain probability.

- If the confidence interval is wide, then the sample mean is a poor estimate of the population mean.
- If the confidence interval is narrow, then the sample mean is a good estimate, i.e. it is a precise estimate of the population mean.

If we have a 95% confidence interval for the mean, then we say that we are 95% certain that the population mean lies within this interval. Strictly, this interpretation is flawed because the population mean is a fixed number and it is the confidence interval that varies from one sample to another. The proper interpretation of the 95% confidence interval is that, if we were to take repeated samples of the same size from the population and calculate the 95% confidence interval from each sample, we would expect 95% of them to contain the true population mean. However, because it is intuitively more appealing, we interpret confidence intervals in this book using the first and more simplistic approach. Typically, we calculate the 95% confidence interval for a parameter but we may sometimes find that 90% or 99% confidence intervals are quoted. A 99% confidence interval will inevitably be wider than a 95% confidence interval because we need to be more confident that the parameter is contained in the interval.

The width of the confidence interval depends on:

- The degree of confidence required.
- The sample size (a larger sample provides a more precise estimate and therefore a narrower confidence interval).
- The variability of the characteristic under investigation (a more variable set of observations provides a less precise estimate and a wider confidence interval).

We develop the uses of confidence intervals in Section 6.6. We summarize the formulae for confidence intervals for frequently used parameters in the tables in Appendix B.

4.5.2 Calculating the confidence interval for the mean

The upper limit of a confidence interval for the mean is calculated by adding a multiple of the standard error to the sample mean; the lower limit is obtained by subtracting that multiple of the standard error from the sample mean. This is the general approach to calculating the confidence interval for most parameters. The difficulty is in deciding which multiple of the standard error to use to determine an interval of a particular confidence.

(a) Where σ is known

Provided we have knowledge of σ, the 95% confidence interval for the mean is $\bar{x} \pm 1.96 \times \text{SEM}$, i.e.

$$\bar{x} \pm 1.96 \frac{\sigma}{\sqrt{n}} = \left(\bar{x} - 1.96 \frac{\sigma}{\sqrt{n}}, \bar{x} + 1.96 \frac{\sigma}{\sqrt{n}} \right)$$

Here, the upper and lower limits of the confidence interval within the bracket are separated by the comma. For the 95% confidence interval, the multiple is 1.96 (often approximated by 2). The multiple is 2.58 for a 99% confidence interval; note that a multiple of 1.00 only gives approximately a 68% confidence interval. The values for the multiples are obtained from Table A.2.

Justification

We know that the sampling distribution of the mean is approximately Normal, and that its mean is equal to the population mean, μ, and its standard deviation is equal to the SEM $= \sigma/\sqrt{n}$ (see Section 4.4.3). Thus, 95% of the sample means in the sampling distribution of the mean are contained in the interval, $\mu \pm 1.96$ SEM (see Box 3.5). An alternative way of saying this is that there is a 95% chance that a sample mean, $\bar{x}$, is contained in the interval $\mu \pm 1.96$ SEM. If we now interchange the μ and the $\bar{x}$, we can say that there is a 95% chance that μ is contained in the interval $\bar{x} \pm 1.96$ SEM or, strictly, that 95% of such confidence intervals on repeated sampling would contain μ. □

(b) Where σ is unknown

Usually we do not know the value of the population standard deviation, σ, so we replace it by the sample estimate

$$s = \sqrt{\frac{\sum (x - \bar{x})^2}{n - 1}}$$

We can no longer use the Normal distribution to determine the multiple (e.g. 1.96) for the confidence interval; instead, we use the t-distribution. Then the 95% confidence interval for the mean is

$$\bar{x} \pm t_{0.05} \frac{s}{\sqrt{n}} = \left(\bar{x} - t_{0.05} \frac{s}{\sqrt{n}}, \bar{x} + t_{0.05} \frac{s}{\sqrt{n}} \right)$$

where the multiple, $t_{0.05}$, is the percentage point of the t-distribution (see Table A.3) with $n - 1$ degrees of freedom; it gives a total tail area probability of 0.05.

Justification

The distribution of the sample mean divided by its estimated standard error follows the t-distribution, provided the observations come from a Normal distribution (see Section 3.6.2). The multiple is affected by the sample size and increases as the sample size decreases. □

We should be aware that the multiple of the standard error obtained from the t-distribution is a slightly larger number than that obtained from the Normal distribution unless n is extremely large. This means that if we need to estimate the standard deviation from the sample, we will obtain a wider confidence interval than if we have knowledge of σ. However, the two intervals are much the same when the sample size is large, because the t-distribution approaches Normality when the degrees of freedom are large (see Section 3.5.4).

Example

In Section 4.4.4 we summarized the results of the milk yields of a sample of 256 Holstein–Friesian cows; the sample mean was 9414 kg and the estimated SEM was 147 kg. From Table A.3, $t_{0.05}$ for $df = 255$ is approximately 1.96. The 95% confidence interval for the true mean milk yield is given by

$$\bar{x} \pm t_{0.05}\frac{s}{\sqrt{n}} = (9414 - 1.96 \times 147, 9414 + 1.96 \times 147)$$

$$= (9125.9, 9702.1)\,\text{kg}$$

Hence we are 95% certain that the mean milk yield for the population of Holstein–Friesian cows lies between 9126 and 9702 kg.

4.6 Sampling distribution of the proportion

4.6.1 Concept of the distribution of sample proportions

The concept of the distribution of sample proportions is the same as that of the distribution of sample means. It is a *hypothetical* distribution whose properties are useful if we want to make statistical inferences about the population proportion.

Suppose we are interested in the **proportion** of individuals in a population, π, who possess a certain attribute. For example, we may want to know the proportion of cattle in an area that has been exposed to *Leptospira* infection. We select a random sample of size n from this population and observe the number, r, with the attribute in the sample. We then take the proportion with the attribute in the sample, $p = r/n$, as our estimate of π. The sampling distribution of the proportion is the distribution of sample proportions that we would obtain if we were to repeat the sampling procedure and take all possible samples, each of the same size, from the population and calculate the proportion from each sample. It is a hypothetical distribution because, in reality, we only take a single sample from the population.

4.6.2 Properties of the sampling distribution of the proportion

The distribution of sample proportions has the following properties:

- Its **distribution** is approximately *Normal* if the sample size is large; in fact, the distribution of a proportion is really a Binomial distribution (see Section 3.4.2) but, as we explained, this is approximately a Normal distribution for large n.
- The **mean** of the sampling distribution of the proportion is the population proportion, π. Thus the sample proportion, p, determined from a single sample, is an unbiased estimate of the population proportion.
- The **standard deviation** of the sampling distribution of the proportion is $\sqrt{\pi(1-\pi)/n}$. It is called the **standard error of the proportion** and is a measure of the precision of p as an estimate of π. It is estimated from the sample by

$$\text{SE}(p) = \sqrt{\frac{p(1-p)}{n}}$$

Even though we estimate π by p, the sampling distribution of the proportion is still approximately Normal for large n.

Note that if we replace the estimated proportion (p) by a percentage ($p\%$), then the estimated standard error of the estimated percentage is

$$\text{SE}(p\%) = \sqrt{\frac{p\%(100-p\%)}{n}}$$

4.7 Confidence interval for a proportion

The confidence interval for the population proportion, π, is calculated by adding to, and subtracting from, the sample proportion, p, a multiple of its standard error. The multiple is obtained from Table A.2 because the sampling distribution of the proportion is approximately Normal (see Section 4.6). In practice, we use the estimated standard error.

The 95% confidence interval for the population proportion is estimated by

$$p \pm 1.96 \, \text{SE}(p)$$
$$= \left(p - 1.96 \sqrt{\frac{p(1-p)}{n}}, \; p + 1.96 \sqrt{\frac{p(1-p)}{n}} \right)$$

The interpretation of this confidence interval is that we are 95% certain that the true population proportion is contained in the interval that spans p by 1.96 times $\text{SE}(p)$. (Strictly, 95% of such confidence intervals contain π in repeated sampling.)

Note that we can modify this formula if we are working with percentages, rather than proportions, by replacing each proportion by the appropriate percentage and replacing the 1 inside each square root by 100.

Example

A sample of 115 cattle is randomly selected from the population in the area. Blood samples from the cattle are tested for the presence of antisera to *Leptospira* and, according to the titres, are classified as either positive or negative. In this sample, there are 36 cattle with positive titres. The estimated proportion of cattle exposed to *Leptospira* is thus $36/115 = 0.31$ (corrected to two decimal places). The estimated standard error of this proportion is

$$\text{SE}(p) = \sqrt{\frac{p(1-p)}{n}} = \sqrt{\frac{0.313(1-0.313)}{115}} = 0.043$$

The 95% confidence interval for the true proportion exposed is given by

$$p \pm 1.96 \, \text{SE}(p)$$
$$= (0.313 - 1.96 \times 0.043, \, 0.313 + 1.96 \times 0.043)$$
$$= (0.228, 0.398)$$

Hence, we are 95% certain that the true proportion of cattle exposed to *Leptospira* lies between 0.23 and 0.40.

4.8 Bootstrapping and jackknifing

Two other approaches to obtaining confidence intervals for parameters are **bootstrapping** and **jackknifing**. Both rely on simulation techniques that are extremely computer intensive and are, therefore, not performed by hand. We might use them to estimate or provide a confidence interval for a parameter when it is difficult or impossible to do so by assuming a known probability distribution for the sampling distribution of the parameter. In each case, we generally start by taking a simple random sample of individuals from our population.

- **Bootstrapping**. We create a set of simple random subsamples (often 999 or more) from our original sample. Each of the subsamples in the set is of the same size as the original sample. This is feasible because the process for each subsample involves *sampling with replacement*; this means that once a particular individual is selected to be in a subsample, it is 'put back' into the original sample so that it is available for reselection, and therefore may occur more than once in that subsample. So a subsample is created by taking a single unit from the original sample, noting it, and then replacing it; a second is taken, it is noted, and so on until the subsample size equals the size of the original sample. Each of the subsamples in the set is produced in this way. A single estimate of the parameter of interest (e.g. the population mean) is determined from each subsample. By considering the distribution of the estimates from all the subsamples, it is possible to obtain an overall estimate of the parameter and its associated confidence interval. In particular, the confidence limits for the parameter are usually taken as the relevant percentiles of the simulated distribution. So they would be the 5th and 95th percentiles for a 90% confidence interval. We discuss an application of bootstrapping in Section 13.6.4(b).
- **Jackknifing**. Here we take a simple random sample of n observations from our population. We then omit a single observation from the original sample to obtain a subsample of size $(n-1)$, and estimate the parameter of interest in this subsample. If we repeat this process, omitting every observation in turn, we produce n subsamples, each containing one observation less than the number of observations in the original sample. We then use the distribution of the n estimates of the parameter from these subsamples

to obtain an overall estimate of the parameter of interest and the relevant confidence interval.   □

Exercises

The statements in questions 4.1–4.3 are either TRUE or FALSE.

4.1 The standard error of the mean:
(a) Measures the accuracy of each observation in the sample.
(b) Is a measure of spread of the observations in the sample.
(c) Is a measure of precision of the sample mean as an estimate of the population mean.
(d) Is always less than the estimated standard deviation of the population.
(e) Decreases as the size of the sample from a given population increases.

4.2 The 95% confidence interval for the mean:
(a) Contains the sample mean with 95% certainty.
(b) Is less likely to contain the population mean than the 99% confidence interval.
(c) Contains 95% of the observations in the population.
(d) Is approximately equal to the sample mean ± 2 × standard deviation.
(e) Can be used to give an indication of whether the sample mean is a precise estimate of the population mean.

4.3 A sample of 14 dogs shows they have a mean plasma potassium of 4.57 mmol/l (see Section 2.6.1(a)), and an estimated SD of 0.32 mmol/l (see Section 2.6.2(d)); the standard error of the mean is thus 0.085 mmol/l. The 95% confidence interval for the mean is 4.42–4.72 mmol/l.

This means that:
(a) There is a 95% chance that a dog's plasma potassium lies between 4.42 and 4.72 mmol/l.
(b) We can be 95% certain that the mean plasma potassium of the population of dogs lies between 4.42 and 4.72 mmol/l.
(c) 95% of sample means of the dogs' plasma potassium levels would lie between 4.42 and 4.72 mmol/l in repeated sampling.
(d) 95% of dogs have a plasma potassium that lies between 4.42 and 4.72 mmol/l.
(e) There is a 5% chance that the sample mean of the dogs' plasma potassium levels lies outside the interval 4.42–4.72 mmol/l.

4.4 Calculate the 95% and 99% confidence intervals for the population means, given the following information:
(a) Analysis of 100 grass samples gave a mean magnesium content of 2.35 mg/kg dry matter with a known population variance of 0.16 $(mg/kg)^2$.
(b) Milk progesterone values in 25 cows taken 24 days after insemination had a sample mean of 34.8 ng/ml and a sample SD of 13.0 ng/ml.

4.5 A representative sample of 60 sows from piggeries in Suffolk showed that five animals had joint lameness.
(a) Calculate the 95% confidence interval for the true proportion of joint lameness in the population of Suffolk sows.
(b) Would you expect the 99% confidence interval for this proportion to be wider or narrower than the 95% confidence interval?
(c) If you had a larger sample of sows, would your 95% confidence interval be wider or narrower than the one you have calculated?

5 Experimental design and clinical trials

5.1 Learning objectives

By the end of this chapter, you should be able to:

- Distinguish between observational and experimental studies.
- Describe what is meant by a clinical trial, longitudinal study, cohort study and case–control study.
- Calculate and interpret the relative risk, various forms of attributable risk, the odds of disease and the odds ratio.
- Explain the need for a 'control' group in a clinical trial.
- Explain the importance of randomization and describe methods for ensuring appropriate random allocation of individuals or groups.
- Explain the importance of 'blinding'.
- Describe the value of replication and blocking in experimental design.
- Explain the terms 'confounding', 'interaction' and 'analysis by intention-to-treat'.
- Describe various approaches to handling confounders.
- Distinguish between different types of missing data and explain ways in which missing data may be handled.
- Distinguish between parallel group designs and cross-over studies.
- Define the term 'outlier' and describe methods to deal correctly with them.

5.2 Types of study

A study of statistics in veterinary and animal science overlaps with **epidemiology**, the study of disease patterns and their determinants in the population. In this chapter, we introduce you to some of the important concepts in epidemiology; they can be explored more fully in specialist texts, such as that by Thrusfield (2005).

Usually, there are restrictions on the availability of cases in studies of clinical conditions in animal populations. This may be because the condition is rare, or the cost of animals is too high, or there are time restrictions in a busy practice or animal industry. In order to make the most of the material available, it is important to design the study in the most productive way. Several different approaches are available.

In the planning stage of your study, you are faced with a number of choices which are dictated by the problem you are investigating. Do you wish to intervene or are you simply going to observe what is there? Do you intend to study your animals at a single point in time or do you wish to follow them over time? Do you want to start with healthy animals and observe whether the disease occurs, or do you start with diseased animals and investigate the causes?

Statistics for Veterinary and Animal Science, Third Edition. Aviva Petrie and Paul Watson.
© 2013 John Wiley & Sons, Ltd. Published 2013 by John Wiley & Sons, Ltd.

5.2.1 Distinction between observational and experimental studies

(a) Observational study

In an **observational study**, we merely observe the animals in the study and record the relevant measurements on those animals. We make no attempt to intervene, for example, by administering treatments or withholding factors that we feel may affect the course of the disease. Clearly, we *cannot* randomly allocate animals to treatment groups in an observational study. A particular type of observational study is a **survey** in which we examine an aggregate of animals in order to derive values for various parameters in the population. This may be one of the following:

- A **population survey** which includes the entire population, e.g. a census.
- A **sample survey** in which we examine a representative sample of animals so that we may draw conclusions about the whole population of animals, as discussed in Section 4.3.

However, many observational studies are concerned with investigating associations. In particular, an *epidemiological* study is concerned with investigating the aetiology of a disease by determining whether various factors (termed *risk factors*) are associated with the occurrence and distribution of the disease. For example, the prevalence of Cushing's syndrome in dogs is greater in toy breeds, a fact established by epidemiological studies comparing breeds.

(b) Experimental study

In an **experimental study**, we intervene in the study by, for example, deliberately applying a preventative measure, such as a treatment, or reducing the exposure of the animal to a factor, such as temperature. We then observe the effect of our intervention on the response of interest, usually with a view to establishing whether a change in response may be directly attributable to our action. Random allocation is an essential design component of an experimental study. Two examples of different types of experimental studies are **laboratory experiments** and **clinical trials**.

In laboratory experiments, the units of investigation may typically be cells, tissues or whole animals, and the interventions can be very varied. For example, we may be concerned with studying the role of growth promoters or hormones on cell processes (e.g. protein phosphorylation or mRNA expression), the effects of feed additives on growth rates of growing animals, or the quality of wound healing with different suture techniques. On the other hand, clinical trials, taken in their widest sense, are concerned with investigating the efficacy of particular treatments or prophylactic measures in resolving or preventing clinical conditions, and the units are generally individual cases. Much, but not all, of what follows is concerned with the design of clinical trials.

A helpful reference for the design of studies, both observational and experimental, is the text by Machin and Campbell (2005).

5.2.2 Distinction between cross-sectional and longitudinal studies

(a) Cross-sectional study

A **cross-sectional study** is one in which we take all our measurements on the animals included in the study *at a given point in time*. In an epidemiological investigation, this means we observe both the values of the risk factors and the disease state for every animal at the same time, within the bounds of practicality. Cross-sectional studies provide only limited information because they do not take into account the temporal relationship between the risk factors and the disease state. However, cross-sectional studies are useful when the aims of the study are essentially descriptive; for example, when we are estimating the point prevalence of a particular disease from a sample survey (Box 5.1).

(b) Longitudinal study

A **longitudinal study** is one in which we investigate changes over time. The clinical trial is an

Box 5.1 The distinction between prevalence and incidence

The *prevalence* and *incidence* of a disease are two terms which are often confused.

- The **prevalence** of a disease relates to the number of cases of the disease that exist at a specific instant in time (point prevalence) or in a *defined interval* of time (period prevalence).
- The **incidence** of a disease relates to the number of new cases of the disease that *develop* in a defined time period.

Both prevalence and incidence are generally expressed as proportions (percentages) of the population at risk (i.e. those individuals who could succumb to the disease) at the midpoint of the study period or at a specified instant in time, as relevant.

example of a longitudinal study; we administer a treatment at one point in time, and observe the effect of that treatment at a later time. There are two types of longitudinal studies, which are defined according to whether the changes over time are investigated **prospectively** (as in most *cohort* studies) or **retrospectively** (as in the case–control study) – see Section 5.2.3.

5.2.3 Distinction between cohort and case–control observational studies

(a) Cohort study

In a **cohort study** of disease aetiology, we start by defining groups (cohorts) of disease-free animals according to the exposure of the animals in the groups to the factor(s) of interest. Generally, we follow these groups forward in time to see which animals develop the disease under investigation. An example of a cohort study is one in which Wilesmith *et al.* (1997), in exploring the mode of transmission of bovine spongiform encephalopathy (BSE), wanted to determine if BSE-positive cows were more likely to produce offspring who developed BSE than those dams who were BSE negative. Their cohort comprised two groups of cows: those that had developed BSE and those that had not shown clinical signs of BSE within 6 years (matched for age and herd). The offspring

of these cows, born in the same calving season, were then followed until their 7th year of life, or until they developed clinical signs of the disease if this occurred earlier. Thus, in this example, the exposure groups were the cows with and without BSE, and the disease outcome assessed was whether the calves developed BSE over a 7-year period.

A cohort study has the advantage that we can use it to collect information on exposure to a wide range of factors, even rare ones, and on different outcomes. However, it is not sensible to embark on a cohort study when the disease outcome is rare and, because its time span can be quite long, it tends to be expensive and may suffer from inconsistencies.

We usually analyse data from cohort studies by estimating the true risk of the disease in the populations of animals that have been 'exposed' and 'unexposed' to the factor. The true **risk of disease** is the proportion of animals in a population of susceptible animals that develop the disease in the time interval under consideration; it represents the probability that an animal will develop the disease in the time period. The disease risk will be greater if the study period is longer as animals will then have more time in which to contract the disease, and so it is essential that the study period is the same for all animals when evaluating risk. The risk of the disease in a particular exposure group is estimated as the proportion of animals in the relevant cohort who develop the disease during the study period.

Relative risk

The **relative risk (RR)**, the *ratio* of the disease risks in the exposed and unexposed groups, provides a measure of the strength of the association between the disease and the exposure to the factor. If the relative risk is unity, then exposure to the factor does not affect the animal's chance of developing the disease. If the relative risk (generally, the risk in the exposed cohort, divided by the risk in the unexposed cohort) is substantially greater than unity, then an animal has an increased risk of developing the disease if it has been exposed to the factor. For example, Wilesmith *et al.* (1997) found that 42 (14.0%) offspring of the 301 animals born to BSE-positive dams developed BSE within the first 7 years of their lives, compared with 13 (4.3%) offspring of the 301 born to BSE-negative dams. This represents an estimated relative risk of 42/13 = 3.23 (95% confidence interval 1.77–5.89, $P < 0.001$), i.e. those calves born to BSE-positive mothers had more than a threefold greater chance of developing BSE than those from BSE-negative mothers. Another way of expressing this is to say that the risk of offspring developing BSE increased by over 200% when the dam was infected. However, these data do not distinguish a possible genetic component from true maternal transmission. (We provide the formula for the confidence interval for the true relative risk in Table B.1, and you can find details of how to test the hypothesis (see Chapter 6) that this relative risk is unity in texts such as Armitage *et al.* (2002). For an explanation of P, see Section 6.3.3.)

Attributable risk

It may be more appropriate in studies relating to veterinary public health, rather than those concerned with disease aetiology, to consider the *difference* in relevant disease risks, and evaluate some form of *attributable risk*. This can be measured in various ways: you may find that the notation and terminology for the different measures is not consistent in different texts.

We may calculate the **population attributable risk (PAR)** which is equal to the difference between the risk in the whole population (estimated by $Risk_{total}$) and the risk in the unexposed group (estimated by $Risk_{unexp}$). It describes the excess risk in the population attributable to the risk factor – see also Table B.1 (for the confidence interval) and Section 16.5.3. In the BSE example, $Risk_{total}$ is the estimated proportion of offspring with the disease in the whole population of dams = (42 + 13)/602 = 0.091 and $Risk_{unexp}$ = 13/301 = 0.043. Hence the PAR is estimated as 0.091 – 0.043 = 0.048 (i.e. approximately 5%), i.e. for every 100 dams in the population, five of the offspring had BSE attributable to the dams being BSE positive. Sometimes, we calculate the PAR as a proportion of the risk in the whole group. This **population attributable fraction (PAF)**, also called the population proportional attributable risk, is estimated as PAR/$Risk_{total}$. It describes the proportion of the disease in the whole popula-

tion attributable to exposure that would be avoided if exposure were removed from the population. The PAF therefore provides a measure of preventable disease. In the BSE example, the PAF is estimated as 0.048/0.091 = 0.527, i.e. 53% of BSE in the offspring is attributable to some of the dams being BSE positive.

Sometimes our focus is on evaluating the effect of a risk factor on individuals who have been exposed to the risk factor rather than evaluating the excess risk in the population. In this case we estimate the **attributable risk (AR)**, also referred to as the **absolute risk reduction (ARR)** or the **risk difference (RD)**. It is equal to the difference in the risks in the exposed and unexposed portions of the population, i.e. it is estimated by $Risk_{exp} - Risk_{unexp}$. It evaluates the increase in the risk of disease in exposed individuals, compared to unexposed individuals, that results from the exposure. In the BSE example, the estimated $Risk_{exp}$ = 42/301 = 0.140, so the estimated AR = 0.140 – 0.043 = 0.097. Hence for every 100 BSE-positive dams, approximately 10 of the offspring were BSE positive as a consequence of the disease status of the dams. Furthermore, the **attributable fraction (AF)**, also called the attributable fraction (exposed) or the proportional attributable risk, is the proportion of disease in the exposed group that would be avoided if the exposure were removed, and is equal to AR/$Risk_{exp}$. The attributable fraction does not take the prevalence of exposure to the risk factor into account so is not very helpful as a public health measure of preventable disease. In particular, when the prevalence of the risk factor is low, exposure to the risk factor will have little effect on the number of animals with the disease, even if the AF is high. In the BSE example, the estimated AF = 0.097/0.140 = 0.693. Thus, 69% of cases of BSE in the offspring of BSE-positive dams is attributed to these dams being BSE positive. It may be of interest to note that the AF = (RR – 1)/RR, where RR is the relative risk.

(b) Case–control study

In a **case–control study** of disease aetiology, we start by defining the groups of diseased and healthy animals; these are the cases and the controls, respectively. Then we assess whether the animals in the two groups have differences in past exposure to various risk factors. Case–control studies are often termed *retrospective* studies because we have to go back in time in order to determine an animal's exposure to the risk factor. There are two types of case–control design which depend on the way in which we select our controls. Either we choose the controls so that each (or more than one) control animal is matched with a case with respect to variables that may be likely to influence the development of disease, such as the animal's breed, sex and/or age; this leads to what is termed a **matched** design. Sometimes, we have **frequency** or **group matching** when the controls are selected so that the potential risk factor is the same, on average, in the groups of cases and controls. On the other hand, we may have an **unmatched** design in which the disease-free or control animals are selected from the population, but without any attempt at matching.

Although a case–control study is relatively quick, easy and cheap to perform, does not suffer from losses to follow-up and can be used when the disease outcome is rare, it may suffer from recall bias (there is a differential ability between carers in remembering relevant facts about cases and controls relating to exposure), and it is not suitable when exposures to the risk factor are rare. Furthermore, we cannot estimate the relative risk directly in a case–control study since the relative risk is a ratio of the risks of the disease in the exposed (to the factor) and unexposed groups of animals. In a case–control study, we start with animals with and without the disease rather than with different exposure groups, so we can only estimate the relative risk indirectly. We do this by calculating what is called the **odds ratio (OR)**, which is the ratio of two odds, usually the odds of disease in the group exposed to the factor divided by the odds of disease in the group not exposed to the factor. The **odds of disease** in a group of animals is the ratio of the probability of having the disease to the probability of not having the disease. Analogous to the relative risk, we can test the hypothesis that the true odds ratio in the population is one (details are given in Armitage *et al.*, 2002) and provide confidence intervals for the odds ratio (see Table B.1). Note that the odds ratio is a reasonable estimate of the relative risk only if the prevalence of the disease

is very low (say, <10%). If the disease is not rare, the odds ratio will be greater than the relative risk if the relative risk is greater than one, and it will be less than the relative risk otherwise.

As an illustration of a case–control study, consider the study (based on Clark *et al.*, 2004) that examined the relationship between the formation of vertical fissures or sandcracks in the hooves of adult beef cattle and the presence of horizontal grooves. At a local abattoir, all four feet were collected from 20 mature beef cows with no vertical fissures present on any claw (the controls) and 20 mature beef cows with a vertical fissure present on at least one claw (the cases). A cow was categorized as suffering from horizontal grooves if one or more hooves showed evidence of a lesion. Of 20 cows classified as having a vertical fissure, 19 had at least one horizontal groove and one cow had no horizontal groove; 13 of the 20 control cows had at least one horizontal groove and seven of the control cows had no horizontal groove. There were therefore a total of 32 cows with at least one horizontal groove and eight cows with no horizontal groove. Thus, the odds of having a vertical fissure in the cows with at least one horizontal groove was estimated as $(19/32)/(13/32) = 1.4615$, and the odds of having a vertical fissure in the cows with no horizontal groove was estimated as $(1/8)/(7/8) = 0.1429$. Hence the odds ratio was estimated as $(1.4615)/(0.1429) = 10.2$ (95% confidence interval 1.1 to 484.7, $P = 0.04$), i.e. the odds of having a vertical fissure was estimated as being 10.2 times greater in a cow with a horizontal groove than in a cow without a horizontal groove. However, the extremely wide confidence interval for the odds ratio indicates that although the true odds of having a vertical fissure could be nearly 500 times greater in a cow with a horizontal groove, there could be very little difference in the two odds.

5.3 Introducing clinical trials

We use the term **clinical trial** to describe any planned experiment that involves human or animal subjects, and is designed to assess the effectiveness of one or more treatments or preventive measures such as vaccines. The term has been expanded from human clinical medicine to include studies in veterinary clinical medicine and animal health sciences; for example, the testing of the efficacy of novel pharmacological agents to control ectoparasites in dogs and cats, or a formal study of a novel method of repair of the anterior cruciate ligament in dogs. You can obtain a full discussion of clinical trials in Hackshaw (2009), Machin *et al.* (2006), Matthews (2006) and Pocock (1983).

In the course of the development of veterinary treatments, there is usually a stage of experiment using laboratory animals to establish safety and efficacy of the treatment. If this is a drug development, this stage would also include pharmacological studies. A treatment that passes these preliminary assessments would then be examined in a clinical trial in which the treatment is applied to the species of interest but with a narrow range of its potential variation, e.g. beagles or Labradors as 'model' dogs. Up to this point, all these trials would usually be carried out in the UK under the Animals (Scientific Procedures) Act 1986 (see Section 15.3.4).

We should distinguish the clinical trial from the **clinical field trial**. The former is a trial that takes place in well-regulated conditions; the clinical field trial is a comparative study involving new treatments or preventive measures applied under natural, field or semi-field conditions. It is usually carried out in the UK under the Veterinary Surgeons Act 1966.

- The clinical field trial introduces elements of variation attributable to the involvement of the owners or stockmen, and these are important in assessing the final efficacy of a treatment in a pragmatic setting. The overall effectiveness of a drug treatment, for example, involves not just the pharmacological action of the drug but the ability of the owner/stockman to administer it correctly, e.g. the use of helminthological treatments under farm conditions.
- The clinical field trial also introduces the full range of genetic and environmental variation in a species, e.g. Chihuahuas to Great Danes kept under a variety of different conditions.

We would like to refer you to the REFLECT statement (see Section 17.3) which is an evidence-based minimum set of items for reporting livestock trials with production, health and food safety outcomes. Following these proposed guidelines may help alleviate the problems arising from inadequate reporting of veterinary randomized controlled trials.

5.4 Importance of design in the clinical trial

We undertake a clinical trial in order to evaluate the benefit to be derived from introducing a new therapy or intervention in given circumstances. Our interest is in projecting the results from the sample of animals studied in the trial to some future population of similar animals suffering from the same condition and treated in comparable circumstances. In order to ensure that this hypothetical future population receives what is truly the best treatment, it is essential that the trial is based on rigorous scientific principles and is free from **bias**, i.e. from an effect that deprives a statistical result of representativeness by systematically distorting it (see also Section 4.4.3). Biases can arise in a clinical trial for a variety of reasons. For example, there may be *selection* bias (the animals in the study are not representative of the population of interest), *observer* bias (say, when one observer tends to over-report a particular variable) or *publication* bias (the tendency for journals to publish only papers with statistically significant results). Two particularly important biases are:

- *Allocation* bias, which may arise if the treatment groups are not comparable when we allocate the experimental animals to the treatment groups.
- *Assessment* bias, which may arise if we are influenced by preconceived ideas about the superiority of one treatment over another when we evaluate the response to treatment.

If we incorporate measures into the trial design that avoid biases arising, we can then contemplate ways in which we can optimize the quality of the estimate of response to treatment, most notably by attempting to maximize its precision.

In the sections that follow, we describe the important features of design that contribute to a worthwhile trial leading to useful and valid conclusions concerning the effectiveness of the treatments or interventions. Note that a competent trial is invariably:

- *Comparative* – comprising more than one treatment group. We are then able to make judgements about the response to the new therapy or intervention in relation to the response that is obtained in the absence of therapy or compared with a standard therapy (see Section 5.5).
- *Randomized* – we assign the animals to the treatment groups by some chance process to ensure that the comparison groups are alike with respect to any variables that may influence response (see Section 5.6).

Incorporating both of these features into a trial leads to a **randomized controlled trial**, often abbreviated to **RCT**.

5.5 Control group

5.5.1 Why do we need a control?

In any experimental investigation, whether a clinical trial or a laboratory investigation, without some basis for comparison we cannot establish, with any degree of certainty, that the new treatment under investigation is preferable to the standard treatment or even to no treatment at all. In a clinical trial, for example, the condition of the animal may improve over a defined period, purely as a consequence of time and the natural curative and healing properties of the body, and irrespective of the treatment the animal receives. Similarly, in a laboratory investigation, changes in the variable under investigation can occur by chance alone. Thus, we cannot make an inference that the new treatment is more beneficial than the standard treatment if we do not have any information about the response to the standard treatment given over the same period to a similar group of animals. Similarly, we may doubt the effectiveness of a new vaccine on a given population if there is no comparable information on a similar population of animals who are not given the vaccine.

Furthermore, in the absence of a comparison or **control group**, we know that every animal is receiving the new treatment (i.e. there is no *blinding* – see Section 5.7), and in our enthusiasm for this treatment, we may compromise the results, particularly if the assessment of response is subjective. A clinical trial which is not comparative is likely to lead to over-optimistic and therefore biased results.

5.5.2 Positive or negative control?

A comparative clinical trial is often termed a **controlled clinical trial**. The choice of control group depends on the exact circumstances of the trial. If a standard therapy exists, then it is ethically unacceptable to conduct the trial without including the standard therapy as the control, which may then be termed a **positive control**. If, however, there is no known effective treatment, or if the condition is not so serious that the absence of treatment does not pose an ethical dilemma, then it is justifiable to have a control group, sometimes described as a **negative control** group, in which the animals receive no active treatment. (NB In some laboratory studies, the term 'positive control' implies a treatment giving a maximum response, e.g. in some immunodetection assays it is usual to include a treatment with cells known to respond positively to the antibody.)

5.5.3 Historical controls

A **historical control** group is one in which the animals have previously been exposed to the control treatment and their results obtained prior to the onset of the trial. Occasionally, we may be tempted to use historical controls instead of **contemporary controls** in an attempt to reduce the number of animals needed in the experiment or from a desire to administer the new treatment to all animals in the trial. The major disadvantage of using historical controls in a retrospective comparison is that the test and control groups may not be truly comparable, both with respect to the type, source and condition of the animal and also to the experimental environment, so that biases may result. The consequence of including historical controls in a clinical trial is, again, a tendency to exaggerate the benefits of the new treatment.

5.6 Assignment of animals to the treatment groups

5.6.1 Need for random assignment

One important potential source of bias in the conduct of a controlled clinical trial is in the allocation of experimental animals to the treatment (test and control) groups. This bias may arise, either consciously or subconsciously, if we exercise personal judgement when we allocate the animals to the treatment groups. If the composition of the test and control groups differs in a systematic fashion (e.g. if one group comprises more severely affected animals), then we may not be able to attribute any differences in response to the effect of treatment. In order to do so, the test and control groups should be as similar as possible and so are balanced in the factors that influence response, known as **covariates** or **prognostic factors**, *whether or not these are known*. However, if they are known and we find that the groups are not comparable at baseline, it may be possible to adjust for the effects of these covariates in the analysis (see Section 5.9.1).

The most appropriate method of removing allocation bias and achieving this balance is the process of **random allocation** or **randomization** of the animals to the test and control groups. In random allocation, we assign the animals to the treatment groups in such a way that:

- All animals have the same chance of receiving any treatment.
- The assigning of one animal to a particular treatment has no influence on the assigning of any other animal.
- We cannot know in advance the treatment that each animal is to receive.

Thus, assigning the animals to the treatment groups in a *systematic* fashion by, for example, alternating the allocation, i.e. test, control, test, control, etc., would *not* comply with this definition. Systematic allocation is more likely to lead to bias than is a strictly random process of allocation. The investigator's knowledge of the allocation sequence may influence the allocation of particular animals to certain treatments.

Randomization has the following advantages:

- It removes bias from the allocation procedure in that the prognostic factors are, in principle, balanced in the different treatment groups.
- We do not require prior knowledge of factors likely to influence response, as the procedure should result in treatment groups which are comparable in unknown, as well as known, factors (apart from the actual treatment being given).
- We do not know in advance the particular treatment that each animal will receive.
- Statistical theory is based on the concept of random sampling. If we construct the treatment groups using random allocation, then the differences between treatment groups are akin to those between random samples. We can, therefore, utilize the process of statistical inference (see Sections 1.10 and 4.3) to evaluate treatment differences.

After the results from the clinical trial have been collected, we should check that randomization has been effective in that the prognostic factors are balanced in the different treatment groups at baseline. To this end, we should scan the results of a table containing the summary statistics for each prognostic factor (e.g. means and standard deviations for Normally distributed numerical variables and proportions for categorical variables) to confirm that any differences in these factors between the treatment groups are negligible. We should *not* compare the groups for each covariate by performing a hypothesis test (see Chapter 6) and providing a P-value. This is because the hypothesis test assesses whether a difference between the groups could be due to chance, and if randomization – a method based on chance – has been used for allocation purposes in a clinical trial, any difference between the baseline values must be due to chance.

As a practical tip, you may find it helpful to mask the allocation sequence by using *sealed envelopes* in the randomization process. These are numbered consecutively; each contains the specification of the treatment regimen (determined by random allocation) to be administered to the next available animal.

5.6.2 Methods of randomization

It is best if you avoid mechanical methods, such as tossing a coin or throwing a die, for allocating the experimental animals to the treatment groups. Although they are probabilistically acceptable procedures that adhere to the definition of randomization, these techniques are cumbersome and cannot be verified.

A common way of employing randomization in the allocation process is to utilize a table of random numbers (see Table A.11). This comprises the digits 0 to 9 generated in a random manner such that each digit occurs the same number of times, and there is no discernible pattern in the arrangement of the digits. If we choose an appropriate allocation scheme, some of which are outlined in the subsections that follow, we can use the table to randomly allocate equal numbers of animals to the different treatments. Alternatively, a random number sequence can be generated on many calculators and computers.

(a) Simple randomization

We may allocate animals to the different treatment groups using **simple randomization** – this is the basic randomization procedure which does not involve any refinements or restrictions. Suppose we have two treatment groups: a test group (T) and a control group (C). We begin by choosing a random starting point, i.e. a digit, in the table of random numbers. Then we follow the row of that digit to the left or the right, or the column of that digit up or down the page. Every number in the sequence of digits obtained in this way is either odd or even (taking 0 as even), the chance of an odd or even number being equal. If

the number is odd, we allocate the next experimental animal in the trial to T, say, and if the number is even, we allocate that animal to C. So the sequence 386674559670 would result in the allocation TCCCTCTTTCTC. We may modify the procedure to accommodate three or more treatments. For example, if there are three treatments, A, B and C, we allocate the animal to A if the digit is 1, 2 or 3; to B if the digit is 4, 5 or 6; to C if the digit is 7, 8 or 9; and we ignore zeros. Then, the above sequence would result in the allocation ACBBCBBBCBC. As you can see, with only 11 animals, the group sizes in this randomization are quite disparate (see Section 5.6.2(c) for a solution to this problem).

(b) Stratified randomization

You should be aware that simple randomization, relying as it does on chance, is not infallible, particularly when the sample size is relatively small. Sometimes, we want to ensure that the treatment groups are similar with respect to one or two key confounding variables, as it is easier to promote comparability at the allocation stage rather than attempting to make adjustments for the confounders (see Section 5.9.1) in the statistical analysis. This may be achieved by **stratified randomization**.

We divide the population into different strata according to the categorization of the key confounding variables. So, for example, for a study of arthritis in dogs, we may create three strata, one for each of large, medium and toy breeds, since the animal's body mass is believed to affect the response to treatment. Then, within each stratum, we randomly (using a different randomization list) allocate the dogs to each of the treatment groups so that the comparison of treatments is not affected by the dogs' body mass.

(c) Restricted randomization

Generally, we aim to have approximately equal numbers of animals in the various treatment groups. We are likely to achieve this with simple randomization if our sample size is large enough, but we may have an undesirable imbalance with a relatively small number of animals. We demonstrated this in the simple randomization example above (see Section 5.6.2(a)) in which the use of a sequence of only 12 digits resulted in one animal being allocated to treatment A, six animals to B and four animals to C. We may overcome this inequality problem by using **restricted** or **blocked randomization**.

We decide (perhaps because of batch variation in the treatment material) that we would like to have a trial in which we are assured of balance in every block of n (e.g. $n = 6, 8, 9$ or 10) animals that enter the trial, where n is a multiple of the number of treatments being compared. Suppose we have two treatment groups, T and C, and that we choose $n = 8$. We follow the sequence of digits in the random number table and allocate the animal to T if the number is odd and to C if the number is even. Once we have allocated four animals to one treatment group (i.e. the block size divided by the number of treatments), then we must allocate the remaining animals in that block of eight to the other treatment group. So, the same sequence as before, 386674559670, would result in TCCCTC after the first six digits, i.e. four animals on C, and only two on T, indicating that we would have to allocate the remaining two animals in that block of eight animals to T: the allocation sequence would then be TCCCTCTT. This procedure, if continued, ensures exact balance after every group of eight animals, and approximate balance when all animals have been entered into the trial if the trial size is not a multiple of eight. It has the added advantage of guarding against imbalances that may result from any time trend in the type of animals admitted to the trial, as well as facilitating balance in any interim analyses (see Section 13.4). Sometimes, as an added safeguard, we can change the block size during the whole allocation process, e.g. sometimes it might be eight and at other times it might be six or four. Stratified randomization usually incorporates restricted randomization within each stratum, provided the overall sample size is large enough.

(d) Group randomization

The **experimental unit** is the smallest unit in an experiment to which a treatment can be assigned, and whose response is independent of the responses of the other units. Generally, in human medicine, clinical trials take the individual person as the experimental unit although, occasionally, clusters of individuals, such as households, are used. However, we often regard the **group** as the most appropriate experimental unit in the veterinary and animal sciences. This is because food, drugs and vaccines are often administered to a group of animals in a litter, pen, paddock or barn, or to a complete herd or to all the fish in a tank. In this case, we apply the randomization procedure to the groups (i.e. **group** or **cluster randomization**), so that all animals or fish within each group receive the same treatment. We have to combine the results of the groups in the appropriate manner to evaluate treatment effects.

A second circumstance that may suggest instituting group randomization is when we *cannot* regard the individual animals within a group (litter, pen, paddock, etc.) as *independent* units. This is likely to arise when we are appraising a vaccine against a parasitic disease; herd immunity and the possibility of vaccine organisms spreading to and protecting the controls would tend to camouflage the effectiveness of the vaccine. If the experimental unit is the animal rather than the group, the protection afforded the vaccinated animals leads to a reduced prevalence of disease in the group environment, resulting in a reduced incidence of disease in the control animals; this is what is meant by **herd immunity**. A similar process may also be applicable when de-wormed and control animals are allowed to graze on the same pasture. Short but useful discussions of group randomization are given by Altman and Bland (1997) and Bland and Kerry (1997).

In group randomization, you must remember:

- To base the *sample size calculations* at the planning stage of the investigation on the number of *groups* that are randomized to the different treatments, and not solely on the number of animals within the groups. The overall sample size in a group or cluster randomized trial will be greater than that required when there is individual randomization if all other factors that affect sample size remain constant. In practical terms, you may find you cannot satisfy a requirement for a large number of groups, for example pens or herds. Suggestions for overcoming the problem are given by Haber *et al.* (1991) and by Halloran and Struchiner (1991). Another useful reference is that by Kerry and Bland (1998).

- To base the *statistical analyses of results* on the group as the experimental unit. We discuss a simple approach in Section 14.5.2 where we explain how the analysis depends on defining an appropriate summary measure for each group. In Section 11.6 we explain how regression methods, such as the use of a random effects model or generalized estimating equations, can be utilized appropriately when there are clustered data such as these. Useful papers in the context of group randomized studies are those by Donner (1987), Donner *et al.* (1981) and Hseih (1988).

If, incorrectly, you take the animal within the group as the experimental unit when you use group randomization, you will underestimate the variation between animals. The lack of independence between these animals will result in less variation, and hence narrower confidence intervals for the parameters of interest, than would be expected if the animals were truly independent. This, in turn, would be likely to lead you to conclude, over-optimistically and erroneously, that there was a statistically significant difference between treatments. Thus, by underestimating the variation between animals, you are likely to overestimate the magnitude of difference between treatments.

5.7 Avoidance of bias in the assessment procedure

We use the randomization process in a clinical trial to ensure that the trial is free from systematic errors of *allocation*. However, biases may arise in the *assessment of response* to treatment because of the preconceived notions of the carer of the animals and/or the assessors as to the benefits of treatment. These biases are most likely to occur when the assessment of response to treat-

ment is subjective, such as the body condition score in sheep or the starkness of coat in cats.

We ensure that our trial is free from assessment bias by making the trial **blind** or **masked**. There are two levels of 'blindness' – double-blind and single-blind.

- Ideally, we should design the trial to be **double-blind** so that neither the carer(s) of the animals nor the assessor of response to treatment (test or control) is aware of which treatment each animal is receiving. If the carers are ignorant of the treatment each animal is receiving (i.e. they are *blind*), it is possible for them to handle the animals impartially and removes from them the temptation to atone, either consciously or subconsciously, for the supposed inferior control regimen. It is essential to keep the assessor blind if the response to treatment is subjective, thus guarding against the tendency to favour or disfavour a particular treatment. Clinical trials should have the maximum attainable degree of blindness in order to remove potential bias in the assessment process. Double-blind trials are desirable but not always achievable.
- In some circumstances, the trial may be **single-blind** in that only one of these two parties, the carer or the assessor, is blind. If the response to treatment is objective, then it may be sufficient to have only the carer blind; if it is possible to distinguish the test and control regimens, perhaps because of experimental procedures, then it may not be feasible to make the carer blind. For example, in a single-blind fertility trial of semen diluent treatments when only one treatment contains egg yolk, the inseminator will be aware of which treatment is used; the assessment of fertility (pregnancy test) must then be performed blind.

In order for the carer to be blind, it is essential that the physical appearance of the test and control treatments, as well as the treatment regimens, should be exactly the same. This may be facilitated by using a **dummy** treatment or **placebo**, a pharmacologically inert substance which is identical in appearance to the test treatment. It forms the baseline against which the effect of the test treatment is measured. The response induced by suggestion on the part of the animal attendants or the animal investigator when the animal receives a placebo is called the **placebo effect**. Placebos are most often used in drug trials; they may, if ethical considerations permit, be used in invasive procedures, e.g. injections of the solvent base (vehicle) for the drug or in sham operations. These are common in experiments that are conducted in the UK under the Animals (Scientific Procedures) Act 1986.

5.8 Increasing the precision of the estimates

5.8.1 Introduction

Our primary concern is with designing a trial that is unbiased; in particular, it should be free from systematic errors of allocation and from biases in the assessment of response to treatment. Our secondary objective is to promote the reliability of our conclusions by maximizing the precision of the estimates of the parameters of interest. Extraneous variations resulting from the inherent variability in the experimental units and from a failure to standardize the experimental technique tend to mask the effects of treatments; we want both to quantify and to minimize these variations.

5.8.2 Replication

We generally choose our trial size to be as large as possible. The greater the number of experimental units in the trial, usually individual animals but sometimes groups of animals (see Section 5.6.2(d)), the greater the precision of the estimates and the greater our chance of detecting a treatment effect, if it exists. However, with an increased awareness of the need to restrict the numbers of animals used in experimental situations, there is a strong encouragement to use only the minimum number of animals consistent with the desired scientific objectives (see Section 15.3.2). We provide a detailed explanation of how to determine the optimal sample size in a trial in Section 13.3.

In addition, we sometimes incorporate **replication** into the trial design so that we can increase the precision of our estimates, and improve the effectiveness of the trial to detect treatment differences. By replication, we mean repeating the number of measurements (i.e. obtain duplicates, triplicates, etc.) of the same type on each experimental unit, for example on each animal. This allows us to segregate the within-animal variability from the variation that is due to biological or treatment differences; it enhances the comparisons of interest, whilst giving us the opportunity to evaluate repeatability (see Section 14.4). We must take care when analysing such data; we have to recognize that k repeated measurements on n experimental units do not provide nk independent observations. For example, if we are observing the number of visits garden birds make to a feeding basket, we may not be sure we are observing different birds at each visit. If a pair of birds each pays 10 visits to the feeder in an hour, this is not the same as 20 birds each making a single visit in the hour. We must not treat these two situations in the same way for statistical analysis, recognizing that they imply quite different behaviour of the bird population. One simple approach often used for the analysis of data that comprise replicate observations is to work with an appropriate summary measure, such as the mean of the replicate observations for each animal (see Section 14.5).

Another form of replication arises when a certain response is measured on several occasions on each experimental unit *over a period of time*. The data from this latter design need to be analysed in a special way, as the time factor may well be of interest, and care must be taken to ensure that treatment comparisons are made within rather than between animals. We discuss some approaches to the analysis of these **repeated measures** or **clustered designs** in Section 14.5; in Section 11.6 we describe how special regression methods can be used to deal with clustered data.

5.8.3 Concept of blocks

We can incorporate careful grouping of the experimental units in a trial as a supplementary technique to reduce the variability in the comparisons of interest. We deliberately separate the experimental units (e.g. animals) into groups, **blocks** or **strata** (e.g. breeds or regions of the country) so that the animals within a block are more homogeneous with respect to the outcome variable than the animals in the population at large. Thus, the random variability *within* each block is smaller than that *between* the blocks. We allocate the animals within each block to the various treatments randomly using a different randomization list for each block (this is stratified randomization – see Section 5.6.2(b)). In the analysis, it is possible to separate the variability in the results due to blocks from that due to treatments, allowing us to obtain a more precise estimate of the treatment effect than if we had not made use of blocks.

We have a **complete randomized block design** when each block contains a complete set of treatments. Other designs, called **incomplete block designs**, in which each block need not contain the entire treatment set, are possible but their complexity is beyond the scope of this book. We refer you to discussion in, for example, Cochran and Cox (1957) or Fleiss (1986).

You should be aware that, sometimes, the use of groups is governed by practical considerations rather than being promoted as a tool for increasing precision. In some situations, we may find it necessary to assemble groups of animals situated on several farms or at several kennels or catteries, with the group defining the animals at a particular location. These groups of animals may be regarded as blocks, but here they introduce an additional source of variation, that attributable to the different locations.

5.8.4 'Between' and 'within' comparisons

For simplicity, suppose that we are comparing just two treatments. There are two basic forms of design:

1. We can randomly assign the animals (the observational units) to the two treatments to create two **independent** groups. There is no relationship between the individual animals in one group and the individual animals in the second group, and the sample sizes may differ. This is a *parallel group design* (see Section 5.9.7) in which the treatment comparisons are made *between* animals. An example is a feeding trial that compares the average gain in weight over a time period in two groups of animals in which only one of the two groups is given a dietary supplement.

2. We can improve our comparison if we deliberately create related or dependent groups. If the observations in the two groups are **paired**, each observation in one group is paired or individually matched with an observation in the other group, and the groups are therefore necessarily of equal size. The treatment comparisons are then made *within* the pairs. There is less variation *within* paired individuals than *between* unpaired individuals, so the treatment effects can be estimated more precisely. Data sets that exhibit dependency in the form of pairing or individual matching should not be analysed as if the data were independent. If we ignore the dependency, we lose information, and this reduces the chance of detecting a treatment difference if one exists.

• The pair may comprise the same animal (**self-pairing**) in different circumstances (see *cross-over trials* in Section 5.9.7), e.g. when two treatments are administered to an animal in random order. An example of self-pairing is when we compare a horse's metabolism on a treadmill and on a normal track (e.g. Exercise 7.3).

You should beware of the common mistake of regarding before and after treatment comparisons on the same animal as suitable for a simple paired analysis; for example, in comparing the heart rate (beats/min) of dogs before and after dosing with a putative cardiac stimulant. Unless the design includes a group of animals for which measurements are made both before and after a control (e.g. placebo) treatment is administered, it is impossible to be sure if a difference in the before and after active treatment measurements can be attributed to the effect of treatment alone. It is more appropriate in these circumstances to compare the two sets of differences, those in the group receiving the control and those in the group receiving the active treatment. Thus, although we pair the observations at the outset, the statistical analysis is a two-sample comparison of differences.

- Another form of pairing often occurs in animal experimentation when litter mates provide the experimental material (**natural pairing**), and the treatments are allocated in such a way that every animal in one group has a litter mate in the other group.
- A third form of pairing occurs when the pair comprises two different animals that have been *matched* with respect to any variables that may be thought to influence response (**artificial pairing**). An example is a study in dogs involving the effect of a drug on haematology values, where animals have been paired for treatment and control on the basis of approximate similarity in age and body size, because these factors were thought to influence response. Bland and Altman (1994) discuss matching in a brief but informative paper.

5.8.5 Use of specific animals

Note that substantial reduction in variability can also be obtained by using microbiologically, genetically or environmentally defined animals. Nevertheless, sufficient animals must be included to give satisfactory estimates. However, the results are only strictly relevant to the type of animal in the trial and may differ from what is found in 'normal' animals. You must exercise care in drawing conclusions on this basis.

5.9 Further considerations

5.9.1 Confounding and interactions

Sometimes, we find that two or more variables are related to each other as well as to the response of interest, so that it is impossible to separate the effects of these variables on the response. The variables are then called **confounders** and the process is called **confounding**.

As a simple example, suppose routine haematology is being done by two laboratories, A and B. Laboratory A is nearby so the samples are delivered by hand and examined almost immediately, whereas Laboratory B is some distance away so the samples have to be sent by post with a delivery time of 2 days. Laboratory A uses old-fashioned equipment and manual counting, while Laboratory B uses a mechanized process and automated counting. We divide specimens and send identical samples to each laboratory over a 3-month period to compare the white blood cell counts, and discover that Laboratory A produces substantially higher counts in the samples. Is the result due to the more thorough and painstaking methods of Laboratory A or to the difference in time of examination in the two laboratories? We cannot separate the effects of the two variables (laboratory, time delay) on the outcome (the count), and the variables are said to be *confounded*. In this example, confounding potentially created a false association between count and laboratory, since the design of the experiment failed to allow for the effect of time delay. Confounding can also obscure a real relationship; for example, if we found that the laboratories were producing similar counts, this could be because any difference in the counts between the laboratories was obscured by the effect of different delay times before haematological analysis. Had we planned the study more carefully we could have separated the time factor from the laboratory by organizing samples to be analysed at the same delay times in each laboratory. The key is in recognizing potential confounding covariates and incorporating them in the original design.

Confounding can occur both in experimental and in observational studies (see Section 5.2.1 for the distinction). It is of less concern in experimental studies if we have used randomization in the allocation process because possible confounding factors should be evenly distributed in the groups being compared, provided the sample size is large enough. However, in observational studies, we should try to identify any possible confounders and adjust for them in the analysis. We can do this in a number of ways:

- We incorporate the confounders as explanatory variables in a **regression model** (see Section 11.3.1(c)).
- We **match** animals on the basis of the confounding variable(s). For example, if gender is the only confounding variable, we identify pairs of animals, so that each member of a pair is of the same gender, and use an appropriate analysis on the variable(s) of interest that takes the pairing into account (e.g. McNemar's test (see Section 9.6) or the paired *t*-test (see Section 7.5)). If there are a number of confounding variables, each pair must be matched on all of them, and this may be impractical. Note that we cannot determine the effects of the matching variable(s) on the outcome.
- We create **subgroups** using stratification (see Section 5.6.2(b)) – i.e. we create strata or subgroups representing the different categories of the confounding variable and examine the relationship of interest in each stratum. For example, if we have categorical data, we can use the **Mantel–Haenszel method** (see, for example, Fleiss *et al.*, 2003), to combine contingency tables in different subgroups to obtain, if appropriate, an overall estimate of the odds ratio. We should be aware, however, that in any subgroup analysis: (i) the subgroups may be small so that they have low power to detect real effects as statistically significant (see Section 6.4.2); to avoid this problem, the subgroups should be identified at the design stage when estimates of optimal sample size (see Section 13.3) are derived for them; and (ii) *P*-values have to be adjusted if we perform at least one hypothesis test in each subgroup to avoid spuriously significant results arising from multiple testing (see Section 8.6.3).
- We use a **propensity score** approach in which a score is determined that describes the chance (propensity) of an animal falling into one of the categories of the (usually binary) explanatory variable (x_1, say) that is of the greatest interest. Often this variable represents 'treatment' if treatments have not been randomly assigned to animals. This score is generated (typically via logistic regression analysis, see Section 11.4) from all the variables associated with x_1, some of which will be the confounding variables that are also associated with the outcome variable. We can use the propensity score in a number of ways, for example by matching or stratifying on the basis of the propensity score, or in a multiple regression analysis (see Section 11.3) where we include x_1 as an explanatory variable in the model together with the propensity score (the latter replacing all the variables used to generate it) and any other covariates of interest. Further details may be found in, for example, Guo and Fraser (2010), Petrie and Sabin (2009) or Stürmer *et al.* (2006).

Confounding between variables should not be confused with there being an **interaction**, sometimes called **effect modification**, between them. When two variables are confounded, it is impossible to separate the effect of each on the outcome of interest. When there is an interaction between two variables, then the variables do not act independently on the outcome of interest. For example, in a study of helminth infestations in bank voles, it was found that total helminth infestation was 20% lower in females than in males in spring, but 5% higher in autumn (Bajer *et al.*, 2005). Thus, the relationship between helminth infestation (the outcome) and gender was dependent on the season, i.e. there was an interaction between gender and season. We explain interactions in the context of analysis of variance in Section 8.5.3, and in Section 11.3.1(d) we describe how to include interaction terms in a multivariable regression model.

5.9.2 Protocol

The protocol is a written document that details all aspects of the rationale, design, conduct and proposed analysis of the trial. Typically, it contains statements relating to the background and objectives of the study, ethical problems, the trial design including methods of randomization, selection of animals, sample size calculations, exclusion criteria, protocol deviations, the potential sources of bias, the variables which will be measured, the measurement techniques, methods of, and forms for, data collection, drug regimens and suppliers, the duration of the trial, the manpower requirements and responsibilities, the statistical analysis and costs.

The protocol is prepared at the outset of the trial, and serves a number of useful functions. It is required for submissions to funding bodies and for ethical committee approval; it is a useful reference document for the study investigators during the progress of the trial; and it is helpful in the final write-up of a study.

5.9.3 Outliers

(a) Identifying the outlier(s)

An **outlier** is an extreme observation that is inconsistent with the main body of the data. We must always check our data at the initial stages of the analysis to determine whether they contain outliers. This is most easily achieved by plotting the data, for example by producing a histogram, a stem-and-leaf plot or a box-and-whisker plot (see Section 2.5.2) for a single continuous variable, or a scatter diagram when we are investigating the relationship between two continuous variables in regression analysis (see Section 10.2). As an alternative strategy, we may look at the range of our sample data to see if any observation in our sample lies outside the range of plausible values. Some statistical software packages contain an automatic procedure for detecting outliers; for example, all values that are greater than 3 standard deviations away from the mean.

The problem with outliers is that they often distort the results and the conclusions drawn from the statistical analysis. This may happen even when there are only one or two outliers in a data set. The real difficulty is in knowing what to do with the outliers. There are four ways in which we can handle them. We can:

- Include them and proceed as originally planned, recognizing that the distribution assumptions of the analysis may not be met.

- Include them in the analysis but adopt a procedure that is appropriate for the data. For example, if the distribution of the variable of interest is skewed (see Section 2.5) because of the presence of outliers, then the median is a better measure of central tendency than the arithmetic mean (see Section 2.6.1), and we may prefer non-parametric methods of statistical analysis (see Chapter 12) for statistical inference. Alternatively we may take an appropriate transformation (see Section 13.2) to mitigate the effect of extreme values.
- Perform a sensitivity analysis by analysing the data both with and without the outliers to determine the effect, if any, of removing them.
- Exclude them from the analysis (this is a high-risk strategy, and, before you do so, you should thoroughly investigate the reason for their presence, see Section 5.9.3(b)). Beware that some computer packages will automatically eliminate outliers from the analysis.

Which of these approaches we choose will depend on the magnitude and the cause of the outlier(s).

(b) Causes of outliers

- Sometimes, we obtain an outlier because the animal on which we are making the measurement is atypical of the population from which it was drawn. We should not exclude an outlier unless there is a justifiable reason for doing so. It may be, for example, that one animal in a group cannot be caught without considerable vigorous activity; this might result in a physiological variable exhibiting an extreme value which could be excluded.
- Alternatively, it may be apparent, on subsequent post-mortem examination, that a particular animal suffered an intercurrent disease that may have caused an outlier during a clinical trial. Again, it is reasonable to omit the outlier from the analysis.
- We may also obtain an outlier because we have made a mistake, perhaps in reading an instrument or in transcribing information. Then it might be possible to correct the mistake, and include the corrected value in the analysis.

5.9.4 Missing data

Despite our best intentions at the start of a study, we may find that our data set is incomplete when we are ready to analyse the data. For example, the carer may have inadvertently lost a reading on an animal, or an animal ear-tag may have been dislodged making identity uncertain, or an animal died in the course of our investigation. It is important that you make a decision about what you will do with missing data before entering your data into the computer. Sometimes you can just leave each missing observation as a blank. Often, however, it is advisable to code the missing observations in some recognizable format, so as to be able to distinguish them from other types of observations. The choice is yours, but you must select a code that is unique and cannot be confused with a real observation. Typically, the numbers 9 (for a variable whose maximum value is less than 9), 99 or 999 are chosen, although some computer programs are prepared to accept an asterisk (*), a bullet (•) or some other symbol. Note that you should remember to distinguish missing data from 'not applicable' results. You could use a specific value for the variable of interest (e.g. age at first litter) to indicate 'not applicable', and you could create a new variable (e.g. animal has or does not have a prior litter) to distinguish those animals that are applicable from those that are not. Mirowsky and Ross (2002) provide an explanation of how to handle the data if you want to ensure that all the observations in the data set are used for estimation when there are a number of variables of interest and some have 'not applicable' results.

We should always investigate the reasons for missing data, to ensure that no biases (see Section 5.4) are likely to arise because of them. For example, if an observation goes beyond the scale of the measuring instrument, it cannot be recorded and may be coded as 'missing'. The failure to record this observation is related to its magnitude, and a bias may well result. Occasionally, missing observations that are left as blanks in the data file may be taken as zeros in the analysis; be warned that this is likely to have a considerable effect on the conclusions. *Always make sure that you know how your software package deals with missing data.*

Some statistical software packages handle missing observations by automatically excluding from the analysis any individual that has a missing observation on at least one variable. This is called **listwise deletion**: it leads to biased and inefficient parameter estimates if there is a considerable quantity of missing data. Others estimate (**impute**) the missing observations, for example, by replacing the missing observation by the average of the remaining observations in the relevant data or the last observation carried forward in a longitudinal analysis. This process is called **simple imputation**. In **multiple imputation**, the missing values for any variable are predicted using existing values from other variables and substituted for the missing values to produce an imputed data set. This process is performed a number of times (typically not more than five times) so that multiple imputed data sets are created. Standard statistical analysis is carried out on each imputed data set and these results are then combined to produce one overall analysis.

Whatever method is used to deal with the missing data, it is important to understand why the data are missing as this will affect the extent to which bias is present when estimating parameters. Consideration should be given to whether the data are:

- **Missing completely at random (MCAR)** – this implies that the probability that the value of a variable for a given individual is missing does not depend on any variable, so that missing cases are no different than non-missing cases and consistent results would be obtained performing the analysis both with and without the missing data. For example, if a dog failed to show up for an examination because its owner was in a car accident, the data for that dog would be missing completely at random.
- **Missing at random (MAR)** – this implies that the probability that the value of a variable for an individual is missing does not depend on that variable, but depends on the known values of the other variables. For example, in monitoring the effects of a prescribed diet for obese

dogs, if poorly-educated dog owners have difficulties in recording the dietary intake of their dogs then the data are missing at random because it is the trouble recording the information and not the diet itself that is accounting for the missing data, i.e. the absence of the data depends on the level of education of the owner.

- **Not missing at random (non-ignorable) (NMAR)** – this implies that the missingness depends not only on the observed data but also on the unobserved (missing) data. For example, in assessing the effect on depression of pet ownership on elderly individuals living by themselves, failing to return the mental health questionnaire because the pet is sick (resulting in a more depressed state for the owner) would constitute not missing at random.

Of particular importance when dealing with missing observations is a **sensitivity analysis** (see Section 10.4.3(d)), that is, we see how our conclusions change as we work through a range of different approaches to dealing with the missing observations.

You can find a full discussion of how to handle missing data in, for example, Allison (2001), Engels and Diehr (2003) and Little and Rubin (2002) and at www.missingdata.org.uk (accessed 15 October 2012). In Section 13.5.2(d), we explain how to use a funnel plot to assess whether there may be missing publications in a meta-analysis.

5.9.5 Analysis by intention-to-treat

One of the greatest problems in the analysis of clinical trials is knowing what to do with the results from animals that do not strictly adhere to the protocol, possibly because they prove too difficult to treat with the treatment that was originally assigned to them. Additionally, some animals may deviate from the original treatment schedule, perhaps because of side effects, and are switched to an alternative treatment or treatment is stopped altogether. Such observations do not count as missing (see Section 5.9.4) if the results are known, but are called **withdrawals** from treatment.

- Provided we have results, the appropriate way of dealing with withdrawals is to analyse them as if they still belonged to the treatment group *to which the animals were originally randomly assigned*. At first glance, you may find this so-called **intention-to-treat** or *pragmatic* approach, aimed at eliciting the effect of treatment in a clinical scenario, difficult to comprehend. You may wonder how you can justify analysing a result as if the observation were made on one treatment when, in fact, it arises from the application of another treatment. Be assured, however, that this is the correct approach.

- The alternative is to analyse the results according to the treatment actually received; this *explanatory* approach is aimed at understanding the processes involved. We do not recommend the explanatory approach as it is more likely to distort the treatment comparisons (and lead to a biased result favouring the new treatment) than the pragmatic approach. Remember that one of the reasons for employing randomization is to aim to have treatment groups that are balanced in the factors that influence response (see Section 5.6). If we use the explanatory approach, then the animals are not analysed in the treatment groups to which they were randomly assigned, and we may disturb this balance of potentially influential factors.

You will find a full discussion in Schwartz *et al.* (1980).

5.9.6 Pilot studies

A **pilot study** is a small-scale preliminary investigation. We conduct pilot studies for a variety of reasons:

- To see whether there is merit in developing a full-scale trial.
- To provide us with an indication of the variability in the results. If we have some idea of the expected variability in the results, we can calculate minimum group sizes to permit detection of real treatment effects in the full-scale trial (see Section 13.3).

- To ensure that the dosing regimen we have chosen for a treatment is appropriate.
- To develop techniques and iron out any difficulties we may experience.

As you will appreciate, a pilot study is well worth the time and resources invested in it, and can save much frustration later, especially if the proposed study breaks entirely novel ground.

5.9.7 Cross-over trials

Most clinical trials are **parallel group designs**; each individual animal receives only one treatment, and treatment comparisons are made between rather than within animals (see also Section 5.8.4). Occasionally, we may conduct a **cross-over trial**. As its name suggests, we apply two or more treatments in succession to each individual animal. The aim is to compare the responses to treatment *within* the animals, rather than *between* animals, thereby enhancing the precision of the estimate of the difference between treatments and reducing the sample size. However, we cannot entirely eliminate individual variation since the treatments are not contemporaneous, and there may be a period effect (when there is a systematic difference in response between the two periods of administration). This may occur, say, when the animals become more accustomed to dosing in the second period and therefore have a different physiological baseline. To minimize the influence of the passage of time and the period effect, the order in which each animal receives the treatments is chosen at random.

This sort of trial is ideally suited to the comparison of palliative treatments of chronic diseases rather than to the comparison of cures, since the condition must return, and be of equal severity, after treatment ceases in order to investigate the other treatments. Suitable examples are the use of dietary restriction or insulin on the control of blood glucose in diabetic dogs, or the use of topical ointments or oral preparations on the control of eczema.

Because of a possible carry-over effect, it is important to establish the question of how long a rest or wash-out period is necessary before instigating the next treatment, since some treatments may have a long lag phase before the effects are eliminated.

The analysis of cross-over trials is a relatively complex subject, and is covered in detail in Senn (2002).

Exercises

The statements in questions 5.1–5.3 are either TRUE or FALSE.

5.1 Animals are randomly allocated to the treatment groups in a clinical trial:
(a) To ensure that there is no assessment bias.
(b) To ensure that all animals have the same chance of receiving any treatment.
(c) So that a control group can be incorporated into the design.
(d) So that the treatment groups are comparable with respect to any variables that are likely to influence response.
(e) So that the trial can be single- or double-blind.

5.2 The wattle reaction of chicks to the injection of phytohaemagglutinin (PHA) is used as an indication of the immune responsiveness. Chicks (3–6 days old) were randomly assigned to four groups, a control and three different monoamine treatments which were suspected of interfering with the immune responses. Thirty minutes after treatment, birds were injected in the wattle with 100 mg PHA-P and wattle thickness was measured prior to the injection and 24 hours later (Lukacs *et al.*, 1987). This is an example of:
(a) An observational study.
(b) A cross-sectional study.
(c) A retrospective study.
(d) A clinical trial.
(e) A sample survey.

5.3 Sedative treatments were administered to 10 ferrets in a cross-over trial, and sedative and cardiovascular responses evaluated (Ko *et al.*, 1998). Diazepam, acepromazine and xylazine were administered to each animal in a random order; a wash-out period was allowed between each treatment. Xylazine produced the longest duration of recumbency on average and was judged most satisfactory as a sedative for ferrets.

(a) The wash-out period allowed the trial to be blind.
(b) The randomization ensured that there was no carry-over effect.
(c) This was an example of a parallel group design.
(d) The treatment comparison was made within animals.
(e) A more precise treatment comparison would be achieved if each ferret received only one treatment, so that the three treatment groups comprised different animals.

5.4 A study was conducted into the influence of spaying of bitches on their subsequent development of urinary incontinence. Young adult bitches presenting for spaying were randomly allocated to immediate ovariohysterectomy or to a deferred operation 6 months later. The bitches were followed during the 6-month period. Was this:

(a) A cross-sectional or a longitudinal study, and why?
(b) An experimental or an observational study, and why?
(c) A cohort study or a case–control study, and why?
(d) Can you propose any other study design to explore this condition and its aetiology?

5.5 In a study of the benefits of surgical intervention in the repair of congenital umbilical hernia, kittens with a visible herniation within 48 hours of birth were randomly allocated to surgery or to a *laissez-faire* approach. At the time of weaning, kittens were assessed for survival rate and hernia resolution. Criticize the choice of control and suggest any improvements.

5.6 Describe an appropriate randomization (simple, stratified, restricted or group) for the following investigations:

(a) Three dose levels (mg/kg) of an acaricide applied to dogs seen at an urban veterinary practice.
(b) Testing the efficacy of a treatment for *Ostertagia* (lungworm) in a herd of cattle in two plots of worm-infested land.
(c) Testing the efficacy of vaccination of kittens against common cat viral diseases by vaccinating litters of kittens at random with one of two different commercial preparations.
(d) The allocation to treatment groups of individual animals in four different farm locations for a study of the effects of lambing indoors in pens or outside in makeshift straw shelters. For an optimal design, equal numbers of animals should be in each treatment group at each location.

5.7 Researchers were concerned with estimating the seroprevalence of Q fever (a zoonosis caused by *Coxiella burnetii*) in commercial dairy goat farms in the Netherlands and wished to identify risk factors for farm seropositivity before mandatory vaccination started. In their cross-sectional study, 2766 ELISA (enzyme-linked immunosorbent assay) test results from goats in 125 farms (each with more than 100 goats) were available. A farm was considered positive when at least one goat tested ELISA positive. Amongst other potential risk factors, they found that a herd size above 800 was a risk factor for Q fever. Thirty-three of the 57 farms that were positive for Q fever had at least 800 goats, and 24 of the 68 farms that were not positive for Q fever had at least 800 goats (based on Schimmer *et al.*, 2011).

(a) Estimate the risk of a farm being positive for Q fever in large and small farms (i.e. those comprising ≥800 and <800 goats, respectively) and the overall prevalence of positive farms.
(b) Estimate and interpret the relative risk (RR) and absolute risk reduction (ARR) of large farms being positive compared with small farms.
(c) Estimate and interpret the odds ratio (OR) of a farm being positive if it is large rather than small. Comment on the similarity or difference between the estimated RR and OR.

6 An introduction to hypothesis testing

6.1 Learning objectives

By the end of this chapter, you should be able to:

- Elaborate the basic concept of hypothesis testing.
- Define the null hypothesis.
- Distinguish between one- and two-tailed tests and decide which is appropriate in any investigative trial.
- Define a test statistic.
- Explain in simple terms the meaning of the term 'degrees of freedom'.
- Interpret the *P*-value.
- Summarize the hypothesis testing procedure.
- Define Type I and Type II errors in hypothesis testing.
- Define the power of a test.
- Distinguish between statistical significance and biological importance.
- Distinguish between the approaches to testing a hypothesis using a test statistic and a confidence interval, identifying the strengths and weaknesses of both.
- Explain the concepts underlying equivalence and non-inferiority studies.

6.2 Introduction

We can categorize statistical theory into two general areas.

1. Firstly, there is **descriptive statistics** which uses the appropriate tools, typically tables, diagrams and/or numerical measures, to describe a data set and provide a summary of its distribution (see Chapter 2).
2. In addition, there is **inferential statistics** which is concerned with drawing conclusions about a population using information obtained from a representative sample selected from it.
   (a) One aspect of statistical inference is the **estimation** of a population parameter by the appropriate sample statistic (e.g. the population mean by the sample mean). The estimation process is complete only when the precision of the estimate, as determined by its standard error (see Section 4.4) or indicated by the confidence interval, is included (see Section 4.5).
   (b) The second aspect of inferential statistics is **hypothesis testing**. In this case, we examine a hypothesis, framed in terms of the parameters in one or more populations. We want to know if the hypothesis about the population(s) is refuted by the sample data.

Estimation is concerned with *description* whereas hypothesis testing is ultimately concerned with *decision*.

6.3 Basic concepts of hypothesis testing

Hypothesis testing is a process that is concerned with making inferences about the population using the information obtained from a sample. We have to recognize that it is impossible to be absolutely certain that our inferences about the population are correct. One randomly selected sample from the population is unlikely to be exactly the same as a second randomly selected sample, and in neither of these is the sample statistic likely to be exactly equal to the population parameter it is estimating and about which we are testing a hypothesis. Because we take a sample, there is an element of uncertainty involved and, therefore, we should accompany the conclusions we draw about the population with a **probability** (see Section 3.2.2). This gives an indication of the chance of getting the observed results if the hypothesis is true. We replace an absolute statement by a probabilistic statement, and this forms the crux of hypothesis testing.

Although the basic concepts of hypothesis testing are not too difficult to grasp, the whole process is shrouded in statistical jargon. It is helpful if you have a proper understanding of this jargon, particularly if you obtain your results from computer output, which may vary in form depending on the particular software package that you are using.

6.3.1 The null hypothesis, H_0

We are concerned with investigating a particular theory or scientific hypothesis, called the *study hypothesis, about the population*. However, it is usually harder to prove a hypothesis than to disprove it. For example, we might have to look at all the goats in Turkey or, at least, a very large number of them in order to prove the hypothesis that all goats in Turkey are Bezoar goats, whereas one goat of a different breed will immediately disprove the hypothesis. Thus, rather than trying to prove that the study hypothesis is true, we proceed in statistical hypothesis testing by attempting to disprove the **null hypothesis**, H_0, which is the converse of the study hypothesis. Usually, our study hypothesis is comparative in nature, involving some numerical **effect** of interest; often this comparison is of different treatments, the measure that compares their responses

being termed the **treatment effect**. This treatment effect is specified by the relevant parameter values in the treatment groups; let us assume, as an illustration, that it represents the difference in means. Then, instead of testing the hypothesis that the study hypothesis is true (i.e. that there is a treatment effect – a difference in means), we test the null hypothesis that there is no treatment effect in the population. Suppose, for example, that we are interested in investigating whether cattle on new spring grass are in danger of hypomagnesaemia (grass staggers). A lower level of plasma magnesium in the outdoor cattle compared with those kept indoors would suggest a risk of grass staggers. We formulate the null hypothesis that the true mean values of plasma magnesium do not differ in the two groups. We examine the sample data to see whether they contradict this hypothesis.

Should the null hypothesis be untrue, an **alternative hypothesis** holds:

- Usually, the alternative hypothesis states that a difference exists between the parameter values but the direction of that difference is not known. It leads to a **two-sided** or a **two-tailed test**. Unless otherwise specified, we assume that a test is two-tailed. In our example, although we might anticipate that eating new grass would reduce the mean plasma magnesium concentration, the alternative hypothesis is merely that the two means differ. We have no prior reason to anticipate that the indoor 'treatment' can *only* be better than the grass 'treatment'.
- Very occasionally, however, we have sound prior knowledge that any difference between the treatments, if it exists, can be in one direction only. This must not be based on hopes or expectations about a novel treatment, but on an absolute certainty that the difference can only be in that direction, if the difference is not zero. This gives rise to a **one-sided** or a **one-tailed test** in which the direction of the difference is specified in the alternative hypothesis.

We must specify both the null and the alternative hypotheses at the outset, before we collect the data. We stress that the alternative hypothesis must be specified *before* the data are collected, and is, therefore, independent of the data. You may be tempted to use a one-sided test because it is more likely than a two-sided test to show a difference! Remember, though, that the prior certainty required for a one-sided test *very rarely exists*.

6.3.2 Getting a feel for the data

Having specified the null and alternative hypotheses, we then **collect** our sample data. It is important that we **look** at the data at this stage and check the *assumptions* inherent in the test. With the advent of computers and easy access to statistical computer software, it is all too easy to overlook the nature of the data, including a lack of awareness of outliers that may be distorting the results, and consequently to draw inappropriate conclusions. A careful, albeit simple, initial look at the data may forestall erroneous judgements.

6.3.3 The test statistic and the *P*-value

From the data we calculate the value of a **test statistic** (an algebraic expression particular to the hypothesis we are testing), usually using a computer or, occasionally, by hand. Attached to each value of the test statistic is a **probability**, called a **P-value**. It describes the chance of getting the observed effect (or one more extreme) *if the null hypothesis is true*. The 'if the null hypothesis is true' is crucial to the correct interpretation of the *P*-value; a common mistake is to omit this phrase, leading to the *erroneous* belief that the *P*-value represents the probability of the sample data arising by chance.

6.3.4 Making a decision using the *P*-value

According to the evidence obtained from our sample, we make a judgement about whether the data are inconsistent with the null hypothesis; this leads to a **decision** whether or not to reject the null hypothesis.

- If the observed results are *not* consistent with what we would expect *if the null hypothesis were true*, we conclude that we have enough evidence to **reject** the null hypothesis. We say that the result of the test is **statistically significant**.
- If, however, the observed results *are* consistent with what we would expect if the null hypothesis were true, we **do not reject** the null hypothesis. We say that the result of the test is **non-significant**.

Although semantically they may appear to be the same, we should note that *not rejecting* the null hypothesis is not synonymous with *accepting* the null hypothesis (see Section 6.8 on equivalence studies). Either we have enough evidence to reject the null hypothesis or we do not have enough evidence to reject it; the latter case does not imply that there is necessarily enough evidence to accept H_0 or, expressed another way, 'absence of evidence is not evidence of absence' (Altman and Bland, 1995). This can be likened to the situation in a law court – an analogy is drawn between the presumption of innocence and the null hypothesis. If there is enough evidence, the defendant will be found 'guilty' of the charge against him. If there is not enough evidence, the defendant will be found 'not guilty'. This does not prove that he is 'innocent', only that there is insufficient evidence to establish his guilt.

The *P*-value allows us to determine whether we have enough evidence to reject the null hypothesis in favour of the alternative hypothesis.

- If the *P*-value is very small, then it is unlikely that we could have obtained the observed results if the null hypothesis were true, so we reject H_0.
- If the *P*-value is very large, then there is a high chance that we could have obtained the observed results if the null hypothesis were true, and we do not reject H_0.

Clearly, distinguishing between large and small *P*-values is crucial to the decision-making process.

We have to decide, *before we collect the data*, what constitutes a large or small *P*-value, i.e. we have to choose a cut-off value, termed the **significance level** of the test. The choice of significance level is dependent on the nature of the data and the circumstances of the investigation.

It makes sense to choose a very low value for the significance level, say 0.01, if we want to err on the side of caution in rejecting H_0. This means that if, from our sample, we obtain a *P*-value which is less than 0.01, we reject the null hypothesis; we say the result is *significant at the 1% level*. For example, in investigating a rather costly novel antibiotic treatment, we would want to be very confident of its benefits over existing, and cheaper, products before introducing it into clinical practice. We might, however, choose a much higher value, say 0.10, in initial testing of the efficacy of a new potential vaccine against a presently incurable infectious disease which is causing great economic loss. This ensures that a marginal benefit is not overlooked.

An arbitrary cut-off point of 0.05 is usually chosen for the significance level such that if $P < 0.05$ then H_0 is rejected, and if $P \geq 0.05$ then H_0 is not rejected (Fisher, 1925). Further distinctions are sometimes made by using asterisks to distinguish between very highly significant (*** representing $P < 0.001$), highly significant (** representing $0.001 < P < 0.01$), significant (* representing $0.01 < P < 0.05$) and non-significant (NS representing $P > 0.05$). *We stress that these values are entirely arbitrary and should not be taken as definitive.* You should avoid the asterisks and, where possible, *quote the exact P-value* invariably provided in computer output for the relevant hypothesis test. Then, conclusions relating to H_0 can be substantiated by the reader. Remember, the smaller the *P*-value, the greater the evidence against H_0.

6.3.5 Deriving the *P*-value

Naturally, a vital link in the whole hypothesis test procedure is the relationship between the value of the **test statistic** and the **P-value**. In the chapters which follow we give the relevant formula for each test statistic corresponding to a specific hypothesis test. It is particularly important, in the context of this general explanatory chapter, that you understand that each test statistic follows a known theoretical probability distribution. This means that its value obtained from a particular set of sample data can be compared with its known distribution to determine the *P*-value (the probability of obtaining the observed value of the test statistic if the null hypothesis is true). Typically, the known distribution of the test statistic is Normal, t, F or χ^2.

If you are performing a computer analysis, you will find the *P*-value you need in the computer output. If necessary, you can obtain the *P*-value by referring the test statistic to the table of its distribution, usually using both tail areas (two-sided test), but occasionally, a single tail area (one-sided test – see Section 6.3.1). You may have to *interpolate* (estimate the value between two tabulated values) when you use the table if the required value is not contained in the table. For example, if the degrees of freedom of the test statistic (see Section 6.3.6) are 35, Table A.3 has tabulated percentage points for degrees of freedom of 30 and 40 only. You would estimate the required percentage point as being midway between that for 30 and that for 40 degrees of freedom.

6.3.6 Degrees of freedom of the test statistic

You will find that the term **degrees of freedom** (*df*) occurs frequently in statistical analysis. If we are using tables to relate the value of the test statistic to the *P*-value, we generally have to know the degrees of freedom of the relevant distribution of our test statistic. The degrees of freedom of a statistic are the number of independent observations contributing to that statistic, i.e. the number of observations available to evaluate that statistic minus the number of restrictions on those observations. The easiest way of calculating the degrees of freedom of any statistic is to take them as the difference between the number of observations we have in our sample and the number of parameters we have to estimate in order to evaluate that statistic.

So, for example, suppose we are estimating a population variance, σ^2, of a variable, x, in a sample of size n by its sample statistic, s^2, given by

$$s^2 = \frac{\sum(x-\bar{x})^2}{(n-1)}$$

We have to estimate the mean in order to evaluate the numerator, and so the degrees of freedom of s^2 are $(n-1)$.

6.3.7 Quoting a confidence interval

The use of a **confidence interval** diminishes, to some extent, the reliance on the P-value and the subsequent significance or non-significance of a test result. We measure the precision of a sample statistic as an estimate of the population parameter by its standard error. This is used in the calculation of the confidence interval for the parameter (see Section 4.5). A small sample leads to a less precise parameter estimate than a large sample, so that its standard error will be larger. Consequently, the confidence interval for a parameter derived from a small sample will be wider than that derived from a large sample. When we have a wide confidence interval, we need to look at the limits carefully and consider their implications, whether or not the test is significant.

Thus, if we want a full statement of the result of a hypothesis test, we should supplement the P-value by an estimate of the effect of interest (e.g. the estimated difference in means if H_0 states that two population means are equal) with the relevant confidence interval. Then we, and others, can make an informed judgement about the results obtained from the hypothesis test. We will have an understanding of what is happening, rather than simply deciding whether or not to reject the null hypothesis.

6.3.8 Summary of the hypothesis test procedure

We can assimilate this whole hypothesis test procedure by generalizing it to a six-step procedure:

1. Specify the **null hypothesis**, H_0, and the **alternative hypothesis** (by default, we adopt a two-sided test unless a different alternative hypothesis is specified).
2. **Collect** the data and **look** at them, diagrammatically if possible, to investigate their distribution(s), check for outliers and get a feel for what they show. Many tests make distributional assumptions about the data: check the assumptions underlying the test.
3. On the computer, select the **appropriate test**, or, by hand, calculate the appropriate **test statistic** using the sample data.
4. Relate the calculated value of the test statistic to a **P-value**.
5. Consider the P-value to judge whether the data are inconsistent with the null hypothesis. Then **decide** whether or not to reject the null hypothesis.
6. If appropriate, calculate the **confidence interval** for the effect of interest, phrased in terms of the parameter specification in the null hypothesis.

We assign significance to the result in the course of this procedure, and therefore this is sometimes called a *significance test*.

As you will see, the choice of test is not always simple – it depends on the nature of the data, the null hypothesis and the assumptions underlying the test. It is a logical procedure, and the flow charts in Appendix E will guide you through the process.

6.4 Type I and Type II errors

6.4.1 Making the wrong decision in a hypothesis test

You must recognize that the final decision whether or not to reject the null hypothesis may be incorrect. As a frame of reference, we discuss the common situation in which we are interested in comparing two population means using independent samples selected from these populations (see Section 7.4.1). The null hypothesis is that the two population means are equal or, equivalently, that the difference between these two population means is zero. Consider the example introduced in Section 6.3.1; we have the plasma magnesium levels for two groups of cattle, one kept indoors and the other put out on spring grass for the past week. A lower level of plasma magnesium in the outdoor cattle would suggest a risk of grass staggers. Our null hypothesis is that the mean values of plasma magnesium do not differ in the two populations from which we have taken our samples.

- We may find that the result of the test is significant. In this case, we reject the null hypothesis at the stated level of significance, and infer that the two population means differ. If this inference is incorrect, and in reality the two means are equal, then we have rejected the null hypothesis when we should not have rejected it (i.e. when it is true). We are making a **Type I error** (Table 6.1).
- Alternatively, we may find that the result of the test is not significant. Then, we do not reject the null hypothesis at the stated level of significance, so we cannot infer that the two population means are different. If this is incorrect, and in reality the two means differ, then we have not rejected the null hypothesis when we should have rejected it (i.e. when it is false). We are making a **Type II error** (Table 6.1).

6.4.2 Probability of making a wrong decision

It is crucial that you understand the importance of these two errors and what each represents as they both play a role in determining the optimal size of an experiment (see Section 13.3) – a critical design consideration.

- The **probability of making a Type I error** is the probability of incorrectly rejecting the null hypothesis, i.e. it is the P-value obtained from

the test. The null hypothesis will be rejected if this probability is less than the significance level, often denoted by α (alpha) and commonly taken as 0.05. Thus the significance level is the maximum chance of making a Type I error. If the P-value is equal to or greater than α, then we do not reject the null hypothesis and we are not making a Type I error. Therefore, by choosing the significance level of the test to be α at the design stage of the study, we are limiting the probability of a Type I error to be less than α.

- The **probability of making a Type II error** is usually designated by β (beta). It is the probability of not rejecting the null hypothesis when the null hypothesis is false. We should decide on a value of β that we regard as acceptable at the design stage of the experiment. β is affected by a number of factors, one of which is the sample size; the greater the sample size, the smaller β becomes (keeping the other factors that affect it constant).

In fact, instead of thinking about β, we usually consider its complement, $1 - \beta$ (often multiplied by 100 and expressed as a percentage). This is called the **power** of the test. It is the probability of rejecting the null hypothesis when the null hypothesis is false, i.e. it is the chance of detecting a treatment effect of a given size if it exists. We want the power of the test to be large or else we will waste our resources when we perform the experiment because we will probably fail to detect a real treatment effect as significant. By 'large', we mean that we should design our experiment so that the power of the test is at least 80% (Cohen, 1988) (see Section 13.3). This has an implication for the size of the study in that larger experiments are more powerful, implying that they have a greater chance of correctly detecting a treatment effect.

6.5 Distinction between statistical and biological significance

We should never consider the result of a hypothesis test expressed by the P-value and the decision whether or not to reject the null hypothesis

Table 6.1 Errors in hypothesis testing.

	Reject H_0	Do not reject H_0
H_0 true	Type I error	Correct decision
H_0 false	Correct decision	Type II error

in isolation. We must relate the result to the biological or clinical implications of the conclusion drawn from the test. A result that is **statistically significant** is not necessarily **biologically** or **clinically important**, and *vice versa*. Biological/clinical importance is a matter of individual judgement, and this may be difficult to discern in borderline cases.

Note that the *power* of a test (representing the ability of the test to detect a real effect, e.g. a treatment difference) is proportional to the *sample size* (see Section 13.3). The larger the sample, the greater the power, so that a large sample has a greater chance of detecting a real treatment difference than a small one. Thus, we may find that even small treatment differences that are biologically unimportant are statistically significant in large samples, whereas we may find that large and biologically important differences in small samples are not statistically significant.

For example, in field trials of modifications of semen diluents for frozen semen it is not uncommon to measure improvements in conception of only a percentage point or two. For such improvements to be statistically significant, many thousands of inseminations must be carried out under controlled conditions. Even then, statistical significance may be borderline. Nevertheless, a consistent improvement in fertility of the order of a percentage point represents a very substantial economic return and may be worth pursuing if the new diluent is not expensive to prepare. Here, then, biological importance may outweigh statistical significance.

In contrast, many anaesthetics used in veterinary medicine are known to cause minor, but consistent, variations in blood pressure. If measured over a sufficiently large sample, these effects would clearly be statistically significant, but normally they are of little biological importance because the effects are slight, and have no practical implications in the healthy animal undergoing elective surgery.

6.6 Confidence interval approach to hypothesis testing

We can use a confidence interval alone to make a decision to reject the null hypothesis about an effect of interest rather than going through the hypothesis testing procedure outlined in Section 6.3.8.

If, for example, we are interested in investigating whether two population means are equal, we first formulate the null hypothesis (that the two means are equal) and the alternative hypothesis (generally, that they are not). We then calculate the appropriate (usually 95%) confidence interval for the difference in the two population means. The 95% confidence interval for the difference in two population means is usually interpreted as the interval within which the true difference in means is contained with 95% certainty (see Section 4.5). It represents the plausible range of values for the difference in population means. Zero is an implausible value for the difference in means if it lies outside the 95% confidence interval. So, if the confidence interval does not span zero, we would conclude that it is unlikely (the chance is at most 5%) that the difference in population means could be zero, and we would reject the null hypothesis that the means are equal at the 5% level of significance.

To summarize, there are two approaches to testing a null hypothesis.

1. We can calculate the appropriate test statistic and determine the associated *P*-value. This represents the probability of obtaining the observed value of the test statistic, or one that is more extreme, if the null hypothesis is true. We reject the null hypothesis if the *P*-value is small, say < 0.05. The whole process is called a hypothesis test or a significance test.
2. We can calculate the 95% (say) confidence interval for the appropriate parameter expression (e.g. the difference in population means, $\mu_1 - \mu_2$, if we are testing $H_0: \mu_1 = \mu_2$). We reject the null hypothesis at the 5% level if the value of the parameter expression under the null hypothesis lies outside the confidence limits. The value of the parameter expression under H_0 is usually zero if we are investigating differences; the value is usually unity if we are investigating ratios such as the odds ratio or relative risk (see Section 5.2.3).

The confidence interval approach to hypothesis testing has the advantage that it is more informative than the corresponding significance test; it provides an interval estimate of the effect of interest as well as allowing us to make a decision to reject the null hypothesis. However, it is more restrictive than the significance test because we are limited to making this decision by considering only one level of significance, e.g. 5% for a 95% confidence interval. The corresponding significance test provides an exact *P*-value, which allows us to make a decision to reject the null hypothesis, as well as indicating the strength of belief we have in the truth of the null hypothesis.

6.7 Collecting our thoughts on confidence intervals

We have now introduced you to the three different uses of a confidence interval:

1. It is an indicator of the precision of the parameter estimate (see Section 4.5). A wide confidence interval indicates poor precision.
2. It provides a means of distinguishing between biological importance and statistical significance (see Section 6.5). The result of a hypothesis test that two means are equal might be significant but the confidence interval for the difference in the two means could be very narrow and its limits only just greater than zero. Here we might have statistical significance but the implications may not be biologically important. Alternatively, the result of the test might be non-significant but the confidence interval could be very wide with the upper limit being very much greater than zero. Here there is the potential for a biologically important difference although there is no statistical significance.
3. It can be used to test a null hypothesis about the parameter of interest (see Section 6.6). For example, the null hypothesis that there is no difference between two treatment means can be rejected if the confidence interval for the difference excludes zero.

A summary of the calculations of confidence intervals is given in Appendix B. A full discussion of confidence intervals appears in Altman *et al.*

(2000). An accompanying computer program (Confidence Interval Analysis) is available for the calculations of confidence intervals for commonly used parameters.

6.8 Equivalence and non-inferiority studies

6.8.1 Approach

All the hypothesis tests used to compare treatments that we describe in this book relate to **superiority trials**. We conduct these studies because we hope to demonstrate statistically the superiority of one treatment over another. In some situations, however, we may be interested in showing that one treatment is clinically *similar* (i.e. equivalent) to or *no worse* than (i.e. not inferior to) another. This may arise if a new treatment is cheaper than the standard treatment, produces fewer side effects and/or its form is more accessible. In such circumstances, the usual superiority trial does not address the relevant question: Can we regard the treatments as equivalent or not inferior in terms of the response of interest? In a superiority trial, our null hypothesis is that there is no treatment effect (e.g. that the mean response is the same in the two treatments in the population). Generally, we do not reject the null hypothesis if $P \geq 0.05$, and then we conclude that there is no evidence to show that there is a treatment effect. However, this is *not* the same as establishing **equivalence** or **non-inferiority**; in the biological sciences, there are many examples where an incorrect inference of equivalence or non-inferiority is drawn. Furthermore, even if $P < 0.05$ so that we reject the null hypothesis, the fact that we have *statistical* significance does not necessarily imply that we have a *clinically* important result; the treatment effect may still be clinically of little interest.

We usually analyse the results of equivalence and non-inferiority studies by defining what is termed an **equivalence interval**. This is the range of values for the effect of interest (e.g. the difference in treatment means) which would be considered of no *clinical* importance. Although the equivalence interval should, if possible, be determined by clinical experts, some regulatory bodies have specified rules for the conduct of **bio-equivalence** studies which are conducted to demonstrate that two formulations of a drug have similar bioavailability (i.e. this is when the same amount of drug gets into the body for each formulation). For example, the US Food and Drug Administration (1992) introduced the 80/20 rule which specifies that a test must have at least 80% power of detecting a 20% difference between the parameters of interest. Then if the (usually 95%) confidence interval for the treatment effect observed in a particular study lies wholly in the equivalence interval, we conclude that the treatment effect is of no clinical importance and the treatments can be regarded as equivalent. If the lower limit of the confidence interval for the treatment effect does not lie below the lower limit of the equivalence interval, then we conclude that the new treatment is not inferior to the other treatment.

The sample size required for an equivalence or non-inferiority trial is generally greater than that required for the comparable superiority trial and is calculated in a different way from that outlined in Section 13.3. Special tables for optimal sample size determination in these studies can be found in Machin *et al.* (2009). You can find further details of equivalence and non-inferiority studies in, for example, Jones *et al.* (1966), Julius (2003), Lesaffre (2008) and Matthews (2006).

6.8.2 Example

Two drugs, meloxicam and flunixin, were compared in their efficiency to control the symptoms of mastitis–metritis–agalactia syndrome in sows by comparison of an overall clinical index score (CIS), ranging from 8 (the best – no pathological findings) to 29 (the worst – highest score for all clinical signs) on day 2 after treatment (Hirsch *et al.*, 2003). Meloxicam (the novel drug) was considered to be *not inferior* to flunixin (the reference drug) if the one-sided 95% confidence limit for the difference (reference minus meloxicam) in mean CIS was greater than the lower equivalence bound of −1.4 score points. As we are only interested in the lower limit of the confidence

interval (our concern is that meloxicam should not be worse than flunixin), it is not unusual to use a one-sided 95% confidence interval, equivalent to a two-sided 90% confidence interval, when testing for non-inferiority at the 5% level.

The study was conducted as a double-blind, randomized, controlled, multicentre, clinical field trial. The mean values (95% confidence interval) of the CIS on day 2 were 15.6 (14.73 to 16.47) for meloxicam and 15.1 (14.31 to 15.89) for flunixin, with sample sizes of 94 and 93, respectively. The difference in mean CIS score in the two treatment groups (flunixin minus meloxicam) was estimated as −0.5 (suggesting that meloxicam is a less effective treatment) with a one-sided 95% confidence interval of −0.67 to 1.67. However, since the lower limit of this confidence interval, −0.67, is greater than the lower equivalence bound of −1.4 score points, meloxicam can be considered to be not inferior to flunixin for controlling the symptoms of mastitis–metritis–agalactia syndrome in sows.

Exercises

The statements in questions 6.1–6.6 are either TRUE or FALSE.

6.1 The null hypothesis for a test to compare two means states that:
(a) The sample means are equal.
(b) There is no difference between the population means.
(c) There is no significant difference between the population means.
(d) The probability of there being a difference between the means is zero.
(e) A difference between the means is not expected.

6.2 A one-tailed test:
(a) Refers only to the right-hand side of a distribution.
(b) Is more powerful than a two-tailed test.
(c) Is the more usual test.
(d) Requires knowledge, independent of the results, that the treatment effect, if it exists, can be in one direction only.
(e) Is used when group sizes are small.

6.3 The *P*-value gives the probability of:
(a) Obtaining a result as, or more, extreme than the one observed.
(b) The null hypothesis arising by chance alone.
(c) The null hypothesis being true.
(d) The observed results arising if the null hypothesis is true.
(e) The discrepancy between the observed values and those under the null hypothesis being due to chance.

6.4 $P < 0.01$ means that:
(a) There is less than a 1/100 chance that the null hypothesis is true.
(b) There is a greater than 99% chance that the alternative hypothesis is true.
(c) The probability of obtaining the observed results if the null hypothesis is true is less than 1%.
(d) The probability that the observed result has arisen by chance is less than 1%.
(e) There is a greater than 99% chance that the null hypothesis is false.

6.5 A test statistic is:
(a) The mean.
(b) The difference between the means.
(c) Assumed to follow a theoretical distribution.
(d) Less than 0.05 if the result of the test is significant.
(e) Only useful if the sample size is large.

6.6
(a) The equivalence of two means can be established at the 5% level of significance if the null hypothesis that two population means are equal is not rejected ($P > 0.05$).
(b) One preparation is not inferior to another if the lower limit of the 95% confidence interval for the effect of interest does not lie below the lower limit of the equivalence interval.
(c) If one treatment is not inferior to another, then the two treatments must be equivalent.

(d) An equivalence interval is equal to the 95% confidence interval for the effect of interest.
(e) The sample size for an equivalence study is generally greater than that required for the comparable superiority study.

6.7 A novel antispasmodic drug is being tested for its effectiveness in preventing smooth muscle contractions (a quantitative variable measured as tension in grams) on pieces of gut in an organ bath. It is tested against a control, which is the vehicle minus the drug. State an appropriate null hypothesis and the alternative hypothesis for the test. How would the null hypothesis and the alternative hypothesis change if the novel drug were to be tested against an existing drug?

6.8 Ponies from the sales need to be broken in. A trainer has his own methods for doing this effectively and wants to demonstrate the advantage of his system. He randomly allocates 15 of his ponies to be trained by his new system, the remaining 12 ponies being trained in the traditional manner. The ponies are tested to see if they will accept a bit and bridle 1 month after starting training. Any animal that refuses the bit and bridle is regarded as failing the test. What is the null hypothesis that you would investigate if you wanted to decide whether to adopt the new system? What is the alternative hypothesis?

6.9 A turkey egg incubator needs to be kept at 37.5°C throughout 'setting', i.e. for 26 days, for good hatchability. A new incubator is to be considered as a replacement for one of the incubators in the hatchery; a test run of 26 days with daily readings performed at the same time of day produced a mean value of 37.3°C with a standard deviation of 0.7°C. Assuming that the distribution of the incubator temperature is approximately Normal, calculate an approximate 95% confidence interval for the true mean temperature of the incubator. Should this incubator be used in the hatchery in future?

7 Hypothesis tests 1 – the *t*-test: comparing one or two means

7.1 Learning objectives

By the end of this chapter, you should be able to:

- Distinguish between one- and two-sample tests.
- Distinguish between the experimental designs that lead to either paired or two-sample *t*-tests.
- List and verify the assumptions that underlie the paired and two-sample *t*-tests.
- Explain what is meant by the treatment effect in the context of the *t*-test.
- Relate the value of the test statistic in the *t*-test to the *P*-value.
- Draw appropriate conclusions from the *t*-test.
- Estimate the magnitude of the treatment effect when comparing means and calculate the relevant confidence interval.

7.2 Requirements for hypothesis tests for comparing means

7.2.1 Nature of the data

The **arithmetic mean**, a summary measure of location for a numerical variable (see Section 2.6.1), is the focus of the hypothesis tests in this chapter. Suppose, for example, we are interested in measuring the stress of transportation of cattle (Nanda *et al.*, 1990). Cortisol is released from the adrenal gland in response to stressful situations; it is of interest to determine whether the mean plasma cortisol (ng/ml) during the transport of dairy cows is different from that of cows at rest.

Before applying the methods described in this chapter and in Chapter 8, we must consider the nature of the data.

- There can be only a *single variable* of interest (e.g. plasma cortisol concentration).
- The variable should be measured on a *numerical* scale (cortisol measurements are in ng/ml).
- A further common feature is the assumption that the variable under investigation is *Normally* distributed (see Section 3.5.3). This is not unreasonable for biological measurements such as plasma cortisol. Note that if the sample size is large, then the sample mean is approximately Normally distributed even if the variable does not follow a Normal distribution (see Section 4.4.3), and we do not have to concern ourselves with the Normality of the data. However, as it is often difficult to distinguish a small sample from a large one, it is safer *not* to ignore this assumption (see also Section 7.2.2).

In fact, the tests we discuss in this chapter are **robust** against a violation of the assumption of Normality; this implies that they are hardly affected if the data show a moderate departure from Normality (this is particularly the case if the sample sizes are equal in the two-sample comparison of means). Thus, in

Statistics for Veterinary and Animal Science, Third Edition. Aviva Petrie and Paul Watson.
© 2013 John Wiley & Sons, Ltd. Published 2013 by John Wiley & Sons, Ltd.

practice, approximate Normality is sufficient. We can verify this with a perfunctory plot of the data, perhaps using a box-and-whisker plot which highlights the median, the interquartile range and the extreme values (see Section 2.5.2(d)). Seldom will you find it necessary to delve into the more formal tests of Normality (see Section 3.5.3(e)) such as the Shapiro–Wilk W or Kolmogorov–Smirnov tests, which are available in many statistical packages. However, if there is a marked departure from Normality, there are two courses of action open to us. Either we can transform the data in an attempt to achieve approximate Normality (see Section 13.2.1), or we can proceed to a suitable non-parametric test, which makes no distributional assumptions (see Chapter 12).

- We assume that we have to use the sample data to estimate any population variances of interest.

7.2.2 Implications of sample size

In many animal investigations, it is not possible to assemble large numbers of subjects either on the grounds of cost or because of low disease prevalence. The question of **sample size** is an important consideration. This section is concerned with the implications of sample size for the choice of hypothesis test. You can find details of how to estimate the sample size you need in Section 13.3.

It is important to realize:

- The distribution of the variable is difficult to establish for *very small* samples, each comprising, perhaps, only five or six observations. We advocate the use of the alternative *non-parametric methods* (see Chapter 12) for very small sample sizes. However, you should be aware of the danger that very small samples may be unrepresentative of the population and, in such circumstances, it may not be sensible to perform hypothesis tests at all.
- If the overall sample size is *small* (say, less than 30), the test statistic follows a Student's *t*-distribution (see Section 3.5.4) provided the

data are approximately Normally distributed (and the variances (see Section 2.6.2(c)) are equal in the two-sample comparison).

- If the overall sample size is *large*, the distribution of the test statistic is approximately Normal. We may take 'large' to be greater than 30 if the data are Normally distributed; alternatively, 'large' may be in excess of, say, 100 if the data are not Normally distributed, but the extent of the deviation from Normality will influence our definition of 'large'.

It is difficult to clarify the distinction between large and small samples in the context of the *t*-test. You will find that many statistics texts distinguish between small and large samples by relating the test statistic either to the *t*-distribution (for small samples, equal variances in a two-sample comparison) or to the Normal distribution (for large samples, equal or unequal variances). Since the *t*-distribution approaches Normality for large sample sizes, the *P*-value is virtually identical using either approach when the sample size is large. We therefore recommend the simpler practice of:

- Checking the data for Normality, and transforming if necessary to achieve approximate Normality.
- Assuming the test statistic follows the *t*-distribution (an exception is the modified approach discussed in Section 7.4.5).

7.2.3 Study designs

A most important aspect of **design** in this chapter is the *grouping* of the data.

- Very occasionally, we find it necessary to investigate the parameter of interest – in this case, the mean – in a **single group** of observations. We may wish to determine whether the mean assumes a particular value in the population. For example, in an investigation of metabolic profiles (total protein, albumin, calcium, phosphate, lactate dehydrogenase) of cattle kept together in a group, we might sample representative animals to estimate their group mean for each variable, which we could then compare with a known value from a larger population. Alternatively, the comparison might be made with a particular set of published values.

- More commonly, however, we are interested in comparing the means of **two groups** of observations, these groups comprising either *independent* or *paired* observations (see Section 5.8.4).
- Sometimes, we may wish to compare the observations in **more than two groups**. The **analysis of variance** (**ANOVA** – see Section 8.5) or **multiple** (also called **multivariable**) **regression techniques** (see Section 11.3) may be used to analyse such data. The distinction between independent and related observations is retained in the analysis even when there are several groups.

7.3 One-sample *t*-test

7.3.1 Introduction

Occasionally, we may be interested in investigating whether the mean of a single group of observations takes a specific value. For example, the pigs in a particular pen on a farm are showing what appears to be a low daily live weight gain compared with the usual growth rate for this farm. We perform a test to assess whether the mean live weight gain of the pigs in this pen contradicts the hypothesis that they are growing at the expected rate for pigs on this farm.

7.3.2 Assumption

The one-sample *t*-test assumes that the sample data are from a Normally distributed population of values and are representative of that population (ideally being chosen by random selection). As we said earlier (see Section 7.2), the test is hardly affected if the data deviate from Normality except in extreme cases where the data are visibly non-Normal. Then we may be able to Normalize the data by an appropriate transformation (see Section 13.2.1), typically a logarithmic transformation, in which case the test statistic is

calculated using the transformed data values. Naturally, we need to convert the confidence limits obtained by using the transformed data back to the original scale of measurement. Alternatively, we can use an appropriate *nonparametric* test such as the **sign test** (see Section 12.3), the **Kolmogorov–Smirnov test** or the **runs test**. We refer you to Siegel and Castellan (1988) for details.

7.3.3 Approach

We present the approach in general terms and illustrate it using the pig example in Section 7.3.4.

1. Specify the **null hypothesis**, H_0, that the true population mean of the variable of interest is equal to a defined value, μ_0. Generally, the **alternative hypothesis** is that the mean is not equal to the specified value and this leads to a *two-tailed* test.
2. **Collect** the data and **display** them by a line plot, a simple histogram, a stem-and-leaf plot or a box-and-whisker plot. From the diagram, check the *assumption* that the data are approximately Normally distributed.
3. Calculate the **test statistic** as the difference between the sample mean ($\bar{x}$) and the specified value of the population mean under test (μ_0), divided by the estimated standard error of the mean ($s/\sqrt{n}$), where s is the estimated standard deviation and n is the sample size. We denote the test statistic by $Test_1$ to distinguish it from the *t*-distribution which it approximates.

$$Test_1 = \frac{\bar{x} - \mu_0}{s/\sqrt{n}} \quad \text{with } n - 1 \text{ degrees of freedom.}$$

4. Obtain the **P-value** by referring the calculated value of the test statistic (ignoring its sign) to the table of the *t*-distribution (see Table A.3).
5. Use the *P*-value to judge whether the data are inconsistent with the null hypothesis. Then **decide** whether or not to reject the null hypothesis. Commonly, we reject the null hypothesis if $P < 0.05$.
6. Quote the **confidence interval** for the mean because it allows you to judge the importance

of the finding (see Section 6.3.7). The 95% confidence interval is

$$\bar{x} - t_{0.05} \frac{s}{\sqrt{n}} \quad \text{to} \quad \bar{x} + t_{0.05} \frac{s}{\sqrt{n}}$$

where $t_{0.05}$ is the critical value obtained from the table of the *t*-distribution with $n - 1$ degrees of freedom; it gives a total tail area probability of 0.05.

7.3.4 Example

Table 7.1 shows the daily live weight gains of a random sample of 36 growing pigs in a rearing unit. The rearing unit expects a mean daily weight gain of 607 g for this stage of growth (weaning to 10 weeks of age) based on current performance indicators. Are these values consistent with a mean daily gain of around 607 g?

1. H_0 is that μ_0, the true mean daily live weight gain, is 607 g. The alternative hypothesis is that it is not.
2. The stem-and-leaf plot in Figure 7.1 shows that the data are approximately Normally distributed.
3. The sample mean is 599.194 g and the estimated standard deviation is 18.656 g. The test statistic is

$$Test_1 = \frac{\bar{x} - m}{s/\sqrt{n}} = \frac{599.194 - 607}{3.109} = -2.51$$

with 35 degrees of freedom.

4. When we ignore the sign of the test statistic, we can see from Table A.3 that $0.01 < P < 0.02$. If we had used the computer, we would have obtained $P = 0.017$; so we have a less than 2% chance of getting a mean daily live weight gain as low as 599.2 g, or lower, if the null hypothesis is true.

5. The null hypothesis is therefore unlikely to be true. We reject H_0, and conclude that the data values are inconsistent with a daily mean gain in weight of 607 g.
6. The 95% confidence interval for the true mean daily live weight gain is 599.194 ± 2.03(3.109) = (592.88, 605.51) g, where 2.03 is the value in the *t* table (see Table A.3) with 35 degrees of freedom, corresponding to a total tail area probability of 0.05.

We could test this hypothesis using only the confidence interval (see Section 6.6). We can see that the range of values, 592.9–605.5 g, between which we expect the true mean daily weight gain to lie with 95% certainty, does not include the value 607 g. Thus we conclude ($P < 0.05$) that the sample is not drawn from a population with a daily mean weight gain of 607 g.

The test reveals that the pigs have a significantly poorer mean daily weight gain than expected. The confidence interval indicates that

Frequency	Stem and leaf
1	55 . 9
1	56 . 5
4	57 . 0478
5	58 . 14689
6	59 . 145668
9	60 . 001235678
5	61 . 25689
3	62 . 137
2	63 . 16

Stem width: 10.00
Each leaf: 1 case(s)

Figure 7.1   Stem-and-leaf plot of average daily live weight gains (g) of pigs.

Table 7.1   Average daily live weight gains (g) of 36 growing pigs.

577 596 594 612 600 584 618 627 588 601 606 559 615 607 608 591 565 586
621 623 598 602 581 631 570 595 603 605 616 574 578 600 596 619 636 589
Mean, $\bar{x} = 599.194$ g
Standard deviation, $s = 18.656$ g
Standard error, $s/\sqrt{n} = 18.66/\sqrt{36} = 3.109$ g

the true mean weight gain may even be as low as 593 g per day. There may be a cause for concern in the unit; an investigation of the causes, whether infectious or environmental, is indicated.

7.4 Two-sample *t*-test

7.4.1 Introduction

The **two-sample *t*-test** (**unpaired *t*-test**) is one of the most frequently used and, perhaps, misused tests in statistics. You risk misusing the test when you have not properly investigated the assumptions on which it is based. The two-sample *t*-test is employed to compare the means in two *independent* groups of observations using representative samples.

7.4.2 Assumptions

The validity of the two-sample *t*-test depends on various assumptions being satisfied. In particular:

- The two samples must be *independent* (i.e. an animal or individual result is unrelated to any other, either within or between groups). They must also be representative of the population(s) of interest (ideally being chosen by random selection). To avoid allocation bias in an experimental study (see Section 5.6), we should randomly allocate each animal to one of the groups.
- Furthermore, the variable of interest should be approximately *Normally* distributed in each population from which the samples are taken. A small departure from Normality is not crucial and leads to only a marginal loss in power (see Section 6.4.2), i.e. the test is *robust* against violations of this assumption.
- In addition, the variability of the observations in each group, as measured by the two *variances*, should be approximately *equal*, in statistical jargon the samples are **homoscedastic**. This assumption is important; we may verify this casually by eye or, more formally, by Levene's test (see Section 8.4) or an *F*-test (see

Section 8.3). (Be warned, however, that the *F*-test is particularly sensitive to non-Normality of the data, whatever the sample sizes.) If the variances do not differ significantly (and the other assumptions are also valid), then we can proceed to the test described in Section 7.4.3. If, however, the variances in the two groups are not equal (i.e. we have heteroscedasticity) we may apply the modified *t*-test, explained in Section 7.4.5.

If we cannot find an appropriate transformation to satisfy the assumptions, there are alternative non-parametric tests to the two-sample *t*-test, such as the **Wilcoxon rank sum test** or the **Mann–Whitney *U* test** (see Section 12.5).

7.4.3 Approach: equal variances

1. Specify the **null hypothesis** that the two population means are equal. Generally, the **alternative hypothesis** is that these means are not equal (i.e. the difference between them can be in either direction) and this leads to a two-tailed test.
2. **Collect** the data and **display** them in a diagram. If the sample size in each group is relatively small, produce a dot diagram (see Section 2.5.2(a)). If the sample size is large, then it may be easier to show the median, interquartile range and extreme values of the response variable for each group in a box-and-whisker plot (see Section 2.5.2(d)). Either way, by studying the diagram, we can assess the approximate distribution of the observations in each group, and check the Normality assumption. We can also make an appraisal of their variability from the diagram; we check the assumption of equal variance by performing an *F*-test (see Section 8.3) or Levene's test (see Section 8.4). Usually, one of these tests will be included in the computer output.
3. The **test statistic** is the difference in the sample means divided by its estimated standard error. The computer package will perform this calculation but it is useful to have its

derivation. The test statistic, which follows the *t*-distribution, is

$$Test_2 = \frac{\bar{x}_1 - \bar{x}_2}{\sqrt{s^2\left(\dfrac{1}{n_1} + \dfrac{1}{n_2}\right)}}$$

with $n_1 + n_2 - 2$ degrees of freedom

where, for the *i*th sample ($i = 1, 2$):

n_i is the number of observations,
$\bar{x}_i$ is the sample mean,
s_i is the estimated standard deviation, and

$$s^2 = \frac{(n_1 - 1)s_1^2 + (n_2 - 1)s_2^2}{n_1 + n_2 - 2}$$

is the pooled estimate of variance.

Note that the denominator of $Test_2$ is calculated assuming that the true variances in the two groups are approximately equal but unknown; we estimate them from the samples as s_1^2 and s_2^2. Sometimes, we find that the two variances are significantly different when we perform an *F*-test or Levene's test. Then we modify the test statistic (see Section 7.4.4).

4. Usually, we obtain the **P-value** from computer output. If you have calculated the test statistic by hand, you can derive the *P*-value by referring the calculated value (ignoring its sign) of the test statistic to the table of the *t*-distribution (see Table A.3).

5. Use the *P*-value to judge whether the data are inconsistent with the null hypothesis. Then **decide** whether or not to reject the null hypothesis. Commonly, although not necessarily, we reject the null hypothesis if $P < 0.05$.

6. Calculate the relevant **confidence interval** (in this instance, for the difference in the two group means) in order to promote understanding (see Section 6.3.7). If the 95% confidence interval for the difference in two means is not included in the computer output, we can calculate it as

$$(\bar{x}_1 - \bar{x}_2) \pm t_{0.05}SE(\bar{x}_1 - \bar{x}_2)$$
$$= (\bar{x}_1 - \bar{x}_2) \pm t_{0.05}\sqrt{s^2(1/n_1 + 1/n_2)}$$

where $t_{0.05}$ is the critical value obtained from the table of the *t*-distribution with $n_1 + n_2 - 2$ degrees of freedom, and s^2 is the combined estimate of variance (assuming the two variances are equal) used in $Test_2$.

As the *sample size increases*, the critical value in the table of the *t*-distribution (see Table A.3) which corresponds to a given probability approaches that in the table of the Standard Normal distribution (see Table A.1). In particular, the tabulated critical value, $t_{0.05}$, in the *t*-distribution table for a two-tailed probability of 0.05 is close to 1.96 (often approximated by 2) when the degrees of freedom are very large, say, greater than about 100.

7.4.4 Example

Consider the comparison of the mean body weights at the time of mating in one group of ewes which have been flushed (put on a high plane of nutrition for 2–3 weeks prior to mating) and another group which have not.

1. The null hypothesis is that the mean body weights in the populations of flushed and control ewes are equal; the two-sided alternative is that they are different.

2. Each ewe in a random sample of 54 ewes is randomly allocated to the flushed or control group. Table 7.2 shows the weights of two samples of 24 flushed and 30 control ewes. We can see from the box-and-whisker plot in Figure 7.2 that the observations in each sample are approximately Normally distributed since, in each case, the median is more or less centrally situated in the box designated by the 25th and 75th percentiles and between the 2.5 and 97.5 percentile values. Furthermore, the range of observations in each sample appears

Table 7.2 Body weights (kg) in a group of 24 flushed ewes and in a control group of 30 ewes.

Controls			Flushed		
62.5	63.9	69.2	70.7	67.8	69.8
66.8	65.7	62.6	71.8	66.8	68.1
69.5	67.2	61.1	64.9	67.0	66.0
64.1	65.2	61.8	68.2	67.1	69.4
65.3	63.5	69.6	69.4	67.6	69.8
65.6	65.3	71.1	64.4	66.1	67.9
66.4	65.1	67.0	66.9	62.7	66.2
66.1	64.8	67.5	69.4	64.6	64.2
68.6	67.4	68.2			
62.5	66.0	63.6			

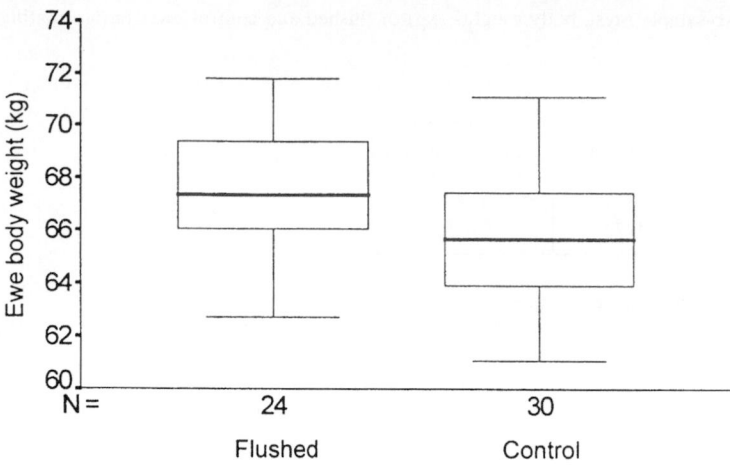

Figure 7.2 Box-and-whisker plot of body weight (kg) in two groups of ewes.

similar, although the median weight of the flushed group is slightly higher than that of the controls. Display 7.1 shows a typical computer output for the results of the two-sample *t*-test. Levene's test (see Section 8.4), a formal hypothesis test for the equality of the two variances, is included and shows that the two variances are not significantly different ($P = 0.62$).

3. The test statistic for the two-sample *t*-test is 2.4 (Display 7.1, equal variances assumed). It is derived as

$$Test_2 = \frac{\text{Difference in means}}{\text{SE (difference in means)}} = \frac{1.5933}{0.655}$$
$$= 2.43 \quad \text{with } 24 + 30 - 2 = 52 \ df$$

where SE (difference in means)

$$= \sqrt{\frac{23(2.52)^2 + 29(2.497)^2}{24 + 30 - 2}\left(\frac{1}{24} + \frac{1}{30}\right)} \ \text{kg}$$

4. The *P*-value shown in Display 7.1 (denoted in SPSS by 'Sig.') is $P = 0.018$, indicating that the chance of obtaining a difference in means at least as large as 1.59 kg is only 1.8% if the null hypothesis is true. Note that if relying on hand calculations, we would refer 2.43 to Table A.3 with 52 degrees of freedom, and find that $0.01 < P < 0.02$.

5. The null hypothesis, that there is no difference in the mean body weights in the two populations, is unlikely to be true. We therefore reject the null hypothesis in favour of the alter-

native hypothesis that there is a difference in the mean body weights. The mean ewe body weights are significantly different, with the estimated mean ewe body weight in the flushed ewes being 1.59 kg greater than that of the control ewes.

6. The 95% confidence interval for the true difference in means is from 0.28 to 2.91 kg. Note that these confidence limits are calculated as $1.59 \pm 2.007 \, (0.655)$ kg, where 2.007 is the value in the table of the *t*-distribution (see Table A.3) corresponding to a two-sided *P* of 0.05 with 52 degrees of freedom. The significantly higher mean body weight of the flushed ewes implies an effect on metabolism and is expected to be associated with an optimal ovulation rate.

The 95% confidence interval for the true difference in means, 0.28 to 2.91 kg, excludes zero. Zero is the value of the parameter specification in the null hypothesis, i.e. H_0 is that the true difference in means is zero. The fact that zero lies outside the 95% confidence limits provides an alternative approach to testing the hypothesis (see Section 6.6), resulting in the decision to reject H_0 at the 5% level of significance.

7.4.5 Modified *t*-test: unequal variances

If the variances in the two groups are *not* equal, then the pooled estimate of variance, s^2, used

Display 7.1 SPSS computer output for the two-sample *t*-test: body weights (kg) of flushed and control ewes before mating (data from Table 7.2).

Group statistics

Group		N	Mean	Std. deviation	Std. error mean
Ewe body weight	Flushed	24	67.3667	2.2525	0.4598
	Control	30	65.7733	2.4972	0.4559

Independent samples test

		Levene's test for equality of variances		*t*-test for equality of means					95% confidence interval of the mean difference	
		F	Sig.	t	df	Sig. (2-tailed)	Mean difference	Std. error difference	Lower	Upper
Ewe body weight	Equal variances assumed	0.253	0.617	2.4	52	0.018	1.5933	0.6551	0.2788	2.9079
	Equal variances not assumed			2.5	51.2	0.017	1.5933	0.6475	0.2935	2.8931

Note: In SPSS, the *P*-value is denoted by 'Sig.' The first line of the *t*-test result (equal variances assumed) is relevant in this instance because the result of Levene's test for the equality of variances indicates that the two variances are not significantly different ($P = 0.617$).

in the denominator of the test statistic, $Test_2$, described in Section 7.4.3, is not appropriate. Some computer packages offer an alternatively derived test statistic in situations where the variances are not equal (see Display 7.1). If you have to resort to hand calculations, you should evaluate a modified test statistic, $Test_3$.

$$Test_3 = \frac{\bar{x}_1 - \bar{x}_2}{\sqrt{\dfrac{s_1{}^2}{n_1} + \dfrac{s_2{}^2}{n_2}}}$$

However, this test statistic does *not* follow the *t*-distribution, so that evaluation of the *P*-value is not straightforward. For large sample sizes (say, greater than 50), $Test_3$ follows an approximately Normal distribution. We can then obtain the relevant *P*-value from the table of the Standard

Normal distribution (see Table A.1). If the sample sizes are not large, we must either transform the data to achieve equal variance or substitute an appropriate *non-parametric* method, such as the **Wilcoxon rank sum test** (see Section 12.5), for the two-sample *t*-test.

7.5 Paired *t*-test

7.5.1 Introduction

We use the **paired *t*-test** when two representative samples from the population comprise *dependent* or *paired* observations. For example, when we compare the preprandial serum glucose levels in dogs with insulin-dependent diabetes mellitus fed low- and high-fibre diets in a randomized cross-over trial (see Section 7.5.4).

The different circumstances for the pairings (see Section 5.8.4) are:

- Self-pairing: each animal is used as its own control.
- Natural pairing: each pair of animals is biologically related (e.g. litter mates).
- Artificial (matched) pairing: each animal is paired with an animal matched with respect to one or more factors that affect response.

To avoid allocation bias (see Section 5.6) in an experiment when there is self-pairing, each animal is randomly allocated to receive one of the two treatments initially; it then receives the other treatment later. If there is natural or matched pairing, one member of the pair is randomly allocated to one of the two treatments and the other member receives the second treatment.

7.5.2 Assumption

The validity of the paired *t*-test is based on the assumption that when we take the *difference* between the observations in each pair, the set of *differences* for all pairs is approximately *Normally* distributed even though the original observations in the groups may not be.

If we suspect that the distribution of the differences is markedly not Normal, and the sample size is adequate, we may take an appropriate transformation of the observations before subtraction to Normalize the distribution of the differences (see Section 13.2.1). We perform the paired *t*-test on the differences of the transformed data.

If we cannot find a suitable transformation to Normalize the data, or if the sample size is small, we should use a *non-parametric test* such as the **Wilcoxon signed rank test** (see Section 12.4).

7.5.3 Approach

1. Specify the **null hypothesis** that the mean of the differences between the paired observations in the population is zero. As there is

likely to be considerably less biological variation exhibited within pairs than between unmatched individuals, it is advantageous to focus the statistical analysis on the differences between the observations within each pair rather than ignoring the matching. Usually, the alternative hypothesis states that this mean difference is not zero, and this leads to a two-tailed test.

Thus, we can see that the hypothesis test is reduced to a *one-sample test of differences* in which the population mean (of differences), μ_0, equals zero. We employ the hypothesis test procedure used in Section 7.3 for the one-sample test on the differences between the pairs. These differences replace the raw data to create a new variable of interest. Consequently, the assumptions on which this test is based relate to the differences and not to the observations in each group.

2. **Collect** and **display** the data. Provided the sample size is manageable, we can display the data in a dot diagram (see Section 2.5.2(a)), similar to that described for the two-sample *t*-test. In addition, we join each pair of points by a line. From the diagram, we are able to discern the average magnitude and direction of the differences. If most of the lines slope in the same direction, either mostly upwards or mostly downwards, then we can surmise that the effect of interest, the mean difference, is unlikely to be zero. If, however, the lines are approximately parallel to the horizontal axis or if they exhibit no consistency in their direction, then it is likely that the mean difference is close to zero. Furthermore, a simple dot plot or, if the sample size is large, a histogram, a stem-and-leaf plot or a box-and-whisker plot of the differences will establish the approximate Normality, or otherwise, of their distribution.

3. When we are using a computer, we have to choose the appropriate test. The **test statistic** is similar in form to that used in the one-sample test. It follows the *t*-distribution, and is given by

$$Test_4 = \frac{\bar{d}}{\text{SE}(\bar{d})} = \frac{\bar{d}}{s_d/\sqrt{n}}$$

with $n-1$ degrees of freedom

where:

n is the number of pairs in the sample,
$\bar{d}$ is the mean of the differences in the sample,
$SE(\bar{d})$ is the estimated standard error of the differences, and
s_d is the estimated standard deviation of the differences.

4. Determine the **P-value** from the computer output. If you have calculated the test statistic by hand, you can ignore the sign of the test statistic and obtain the P-value from the table of the t-distribution (see Table A.3).
5. Use the P-value to judge whether the data are inconsistent with the null hypothesis. Then **decide** whether or not to reject the null hypothesis. Commonly, we reject H_0 if $P < 0.05$.
6. Derive a **confidence interval** for the true mean difference. The 95% confidence interval is given by

$$\bar{d} \pm t_{0.05} SE(\bar{d}) = \bar{d} \pm t_{0.05}\left(s_d / \sqrt{n}\right)$$

where $t_{0.05}$ is the entry in the table of the t-distribution (see Table A.3) with $n - 1$ degrees of freedom, corresponding to a two-tailed probability of 0.05.

7.5.4 Example

Nelson *et al.* (1998) conducted a randomized cross-over trial (see Section 5.9.6) of two diets in 11 insulin-dependent diabetic dogs; they measured serum glucose as the variable indicating the quality of diabetic control. The diets contained either low insoluble fibre (LF) or high insoluble fibre (HF). Each dog was randomly allocated to receive a particular diet first. The dogs were adapted to the diet for 2 months and then fed it for 6 months: evaluation was performed at 6-week intervals. As the study ran over 16 months of each dog's life, we might expect changes in the animal's metabolic responses to diabetes during the course of the trial, irrespective of diet. This would reduce the value of a cross-over design since there might be considerable variability in the within-dog comparisons even without a change in diet. However, as the order in which

Table 7.3 Preprandial serum glucose levels (mmol/l) in dogs with insulin-dependent diabetes mellitus fed a low- and high-fibre diet (based on summary data from Nelson *et al.*, 1998).

Dog	Low-fibre diet (LF)	High-fibre diet (HF)
1	9.44	9.28
2	17.61	8.67
3	8.89	6.28
4	16.94	12.67
5	10.39	6.67
6	11.78	7.28
7	15.06	15.39
8	7.06	5.61
9	19.56	11.94
10	8.22	5.11
11	23.17	17.33

the dogs received the diets was determined randomly, the results should not be biased.

Table 7.3 has been developed from the authors' summary results and gives the mean morning preprandial serum glucose concentrations (mmol/l) for each dog in each 6-month period.

1. The null hypothesis states that the true mean difference in the preprandial serum glucose levels between the low-fibre and high-fibre diets is zero; the two-sided alternative is that it is not zero.
2. We can see from Figure 7.3 that there is a tendency for the lines to slope downwards, indicating that the dogs' serum glucose concentration is lower on the high-fibre diet. For each dog, the difference (LF – HF) in serum glucose is calculated. Figure 7.4 is a dot diagram of these differences; the distribution may be regarded as approximately Normal for this test.
3. Display 7.2 shows a typical computer output for the paired t-test. The value of the test statistic, ignoring its sign, is $Test_4 = 4.37$ (which is the mean difference, 3.808 mmol/l, divided by its standard error, 0.872 mmol/l) which follows the t-distribution with 10 degrees of freedom.
4. The P-value is 0.001 (called 'Sig. (2-tailed)' in Display 7.2). Hence, if the null hypothesis is true, we have only a 0.1% chance of observing a mean difference at least as large as

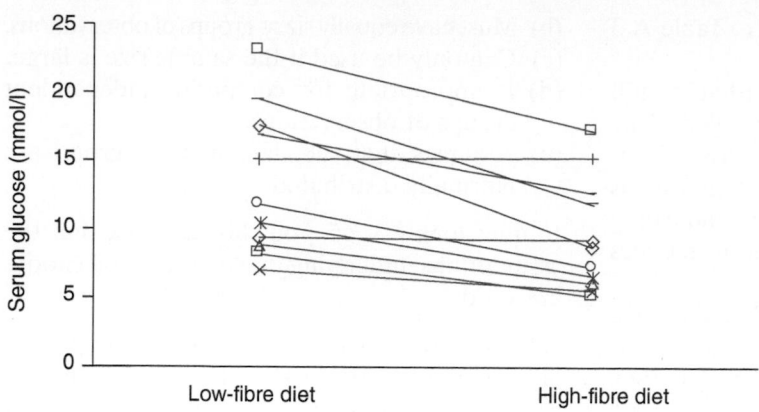

Figure 7.3 Preprandial serum glucose concentration in 11 dogs with insulin-dependent diabetes mellitus on different diets (based on summary data from Nelson *et al.*, 1998).

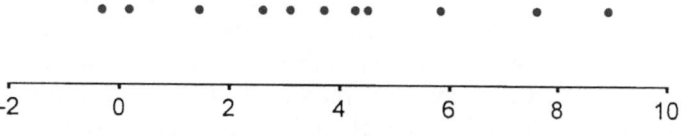

Figure 7.4 Dot diagram of the differences in preprandial fasting serum glucose concentrations (mmol/l) in dogs fed low-fibre (LF) and high-fibre (HF) diets (based on summary data from Nelson *et al.*, 1998).

 Display 7.2   SPSS computer output for the paired *t*-test: preprandial serum glucose (mmol/l) in dogs with insulin-dependent diabetes mellitus fed a low-fibre and a high-fibre diet (data from Table 7.3).

Paired samples statistics

		Mean	N	Std. deviation	Std. error mean
Pair 1	HF	9.657273	11	4.125271	1.243816
	LF	13.465455	11	5.301857	1.598570

Paired samples test

	Paired differences							
				95% confidence interval of the difference				Sig.
	Mean	Std. deviation	Std. error mean	Lower	Upper	*t*	*df*	(2-tailed)
Pair 1 LF – HF	3.808182	2.891563	0.871839	1.865603	5.750760	4.368	10	0.001

3.81 mmol/l. Note, referring 4.37 to Table A.3 gives $0.001 < P < 0.01$.

5. The data are not consistent with the null hypothesis, which we therefore reject. The mean of the preprandial serum glucose differences (LF − HF), estimated as 3.81 mmol/l, is significantly different from zero, indicating that the high-fibre diet significantly reduces fasting blood sugar.

6. We can see from Display 7.2 that the 95% confidence interval for the true mean difference has limits equal to 1.87 and 5.75 mmol/l. Because the sample size is relatively small, this confidence interval is wide. If you are calculating the limits by hand, they are $3.8082 \pm 2.228 \times 0.872$, where 2.228 is the value obtained from the table of the t-distribution (see Table A.3) corresponding to a two-sided P of 0.05 with $11 - 1 = 10$ degrees of freedom, and the standard error of the mean difference is 0.872 mmol/l.

Note that zero, the value against which the mean difference is tested in the specification of the null hypothesis, is less than the lower limit, 1.87 mmol/l, of the 95% confidence interval. This provides an alternative approach to testing H_0 (see Section 6.6) leading to the same conclusion to reject H_0.

Exercises

The statements in questions 7.1 and 7.2 are either TRUE or FALSE.

7.1 The two-sample t-test:
(a) Must have equally sized groups of observations.
(b) Is used on dependent groups of observations.
(c) Tests the null hypothesis that two sample means are equal.
(d) Assumes that the variances are not significantly different in the two groups.
(e) Is preferred to the paired t-test when the sample size is large.

7.2 The paired t-test:
(a) Tests the null hypothesis that the mean of the differences in the population is zero.

(b) Must have equally sized groups of observations.
(c) Can only be used if the sample size is large.
(d) Is appropriate for comparing independent groups of observations.
(e) Assumes that the data in each group are Normally distributed.

In questions 7.3–7.5, you should check that the assumptions underlying the tests that you choose are valid.

7.3 A study was made to compare the plasma lactate concentration in Dutch Warmblood horses cantering at a constant speed either on a track or on an inclined treadmill. The speed was chosen as the horse's own comfortable speed on the track. Samples were taken after 5 minutes' cantering on the track and treadmill, the order of which was randomized for the 10 horses, and we show the plasma lactate concentrations (mmol/l) (developed from data presented by Sloet van Oldruitenborgh-Oosterbaan and Barneveld, 1995, with permission from BMJ Publishing Group Ltd):

Horse	1	2	3	4	5	6	7	8	9	10
Track	2.0	7.7	4.7	4.7	2.9	2.5	5.3	4.8	3.1	3.9
Treadmill	3.5	7.2	4.6	5.7	5.5	4.4	5.6	4.6	3.5	4.9

(a) What design is this?
(b) State the hypothesis you would test to investigate whether the exercise exerted by the horses can be considered to be of similar metabolic demand in both situations.
(c) Conduct a test of this hypothesis.
(d) What conclusion do you draw?

7.4 Observe the sperm numbers obtained either by electroejaculation (EE) or artificial vagina (AV) from 23 adult tom cats. The tom cats were randomly assigned to one of the two methods.

Sperm numbers ($\times 10^6$):

AV	61, 19, 51, 108, 34, 44, 57, 58, 73, 74, 85, 94, 67
EE	41, 11, 76, 23, 39, 34, 45, 49, 55, 66

(a) What design is this?
(b) State the hypothesis you would test to investigate whether the sperm numbers obtained from the two methods are similar.

(c) Conduct a test of this hypothesis.

(d) What conclusion do you draw?

7.5 Plasma urea and creatinine are routinely measured to evaluate renal function and, in healthy cats, the mean urea value in a given pathology laboratory is 7.5 mmol/l. Plasma urea values in a random sample of 140 healthy cats in January were measured to verify the assay. The data were approximately Normally distributed with a mean urea content of 9.7 mmol/l and an estimated standard error of 0.22 mmol/l. Is there any evidence to indicate that the assay performance in this laboratory changed in January?

7.6 Hiraga *et al.* (1997) performed cardiorespiratory tests on 12 Thoroughbred yearling horses before and after an 8-week breaking programme. Paired *t*-tests of a number of variables, comparing the effects before and after the breaking programme, showed that cardiopulmonary function was significantly higher after the breaking period. However, the authors conclude that whether this was due to the exercise during breaking or to physical growth of the horses is unclear. Criticize the experimental design, and provide a design that can separate the possible causes.

7.7 Investigators were interested in comparing the pharmacokinetics (in basic terms, the study of what the body does to the drug) of tripelennamine in horses and camels following intravenous administration of a dose of 0.5 mg/kg body weight. Wasfi *et al.* (2000) found that in the six healthy horses (four cross breeds and two Arabian breeds) and five healthy Arabian camels in their study, the mean (SEM) percentage of protein binding was 73.6% (8.5%) and 83.4% (3.6%) for the horses and camels, respectively. The difference in the mean percentage of protein binding in the two groups of animals was 9.8% (95% confidence interval −12.7% to 32.3%). The authors inferred from these results that their study demonstrated that the mean percentage of protein binding was the same in horses and camels.

Suppose (hypothetically) that other investigators later conducted a similar study on 25 horses and 19 camels; the results of the SPSS statistical analysis of these data are shown in Figure 7.5 and Display 7.3.

(a) What should Wasfi *et al.* have concluded from their results about the difference in the mean percentage of protein binding in horses and camels? Explain your answer fully.

(b) What kind of *t*-test was used on the hypothetical data to compare the mean percentage of protein binding in horses and camels and what is the null hypothesis for this test?

(c) What are the assumptions underlying this test?

(d) Are these assumptions of the test satisfied? Explain your answer fully.

(e) What is the magnitude of the *P*-value for the null hypothesis specified in (b) and what do you conclude about the null hypothesis from this *P*-value?

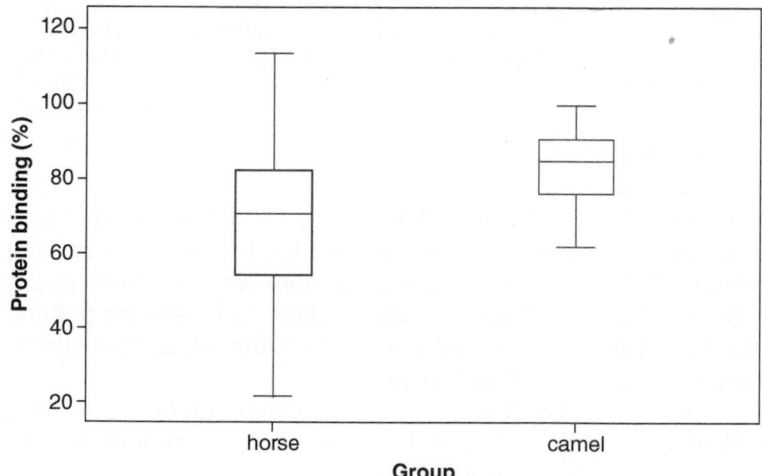

Figure 7.5 Box-and-whisker plot of percentage of protein binding in horses and camels (hypothetical data).

Display 7.3 SPSS computer output for the two-sample *t*-test: protein binding (%) in horses and camels following intravenous administration of tripelannamine.

Group Statistics

	Group	N	Mean	Std. deviation	Std. error mean
Protein binding (%)	horse	25	68.5999	21.88507	4.37701
	camel	19	82.9979	9.93146	2.27843

Independent samples test

		Levene's test for equality of variances		*t*-test for equality of means					95% confidence interval of the difference	
		F	Sig.	t	*df*	Sig. (2-tailed)	Mean difference	Std. error difference	Lower	Upper
Protein binding (%)	Equal variances assumed	7.897	.007	−2.661	42	.011	−14.39806	5.40999	−25.316	−3.480
	Equal variances not assumed			−2.918	35.31	.006	−14.39806	4.93452	−24.413	−4.384

(f) Is this conclusion the same as that which you drew from the results of Wasfi *et al.*? If not, explain why they differ.

(g) Interpret the confidence interval for the difference in the mean percentage of protein binding given in Display 7.3.

7.8 The mercury concentration in secondary and tail feathers of different species of birds in southwest Iran was measured between April and October 2005. The summary measures in the table that follows (based on Zolfaghari *et al.*, 2007) show, for nine tawny owls (*Strix aluco*) and eight eagle owls (*Bubo bubo*), the mean (95% confidence interval) feather mercury (Hg) in mg/kg dry weight of: (i) the secondary feathers; (ii) the tail feathers; and (iii) the differences between the tail and secondary feathers (where each difference is obtained from a single owl of either species).

	Secondary feathers	Tail feathers	Tail − secondary feathers
Tawny owls (*n* = 9)	0.556 (0.535 to 0.577)	0.840 (0.819 to 0.862)	0.284 (0.257 to 0.311)
Eagle owls (*n* = 8)	0.307 (0.263 to 0.352)	0.713 (0.708 to 0.718)	0.406 (0.360 to 0.451)

(a) Name two appropriate statistical hypothesis tests that can be used to assess whether, on average, there is more Hg in the tail feathers than in the secondary feathers in the population of tawny owls from which this sample was selected.

(b) What is/are the assumption(s) underlying each of these tests that you mention in your answer to (a)?

(c) Describe how you can use the relevant confidence interval to assess whether there is significantly more feather Hg in the tail feathers than in the secondary feathers of (i) tawny owls and (ii) eagle owls. Provide a relevant *P*-value for each species of owl and draw appropriate conclusions.

(d) What conclusion do you reach, if any, about whether the mean of the difference between the tail feather Hg and secondary feather Hg is significantly greater in eagle owls than in tawny owls? Explain your reasoning.

(e) Name two statistical tests that are appropriate to use to assess whether, on average, the difference in secondary feather Hg and tail feather Hg is greater in eagle owls than in tawny owls.

8 Hypothesis tests 2 – the *F*-test: comparing two variances or more than two means

8.1 Learning objectives

By the end of this chapter, you should be able to:

- List and verify the assumptions that underlie the *F*-test.
- Explain the principles underlying the *F*-test for equality of variances.
- Elaborate the use of Levene's test.
- Explain the circumstances in which an analysis of variance would be appropriate.
- List and verify the assumptions that underlie the one-way analysis of variance.
- Interpret a computer output of a one-way analysis of variance, and explain the result.

8.2 Introduction

In Chapter 7 we considered hypothesis tests, based on the *t*-distribution, that are used to compare means. For example, in Section 7.4, we performed a two-sample *t*-test to compare the mean body weight of flushed and control ewes. For this test to be valid, we needed to be sure that the two groups had similar variances.

In this chapter we review some tests whose test statistics follow the *F*-distribution (see Section 3.5.4), and which compare variances. These *F*-tests can be used in a wider context, as part of the analysis of variance, to compare two or more means – a not uncommon situation in veterinary and animal science.

Suppose, for example, we have four groups of observations to compare. Spurious *P*-values are likely to result if the difference in means (using a two-sample *t*-test) is investigated for every combination of pairs of groups. Four groups would result in six possible *t*-tests, and the more tests that we perform the more likely it is that we will obtain a significant *P*-value on the basis of chance alone. If we perform 20 tests at the 5% level of significance, it is likely that one will be falsely significant and therefore lead to the erroneous conclusion that the means of these groups differ (see also Section 8.6.3). This is the Type I error discussed in Section 6.4.1. We can use the analysis of variance to address this problem.

As in the last chapter, the tests in this chapter apply to a single numerical variable which is assumed to follow a Normal distribution.

8.3 The *F*-test for the equality of two variances

8.3.1 Rationale

The two-sample *t*-test and the analysis of variance (see Section 8.5) make the assumption of *homoscedasticity*, i.e. of equal variances in groups of data. The **F-test**, often called the **variance ratio test**, may be used to investigate the homoscedasticity of two data sets. **Levene's test** may be used to compare two or more variances (see Section 8.4).

Statistics for Veterinary and Animal Science, Third Edition. Aviva Petrie and Paul Watson.
© 2013 John Wiley & Sons, Ltd. Published 2013 by John Wiley & Sons, Ltd.

Suppose that we select two independent random samples of data from populations 1 and 2, and that we calculate s_1^2 and s_2^2 as estimates of the population variances, σ_1^2 and σ_2^2, respectively. We consider the ratio of these estimated variances and, by convention, we divide the larger by the smaller.

- If we find that the ratio is unity, or close to it, then we would conclude that the two population variances are probably equal.
- If, however, we find that the ratio of these estimated variances is much greater than one, then it is unlikely that the populations, from which we have selected our samples, have equal variances. We have to make a decision whether or not the population variances are likely to be different. This means that we need a cut-off for the variance ratio; if the variance ratio exceeds this cut-off value, we will conclude that the variances are unequal.

We determine this cut-off value formally, under the *null hypothesis* that the two population variances are equal, by referring the ratio to the table of the *F*-distribution (see Table A.5). The *degrees of freedom* are $n_1 - 1$ in the numerator (the larger variance) and $n_2 - 1$ in the denominator (the smaller variance), where n_1 and n_2 represent the two sample sizes.

Note that this is actually a two-tailed test because the alternative hypothesis states that the two variances are not equal, rather than specifying which is the greater. However, the table of the *F*-distribution (see Table A.5) shows tail area probabilities in only the upper tail, when the *F*-ratio is greater than one. For the required significance level in a two-tailed test, therefore, we must halve this tail area. So, for a two-tailed test at the 5% level of significance, we have to relate the test statistic to $P = 0.025$. For convenience, we give the upper percentage points corresponding to $P = 0.025$ and $P = 0.005$ (relating to two-tailed *P*-values of 0.05 and 0.01, respectively) in separate tables, Tables A.5a and A.5b.

8.3.2 Assumptions

This hypothesis test is dependent on the assumptions that the independent samples are selected from Normally distributed populations and are representative of these populations (ideally having been chosen by random selection). It is particularly sensitive to departures from Normality.

8.3.3 Approach

1. Specify the **null hypothesis** that the two population variances, σ_1^2 and σ_2^2, are equal, and specify the alternative hypothesis, usually that the variances are not equal.
2. **Collect** and **examine** the data by constructing a dot plot, a histogram or a box-and-whisker plot (see Section 2.5.2). Check the Normality assumption.
3. Select the appropriate test on the computer, or calculate by hand the **test statistic**. This is the ratio of the larger (s_1^2) to the smaller (s_2^2) estimated population variances derived from the samples. It follows the *F*-distribution and is given by

$$Test_5 = \frac{s_1^2}{s_2^2}$$

with $n_1 - 1, n_2 - 1$ degrees of freedom

The degrees of freedom for the *F*-test are, by convention, written in the order shown above, with the degrees of freedom for the numerator preceding those for the denominator. In this case, they are $n_1 - 1$ in the numerator (the larger variance) and $n_2 - 1$ in the denominator (the smaller variance), where n_1 and n_2 represent the two sample sizes.

4. Determine the **P-value**. You may find this in the computer output or, alternatively, turn to the *F*-table (see Table A.5b). You will see that both Table A.5a and Table A.5b have columns and rows that correspond to the degrees of freedom for the numerator and the denominator, respectively, of the *F*-ratio. The *P*-value for a two-sided *F*-test is obtained by consulting $P/2$ in Table A.5b (see Section 8.3.1), i.e. for a *P*-value of 0.05, consult $P = 0.025$ in Table A.5b.
5. Use the *P*-value to judge whether the data are inconsistent with the null hypothesis. Then **decide** whether or not to reject the null

hypothesis. Commonly, we reject the null hypothesis if $P < 0.05$.

Usually, we perform this test to check the assumption of equality of variance in other tests, such as the two-sample t-test. It is, therefore, unlikely that we will need to consider the confidence interval for the ratio of the two variances. The confidence interval for a variance ratio is based on the F-distribution; you will find details in more advanced texts such as Armitage *et al.* (2002).

8.3.4 Example

We illustrated the two-sample t-test by comparing the mean weights of 54 ewes that were randomly assigned to one of two 'treatment' groups, the ewes being either flushed or not flushed before mating (see Section 7.4.4).

1. One of the assumptions underlying the t-test is that the true variances of these two groups are equal. The null hypothesis for the test which follows is that the variances of the weights in the two populations from which the ewes are selected are equal. The alternative hypothesis is that they are unequal (direction unspecified), leading to a two-tailed test.
2. Figure 7.2 indicates that both samples are approximately Normally distributed.
3. We test the hypothesis of equal variances by finding the ratio of the two estimated variances. Display 7.1 shows that the two estimated standard deviations are 2.252 kg and 2.497 kg for the 24 flushed and 30 control ewes, respectively. The estimated variances are thus 5.072 kg^2 and 6.235 kg^2, so that the ratio of the larger to the smaller estimated variance is $6.235/5.072 = 1.23$.
4. We refer this quotient to the table of the F-distribution (see Table A.5b) with 29 (in the numerator) and 23 (in the denominator) degrees of freedom. There is no column for $29\,df$ or row for $23\,df$. However, we can see that our value (1.23) is less than the tabulated value (2.09) for infinity df in the numerator and $20\,df$ in the denominator for $P/2 = 0.025$.

Thus, $P > 0.05$ (in fact, the exact P-value is $P = 0.62$).
5. There is no evidence of inequality between the variances, and we can proceed with the t-test assuming homoscedasticity.

8.4 Levene's test for the equality of two or more variances

When you use the computer to analyse your data, you may encounter an alternative test of homogeneity of variance, called **Levene's test**. It may be used to *compare two or more variances*, and has the considerable advantage that it is less dependent on the assumption that the data come from Normal populations than most homogeneity of variance tests. It is particularly useful in the context of the analysis of variance. A test statistic is calculated in Levene's test which follows the F-distribution. Since it is most unlikely that you will use this test other than when you are doing a computer analysis, we omit details of the calculation.

Note that Display 7.1, an SPSS computer output for the two-sample t-test, includes Levene's test for the equality of variance. This test gives $P = 0.617$, and it therefore is in agreement with the result we obtained by calculating the ratio of the variances (see Section 8.3.4). Note that, should Levene's test be significant, the SPSS computer output offers a modified t-test allowing a comparison of means even when the two groups have unequal variances.

8.5 Analysis of variance (ANOVA) for the equality of means

8.5.1 Rationale

The analysis of variance (ANOVA) is an expression used to describe a set of techniques that compare the *means* of two, three or more groups by investigating relevant variances. The analysis is based on the variance ratio test, i.e. an F-test, which compares two variances by examining their ratio and relating it to the F-distribution (see Section 8.3).

The principle underlying the analysis of variance is that the total variability in a data set is partitioned into its component parts. Each component represents a different source of variation. The variation is expressed by its variance. The sources of variation comprise one or more **factors**, each resulting in variability which can be accounted for or *explained* by the **levels** or categories of that factor (e.g. the two levels, 'male' and 'female', defining the factor 'sex', or three dose levels for a given drug factor), and also *unexplained* or *residual* variation which results from uncontrolled biological variation and technical error. We can assess the contribution of the different factors to the total variation by making the appropriate comparisons of these variances.

Consider the simple case in which there is only one factor of interest, the levels of this factor defining different groups to which, in the experimental situation, individuals are assigned at random (this leads to a one-way ANOVA – see Section 8.6). We want to know if all the observations come from a single population. If this is the case, the levels of the factor do not affect the variation (i.e. the variation between the group means would be the same as that of the observations within the groups), and we would not expect the group means to differ. We therefore investigate the null hypothesis that all the group means are equal in the population. If there appears to be significantly more variation between the groups than would be expected under the null hypothesis, we reject the null hypothesis in favour of the alternative hypothesis, and conclude that the group means are different. Thus, despite its name, the analysis of variance is a device for comparing two or more means. Note that the alternative hypothesis is that there is *more* variation between the group means than within the groups – i.e. it is a one-tailed test, so we look up the *P*-values directly in Table A.5a (because we are comparing variances using an *F*-test), without any adjustment.

8.5.2 The ANOVA table

Although the basic concepts of the analysis of variance can be expressed in relatively simple terms, the mathematical details are cumbersome and best avoided. We refer you to books such as Cochran and Cox (1957), Doncaster and Davey (1997) and Gardiner and Gettinby (1998) for the underlying theory. It is more relevant, in this day and age, that you understand the computer output resulting from the analysis of variance. This comprises an **analysis of variance table** which lists the various sources of variation, for example see Display 8.1. For each source of variation, you will find values for the **sum of squares** and the **degrees of freedom** (see Section 6.3.6); the sum of squares divided by the degrees of freedom determines the **mean square**, which provides an estimate of the relevant variance. Finally, the appropriate mean squares are compared using an *F*-test (see Section 8.3). For each factor (source of explained variation), the null hypothesis states that the population means of the groups defined by the levels of that factor are equal.

8.5.3 Particular forms of ANOVA

The considerations of ANOVA that underlie the experimental design and subsequent handling of the data can be exceedingly complicated. In this section, we outline some of the common designs to give you an indication of the potential of ANOVA. You can skip this section without loss of continuity if you find it difficult.

The analysis of variance encompasses a broad spectrum of experimental designs ranging from the simple to the complex. In each case, the appropriate mathematical model is constructed, based on the structure or pattern of the experimental design. This model takes the form of a regression equation (see Chapters 10 and 11) so that it is possible to analyse the data using regression techniques directly (see Section 11.3.1(b)) rather than relying on the ANOVA software provided by many computer packages. Furthermore, the ANOVA model assumptions may be checked by studying the residuals, as in multiple regression analysis (see Section 11.3.2(a)). The essential forms of some simple designs are illustrated in Figure 8.1.

- We may regard the **one-way ANOVA** (the simplest form of ANOVA) as an extension of the *two-sample t-test* when we compare the means of more than two groups (see Section 8.6). They give identical *P*-values when there are two groups.

  For example, in order to determine whether the build-up of calculus on dogs' teeth is affected by diet, Stookey *et al.*

One-way ANOVA

Diet group		
Control	Diet 1	Diet 2
x	x	x
x	x	x
x	x	x
x	x	x
x	x	x
x		x
x		
x		

One-way repeated measures ANOVA

	Treatment groups		
Beagles	Control	Dose 1	Dose 2
1	x	x	x
2	x	x	x
3	x	x	x
.	.	.	.
.	.	.	.
.	.	.	.
k	x	x	x

Two-way ANOVA

	Daily feeding schedule		
	1 portion	2 portions	3 portions
Feed 1	x x x x x x x	x x x x x x x	x x x x x x x
Feed 2	x x x x x x x	x x x x x x x	x x x x x x x

Figure 8.1 Diagrams of the most common forms of experimental designs analysed by ANOVA.

(1995) randomly allocated 26 dogs to one of three diets. One-way ANOVA was used to test the null hypothesis that the mean calculus accumulation was equal in the three diet groups after 4 weeks on the diet. We give full details in Section 8.6.4.

- The **one-way repeated measures ANOVA** may be regarded as an extension of the *paired t-test*, for example when the data are longitudinal and are measured on each individual at successive time points, or when the within-subject/ animal comparison is between three or more treatments. We say that we have repeated measures of a particular factor if each individual has measurements at every level of that factor. We describe a simple approach to analysing repeated measures data (as an alternative to ANOVA) in Section 14.5.2.

As an example of this ANOVA approach, Burton *et al.* (1997) compared the effects of three treatments (control, and two dose levels of a sedative drug, medetomidine) on the insulin concentrations of healthy adult Beagles in a trial in which each dog received all three treatments. Each dog was used as its own control in a randomly allocated sequence of treatments. The ANOVA showed that the mean serum insulin values in the three treatment groups were significantly different when measured 60 minutes after administration of treatment (further investigation indicated that both of the doses of medetomidine significantly decreased the serum insulin when compared with the control).

- The **two-way ANOVA** examines the effect of two factors on a response variable, when each of these factors pos-

sesses two or more levels. We create a two-way table in which the rows and the columns represent the levels of each of the two factors; every cell in the table represents a unique combination of particular levels of the two factors. Each individual is randomly assigned to one of the different levels of each factor. Providing there is no replication in any cell of the table, the design is often called a **randomized block**. If there is replication in the cells, then it is possible to study the **interaction** between the factors (see Section 5.9.1); this is when the differences in the levels of one factor are not consistent for the various levels of the other factor.

Suppose, for example, two different feed formulations for optimal growth promotion of kittens are to be compared, with the daily ration administered in one, two or three divided portions. This gives six unique treatment combinations; 42 animals are randomly allocated to one of these feeding regimens with seven animals (replications) in each cell of the table, and their weight gain (growth) is monitored over a 3-month period. The ANOVA would allow us to investigate whether there is any difference in the mean weight gain between the two different feeds, and between the number of daily portions. An interaction between the factors would imply that the difference observed in the mean weight gain between the feed formulations is not consistent for each of the three forms of administration of the feed (one, two or three daily portions).

- More complex experimental designs may involve hierarchical (nested) or cross-classifications of a number of factors (each at various levels), perhaps with repeated measures. These include the *Latin square*, *split plot* and the more general *factorial designs* which reflect the flexibility of ANOVA. Details of each design are to be found in books such as Cochran and Cox (1957), Doncaster and Davey (1997) and Gardiner and Gettinby (1998).

In Section 8.6 we use the one-way ANOVA to illustrate the general approach; the principles underlying more complicated ANOVA are similar. □

8.6 One-way analysis of variance

8.6.1 Assumptions

We apply the analysis of variance when the variable of interest is numerical; the results are reliable only if the assumptions on which it is based are satisfied. The one-way ANOVA is concerned with several levels or categories of a single factor, where each level comprises a group of observations. For example, the levels may represent different treatments as in a comparison of, say, a dry feed formula, a formulated tinned feed and a raw meat diet for dogs. Alternatively, they can be different treatment dose levels of a drug, one of which is a placebo representing simply the drug vehicle, while the others are, say, 50%, 100% and 200% of the presumed effective dose. In the experimental situation, the animals should be randomly allocated to one of the levels of the factor, i.e. to one of the groups, in order to avoid allocation bias (see Section 5.6).

The assumptions of the one-way ANOVA are that the samples representing the levels are *independent* and the observations in each sample come from a *Normally distributed* population with variance σ^2; this implies that the group variances are the same. Approximate Normality may be established by drawing a histogram; moderate departures from Normality have little effect on the result. Constant variance, the more important assumption, may be established by Levene's test (see Section 8.4).

If we are concerned about the assumptions, we can take an appropriate transformation of the data (see Section 13.2) or use an alternative non-parametric method such as the **Kruskal–Wallis one-way ANOVA** (see Section 12.6.2). As a point

of interest, we can use the **Friedman two-way ANOVA** as a non-parametric alternative to the two-way ANOVA (see Section 12.6.3).

8.6.2 Approach

1. Specify the **null hypothesis** that the population group means do not differ, i.e. the groups represent a single population. Generally, the alternative hypothesis is that at least one of the group means is dissimilar.
2. **Collect** the data and **display** them in exactly the same way as for the two-sample *t*-test (see Section 7.4) except that here there are more than two groups. Check the assumptions of Normality and homogeneity of variance.
3. Use the computer to calculate the **test statistic**, which is found in the ANOVA table. It is the ratio of the between-groups to the within-groups mean squares (*F*-ratio). This *F*-ratio follows the *F*-distribution with $k - 1$, $n - k$ degrees of freedom, where k = number of groups and n = total number of observations in the sample.
4. Look at the **P-value**; it is usually given in the ANOVA table of the computer output. If you want to determine it for yourself, you have to refer to the table of the *F*-distribution (see Table A.5a). You can read the appropriate degrees of freedom that you need for Table A.5a from the ANOVA table: use $k - 1$ for the numerator (the between-groups degrees of freedom); use $n - k$ for the denominator (the within-groups (residual) degrees of freedom).
5. Use the *P*-value to judge whether the data are inconsistent with the null hypothesis. Then **decide** whether or not to reject the null hypothesis; usually, but not necessarily, we reject H_0 if $P < 0.05$. If we reject the null hypothesis, we may need to establish which group means differ (see Section 8.6.3).
6. Derive the **confidence intervals** for differences between group means, in essentially the same way as for the two-sample *t*-test (see Section 7.4.3). However, the combined estimate of variance used in the calculation of the confidence interval is the within-group (residual) mean square in the ANOVA table.

8.6.3 Multiple comparisons

If we reject the null hypothesis in the one-way ANOVA (see Section 8.6.2), then we need to establish which group means differ. This will involve conducting a number of tests, but the more tests that we perform, the more likely it is that we will obtain a significant *P*-value on the basis of chance alone. We have to approach this problem of **multiple comparisons** in such a way that we avoid spurious *P*-values. Formal multiple comparison techniques should be used, such as **Duncan's multiple range test**, **Least significant difference (LSD) test**, **Bonferroni's correction**, and **Scheffe's, Tukey's** or **Newman–Keuls tests**, often termed procedures. Be aware: they often produce slightly different results!

The Bonferroni approach is relatively simple, even without the aid of a computer; we concentrate on comparing those groups that are of particular interest, and then employ Bonferroni's correction. The procedure involves modifying the *P*-value obtained from any one comparison by multiplying it by the number of tests or comparisons that are to be performed. So, if we plan to undertake three *t*-tests, we should multiply the *P*-value (p_1, say) obtained from a single *t*-test by 3 to produce an amended *P*-value of $3p_1$ which we can assess for significance in relation to our pre-specified significance level, typically 0.05. If we intend to use the two-sample *t*-test to make pairwise comparisons after performing a one-way ANOVA, we should modify the denominator of the test statistic by using the pooled estimate of variance from all the groups, i.e. the residual mean square (variance) in the ANOVA table, and we should use this, too, in any calculations of confidence intervals. This Bonferroni approach works reasonably well if the number of comparisons is less than about five, but for more comparisons it is too conservative.

You may be tempted to rely solely on these multiple comparison methods, but it is sensible to start your analysis with the ANOVA when there are three or more levels of any one factor and/or when more than two factors are to be investigated. The ANOVA may act as a buffer, precluding 'fishing' expeditions to discover treatment differences. It therefore precedes, and perhaps even obviates the need for, pairwise comparisons of groups. *You only proceed to investigate differences between pairs of means if the P-value for that factor in the ANOVA is significant.*

You should be aware that this problem of multiple testing also arises in other circumstances, not just in relation to the comparisons in this simple ANOVA design. Examples are when we have multiple outcome measurements, and when we subdivide our sample into subsets and investigate differences in these subgroups. Another particular example arises when we have repeated measurements on the same individual; you will find more information to deal with this situation in Sections 11.6 and 14.5.2. In all such cases, you should attempt to avoid spurious *P*-values. This may not be a simple process and we recommend that you seek the advice of a statistician.

Furthermore, remember never to compare P-values as a way of judging the magnitude of different effects. Instead, obtain quantitative measures of the effects of interest (e.g. the differences in the treatment means) and use these for comparative purposes. It is incorrect to compare the *P*-values as they are dependent on considerations such as the sample size, the power of the test and the variability of the observations.

8.6.4 Example

Dogs were fed a dry diet coated with different agents that were believed to affect the build-up of calculus on the teeth. Calculus accumulation was measured by an index that combined estimates of both the proportion of the teeth covered by the deposit and the thickness of the deposit. Twenty-six dogs were randomly allocated to three treatments: control, soluble pyrophosphate (P_2O_7) and sodium hexametaphosphate (HMP). The calculus accumulation index was measured on each dog 4 weeks after it received treatment. The data are presented in Table 8.1; they are developed from the summary results presented by Stookey *et al.* (1995). Display 8.1 contains the ANOVA results from an SPSS computer analysis.

	Dog	Control	Dog	P_2O_7	Dog	HMP
	1	0.49	10	0.34	19	0.34
	2	1.05	11	0.76	20	0.05
	3	0.79	12	0.45	21	0.53
	4	1.35	13	0.69	22	0.19
	5	0.55	14	0.87	23	0.28
	6	1.36	15	0.94	24	0.45
	7	1.55	16	0.22	25	0.71
	8	1.66	17	1.07	26	0.95
	9	1.00	18	1.38		
Sample size	9		9		8	
Mean	1.09		0.75		0.44	
SD	0.42		0.37		0.29	
SEM	0.14		0.12		0.10	
95% CI*	(0.81, 1.37)		(0.46, 1.03)		(0.13, 0.74)	

Table 8.1 Index of calculus formation on the teeth of dogs fed a control diet or one supplemented with soluble pyrophosphate (P_2O_7) or sodium hexametaphosphate (HMP) (based on summary data from Stookey *et al.*, 1995).

*These are the 95% confidence intervals for each mean (calculated using the residual mean square = 0.1353 from the ANOVA table as the combined estimate of variance).

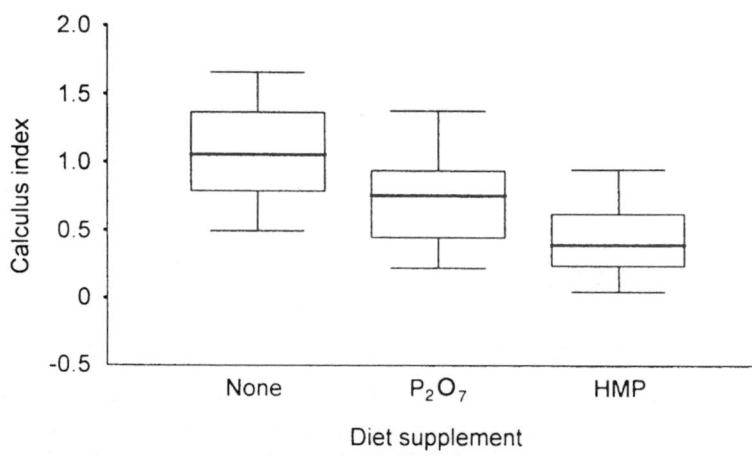

Figure 8.2 Box-and-whisker plot of the calculus index of teeth in three groups of dogs (based on summary data from Stookey *et al.*, 1995).

1. The null hypothesis is that the true mean calculus indices in the three treatment groups are equal; the alternative hypothesis is that they are not all equal.
2. We can see from Figure 8.2 that the data are approximately Normally distributed in each group; Levene's test (Display 8.1) indicates that the variances of the observations in the three groups are not significantly different ($P = 0.44$).
3. The *F*-ratio in the ANOVA table (Display 8.1) produces $P = 0.005$.
4. It is therefore unlikely that all the three means are equal and we reject the null hypothesis.
5. The means and their associated confidence intervals are shown in the descriptives table in Display 8.1. Further examination by *post hoc* Bonferroni tests (see the multiple comparisons table in Display 8.1) indicates that the mean calculus index is significantly greater

Display 8.1 SPSS computer output for analysis of variance of calculus data on three groups of dogs (data from Table 8.1).

Descriptives

		N	Mean calculus	Std. deviation	Std. error	95% confidence interval for mean	
						Lower bound	Upper bound
Treat group	None	9	1.0889	0.4225	0.1408	0.7641	1.4137
	P₂O₇	9	0.7467	0.3695	0.1232	0.4626	1.0307
	HMP	8	0.4375	0.2907	0.1028	0.1945	0.6805
	Total	26	0.7700	0.4435	8.697E-02	0.5909	0.9491

Note: E-02 means $\times 10^{-2}$.

Test of homogeneity of variances

	Levene statistic	df1	df2	Sig.
Calculus	0.855	2	23	0.438

ANOVA

		Sum of squares	df	Mean square	F	Sig.
Calculus	Between groups	1.805	2	0.902	6.668	0.005
	Within groups	3.112	23	0.135		
	Total	4.917	25			

Multiple comparisons

Dependent variable: Calculus
Bonferroni

(I) group	(J) group	Mean difference (I – J)	Std. error	Sig.	95% confidence interval	
					Lower bound	Upper bound
None	P₂O₇	0.3422	0.173	0.182	−0.1055	0.7899
	HMP	0.6514*	0.179	0.004	0.1899	1.1129
P₂O₇	None	−0.3422	0.173	0.182	−0.7899	0.1055
	HMP	0.3092	0.179	0.291	−0.1523	0.7707
HMP	None	−0.6514*	0.179	0.004	−1.1129	−0.1899
	P₂O₇	−0.3092	0.179	0.291	−0.7707	0.1523

*The mean difference is significant at the 0.05 level.

($P = 0.004$) in the control group of dogs (mean index = 1.09; 95% CI 0.76 to 1.41) than in the group of dogs receiving HMP (mean index = 0.44; 95% CI 0.19 to 0.68). We estimate the difference between these means as 0.65; the 95% confidence interval for the true difference in means is 0.19 to 1.11. The two other comparisons of means are not significant ($P > 0.05$); the relevant differences between these means and their associated confidence intervals are given in Display 8.1.

Exercises

The statements in questions 8.1 and 8.2 are either TRUE or FALSE.

8.1 In a one-way analysis of variance to compare the means of four groups of observations:
(a) The observations in each group should be Normally distributed.
(b) There should be the same number of observations in each group.
(c) The group variances should be equal.
(d) The groups should comprise matched individuals or the same individuals in different circumstances.
(e) The null hypothesis states that the sample means are all the same.

8.2 The *F*-test used on two groups of observations:
(a) Assumes that the means of the two groups are the same.
(b) Assumes that the data in each group are Normally distributed.
(c) Tests the null hypothesis that the two population variances are equal.
(d) Can be used instead of the paired *t*-test to investigate the mean difference.
(e) Should always be followed by a two-sample *t*-test.

In questions 8.3 and 8.4, you should check that the assumptions underlying the test that you choose are valid.

8.3 The following data show the liver weights (kg) taken from randomly selected cattle in two farms in southwest England during outbreaks of

liver fluke disease. As a preliminary to testing the null hypothesis that the mean liver weights of the cattle in the two farms are the same, check that the variability of the observations in the two groups is similar.

Group 1:	18.0, 18.5, 18.9, 18.2, 17.9, 15.9, 16.8, 18.2, 17.3, 17.5, 17.7, 17.8, 17.1, 17.0, 16.3
Group 2:	14.3, 13.2, 17.3, 14.9, 16.4, 16.0, 18.6, 17.3, 15.5, 16.8, 15.7, 18.0, 15.2

8.4 Look at the measurements of the mean fluorescence intensity of sperm cells stained with a fluorescent marker, 1-anilinonaphthalene-8-sulphonate (ANS), showing the effect of the presence of egg yolk in the diluent solution (Table 8.2). ANS fluoresces only when bound to the sperm membrane. Each value represents the mean of 10 individual spermatozoa and is estimated by a densitometer from photographic film.

What evidence is there that the egg yolk affects the binding of the fluorophore to the sperm membrane? If you have the appropriate computer software, analyse the data yourself and see if you get the same ANOVA table as shown (Display 8.2). If you do not have the software, you can use the ANOVA table to help you answer this question.

8.5 The pharmacokinetic behaviour of two antiparasitic drugs, doramectin and moxidectin, were compared after a single subcutaneous administration in goats at a dosage of 0.2 mg/kg,

Table 8.2 The effect of egg yolk in the medium on the fluorescence intensity of spermatozoa labelled with a fluorescent probe. Data are in arbitrary densitometry units (based on Watson, 1979).

Egg yolk content		
1%	5%	25%
0.944	0.865	0.811
1.048	1.000	0.862
1.026	1.001	0.910
1.007	0.900	0.799
0.933	0.923	0.837
0.998	0.876	0.854
1.035	1.046	
	0.990	

Display 8.2   ANOVA table of data in Table 8.2.

		Sum of squares	*df*	Mean square	*F*	Sig.
Fluoresc	Between groups	7.832E-02	2	3.916E-02	13.659	0.000*
	Within groups	5.160E-02	18	2.867E-03		
	Total	0.130	20			

Note: E-02 means $\times 10^{-2}$, E-03 means $\times 10^{-3}$.
*Implies $P < 0.0005$, therefore we can say $P < 0.001$.

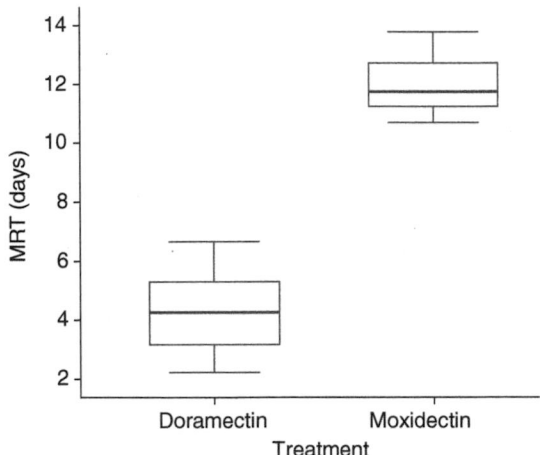

Figure 8.3 Box-and-whisker plot of mean residence times (MRT) of drugs in two groups of goats (see Exercise 8.5).

Display 8.3   SPPS output of summary statistics and test results for mean residence times (MRT) of drugs in two groups of goats (see Exercise 8.5).

Group statistics

	Treatment	*N*	Mean	Std. deviation	Std. error mean
MRT	Doramectin	20	4.2220	1.26674	0.28325
	Moxidectin	20	11.9873	0.91536	0.20468

Independent samples test

		Levene's test for equality of variances		*t*-test for equality of means						95% confidence interval of the mean difference	
		F	Sig.	*t*	*df*	Sig. (2-tailed)	Mean difference	Std. error difference		Lower	Upper
MRT	Equal variances assumed	3.016	0.091	−22.221	38	0.000*	−7.76529	0.34947		−8.47275	−7.05784
	Equal variances not assumed			−22.221	34.591	0.000*	−7.76529	0.34947		−8.47504	−7.05554

*Indicates $P < 0.001$.

with 20 goats being randomly assigned to each of the two drug regimens (based on summary data of Escudero *et al.*, 1999). The drug plasma concentration–time data were analysed by compartmental pharmacokinetics and non-compartmental methods. We are interested in comparing the mean residence times (MRT in days) in the two groups of goats. Some SPSS computer output, produced by a statistical analysis of our data, is shown in Figure 8.3 and Display 8.3.

(a) What aspects of the distribution of the data does the box-and-whisker plot show?

(b) What is the full name of the statistical test that the investigators have used to compare MRT in the two groups?

(c) What is the null hypothesis of this test?

(d) What are the assumptions underlying this test?

(e) Are the assumptions satisfied (explain your reasoning using both the diagram and the second table of results, as appropriate)?

(f) Explain where you find the *P*-value from the test comparing the average MRT in the two groups. What is this *P*-value, and what do you conclude as a consequence?

(g) What is the estimated effect of interest and what is its associated confidence interval?

9 Hypothesis tests 3 – the Chi-squared test: comparing proportions

9.1 Learning objectives

By the end of this chapter, you should be able to:

- Explain how to test a hypothesis about a single proportion.
- Outline the steps involved in comparing two proportions.
- Construct a 2×2 contingency table of observed frequencies.
- Explain the meaning of 'expected frequency' in a contingency table.
- Use the Chi-squared test to analyse data in a 2×2 contingency table.
- Analyse frequencies in an $r \times c$ contingency table.
- Describe the situations in which the Chi-squared test is not appropriate in the analysis of a contingency table.
- Describe the situation in which McNemar's test is appropriate.
- Compare two proportions using McNemar's test.
- Perform a Chi-squared goodness-of-fit test.

9.2 Introduction

In Chapters 7 and 8 we discussed hypothesis tests for the *arithmetic mean*, a summary measure of location for a numerical variable. In this chapter we describe some of the hypothesis tests for the **proportion**, a parameter that summarizes the observations of a binary variable. In addition, we explain how to analyse data when the categorical variable has more than two categories.

You will recall that a **binary variable** is a categorical (qualitative) variable with only two categories of response, often termed *success* and *failure* (see Sections 1.6 and 3.4.2). For example, Little *et al.* (1980) investigated the influence of *Leptospira* infection on the incidence of abortion in cattle. The test which they used for the presence of leptospiral antibodies gives a binary response, either positive (success) or negative (failure). They compared the proportions of cows that were positive for *Leptospira* infection in two groups, those which aborted and those which calved normally.

In Section 7.2.3 we explained that when we test hypotheses about means, we improve our comparisons and measure our treatment effects more precisely if we give due consideration to the design of the study. Do we have a single group of observations, or do we have two or more groups of observations? Do these groups comprise independent or paired values? We should also be asking these questions when we test hypotheses about proportions.

9.3 Testing a hypothesis about a single proportion

9.3.1 Approach

In Section Section 4.6 we defined the properties of the sampling distribution of a proportion.

Statistics for Veterinary and Animal Science, Third Edition. Aviva Petrie and Paul Watson.
© 2013 John Wiley & Sons, Ltd. Published 2013 by John Wiley & Sons, Ltd.

We know that its distribution is approximately Normal if the sample size, n, is large; that the sample proportion, p, is an unbiased estimate of the population proportion, π; and that the standard error of the proportion is estimated in the sample by $\sqrt{p(1-p)/n}$. We use this information to test a hypothesis about the proportion of successes in a single population using the following approach:

1. Specify the **null hypothesis** that the proportion of successes in the population is equal to a specified value, π_1. Specify the alternative hypothesis – generally, that the population proportion is not equal to π_1.
2. **Collect** the sample data and classify each individual as a success or a failure.
3. Calculate the **test statistic**, which approximates the Normal distribution. It is

$$Test_6 = \frac{|p - \pi_1| - \frac{1}{2n}}{\sqrt{\frac{\pi_1(1-\pi_1)}{n}}}$$

where p is the observed proportion of successes and n is the number of individuals in the sample. The vertical lines to either side of the difference in proportions indicate that we ignore the sign of the difference. We subtract $1/(2n)$, called a **continuity correction**, from this difference to make an allowance for the fact that we are using the continuous Normal distribution to approximate the discrete Binomial distribution. The effect of the continuity correction is negligible when the sample size is large.

4. Determine the **P-value** by referring the calculated value of the test statistic, ignoring its sign, to the table of the Standard Normal distribution, Table A.1.
5. Make a **decision** whether or not to reject the null hypothesis according to the P-value. You may have decided that you would reject the null hypothesis if $P < 0.05$.
6. Calculate the **confidence interval** for the proportion of successes. The 95% confidence interval for π is given by $p \pm 1.96\sqrt{p(1-p)/n}$ (see Section 4.7).

9.3.2 Example

Suppose we are investigating the sex ratio in wild rabbits. In the present season, we notice that the sex ratio of live births is distorted in favour of females. Our records show that in a random sample of 297 live births, 167 were female. Is this a chance deviation or do we have evidence of some factor (e.g. a genetic mutation which predisposes to higher embryonic mortality in males) affecting the sex ratio?

1. The null hypothesis is that the proportions of female and male live births in this wild rabbit population are identical and equal to 0.5. The alternative hypothesis is that they are unequal.
2. The proportion of females in the random sample of 297 live births is $167/297 = 0.562$.
3. The test statistic is:

$$Test_6 = \frac{|0.562 - 0.5| - 1/(594)}{\sqrt{0.5(1-0.5)/(297)}} = 2.08$$

4. Referring to Table A.1, we find $P = 0.0375$ (corrected to two decimal places, $P = 0.04$).
5. There is evidence to reject the null hypothesis at the 5% level of significance.
6. The 95% confidence interval for the true proportion of female live births is $0.562 \pm 1.96\sqrt{0.562(1-0.562)/(297)} = 0.51$ to 0.62.

Although $P = 0.04$ leads us to reject the null hypothesis, the lower limit of the confidence interval only just exceeds 0.5, an equal proportion of males and females. We should be cautious in putting too much emphasis on the conclusion that some factor is affecting the sex ratio. This is an example where the confidence interval leads us to be more circumspect about the significance test's implications.

9.4 Comparing two proportions: independent groups

9.4.1 Introduction

Hawkins *et al.* (1993) investigated the effect of neonatal castration on the prevalence of diabetes in mice. Mice were randomly allocated to receive either active (castration) or control (sham operation) treatment. The investigators were interested in comparing, after a given time period, the proportions of diabetic animals ('successes') in these two independent groups of observations.

In an analysis of this sort, we regard these groups as samples from two populations, and use the sample proportions, p_1 and p_2, to estimate the population proportions, π_1 and π_2. We can test the hypothesis that the population proportions are the same in one of two ways.

- We can use the Chi-squared test, described in Section 9.4.3, which is based on the Chi-squared distribution (see Section 3.5.4).
- The other way of proceeding is to use the Normal approximation to the Binomial distribution (see Section 3.6.1), and derive a test statistic that approximates a Normal distribution.

As you will probably be using the computer to compare the two proportions, we do not feel that it is necessary to give details of both approaches. We expand on the Chi-squared test because it can be extended to compare more than two proportions (see Section 9.5) and other investigations of categorical data. In fact, the two tests produce identical P-values; the square of the test statistic approximating the Normal distribution is equal to the test statistic used in the Chi-squared test.

9.4.2 The 2 × 2 contingency table (the fourfold table)

We can summarize the results of the example introduced in Section 9.4.1 by presenting the *frequencies* in what is called a two-way **frequency** or **contingency table**. If each row (say) designates an outcome (success or failure), and each column (say) designates one of the two groups, then each of the four cells of the table contains the number or frequency of animals in a particular group that have the stated outcome. This type of contingency table is often called a **fourfold** or **two-by-two** (2 × 2) contingency table because it has two rows and two columns. The $r \times c$ contingency table has r rows and c columns. We show the general form of a 2 × 2 contingency table in Table 9.1a (a numerical example is shown later in Table 9.2).

9.4.3 Comparing two proportions in a 2 × 2 table using the Chi-squared test

(a) Rationale

If there is no association between the outcome and the group, then we would expect the proportions of successes to be the same in the two groups. Thus, we can compare the two proportions by investigating the association between the two factors that define the contingency table (Table 9.1a). A **factor**, in this context, is a variable with two or more mutually exclusive categories into which individuals can be classified. Our null hypothesis is that there is no association between the two factors (outcome, group), equivalent to the null hypothesis that the two population proportions are equal.

In order to calculate the test statistic using this approach, we have to compare the frequency we *observe* in each cell of the contingency table with the frequency we would *expect* in that cell *if the null hypothesis were true*. The null hypothesis is that the proportions of successes in the two populations are equal. If the null hypothesis is true, we would expect the overall proportion of successes, $(a + b)/n$, to apply to each of groups 1 and 2. The expected successes under the null hypothesis are $(a + c) \times (a + b)/n$ in group 1 and $(b + d) \times (a + b)/n$ in group 2. The remaining numbers in each group are expected failures. Thus, we can build a table so that in each cell of the table there is an expected frequency corresponding to each observed frequency (see Table 9.1b).

If we find that the discrepancy between the observed and expected frequencies is large, we reject the null hypothesis. We decide whether the discrepancy is large by calculating the appropriate test statistic which approximates the Chi-squared distribution (see Section 3.5.4(b)); we refer the test statistic to Table A.4 to determine the P-value.

(a) Observed frequencies.

Table 9.1 The 2×2 table of frequencies.

Outcome	Group 1	Group 2	Row marginal total
Success	a	b	$a + b$
Failure	c	d	$c + d$

			Overall total
Column marginal total	$n_1 = a + c$	$n_2 = b + d$	$n = a + b + c + d$
Observed proportion of successes	$p_1 = \dfrac{a}{a+c}$	$p_2 = \dfrac{b}{b+d}$	$p = \dfrac{a+b}{a+b+c+d}$

(b) Expected frequencies in the four cells of the table.

Outcome	Group 1	Group 2
Success	$\dfrac{(a+c)(a+b)}{n}$	$\dfrac{(b+d)(a+b)}{n}$
Failure	$\dfrac{(a+c)(c+d)}{n}$	$\dfrac{(b+d)(c+d)}{n}$

(b) Assumptions

In the Chi-squared test of association in a contingency table with two columns (e.g. defining groups) and two rows (e.g. defining outcomes), we assume that each individual is represented only once (i.e. the individual belongs to only one group and has only one outcome). In the experimental situation, we have the responsibility of randomly allocating each individual to one of the two levels of the factor defining the groups (e.g. in the diabetic mice example, to castrated or sham-operated). In the observational situation, the attribution of an individual to a group is determined for us (e.g. the *Leptospira* example in Section 9.2). The data are collected in the form of frequencies which indicate the number of successes and failures in each sample. The Chi-squared test of association in a 2×2 table is invalid if the *expected* frequency in any one of the four cells is less than 5. If this is the case, we employ **Fisher's exact test** which does not make any assumptions; it involves calculating the exact probability of our particular table arising if we

consider all possible 2×2 tables that have the same marginal totals as our observed table. These calculations are cumbersome and are best left to computer analysis.

(c) Approach

1. Specify the **null hypothesis** that the two population proportions are equal or, equivalently, that there is no association between the two factors of interest. Specify the alternative hypothesis, generally that the two proportions are not equal or that there is an association between the two factors.
2. **Collect** the data. **Display** the observed frequencies in a 2×2 contingency table (see Table 9.1a).
3. Use the appropriate command(s) to select the **Chi-squared test** on the computer. If performing the test by hand, calculate the frequencies that you would *expect* in every cell of the table *if the null hypothesis is true*. Note that the expected frequency for each cell is the product of the observed frequencies for the

row marginal total and the column marginal total for that cell, divided by the observed overall total (see Table 9.1b). Then calculate the **test statistic**, which approximately follows the Chi-squared distribution. It is

$$Test_7 = \sum \frac{(|O - E| - 0.5)^2}{E}$$

with one degree of freedom,

where O and E represent the observed and expected frequencies of a given cell, and the vertical lines surrounding them indicate that you take the absolute value of their difference, i.e. ignore its sign. The calculation $\{(|O - E| - 0.5)^2 / E\}$ is computed for each cell of the table, and the summation is over all four cells of the table. The 0.5 in the numerator is known as **Yates' correction**, a continuity correction included to remove bias. This bias arises because we are assuming the test statistic approximates the continuous Chi-squared distribution although it has a discrete distribution.

A formula for calculating the test statistic, which is identical to $Test_7$ when the contingency table has only two rows and two columns, but quicker to evaluate, is

$$Test_7' = \frac{n(|ad - bc| - 0.5n)^2}{(a+b)(c+d)(a+c)(b+d)}$$

4. Obtain a **P-value**, usually from the computer output, but you can derive it by referring the calculated value of the test statistic to the table of the Chi-squared distribution, Table A.4. The test statistic has 1 degree of freedom – equivalent to the number of rows minus 1 (i.e. $2 - 1 = 1$) times the number of columns minus 1 (i.e. $2 - 1 = 1$).
5. Make a **decision** whether or not to reject the null hypothesis. Usually, we reject the null hypothesis of no association if $P < 0.05$. Remember, in an observational study, association does not imply causation, so that even if you reject the null hypothesis, you cannot necessarily infer that the effect on one factor is actually caused by a particular level of the other factor.
6. Calculate the relevant **confidence interval** for the difference in the two proportions. If the computer output does not provide this information, you can calculate the 95% confidence interval as $(p_1 - p_2) \pm 1.96\, SE(p_1 - p_2)$, i.e.

$$(p_1 - p_2) \pm 1.96 \sqrt{\frac{p_1(1-p_1)}{n_1} + \frac{p_2(1-p_2)}{n_2}}$$

9.4.4 Example

The non-obese diabetic (NOD) mouse develops an autoimmune diabetes that can be used as a model for human juvenile insulin-dependent diabetes. In the colony of Hawkins *et al.* (1993), the incidences for male and female NOD mice were 24% and 73%, respectively. Hawkins *et al.* investigated the causes of this sex difference by considering the effect of early castration on the incidence of diabetes in male NOD mice. (The following is based on their findings.) Fifty mice were randomly selected from 100 male mice and were castrated 1 day after birth; they were compared with the remaining 50 sham-operated mice. The mice were maintained for 140 days, and blood samples were collected biweekly starting at 42 days old. Diabetes was determined by three consecutive blood glucose levels greater than 200 mg/dl. It was shown that neonatal castration more than doubled the incidence of diabetes (52%) when compared with controls (24%) at day 112. But is this difference significant?

1. The null hypothesis is that the proportions of mice with diabetes are equal in the control and castrated populations. The alternative hypothesis is that they are not equal.
2. The data are displayed in Table 9.2a.
3. Table 9.2b shows the expected frequency corresponding to each observed frequency for each of the four cells of the table.

$$Test_7 = \sum \frac{(|O - E| - 0.5)^2}{E}$$

$$= \frac{(|26 - 19| - 0.5)^2}{19} + \frac{(|12 - 19| - 0.5)^2}{19}$$

$$+ \frac{(|24 - 31| - 0.5)^2}{31} + \frac{(|38 - 31| - 0.5)^2}{31}$$

$$= 2.2237 + 2.2237 + 1.3629 + 1.3629$$

$$= 7.17$$

Alternatively, we could have used the formula

$$Test_7' = \frac{100(|26 \times 38 - 12 \times 24| - 50)^2}{38 \times 62 \times 50 \times 50} = 7.17$$

4. We refer the value 7.17 to Table A.4 with 1 degree of freedom, and find that $0.001 < P < 0.01$ (in fact, a computer analysis, the results of which are shown in Display 9.1, gives $P = 0.007$).

5. The data are not consistent with the null hypothesis that the true proportions of mice with diabetes are equal in the control and cas-

Table 9.2 Frequencies of mice with and without diabetes.

(a) Observed frequencies (based on summary data from Hawkins *et al.*, 1993).

	Castrated mice	Control mice	Total
With diabetes	26	12	38
Without diabetes	24	38	62
Total	50	50	100

(b) Expected frequencies.

	Castrated mice	Control mice
With diabetes	$\frac{50 \times 38}{100} = 19$	$\frac{50 \times 38}{100} = 19$
Without diabetes	$\frac{50 \times 62}{100} = 31$	$\frac{50 \times 62}{100} = 31$

NB Identical expected frequencies in the rows of (b) arise because the group sizes in (a) are equal.

trated groups. There is evidence to indicate that neonatal castration is linked with the incidence of diabetes in NOD mice. This suggests that the difference in incidence of diabetes in male and female mice may be associated with the concentration of testosterone in the blood circulation.

6. The 95% confidence interval for the true difference in the proportions of mice with diabetes in the two groups is

$$(p_1 - p_2) \pm 1.96 \sqrt{\frac{p_1(1-p_1)}{n_1} + \frac{p_2(1-p_2)}{n_2}}$$

$$= (0.52 - 0.24)$$

$$\pm 1.96 \sqrt{\frac{0.52 \times 0.48}{50} + \frac{0.24 \times 0.76}{50}}$$

$$= 0.28 \pm 1.96 \times 0.0929$$

$$= 0.098 \text{ to } 0.462$$

Thus, although castration is associated with an increased incidence of diabetes, estimated as 28%, the true effect could be as low as 10% or as high as 46%.

9.5 Testing associations in an $r \times c$ contingency table

9.5.1 Introduction

We can extend the Chi-squared test of association in a 2×2 table to the larger contingency

Chi-square test

	Value	df	Asymp. sig. (2-sided)	Exact. sig. (2-sided)	Exact sig. (1-sided)
Pearson Chi-square	8.319*	1	0.004		
Continuity correction†	7.173	1	0.007		
Fisher's exact test				0.007	0.004
No. of valid cases	100				

Display 9.1 SPSS computer output for analysis of mice castration data from Table 9.2a.

*Zero cells (0.0%) have an expected count of less than 5. The minimum expected count is 19.00.
†Computed only for the 2×2 table.

table which has r rows and c columns, where either r or c or both are greater than 2. We are interested in determining whether the two variables that define the rows and columns of the table are related in some way. We test the null hypothesis of no association by calculating a Chi-squared test statistic.

9.5.2 Assumptions

We assume that the two variables are categorical, and that the data contained in the cells of the contingency table are frequencies. The data should be independent in that no animal/individual may be represented more than once in the table. No more than 20% of the cells of the table should have an expected frequency (calculated under the null hypothesis) whose value is less than 5. If necessary, we can reduce the contingency table in size by combining appropriate rows and/or columns to accommodate this latter assumption. Note that this requirement means that all cells must have expected frequencies that are at least 5 in a 2×2 table (see Section 9.4.3(b)). Alternatively, many statistical packages now have the facility to perform a Fisher's exact test on frequencies contained in a contingency table that has more than two rows and/or columns; this test does not make any assumptions.

9.5.3 General approach

The approach to testing the null hypothesis, that there is no association in the population between the two categorical variables (i.e. factors) defining the $r \times c$ contingency table, is almost identical to that for the 2×2 table (see Section 9.4.3).

1. Specify the **null hypothesis** and the alternative hypothesis.
2. **Collect** the data and **present** them in a contingency table.
3. Select the **Chi-squared test** on the computer, or, by hand, calculate the **test statistic** which approximates the Chi-squared distribution. It is

$$Test_8 = \sum \frac{(O-E)^2}{E}$$

with $(r-1)(c-1)$ degrees of freedom,

where O and E represent the observed and expected frequencies of a given cell, and the summation is over all $r \times c$ cells of the table. Each expected frequency is evaluated under the assumption that the null hypothesis is true; for a given cell, it is calculated as the product of the marginal totals for that cell, divided by the overall total. You will note that the components of this test statistic are almost identical to those of $Test_7$, the test statistic for the 2×2 table; the discrepancy is in the continuity correction (the subtraction of 0.5 in the numerator). The continuity correction has a negligible effect on the test statistic when the sample sizes are large, and is only necessary in the 2×2 table.

4. We determine the **P-value**, if it is not contained in the computer output, by referring the test statistic to the table of the Chi-squared distribution, Table A.4.
5. Make a **decision** whether or not to reject the null hypothesis by considering the P-value, often rejecting the null hypothesis if $P < 0.05$. Note that since we do not estimate an effect, we cannot calculate a confidence interval for it.

9.5.4 Example

Following staff training in insemination techniques in cattle, an artificial insemination centre compared three training methods. The cows were randomly assigned to a particular training method, each cow was inseminated once and the proportion of cows that became pregnant in each group is given in Table 9.3. Is there any evidence for believing that the training methods show different proportions of pregnant animals?

1. The null hypothesis is that the true proportions pregnant are the same for the three methods. Another way of expressing this null hypothesis is that there is no association between the training methods and the

	Method I	Method II	Method III	Total
Pregnant	275 (258.8)	192 (187.7)	261 (281.5)	728
Not pregnant	78 (94.2)	64 (68.3)	123 (102.5)	265
Total	353	256	384	993
Proportion pregnant	0.78	0.75	0.68	0.73
95% CI for true proportion	0.73 to 0.82	0.69 to 0.80	0.63 to 0.73	

Table 9.3 Observed frequencies of pregnant and non-pregnant cows (expected frequencies in brackets).

CI, confidence interval.

pregnancy state of the cows. The alternative hypothesis is that the proportions pregnant are not equal.

2. The data are displayed in Table 9.3.
3. The expected frequencies, which are required if the test is to be performed by hand, are shown in brackets in Table 9.3. The expected number of pregnant cows for Method I is $(353 \times 728)/(993) = 258.80$, and so on for the other methods. The test statistic is

$$Test_8 = \frac{(275-258.80)^2}{258.80} + \frac{(78-94.20)^2}{94.20}$$
$$+ \frac{(192-187.68)^2}{187.68} + \frac{(64-68.32)^2}{68.32}$$
$$+ \frac{(261-281.52)^2}{281.52} + \frac{(123-102.48)^2}{102.48}$$
$$= 1.015 + 2.787 + 0.099 + 0.273$$
$$+ 1.496 + 4.110$$
$$= 9.78$$

4. Referring this value to the Chi-squared distribution (see Table A.4) with $(3-1)(2-1) = 2$ degrees of freedom, we obtain $0.001 < P < 0.01$ (a computer analysis gives $P = 0.008$).
5. Hence we have evidence to reject the null hypothesis that the proportions pregnant are the same for the three methods. In this instance, because one of the variables is binary, we can estimate the proportion of successes for each of the methods, and evaluate the confidence interval for the true proportion (see

Section 4.7) in each case. These quantities are shown in Table 9.3.

Further analysis by Chi-squared tests comparing the proportions of pregnancies obtained by any two methods shows that Method III has a significantly lower proportion of cows pregnant than Method I (test statistic = 8.66, $P = 0.009$ after employing Bonferroni's correction for multiple comparisons, see Section 8.6.3) but no other comparison is significant ($P > 0.05$).

9.5.5 Particular circumstances

We have explained the general approach to analysing $r \times c$ contingency tables in Section 9.5.3. There are, however, special considerations that we should afford the analysis when at least one of the categorical variables defining the table is **ordered** in some way (e.g. body condition score or age categories), or when we want to **combine** contingency tables. We only outline some of the approaches to the analyses in the different circumstances described below. You can obtain details in more advanced statistical texts, such as Armitage *et al.* (2002).

- *The $2 \times c$ contingency table in which the variable defining the columns comprises c ordered categories.* We are interested in comparing the proportions of successes in c ordered groups, and would expect any differences in the proportions, if they exist, to be related to the ordering. We can perform the **Chi-squared test**

for trend to test the null hypothesis that there is no trend in the proportions.

- *The r × c contingency table in which one of the two variables defining the contingency table is ordered.* Firstly, we assign scores to the categories of the ordered variable. Then we can evaluate a test statistic, approximating the Chi-squared distribution, that tests whether the mean scores of the ordered variable are the same in the different categories of the other variable. Alternatively, we can apply the non-parametric Wallis test (see Section 12.6) to compare the categories of the unordered variable.

- *The r × c contingency table in which both of the variables defining the contingency table are ordered.* We assign scores to the categories of each of the two variables, and then regress one set of variables on the other (see Chapter 10). Alternatively, we can calculate the non-parametric **Spearman's rank correlation coefficient** (see Section 12.7) between the two variables.

- *Frequencies are available for various groups in a number of 2 × 2 contingency tables, each defined by the same two variables.* These groups may represent different subgroups or strata of the population (e.g. different sexes or different age groups); alternatively, they may represent different studies, each investigating the relationship between the same two variables. We should like to know how best to use all the information to determine whether there is an association between the two variables. *Do not be tempted to pool the frequencies in the corresponding cells of the tables, and thereby obtain a single 2 × 2 table containing all the frequencies – you can come to quite the wrong conclusions.* Instead, analyse the data using the **Mantel–Haenszel method** (details in, for example, Armitage *et al.*, 2002) which combines, in an appropriate manner, the information from each table. This approach can also be extended to combine a number of *r × c* tables. An alternative approach is to use **logistic regression** analysis (see Section 11.4) in which the association between a binary outcome and a number of exposure variables can be investigated.

9.6 Comparing two proportions: paired observations

9.6.1 Introduction

Sometimes we are interested in comparing two proportions when we have pairs of results on a binary variable. An analogy is the comparison of two means in related samples leading to the paired *t*-test (see Section 7.5).

Suppose our random sample comprises *m* animals, each animal being investigated in two ways. We observe whether the response for each member of a pair results in a success or a failure – the two possible outcomes of the binary variable of interest. For example, Schönmann *et al.* (1994) compared the efficiency of diagnosis of two methods to detect *Tritrichomonas foetus* in bulls. A sample was taken from each bull and classified by each of the two methods as positive (success) or negative (failure). The investigators determined the number of pairs in which both methods yielded a success, both methods were a failure, and where one was a success and the other a failure.

In Table 9.4a we use a general notation to show the frequencies of the four types of pairs from two samples. We exhibit the same results in a slightly different format in Table 9.4b. We use **McNemar's test** to test the null hypothesis that the true proportions of successes using the two methods are equal. These are estimated by $p_1 = (e + f)/m$ in Method 1 and $p_2 = (e + g)/m$ in Method 2. Their difference, $p_1 - p_2 = (f - g)/m$, focuses only on the discordant pairs, as does McNemar's test statistic; the frequencies relating to the concordant pairs are of no relevance in the analysis. McNemar's test is based on the observed frequencies, f and g, and their corresponding expected frequencies, calculated under the null hypothesis. These are incorporated into a test statistic, $\Sigma\{(O - E)^2/E\}$, which approximately follows a Chi-squared distribution.

9.6.2 Assumptions

We assume there are two possible outcomes (success and failure) to the variable of interest,

(a) Observed frequencies.

Type	Outcome using method 1	Outcome using method 2	Frequency
1	Success	Success	e
2	Success	Failure	f
3	Failure	Success	g
4	Failure	Failure	h
Total			m

Table 9.4 Two layouts to show the frequencies of the four types of pair in paired samples when there are two possible outcomes – success and failure.

(b) Two-way contingency table of observed frequencies.

Method 1	Method 2 Success	Method 2 Failure	Total No. of pairs
Success	e	f	$e + f$
Failure	g	h	$g + h$
Total no. of pairs	$e + g$	$f + h$	$m = e + f + g + h$

and that we observe the outcome on each member of a pair. The pair may comprise matched individuals, each assessed in one of two circumstances, or it may comprise the same individual assessed twice. McNemar's test is inappropriate if the number of discordant pairs $(f + g)$ is less than about 10.

9.6.3 Approach

1. Specify the **null hypothesis** that the proportions of successes in the two populations are equal. Specify the alternative hypothesis, generally that the two proportions are unequal.
2. **Collect** the data and **display** them in a frequency table, as shown in Table 9.4b.
3. Select *McNemar's test* on the computer or, by hand, calculate the **test statistic**, which approximately follows the Chi-squared distribution. It is

$$Test_9 = \frac{(|f - g| - 1)^2}{f + g}$$

with one degree of freedom.

Sometimes, you may find that McNemar's test uses the related test statistic, $\sqrt{Test_9}$, which approximates the Standard Normal distribu-

tion. The 1 in the numerator of $Test_9$ is a continuity correction which is subtracted from the absolute difference (without regard to sign) between f and g to adjust for approximating a discrete distribution by the continuous Chi-squared distribution.

4. Obtain the **P-value**, either from computer output or by referring the test statistic to the table of the Chi-squared distribution, Table A.4, with 1 degree of freedom.
5. Make a **decision** whether or not to reject the null hypothesis by considering the P-value. Usually, we reject the null hypothesis if $P < 0.05$.
6. Calculate the **confidence interval** for the difference in the two proportions of successes, estimated by $p_1 = (e + f)/m$ in sample 1 and $p_2 = (e + g)/m$ in sample 2. The approximate 95% confidence interval for the true difference in the proportions is given by

$$\frac{f - g}{m} \pm 1.96 \frac{1}{m} \sqrt{f + g - \frac{(f - g)^2}{m}}$$

9.6.4 Example

In the example introduced earlier, Schönmann *et al.* (1994) compared two methods of culture of

Table 9.5 Numbers of the organism, *Tritrichomonas foetus*, detected in bovine preputial washings using two different methods (reproduced from Schönmann *et al.*, 1994, with permission from BMJ Publishing Group Ltd).

	Claussen's positive	Claussen's negative	Total
Commercial positive	59	14	73
Commercial negative	2	8	10
Total	61	22	83

Tritrichomonas foetus in the washings of the prepuce of infected beef bulls to determine the best method for detection of the organism. In comparing the methods of culture, Claussen's medium detected the organism in 61 of 83 samples whereas a commercial system detected the organism in 73 of the same 83 samples.

1. The null hypothesis is that the true proportions detected are the same using Claussen's medium and the commercial system. The alternative hypothesis is that the two proportions are different.
2. The data are displayed in Table 9.5.
3. The test statistic is

$$Test_9 = \frac{(|14-2|-1)^2}{14+2} = 7.56$$

This approximates the Chi-squared distribution with 1 degree of freedom.
4. Reference to Table A.4 gives $0.001 < P < 0.01$ (a computer analysis gives $P = 0.006$).
5. We have evidence to reject the null hypothesis; we conclude that the commercial system has the ability to detect the greater proportion of organisms.
6. We estimate the proportions of organisms detected by Claussen's medium and the commercial system to be $61/83 = 0.735$ and $73/83 = 0.880$, respectively. The approximate confidence interval for the true difference in the proportions of organisms detected by the two methods, taking into account the pairings, is

$$\frac{14-2}{83} \pm 1.96 \frac{1}{83} \sqrt{14+2-\frac{(14-2)^2}{83}}$$
$$= 0.1446 \pm 0.0892$$
$$= 0.055 \text{ to } 0.234$$

In other words, although Claussen's medium detected 74% of infected samples and the commercial system detected 88%, a difference of 14%, this difference could, with 95% certainty, be as low as 6% or as high as 23%. We must judge, in the particular circumstances, whether 6% constitutes an important difference.

9.7 Chi-squared goodness-of-fit test

9.7.1 Introduction

We may be interested in establishing whether a set of observed data comes from a population that follows a particular theoretical distribution. The discrete or continuous distribution may be one of those to which we have already referred, such as the Binomial, Poisson or Normal (see Sections 3.4 and 3.5, but note that there are easier ways of establishing Normality, as discussed in Section 3.5.3(e)). Alternatively, it may reflect an expected distribution determined by the biological circumstances. Particular examples of these arise in genetics, where the assumed pattern of segregation of the alleles of a gene will lead to specific expectations of genotype (and perhaps phenotype) in the offspring.

The observed frequencies in each category of response (e.g. a genotypic class or an interval for a continuous variable) can then be compared with the number expected in that category if the data followed the theoretical distribution. This gives rise to a test statistic that approximates the Chi-squared distribution. Note that, in this text, we have not provided the equations for the Binomial or Poisson distributions from which expected numbers can be derived; they can be found in, for example, Armitage *et al.* (2002).

9.7.2 Assumptions

In the **goodness-of-fit test**, we assume that the sample is representative of the population and the responses are independent and are categorized into distinct classes or intervals. The approximation to the Chi-squared distribution is poor if the expected frequency is less than 5 in more than 20% of the categories.

9.7.3 Approach

1. Specify the **null hypothesis** that the distribution of the variable in the population follows the specified theoretical distribution. The alternative hypothesis is that it does not.
2. **Collect** the data and **display** them in a frequency table.
3. Calculate the expected frequency in each category, and determine the **test statistic**, either by computer or by hand.

$$Test_8 = \sum \frac{(O-E)^2}{E}$$

where O and E represent the observed and expected frequencies in a given category, and the sum is over all categories. This test statistic approximates the Chi-squared distribution with degrees of freedom = (number of categories) − (number of parameters that have to be estimated in order to calculate the expected values) − 1. For example, the mean is the only parameter that has to be estimated in the Poisson distribution.
4. Obtain the **P-value** from the computer output or by referring the test statistic to Table A.4.
5. Make a **decision** whether or not to reject the null hypothesis. Usually, but not necessarily, we reject the null hypothesis if $P < 0.05$. Note that, since the null hypothesis does not relate to an effect of interest, which we would estimate from the sample data, we do not calculate a confidence interval.

9.7.4 Example

The offspring of a random sample of roan Shorthorn cattle were classified according to coat colour: red 82, roan 209 and white 89. Is this distribution inconsistent with the hypothesis that coat colour is determined by a single pair of alleles with co-dominance? Co-dominance implies that neither allele is dominant, and the heterozygote exhibits the effect of both alleles.

Table 9.6 Observed and expected frequencies of colour categories for Shorthorn cattle.

Colour	Observed frequency O	Expected frequency E	$O-E$
Red	82	380/4 = 95	−13
Roan	209	380/2 = 190	19
White	89	380/4 = 95	−6
Total	380	380	

1. The null hypothesis is that coat colour is determined by a single pair of alleles with co-dominance. If this is so, then the offspring would be expected to display coat colours in the ratio of $1:2:1$. The alternative hypothesis is that coat colour is not determined by a single pair of alleles with co-dominance.
2. The data are displayed in Table 9.6.
3. The Chi-squared test statistic is

$$Test_8 = \frac{(-13)^2}{95} + \frac{(19)^2}{190} + \frac{(-6)^2}{95} = 4.06$$

This approximates the Chi-squared distribution on $(3-1)$ degrees of freedom. Note that, in this example, we have not had to estimate any parameters in order to calculate the expected frequencies.
4. Reference to Table A.4 gives $P > 0.05$ (computer analysis gives $P = 0.131$).
5. There is insufficient evidence to reject the null hypothesis that coat colour is determined by a single pair of alleles with co-dominance.

It should be noted that, while this is a straightforward test of a simple segregation hypothesis, more complicated segregation involving multiple genes leads to complex hypotheses which are the domain of the trained geneticist (see Section 15.6). Moreover, corrections need to be built into the analysis if the data are not a random selection because of potential biases. Nicholas (2010) covers these situations in more detail.

Exercises

The statements in questions 9.1 and 9.2 are either TRUE or FALSE.

9.1 An investigator is interested in whether there is a breed-related basis for incidence of hip dysplasia in dogs. She selects samples of adult Greyhounds and adult German shepherd dogs. From pelvic X-ray examination, the number of animals having shallow or abnormal coxo-femoral joints in each group is recorded. An appropriate test for the null hypothesis that there is no association between breed and the frequency of hip dysplasia in the population is:
(a) the two-sample *t*-test.
(b) the *F*-test.
(c) the Chi-squared test for the difference in two proportions.
(d) McNemar's test.
(e) the Chi-squared goodness-of-fit test.

9.2 In a study of the influence of artificial insemination on the occurrence of uterine infection in gilts, data were collected on the occurrence of bacteria in cervical swabs in two samples of gilts randomly allocated to either washing of the vulva or faecal contamination of the vulva before sham insemination. The results are presented in a 2 × 2 table; the proposed Chi-squared test for the difference in the proportions with uterine infection in the two groups:
(a) Is only valid if the observed frequency is greater than 5 in each cell of the table.
(b) Has degrees of freedom equal to 2.
(c) Tests the null hypothesis that there is no association in the population between uterine infection and the condition of the vulva.
(d) Tests the null hypothesis that there is a difference between the true proportions with uterine infection in the two groups.
(e) Is only valid if the data are Normally distributed.

9.3 The local National Farmers' Union Committee have just received the Ministry of Agriculture, Forestry and Fisheries national figures for cattle numbers in England. They show that nationally the proportion of dairy cows in the national herd is 0.29. The committee express some surprise at this figure, which they believe does not reflect their area, and they decide to do their own local survey. They take a random sample of the cattle holdings in their area, and in these 1375 cattle they discover there are 359 dairy cows. Is there evidence that the proportion of dairy cows in their area differs from the national figure?

9.4 Medroxyprogesterone (MPA) used to be administered to bitches to suppress oestrus. Researchers investigated the effect of administration of MPA to older bitches, aged 6 years and above, on the chance of them developing mammary nodules (early signs of mammary changes which may develop into malignant tumours). The results of their 4-year prospective cohort study indicated that 21 of the 33 bitches that received MPA developed mammary nodules on clinical examination, whereas 13 of the 39 bitches that did not receive MPA developed mammary nodules (based on data from Støvring *et al.*, 1997). Is there evidence for there being a greater risk of mammary nodules in the event of being administered MPA?

Display the data in a frequency table. Formulate the null hypothesis, and calculate the expected frequency in each cell of the table. Conduct a suitable analysis to test this null hypothesis.

9.5 *Fasciola hepatica* (liver fluke) infestation in beef cattle is present if the animal sheds *F. hepatica* eggs. Welch *et al.* (1987) were interested in determining whether a positive reaction to an enzyme-linked immunosorbent assay (ELISA) could be used as an alternative test for liver fluke infestation. They investigated 143 calves from a number of beef cattle herds in central and southern Louisiana. Of 55 calves that were ELISA positive, 39 were shedding eggs; of 53 calves that were shedding eggs, 14 were ELISA negative. Present these results in a contingency table, and use them to test the null hypothesis that the two procedures are equally effective in detecting liver fluke infestation.

9.6 One hundred and twenty young adult female Beagles were given 0.026–106 kBq plutonium (^{239}Pu) per kg by intravenous injection and compared with 63 comparable female control Beagles with a view to determining whether ^{239}Pu deposit in bone affects the appearance of mammary tumours (based on Lloyd *et al.*, 1995). Forty-five (71.4%; 95% CI 60.2% to 82.6%) of the control dogs developed mammary tumours of any kind (benign or malignant) whereas 67 (55.8%; 95% CI 46.9% to 64.7%) of the dogs given ^{239}Pu developed mammary tumours of any kind. There was no significant difference between the percentages developing mammary tumours in the two groups ($P = 0.06$).

(a) Criticize the design of the experiment.
(b) Draw up a contingency table of the results.
(c) Which test should the authors have used to compare the percentages developing mammary tumours in the two groups?
(d) What are the assumptions underlying this test?
(e) Interpret the confidence interval for the percentage of control Beagles developing tumours.
(f) Using only the confidence intervals provided, is it possible to assess whether there is a significant difference between the percentages developing mammary tumours in the two groups? Explain your reasoning.
(g) The authors write 'There were 45 controls (71.4%) with any tumor vs. 67 dogs (55.8%) given Pu (95% CI 46.9% to 82.6%).' To what do the lower and upper limits of their 'confidence interval' relate? Why is this not actually a confidence interval?
(h) Which single confidence interval would be a useful summary of the effect of ^{239}Pu on mammary tumour development?

9.7 In a study to gauge the pregnancy rate in a large mob of sheep on an Australian sheep farm, a sample of 272 sheep were taken for ultrasound scanning. For ease of handling, they were taken in groups of eight and the number of pregnant animals recorded for each group. The results of the ultrasound scanning are shown in Table 9.7. At lambing 64% of the mob gave birth to lambs. The table shows the numbers of pregnant ewes per group of eight expected if they followed a Binomial distribution with $\pi = 0.64$. Ignoring the difference in the proportions pregnant between ultrasound scanning and parturition and assuming that each ewe has the same chance of getting pregnant, use the Chi-squared analysis to assess whether the observed distribution conforms to the stated Binomial distribution.

Table 9.7 Thirty-four groups of eight sheep sampled for pregnancy status from a large mob of sheep in Australia.

No. of pregnant ewes per sample	Observed frequency of occurrence	Expected No. for a Binomial distribution ($\pi = 0.64, n = 8$)
0	0	0.010
1	1	0.136
2	3	0.850
3	4	3.019
4	7	6.708
5	9	9.537
6	7	8.480
7	2	4.308
8	1	0.955

9.8 A pet shop owner was considering stocking a new cat collar that was fastened by a quick release catch which she considered a bit insecure. So she set up a small test to try to assess its security compared with a regular collar fastened with a standard buckle. Thirty-five cats were randomly allocated to be fitted with one of the collars first and then after 2 months they were fitted with the alternative collar. After the second period of 2 months, she registered how many of the collars had been lost or retained in place for each 2-month test period. Six of the cats lost both types of collar, whereas eight of them retained both types and two cats retained the new collar but lost the standard collar.

(a) Draw up a contingency table to show the results.
(b) What percentage of cats lost the new collar and what percentage of cats lost the old collar?
(c) What is the name of the appropriate test to compare these percentages?
(d) What is the null hypothesis for this test?
(e) What is the two-sided alternative hypothesis for this test?
(f) Explain what is meant by the significance level of the test.
(g) How is the significance level related to the Type I error?
(h) The test result gave $P = 0.0005$. Interpret this P-value.
(i) On the basis of this result, what would the pet-shop owner have concluded?

10 Linear correlation and regression

10.1 Learning objectives

By the end of this chapter you should be able to:

- Recognize a linear relationship in a scatter diagram.
- Interpret Pearson's correlation coefficient.
- Explain the value of r^2.
- Test the null hypothesis that the correlation coefficient is zero.
- Elaborate circumstances when it would be improper to calculate the correlation coefficient.
- Identify data sets that are suited to linear regression analysis.
- Distinguish between the outcome and explanatory variables in regression analysis.
- Check the assumptions in a linear regression analysis.
- Interpret a linear regression equation.
- Test the null hypothesis that the slope of the regression line is zero.
- Decide whether the regression line is a good fit to the data.
- Use the regression equation for prediction.
- Explain what is meant by regression to the mean.

10.2 Introducing linear correlation and regression

10.2.1 Types of variable

In Chapter 9 we examined the relationship between two *categorical* variables by considering the Chi-squared test of the null hypothesis that there is no association between the two variables. In this chapter, we describe the statistical techniques that we can use to investigate the association between two *numerical* variables, x and y, for example the chest girth and live weight of sheep. The two techniques that we discuss are **linear correlation** and **linear regression analysis**, each of which has a defined role.

10.2.2 Aims of linear correlation and regression

- In **linear correlation** we are concerned with determining whether there is a linear relationship between two numerical variables, and with measuring the degree of that relationship. We would like to know how well a straight line

Statistics for Veterinary and Animal Science, Third Edition. Aviva Petrie and Paul Watson.
© 2013 John Wiley & Sons, Ltd. Published 2013 by John Wiley & Sons, Ltd.

describes the linear association between the two variables when one variable is plotted against the other (see Section 10.2.3). We derive a measure, called the *correlation coefficient*, that reflects the closeness of the points to the straight line. In correlation analysis, we make no distinction between the two variables. We can interchange x and y, and we will still obtain the same value for the correlation coefficient.

- The purpose of **linear regression** is to describe the linear relationship between the two variables by determining the mathematical equation that relates the variables. We often use this equation to predict the value of one variable (called the outcome, dependent or response variable) from a value of the other variable (called the explanatory, independent or predictor variable). By convention, we take the y variable as the outcome variable, and the x variable as the explanatory variable. We assume that y is influenced by x (rather than the other way round). *We cannot interchange x and y in regression analysis.* As an example, think about the standard curve prepared for a protein assay; the colour development (y) is plotted against the predetermined concentrations of protein (x), and the linear regression line is calculated as the line of best fit.

We give details of linear correlation and regression in the sections that follow. Note that the assumptions underlying the inferential procedures are different in correlation and regression.

10.2.3 Scatter diagram

The first stage, though, before we attempt any formal analysis, is to plot the data on a rectangular co-ordinate system so we can see what, if any, is the relationship between the two variables. If we represent the two variables under investigation by x and y, then each of the n animals in our random sample has a value for the x variable and a value for the y variable. Our sample data therefore consist of a series of n independent pairs of x and y values, $\{(x_1, y_1), (x_2, y_2), (x_3, y_3), \ldots, (x_n, y_n)\}$.

Conventionally, we plot the data with the x values on the horizontal axis and the y values on the vertical axis (see Figure 10.6 in which x = chest girth (cm) and y = live weight (kg) of sheep). Every pair of observations is marked by a point on the diagram, and once we have plotted all the observations, we have a scatter of points. Hence the term **scatter diagram** is used to describe the visual display of the data.

Before we are to proceed with either linear correlation or linear regression analysis, we must consider the 'curve' that approximates the data points. This line does not 'link' all the points, but is a line drawn through the midst of the points, illustrating the general 'drift'. If this is a straight line, then we can conclude that a linear relationship exists between the two variables, and can use the appropriate statistical technique to investigate that relationship. For example, we may be interested in using the linear relationship to predict the live weight of sheep from their chest girth. (Sometimes it is possible to linearize a nonlinear relationship by transforming the data – see Section 13.2.2)

10.3 Linear correlation

10.3.1 Correlation coefficient

If we believe that there is a linear relationship between two numerical variables with a change in one variable being associated with a change in the other, we may be interested in determining the strength of that relationship. We do not actually draw the line in correlation analysis (this is part of regression analysis), but we can imagine the line that approximates the data most closely. Are the points in the scatter diagram close to this line or are they widely dispersed around it? Provided a linear relationship exists between the two variables, the closer the points are to the line, the stronger the linear association between the two variables.

We measure the degree of association by calculating **Pearson's product moment correlation coefficient**, usually just called the **correlation coefficient** or, sometimes, the **linear correlation coefficient**. It can take any value from −1 to +1.

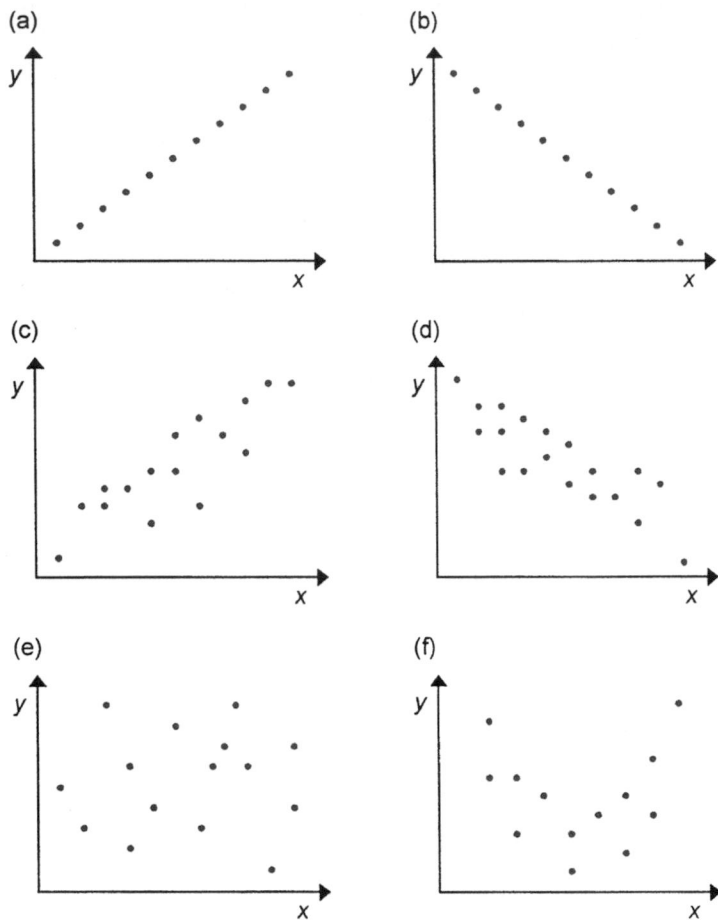

Figure 10.1 Data with different correlation coefficients: (a) perfect positive association, $r = +1$; (b) perfect negative association, $r = -1$; (c) positive association, $r = +0.86$; (d) negative association, $r = -0.85$; (e) no association, $r = 0$; (f) no linear association, $r = 0$.

- We say that we have *perfect correlation* if all the points lie on the line; in this case, the value of the correlation coefficient takes one of its extreme values, either +1 or −1 (Figure 10.1a and b).
- We have *positive correlation* if the sign of the correlation coefficient is positive; then there is a direct relationship between the two variables so that as one variable increases in value, the other variable increases (Figure 10.1a) or there is a tendency for it to do so (Figure 10.1c).
- We have *negative correlation* if the sign of the correlation coefficient is negative; then there is an inverse relationship between the two variables so that as one variable increases in value, the other variable decreases (Figure 10.1b) or there is a tendency for it to do so (Figure 10.1d).

- We have no linear association (i.e. the variables are *uncorrelated*) if the correlation coefficient is zero; then there is a random scatter of points with no indication of a linear relation between the variables (Figure 10.1e). Note that a non-linear relationship between the variables can also give a correlation coefficient of zero (Figure 10.1f).

The closer the value of the correlation coefficient is to either of its extreme values, the stronger the relationship between the variables, and the nearer the points are to the line.

We give the rather cumbersome formula for calculating the correlation coefficient, even though you will probably use the computer to obtain its value. If we take a random sample of

n independent pairs of observations $\{(x_1, y_1), (x_2, y_2), (x_3, y_3), \ldots (x_n, y_n)\}$ on two numerical variables, x and y, then we estimate the correlation coefficient, ρ (the Greek letter rho), in the population by the sample correlation coefficient

$$r = \frac{\sum (x-\bar{x})(y-\bar{y})}{\sqrt{\sum (x-\bar{x})^2 \sum (y-\bar{y})^2}}$$

Note that:
- The correlation coefficient is independent of the units of measurement of the two variables, i.e. it is dimensionless.
- We can interchange x and y without affecting the value of the correlation coefficient.
- The correlation coefficient is only valid within the limits of the data in the sample.
- The absolute value of the correlation coefficient (i.e. ignoring its sign) tends to increase as the range of values of x and/or y increases, i.e. it tends to become more extreme (i.e. closer to +1 if positive and closer to −1 if negative).

10.3.2 Testing a hypothesis that the correlation coefficient is zero

The correlation coefficient provides a measure of the strength of the linear association between two variables. There is no linear association between the variables if the correlation coefficient is zero, and so testing the hypothesis that $\rho = 0$ is a useful exercise in correlation analysis. Note, however, that even if the correlation coefficient is deemed significantly different from zero, this does *not* provide evidence of a *causal* relationship between the two variables; it merely indicates that they vary together.

(a) Assumptions

There are certain assumptions that have to be satisfied if we are to test a hypothesis about the correlation coefficient, or determine the confidence interval for it. In particular:

- Both of the variables, x and y, are numerical.
- The hypothesis test that the true population correlation coefficient is zero only requires *at least one* of the two variables to be Normally distributed in the population (strictly, one variable is Normally distributed with constant variance for any given value of the other variable).
- If we calculate the confidence interval for the population correlation coefficient by taking a random sample of pairs of independent observations $\{(x_1, y_1), (x_2, y_2), (x_3, y_3), \ldots (x_n, y_n)\}$ on two variables, x and y, then *both x and y* should be Normally distributed in the population (strictly, they should come from a bivariate Normal distribution, i.e. y is Normally distributed with constant variance for any given value of x, and x is Normally distributed with constant variance for any given value of y). If the data come from a bivariate Normal distribution, the scatter of points will be elliptical, although this will be difficult to discern if the correlation coefficient is close to either of its extremes.

If the data are measured on an ordinal scale or if we are concerned about the distributional assumptions in other circumstances, we calculate **Spearman's rank correlation coefficient** (see Section 12.7), a non-parametric equivalent to Pearson's product moment correlation coefficient.

(b) Approach

1. Specify the **null hypothesis** that the population correlation coefficient, ρ, is equal to zero. Generally, we adopt the alternative hypothesis that the correlation coefficient is not equal to zero.
2. **Collect** the data and **display** them in a scatter diagram from which we can discern whether a linear relationship exists between the two variables. Check the assumption that at least one (or both if a confidence interval is to be calculated) of the variables is Normally distributed.
3. Calculate the sample correlation coefficient, preferably using a computer. You may find that the computer calculates a **test statistic** which has a t-distribution on $n - 2$ degrees of freedom.

The test statistic is

$$Test_{10} = r\sqrt{\frac{(n-2)}{(1-r^2)}}$$

where r is the sample correlation coefficient, and n is the number of pairs of observations in the sample. It is not difficult to calculate $Test_{10}$ by hand, but this is seldom required as there is a table (see Table A.6) that relates the values of r directly to the P-values.

4. Obtain the **P-value**, generally from the computer output. You can refer r directly to Table A.6. Alternatively, you could refer $Test_{10}$ to the table of the t-distribution, Table A.3, with $n - 2$ degrees of freedom.
5. Make a **decision** whether or not to reject the null hypothesis by considering the P-value. Usually, although not necessarily, we reject the null hypothesis if $P < 0.05$.
6. Calculate the **confidence interval** for the true correlation coefficient. Your computer package may do this automatically but, if not, we explain how to perform the calculation manually. Although the sampling distribution of r is not Normal, the distribution of a transformed variable, $z = 0.5\log_e\{(1 + r)/(1 - r)\}$, follows the Normal distribution, and we use this information to enable us to calculate the confidence interval for ρ.

It can be shown that the approximate 95% confidence limits for z are $z_1 = z - 1.96/\sqrt{n-3}$ and $z_2 = z + 1.96/\sqrt{n-3}$. We then back-transform, by taking exponentials, to get a confidence interval for ρ. Thus, the approximate 95% confidence interval for ρ is

$$\frac{e^{2z_1} - 1}{e^{2z_1} + 1} \quad \text{to} \quad \frac{e^{2z_2} - 1}{e^{2z_2} + 1}$$

(c) Using the correlation coefficient as an aid to understanding

You should not rely solely on the magnitude of the correlation coefficient to judge the biological importance of the relationship between the two variables. You will see, if you look at Table A.6, that when the sample size is large we reject the null hypothesis that the population correlation coefficient is zero, even though the value of the sample correlation coefficient is quite close to

zero. For example, we reject the null hypothesis at the 5% level of significance if r is greater than 0.29, 0.20 and 0.16 for sample sizes of 45, 100 and 150, respectively. Furthermore, even when the sample size is much smaller (20, say), the result of the test is significant for quite low values of r ($P < 0.05$ if $r > 0.44$). A statistically significant result indicates only that there is a linear relationship between the two variables. We need to gauge the importance of a significant result, and, clearly, we cannot do so by assessing the magnitude of the correlation coefficient.

Instead, we calculate the **square of the correlation coefficient**, r^2. It represents the proportion of the total variance in one variable that can be explained by or is attributed to its linear relationship with the other variable. It is usually multiplied by 100 and expressed as a percentage. So, if the correlation coefficient obtained from a sample of size 45 is 0.30, from which we can deduce that the true correlation coefficient is significantly different from zero ($P < 0.05$), its square is 0.09. Hence, even though the test of the correlation coefficient is significant, only 9% of the total variance of one variable is explained by its linear relationship with the other variable; the remaining 91% is unexplained by the relationship.

We advise you to calculate and interpret the value of r^2 routinely whenever you estimate the correlation coefficient. It is a great aid to understanding the strength of the underlying linear relationship between the two variables.

(d) Example

Jackson *et al.* (1996) developed a novel specific assay for measuring bone alkaline phosphatase activity, an enzyme which reflects bone metabolism. They were interested to know whether this measure, the wheatgerm lectin precipitated bone alkaline phosphatase activity (wBAP), was correlated with an independent marker of bone formation, the carboxy-terminal propeptide of Type I collagen (PICP). Table 10.1 is based on the results they obtained from a random sample of 46 adult horses. The data are plotted in Figure 10.2, a scatter diagram in which both of the axes have logarithmic scales (this is an example of data transformation – see Section 13.2 – the two variables being log transformed to Normalize the data). The relationship appears approximately linear, and we calculate the sample correlation coefficient as $r = 0.785$. Note that $r^2 = 0.62$, indicating that a substantial proportion, 62%, of the variance in log PICP is explained by its linear relationship with log wBAP. In order to test the null hypothesis that the true correlation coefficient is zero we need to follow these steps:

1. We specify H_0: there is no linear association between PICP and wBAP, i.e. $\rho = 0$; the alternative hypothesis is that $\rho \neq 0$.
2. The data are displayed in Figure 10.2, which exhibits a positive linear relationship between the two variables when each is represented on a log scale. Separate histograms for log PICP and log wBAP reveal that each is approximately Normally distributed. Furthermore, the scatter of points suggests an ellipse, indicating that the data on the log scales are approximately bivariate Normal.
3. $r = 0.785$; note that we could calculate $Test_{10} = 0.785 \sqrt{(44)/(0.3838)} = 8.41$.
4. When we refer 0.785 to Table A.6 with a sample size of 46, we find that $0.785 > 0.4742$ and that $0.785 > 0.4514$ (the entries in the table for sample sizes of 45 and 50), so $P < 0.001$. Note that we also obtain $P < 0.001$ if we refer $Test_{10}$ to Table A.3 with $46 - 2 = 44$ degrees of freedom.
5. We have strong evidence to reject the null hypothesis.
6. $z = 0.5\log_e(1.7846/0.2154) = 1.0572$. Hence $z_1 = 1.0572 - 1.96/\sqrt{43} = 0.7583$ and $z_2 = 1.0572 + 1.96/\sqrt{43} = 1.3561$. Thus the 95% confidence interval for ρ is:

$$\frac{e^{1.5166} - 1}{e^{1.5166} + 1} \text{ to } \frac{e^{2.7122} - 1}{e^{2.7122} + 1}$$

$$= \frac{3.5567}{5.5567} \text{ to } \frac{14.0624}{16.0623} = 0.64 \text{ to } 0.88$$

Table 10.1 Two measures of bone activity in 46 adult horses (based on summary data from Jackson *et al.*, 1996, with permission from Elsevier).

wBAP (μg/l)	PICP (U/l)	wBAP (μg/l)	PICP (U/l)	wBAP (μg/l)	PICP (U/l)
20	190	30	400	52	1005
31	186	36	380	61	1100
31	190	50	405	61	1070
22	205	54	370	57	810
18	210	31	490	59	720
16	290	35	470	63	740
18	306	39	470	65	700
55	1000	36	580	62	750
28	170	36	540	61	700
32	180	40	520	70	570
33	300	36	700	71	1300
38	303	34	800	88	1050
34	320	41	800	90	1100
21	360	48	850	90	1200
41	340	50	980	110	940
				34	360

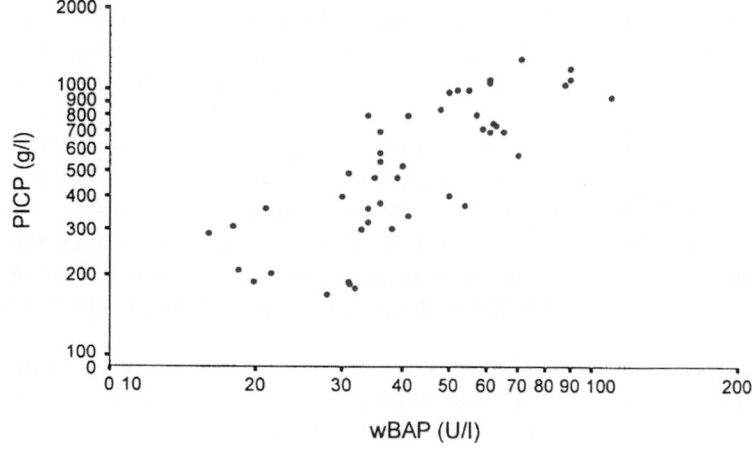

Figure 10.2 Scatter diagram of the relationship between two measures of bone formation, bone alkaline phosphatase activity (wBAP) and Type I collagen concentration (PICP). Note that the variables are plotted on log scales (redrawn from Jackson *et al.*, 1996, with permission from Elsevier).

(a)

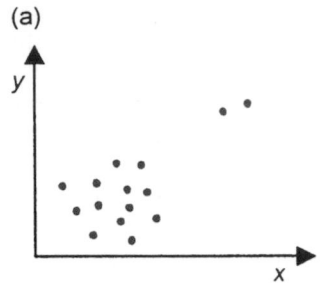

(b)

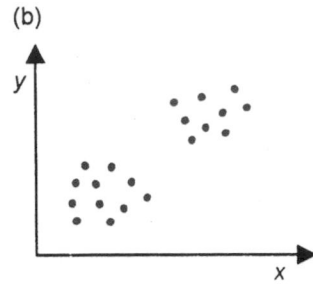

Figure 10.3 Two circumstances in which the correlation coefficient should not be calculated: (a) data with outliers, and (b) data from subgroups.

The correlation coefficient is significantly different from zero, and even the lower limit of the confidence interval is indicative of a fairly strong linear association between the two measures; it would seem that the novel measurement of bone alkaline phosphatase activity indeed reflects the metabolic activity of bone tissue.

10.3.3 Misuse of the correlation coefficient

Unfortunately, the correlation coefficient is a frequently misused statistic. You must remember that a significant correlation coefficient does not provide evidence of a causal relationship between two variables. For example, just because the annual pet food consumption in the UK is correlated with the number of air-miles flown by UK residents, this does not suggest that pets are using food as a comfort substitute for absentee owners! Another example of misuse is when the correlation coefficient is relied upon to assess the repeatability of a technique or the agreement between two methods (see Section 14.4.2(c)).

We have discussed the assumptions underlying the test of significance and the calculation of the confidence interval for the correlation coefficient (see Section 10.3.2(a)). Clearly, you must ensure that these assumptions are satisfied in the relevant circumstances, but remember that you *should not even calculate the correlation coefficient* when:

- There is an underlying relationship between the two variables, but it is not linear (see Figure 10.1f).

- The observations are not independent; for example, when there is more than one observation on some or all of the experimental units.
- In the presence of outliers (see Section 5.9.3) when one or two extreme observations may distort the value of r (Figure 10.3a).
- The data consist of subgroups of animals if these subgroups differ in their average response to one of the variables (Figure 10.3b).

10.4 Simple (univariable) linear regression

10.4.1 Equation of the regression line

In simple **linear regression analysis**, we describe the relationship between two numerical variables, x and y, by determining the straight line that approximates the data points on a scatter diagram most closely. We regard the x variable as one whose values can be measured without error or which are predetermined by the experimenter; so, for example, it may represent doses, ages, weights or concentrations at predetermined values. On the other hand, the y variable is a random variable which is subject to experimental variation, such as systolic blood pressure, haemoglobin concentration or colour intensity. We assume that y is *dependent* on x (rather than the other way round) so that if we change the value of x, this will lead to a change in the value of y.

- We call y the **outcome**, **dependent** or **response variable** and we represent this on the vertical axis of the scatter diagram.

- We call x the **explanatory**, **independent** or **predictor variable** or the **regressor** and we represent this on the horizontal axis. Since there is only one explanatory variable, the regression is usually referred to as **simple linear regression**, sometimes described as **univariable**. We discuss *multivariable* regression models, when there is more than one explanatory variable, as well as *centring* and *scaling*, which involve transformations of the explanatory variable to aid interpretation, in Chapter 11.

We could draw 'by eye' what we believe to be the 'line of best fit' but this would be a subjective approach and not very satisfactory. Instead, we use an *equation* to describe the straight line relationship between x and y. This equation defines a particular mathematical **model** which, in general terms, is a simplified representation of a real-world situation or process that occurs in the population. If we imagine that, for each value of x, there is a *population* of y values, the equation would be:

$$Y_{\text{pop}} = \alpha + \beta x$$

where:

- Y_{pop} is the predicted, expected, fitted or mean value of y for a given value of x.
- α is the constant term that represents the *intercept* of the line; it is the value of y when x is equal to zero.
- β is the *slope* or *gradient* of the line and represents the mean change in y for a unit change

in x, i.e. it describes by how much y changes on average when x increases by one unit.

α and β are the parameters that define the line. They are both called **regression coefficients** although, frequently, you may find that this description is reserved only for β.

We have to *estimate* the two parameters α and β (by a and b, respectively) from our random sample of n pairs of observations, $\{(x_1, y_1), (x_2, y_2), (x_3, y_3), \ldots, (x_n, y_n)\}$, in such a way that the line 'fits' the points as closely as possible.

- Generally, we approach the problem by requiring the deviations of the points from the line to be as small as possible. We take the deviation of a point from the line as the *vertical* distance of the point from the line, i.e. in the direction parallel to the y axis. We look at deviations in this direction because we believe that only the y variable is subject to experimental variation; we regard the x variable as measured without error. Each deviation, the difference between an *observed* value of y and its *predicted* or *fitted* value for a given value of x, is called a **residual** (Figure 10.4).
- Since some of the points are above the line and the corresponding residuals are positive, and others are below the line with negative residuals, if we were to add the residuals, the positive and negative values would cancel each other out. We overcome this difficulty by determining a and b in such a way that the sum of the

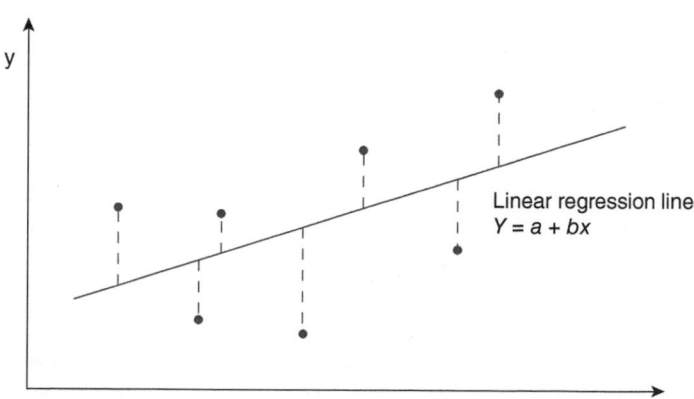

Linear regression line
$Y = a + bx$

Figure 10.4 Scatter diagram showing the fitted regression line (solid line) and residuals (dashed lines).

squared deviations is as small as possible (i.e. is minimized). Remember, the square of both negative and positive numbers is always positive. Hence the terminology, the **method of least squares**, to describe the technique for estimating α and β.

We generally do not need to concern ourselves with the formulae for calculating a and b since we will probably use the computer or the appropriate function buttons on a calculator. However, if we have to resort to hand calculations, the minimization procedure produces the following statistics

$$b = \frac{\sum(x - \bar{x})(y - \bar{y})}{\sum(x - \bar{x})^2} \quad \text{and} \quad a = \bar{y} - b\bar{x}$$

Then we estimate the best fitting line, called the **regression equation of y on x**, from our sample of observations as

$$Y = a + bx$$

where (Figure 10.5):

- Y is the estimated predicted (fitted) or mean value of y for a given value of x.

- a is the estimated intercept of the line.
- b is the estimated slope.

We can *draw* the line on the scatter diagram by hand if we choose two or, preferably (just to play safe), three values of x along the range of values of x. By substituting these values of x in the equation of the line, we can calculate the corresponding predicted Y values. We plot these points on the scatter diagram and join them by a straight line. *The line must **not** be extrapolated beyond the limits of the data.*

10.4.2 Example

It is necessary from time to time to estimate the body weight of sheep; for example, for accurate drug dosing or for predicting market dates. Unfortunately, weighing sheep is difficult, so it is helpful to be able to estimate the sheep's weight from some other, more easily obtained, measure. A study was conducted to investigate the relationship between the sheep's live weight and its chest girth. Table 10.2 shows the measurements of a random sample of 66 sheep studied whose chest girth lay between 60 and 90 cm (based on data from Warriss and Edwards, 1995). Figure 10.6a is a scatter diagram that shows the relationship between the live weight (kg) and

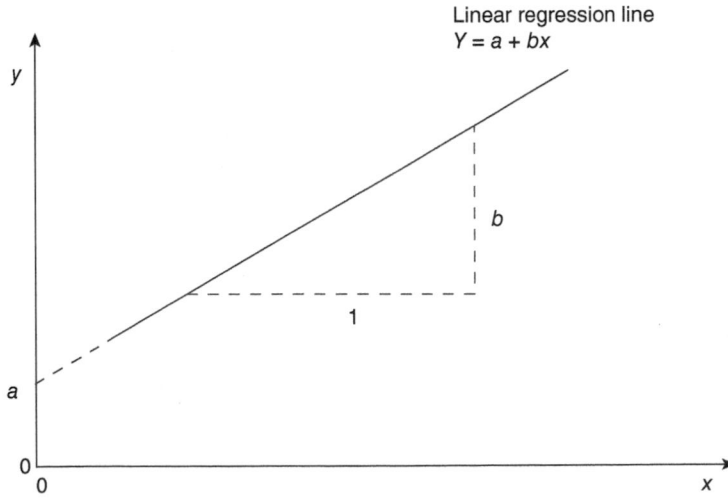

Figure 10.5 Estimated linear regression line showing the intercept, a, and the slope, b.

LW	CG	LW	CG	LW	CG	LW	CG	LW	CG	LW	CG
30	76	20	63	28	77	29	73	18	62	19	67
24	71	28	70	25	71	30	74	28	70	27	69
20	63	22	65	27	72	21	64	27	71	31	74
25	69	28	72	28	74	28	74	30	73	23	67
25	67	25	67	25	65	48	89	28	72	22	63
19	62	20	62	20	64	17	60	22	69	35	75
35	77	35	78	35	78	46	86	48	90	44	84
37	84	43	81	32	73	43	84	31	73	31	73
39	78	36	81	33	80	44	82	39	80	45	86
43	88	41	87	36	82	43	80	33	79	35	78
38	78	36	76	35	74	39	81	34	74	39	76

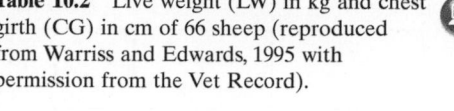

Table 10.2 Live weight (LW) in kg and chest girth (CG) in cm of 66 sheep (reproduced from Warriss and Edwards, 1995 with permission from the Vet Record).

(a)

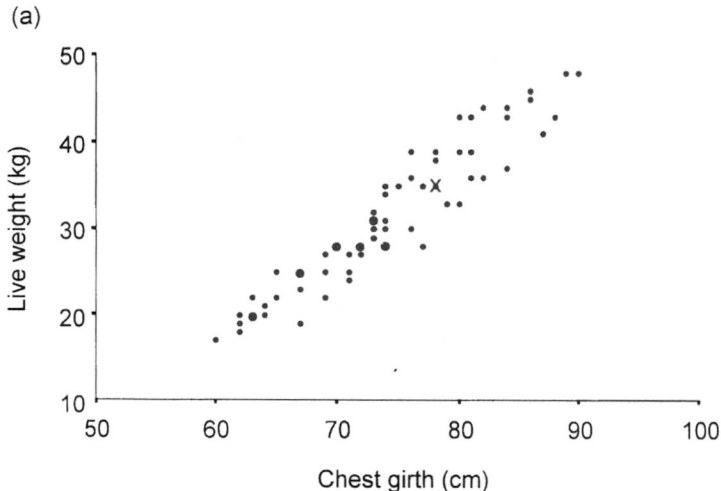

(b)

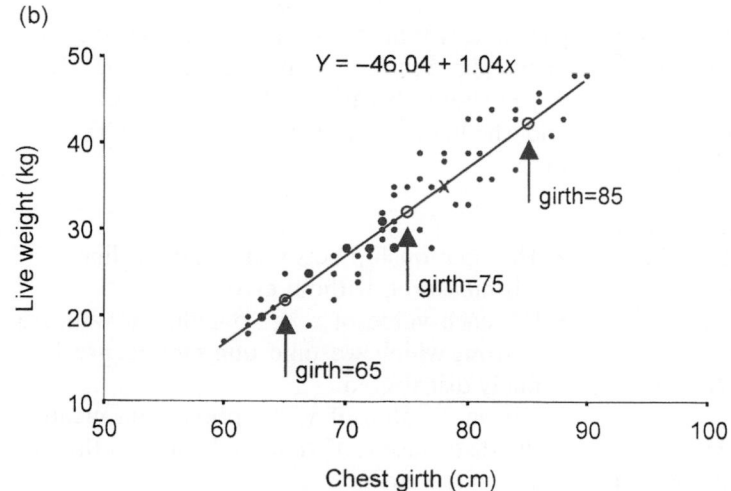

$Y = -46.04 + 1.04x$

Figure 10.6 Scatter diagram of (a) sheep chest girth and live weight, and (b) the same data with a fitted regression line as discussed in Section 10.4.2. A large solid circle (•) shows duplicate points, a cross (×) shows triplicate points and an open circle (o) shows a calculated point (reproduced from Warriss and Edwards, 1995 with permission from the Vet Record).

ANOVA

	Sum of squares	df	Mean square	F	Sig.
Regression	3972.930	1	3972.930	562.113	0.000*
Residual	452.342	64	7.068		
Total	4425.272	65			

Predictors: (Constant), CHESTGTH.
Dependent variable: LIVEWT.
*Indicates $P < 0.001$.

Coefficients

	Coefficients				95% confidence interval for B	
	B	Std error	t	Sig.	Lower bound	Upper bound
(Constant)	−46.04	3.281	−14.03	0.000*	−52.60	−39.48
CHESTGTH	1.04	0.044	23.64	0.000*	0.95	1.13

Dependent variable: LIVEWT.
Note that the entries for B in the penultimate and final rows of the table represent the intercept, a, and the slope, b, in the estimated regression equation. Coefficients (and CI) are corrected to two decimal places.
*Indicates $P < 0.001$.

Display 10.1 SPSS computer output for the simple linear regression analysis of the sheep girth data described in Table 10.2.

chest girth (cm) in the 66 sheep. The estimated regression equation of live weight (y) on chest girth (x) is shown by a computer analysis (Display 10.1) to be

$$Y = -46.04 + 1.04x$$

The estimated slope indicates that a sheep's live weight increases on average by 1.04 kg as its chest girth increases by 1 cm. This estimated regression line is valid only in the specified range of values of chest girth (i.e. 60–90 cm) and should not be extrapolated beyond these limits. We have drawn the line by substituting three values of chest girth (65, 75 and 85 cm) into the equation to obtain the three corresponding values of live weight (21.56, 31.96 and 42.36 kg, respectively), plotting these points and joining them (Figure 10.6b).

10.4.3 Regression diagnostics

Regression diagnostics are the procedures that we use to check the underlying assumptions of a regression analysis and to assess the influence exerted by particular points on the estimated parameters.

(a) What are the assumptions?

Before you go on to make inferences about the parameters that define the regression equation, or use the equation to predict values of y from x, you should be aware of the assumptions that underlie linear regression (Figure 10.7). They are that:

- The relationship between x and y is linear.
- x is measured without error.
- For each value of x, the population values of y, from which we take our sample, are Normally distributed.
- For each value of x, the population mean of the distribution of values of y lies on the line, $Y_{pop} = \alpha + \beta x$.

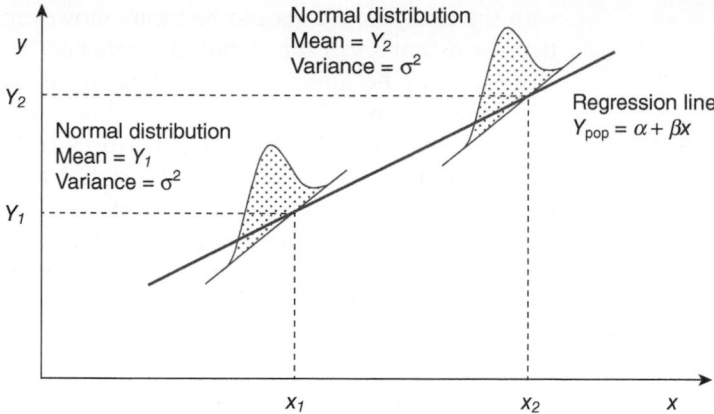

Figure 10.7 Diagram illustrating assumptions underlying regression analysis.

- The population variance of the distribution of values of y is constant for each value of x.
- The observations are independent; this implies that each individual is represented once in the random sample.

(b) How do we check the assumptions?

It is essential to check the underlying assumptions in linear regression analysis; this is an often overlooked process. Although we can sometimes get an indication of whether the assumptions are satisfied by plotting the data and drawing the best fitting line, the most efficient approach is to study the *residuals*. Remember, for each value of x, the residual is the difference between its observed and predicted values of y. We can only obtain the residuals once we have estimated the parameters of the line using the sample data. You may have to request the residuals from your computer package, although many packages produce them automatically.

If the assumptions underlying linear regression are satisfied, then, in addition to the requirements that *x is a variable measured without error* and the *observations are independent, the residuals are Normally distributed with a mean of zero, and their variability is constant throughout the range of the fitted values of y*. We can check assumptions by producing appropriate plots of the residuals. In particular, using the sheep girth data discussed in Section 10.4.2 for illustrative purposes, we can verify that:

- *The relationship between x and y is linear* by plotting the residuals against the values of x. If the relationship between x and y is linear, the residuals should be randomly scattered around zero, and there should be no apparent trend in the residuals for increasing or decreasing values of x (Figure 10.8a). Alternatively, we can simply plot y against x and observe whether the approximating curve is a straight line.
- *The residuals are Normally distributed* by producing either a histogram or a Normal plot (see Section 3.5.3(e)) of the residuals (Figure 10.8b).
- *The variability of the residuals is constant throughout the range of fitted values of y* by plotting the residuals against the fitted values. If the assumption is satisfied, we should expect a random scatter of residuals (Figure 10.8c). If we can discern a funnel or cone effect, with the variability of the residuals appearing to increase (or decrease) with increasing fitted values, then the constant variance assumption is not satisfied.

(c) What do we do if the assumptions are not satisfied?

The linearity and independence assumptions are the most crucial. Sometimes a simple transformation of x or y will achieve linearity (see Section 13.2.2). If the linearity assumption is in doubt, we may decide that another form of relationship, such as a quadratic, is more appropriate

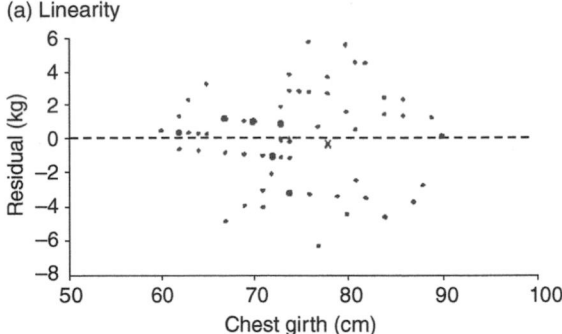

(a) Linearity

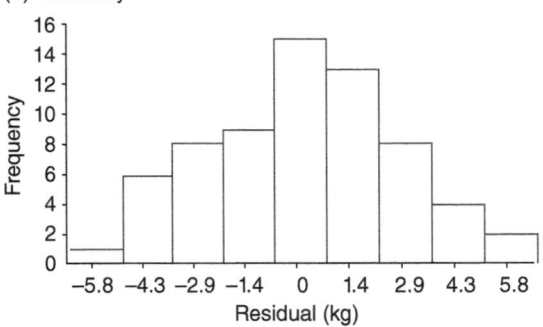

(b) Normality

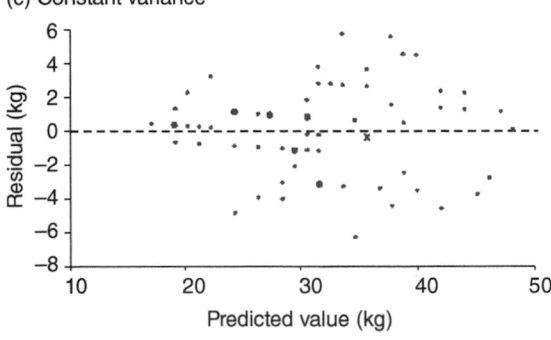

(c) Constant variance

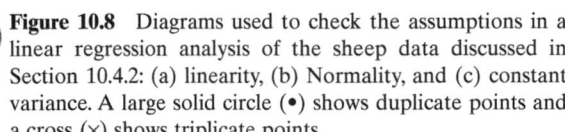

Figure 10.8 Diagrams used to check the assumptions in a linear regression analysis of the sheep data discussed in Section 10.4.2: (a) linearity, (b) Normality, and (c) constant variance. A large solid circle (•) shows duplicate points and a cross (×) shows triplicate points.

than a straight line (see Section 11.3.1(d)). A simple linear regression analysis would then be inappropriate.

If the residuals are not Normally distributed and/or do not have constant variance, we have two choices. Provided there are only moderate departures from the assumptions, we can proceed

with the analysis. We should be aware, however, that the estimates of the standard errors and the *P*-values may be affected by a failure to satisfy the assumptions. Alternatively, and this is the only option if there are gross departures from the assumptions, we take an appropriate transformation (see Section 13.2), either of *x* or of *y* or of both of them. For example, we often find that a logarithmic transformation of the *x* variable is suitable. We then repeat the analysis by calculating another regression line of *y* on the transformed *x*, and check that the assumptions underlying this new line are satisfied.

(d) Identifying outliers and influential points

An **outlier** is an observation that does not belong to the main body of the data. Such an observation may adversely affect the validity of the assumptions underlying a regression analysis. If the outlier is an **influential point**, then it has a large effect on one or more of the estimates of the regression parameters and/or their standard errors. We can establish whether or not a point is influential by estimating the regression parameters both with and without the point, and observing the effect, if any, on each of the estimates. This is a form of **sensitivity analysis** in that we are assessing how sensitive our **linear regression equation** is to individual observations.

We may be able to identify an outlier if it has one or both of the following:

- A **large residual**, the residual being the difference between the observed and predicted values of the outcome variable, *y*, for that individual. We can use the residual plots described in Section 10.4.3(b) to identify outliers.
- **High leverage**, which implies that an individual's value of *x* for a particular value of *y* is a long way from the mean of the *x* values. It is suggested that any point which has a leverage greater than 4/*n*, where *n* is the number of pairs of observations in the sample, is regarded as having high leverage (being disparate from the mean leverage of 2/*n*) and should be investigated.

In addition, there are a number of statistics that provide an overall measure of influence for each point. One of the most well known of these is **Cook's distance** which yields, for each point, a standardized measure of the change in the parameters of the regression equation if the particular point were omitted. If Cook's distance is greater than one, the associated point should be scrutinized as it may well be influential. Comprehensive statistical software will provide output containing the residual, leverage and Cook's distance for each point, so that we can examine them and investigate points that are flagged by these measures.

10.4.4 Residual variance and the ANOVA table

Corresponding to each observation is a residual, which is the difference between the observed value of y and its estimated predicted or fitted value, Y, where $Y = a + bx$. The variance of the residuals is estimated in a sample of size n by

$$s_{res}^2 = \frac{\sum (y - Y)^2}{(n - 2)}$$

and is usually called the **residual mean square** or the **residual variance**. The residual variance is incorporated into the formulae used for testing hypotheses about the parameters of the line and for calculating confidence intervals.

Instead of determining the residual variance using the formula given by s_{res}^2, we can use the residual mean square in the computer-generated **analysis of variance (ANOVA) table** (see Section 8.5.2).

Justification

In the ANOVA table for linear regression analysis, the total variation of y is partitioned into two components: the variation that is *explained* by the linear relationship of y on x, and the *residual variation* that is *unexplained* by the relationship. To understand this dichotomy, consider what happens if there is a perfect positive relationship between x and y; then every point lies on the line, and all the variation in y is explained by the relationship. This is an ideal circumstance; more usually, y tends to increase as x increases.

Thus, only some of the variation in y occurs because of the relationship between y and x, and this is the variation explained by the relationship. The remainder of the variation in y, that which is left over or residual, is unexplained by the relationship. Since the mean squares in an ANOVA table represent variances, the *residual variance is the mean square of the source of variation that is unexplained by the regression.*

The source of variation in the ANOVA table that is explained by the regression is sometimes called that which is *due to regression, explained by regression* or simply *regression*; the source of variation that is unexplained by the regression is sometimes called that which is *unexplained* or *residual*. We show the ANOVA results for the sheep girth data in the ANOVA table in Display 10.1. From this table, we can see that the residual variance is estimated as 7.068 kg². □

10.4.5 Assessing goodness-of-fit

The usual way of establishing whether the line is a good fit is to determine the proportion of the total variation in y which is explained by the linear relationship of y on x; it is often denoted by R^2 and is sometimes called the **coefficient of determination**. This proportion is the sum of squares explained by the regression divided by the total sum of squares, both sums of squares being obtained from the ANOVA table. *In simple linear regression, it is the square of the correlation coefficient, r^2* (see Section 10.3.2(c)).

In the ANOVA table in Display 10.1, the proportion of the variation explained by the regression is (3972.930)/(4425.272) = 0.898. Thus, approximately 90% of variation in the sheep's live weight is explained by its linear relationship with chest girth; this indicates that the line is a good fit in the specified range. Note that the estimated correlation coefficient between the sheep's live weight and chest girth is the square root of this quantity, i.e. $r = \sqrt{0.898} = 0.95$.

10.4.6 Investigating the slope

(a) Approach

Once we have determined the equation of the best fitting line, we usually proceed to investigate the parameters that define the line. Invariably, our primary interest lies with the slope of the line. The slope shows by how much y changes on average as we increase x by one unit. If there is no linear relationship between x and y, then as we increase x by one unit, the value of y is equally likely to increase or decrease, i.e. its average is zero. Thus, we can test the null hypothesis that the true slope, β, is zero if we want to decide whether or not a linear relationship exists. The approach is:

1. Specify the **null hypothesis** that the true slope, β, is zero. Specify the alternative hypothesis, generally, that the slope is not equal to zero.
2. **Collect** the data and **display** them in a scatter diagram. Determine the best fitting line, $Y = a + bx$, where Y is the estimated fitted value corresponding to a given value of x, and the statistics, a and b, estimate the parameters, α and β, respectively. Check the assumptions underlying linear regression by studying the residuals (see Section 10.4.3).
3. Select the **appropriate test** on the computer or calculate the **test statistic** by hand. This test statistic follows the t-distribution and is given by

$$Test_{11} = \frac{b}{SE(b)} \text{ with } n - 2 \text{ degrees of freedom}$$

where $SE(b) = \dfrac{s_{res}}{\sqrt{\sum(x - \bar{x})^2}}$, and s_{res} is the standard deviation of the residuals.

The alternative approach is to refer to the ANOVA table in regression analysis (see Section 10.4.3) which is used to test the same null hypothesis, namely that β is zero. Then the test statistic is the F-ratio which is the 'due to regression' mean square divided by the residual mean square; it follows the F-distribution with 1 degree of freedom in the numerator and $n - 2$ degrees of freedom in the denominator. Note that the two tests produce the same P-value since the square of $Test_{11}$ is equal to the statistic derived from the ANOVA table.

4. Determine the **P-value**. Usually the computer will do this for you. Alternatively, you can refer your test statistic to the table of the t-distribution (see Table A.3) or F-distribution (see Table A.5), as appropriate.

5. Make a **decision** whether or not to reject the null hypothesis; usually, but not necessarily, reject H_0 if $P < 0.05$. Note that when there is no linear relationship between the two variables, both the slope, β, and the correlation coefficient, ρ, are equal to zero.
6. Derive the **confidence interval** for the true slope, β. If the computer output does not contain this information, you can calculate the 95% confidence interval as

$$b \pm t_{0.05} \, SE(b)$$

where $t_{0.05}$ is the critical value or percentage point (giving a tail area probability of 0.025 in each tail) obtained from the table of the t-distribution with $n - 2$ degrees of freedom, and $SE(b) = s_{res} / \sqrt{\sum(x - \bar{x})^2}$.

(b) Example

In the sheep girth example of Section 10.4.2:

1. The null hypothesis is that the true slope, β, of the linear regression of live weight on chest girth is zero. The alternative hypothesis is that it is not zero.
2. The data are displayed in Figure 10.6b in which the best fitting line, $Y = -46.04 + 1.04x$, is drawn. The assumptions underlying the regression analysis have been investigated in Section 10.4.3 by studying the residuals displayed in Figure 10.8, and are valid.
3. A typical computer output which shows both the estimated regression coefficients and the test statistic (equal to $(1.043)/(0.044) = 23.70$) is shown in the Coefficients table in Display 10.1. Note that we could also use the F-ratio in the ANOVA table in Display 10.1, which has a value of 562.11, to test the null hypothesis. Apart from rounding errors, $t^2 = F$.
4. The P-value (i.e. Sig. = 0.000) from the computer output in both the ANOVA table and the Coefficients table in Display 10.1 indicates that $P < 0.001$. We could obtain this P-value by referring the value of 23.64 to Table A.3 of the t-distribution with 64 degrees of freedom (df), or the value of 562.11 to Table A.5a of

the *F*-distribution with 1 *df* in the numerator and 64 *df* in the denominator.

5. The data do not appear to be consistent with the null hypothesis ($P < 0.001$), which we therefore reject. We have evidence which indicates that the true slope of the line is not equal to zero.

6. The 95% confidence interval for the true slope, shown in Display 10.1, is from 0.95 to 1.13 kg/cm. We can calculate it as

$$1.04 \pm 2.00 \times 0.044$$

where the value 2.00 is the approximate percentage point from the *t*-distribution (see Table A.3) with $66 - 2 = 64$ *df*. This confidence interval excludes zero, as expected, since the slope is significantly different from zero.

10.4.7 Predicting *y* from a given *x*

We often use the regression line, once we have established that there is a linear relationship between *x* and *y* (i.e. that the slope is significantly different from zero), to **predict the mean value of** *y* that we expect for individuals or animals who have a specified value of *x*, say x_1. To obtain the predicted value is straightforward; we substitute the value of *x* in the equation, $Y = a + bx$, so that our estimated mean predicted value is $Y_1 = a + bx_1$. In the sheep girth example of Section 10.4.2, we predict that sheep which have a chest

girth of 73.2 cm would be expected on average to weigh 30.09 kg (i.e. if $x_1 = 73.2$, $Y_1 = -46.04 + 1.04 \times 73.2 = 30.09$).

We have to recognize, however, that because we only have a sample of observations, there is sampling error associated with this estimated mean predicted value. It is possible to quantify the error and therefore calculate a confidence interval for the mean predicted value. The formulae are not easy and we refer you to Armitage *et al.* (2002) for details.

Sometimes we wish to determine a region, over the range of values of *x*, within which we expect the *true regression line* to lie with a certain probability (say, 0.95). This **confidence band, region or interval for the line** is obtained, usually on the computer, by determining the 95% confidence intervals for the mean predicted values of *y* for various values of *x*. Each confidence interval has an upper limit above the regression line, and a lower limit below the regression line. The required band is obtained by connecting all the upper limits and, similarly, all the lower limits (Figure 10.9). The confidence band is generally narrower in the middle of the range of values of *x* than at the extremes, reflecting the fact that we have less confidence in the prediction of the mean of the *y*-values as we move towards the extremes.

It may be that you see a wider band illustrated (Figure 10.9). This relates to the scatter of the data points and is the region that contains

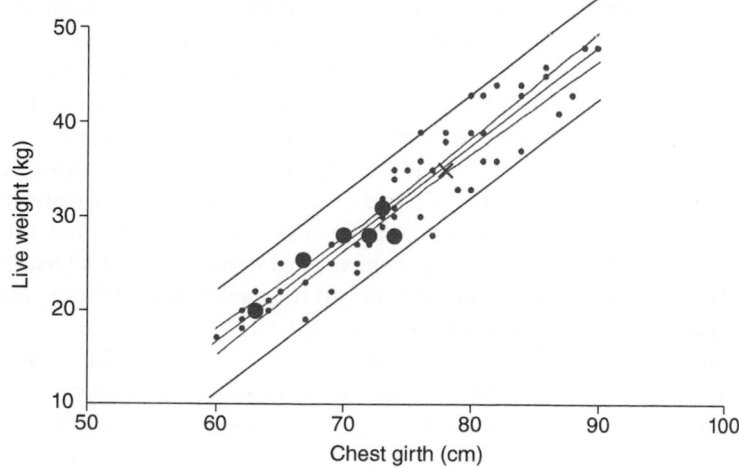

Figure 10.9 Ninety-five per cent confidence limits for the regression line (the inner limits on either side of the regression line) and the individual points (the outer limits). A large solid circle (•) shows duplicate points and a cross (×) shows triplicate points. (Data from Table 10.2.)

approximately 95% of the *individual population values* (for a 95% confidence band).

10.5 Regression to the mean

The concept of **regression to the mean** derives from Sir Francis Galton's studies of inheritance in 1889. He observed that, in many instances, although one might expect that sons would inherit the characteristics of their fathers, the measurements on sons tend to be closer to those of the general population of men than to those of their fathers. This phenomenon can be demonstrated by considering the relationship between a man's height and his son's height. Although, as we would expect, tall fathers tend to have tall sons, when we look at the heights of the sons of tall fathers, they are, *on average*, less than those of their fathers. There is a regression, or going back, of the sons' heights towards the average heights of all men. The regression coefficient, when we regress the son's height on the father's height, is substantially less than one. It is important to recognize that the regression to the mean height does not relate to a particular son, but rather to the whole group of sons.

Another instance in which regression to the mean can be demonstrated is when a variable is measured on two occasions on every animal in a group. For example, suppose we want to investigate the effects of a beta-blocking agent on tachycardia (elevated heart rate) in cats. We select for our trial a group of cats whose resting heart rates are all above the upper limit of normal, i.e. above 180 beats/min. Were we to record their heart rates a second time, *before* treatment, we should most likely find that their average heart rate was lower than before, perhaps even within the reference range; this is due to regression to the mean. However, if, unaware of this phenomenon, we had treated the animals and then measured their heart rates, we could falsely attribute the decrease in heart rate to the action of the drug. Regression to the mean is therefore especially relevant in screening procedures. A way of dealing with regression to the mean in such circumstances is to ensure that sufficient measurements are taken on each animal to obtain a true reflection of its condition.

Exercises

The statements in questions 10.1 and 10.2 are either TRUE or FALSE.

10.1 Pearson's correlation coefficient:
(a) Must always be positive.
(b) Cannot be calculated if at least one of the two variables is not Normally distributed.
(c) Measures how well a straight line describes the relationship between two variables.
(d) Is zero if there is no relationship between the two variables.
(e) Measures the average change in one variable for a unit increase in the other.

10.2 A simple linear regression equation:
(a) Measures the degree of the relationship between two variables.
(b) Predicts the dependent variable from the independent variable.
(c) Describes the straight line relationship between two variables.
(d) Assumes that both of the variables are Normally distributed.
(e) Makes no distinction between the two variables.

10.3 Lake *et al.* (unpublished data) obtained blood samples on a random sample of 124 donkeys in the Ngamiland area of Botswana, some of which were suffering from dourine, a venereal disease of Equidae caused by *Trypanosoma equiperda*. The researchers were interested to know whether the enzyme-linked immunoadsorbent assay (ELISA) and complement fixation test (CFT) results on these donkeys were associated, and whether it would be possible to describe a linear relationship between them. High values of both CFT and ELISA are indicative of dourine. The output for the regression analysis that they performed is shown in Figure 10.10 and Display 10.2. Use this output to answer, with full explanations, the following questions.
(a) Do you think, by examining the scatter plot (Figure 10.10a), that it is reasonable to assume a linear relationship between CFT and ELISA?

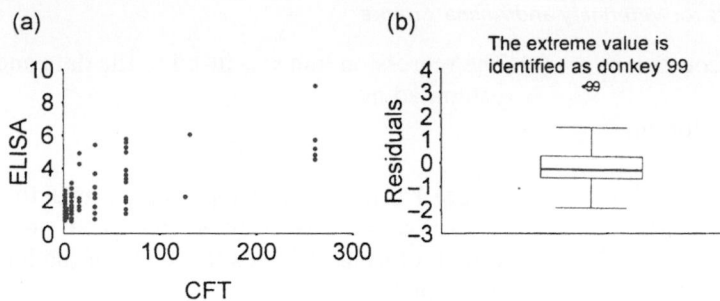

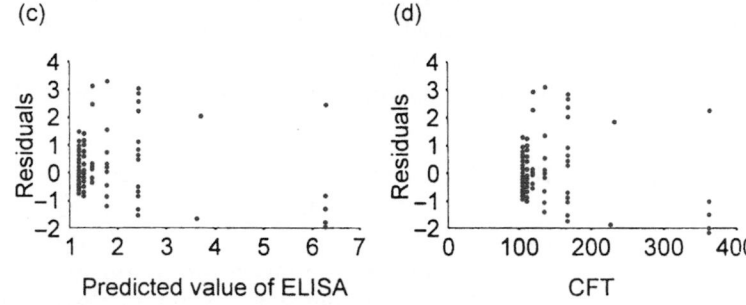

Figure 10.10 Diagrams for checking the assumptions of linear regression analysis of data relating to a complement fixation test and an ELISA test for dourine infection (data described in Exercise 10.3 from Lake *et al.*, unpublished).

Display 10.2 SPSS computer output of data described in Exercise 10.3 and Figure 10.10a.

Model summary*

Model	R	R square	Adjusted R square	Std. error of the estimate
1	0.737[†]	0.543	0.539	0.974267

*Dependent variable: ELISA.
[†] Predictors: (Constant), CFT.

ANOVA*

Model		Sum of squares	df	Mean square	F	Sig.
1	Regression	137.467	1	137.467	144.824	0.000[†,‡]
	Residual	115.802	122	0.949		
	Total	253.269	123			

*Dependent variable: ELISA.
[†] Predictors: (Constant), CFT.
[‡] Indicates $P < 0.001$.

Coefficients*

Model		Coefficients				95% confidence interval for B	
		B	Std error	t	Sig.	Lower bound	Upper bound
1	(Constant)	1.207	0.096	12.513	0.000[‡]	1.016	1.398
	CFT	1.982E-02	0.002	12.034	0.000[‡]	0.017	0.023

*Dependent variable: ELISA.
[‡] Indicates $P < 0.001$.
E-02 means $\times 10^{-2}$.

(b) What is the estimated correlation coefficient between CFT and ELISA?
(c) What is the estimated linear regression line?
(d) Is the regression line a good fit?
(e) Are the assumptions underlying the regression analysis satisfied (Figure 10.10b–d)?
(f) What can you conclude from the results of the ANOVA table?
(g) Interpret the slope of the linear regression line.
(h) Is the slope of the regression line significantly different from zero?

10.4 Several disease states in dogs lead to alterations of the thickness of the gastric rugal folds. However, there may be a relationship between rugal fold thickness and body size, and this must be investigated before rugal fold thickness can be used as a determinant of disease. Jakovljevic and Gibbs (1993) studied 29 dogs without known gastric lesions. The measurements (in mm) of the dogs' mucosal folds were determined radiographically and then related to their body weights (kg). The correlation coefficient between rugal fold thickness and body weight was 0.71 ($P < 0.001$).
(a) Explain what the correlation coefficient is measuring.
(b) What does the *P*-value tell you?

(c) The regression line was fitted to the data and estimated as

$$Y = 2.064 + 0.069x$$

where Y is the estimated predicted rugal fold thickness and x is body weight. What additional information does the slope of the line give you?
(d) What fraction of the total variability of rugal fold thickness (y) is explained by the dog's body weight (x)?
(e) What do you conclude from your answer to (d)?

10.5 The number of cases of lameness in cattle in relation to fortnightly rainfall (mm) was recorded on a farm in England in 1977 (quoted in Thrusfield, 2005, and used with permission). It was of interest to determine whether there was a linear relationship between the two variables. The SPSS computer output of a linear regression analysis of the data is shown in Display 10.3.
(a) What is the correlation coefficient between the number of lameness episodes and the amount of rainfall in a fortnight?
(b) In the regression analysis, which is the outcome variable and which is the explanatory variable? Why were they chosen in this way?

Model summary

Model	R	R square	Adjusted R square	Std. error of the estimate
1	0.158(a)	0.025	−0.016	14.04089

(a) Predictors: (Constant), rainfall.

Display 10.3 SPSS output for data described in Exercise 10.5.

Coefficients[a]

Model	Coefficients B	Std error	t	Sig.	95% confidence interval for B Lower bound	Upper bound
1 (Constant)	31.235	4.878	6.403	0.000[‡]	21.167	41.303
Rainfall	0.081	0.103	0.782	0.442	−0.133	0.294

[a] Dependent variable: lameness.
[‡] Indicates $P < 0.001$.

(c) What is the estimated linear regression equation?

(d) Interpret both the estimated slope of this line and its associated confidence interval.

(e) What is the null hypothesis that relates to the slope? What are the test statistic and the P-value for the test of this null hypothesis? What do you conclude from this result?

(f) Does the regression line fit the data well? Explain your answer.

10.6 Approximately 80% of the avian biomass (the total living biological material of a biological community or group in a given area) in the Antarctic region is composed of Macaroni penguins (*Eudyptes chrysolophus*), which are thought to be significant consumers of the marine food resources required by several species including the Antarctic fur seal (*Arctocephalus gazella*). Investigators were interested in knowing whether there was a linear relationship between the heart rate (beats/min) of a Macaroni penguin and its metabolic rate (i.e. the mass-specific rate of oxygen consumption in ml/min/kg). If there was, they hoped to provide estimates of energy expenditure that could give the investigators an indication of food consumption. They analysed the data from each of 24 penguins which were exercised on a variable speed treadmill. The estimated correlation coefficient (based on Green *et al.*, 2001) for one of the penguins whose heart rate lay in the range 125–225 beats/min was 0.904 ($P < 0.001$).

(a) What are the units of measurement of the correlation coefficient?

(b) In general, what happens to the penguin's rate of oxygen consumption as its heart rate increases?

(c) What is the null hypothesis that relates to the P-value that has been provided?

(d) Interpret the 95% confidence interval for the correlation coefficient which is estimated as being from 0.703 to 0.971. (For practice, you could calculate this 95% confidence interval using the formula in Section 10.3.2(b).)

(e) How much of the variation in oxygen consumption can be attributed to its linear relationship with heart rate?

(f) What assumption(s) is(are) made in performing the hypothesis test for the Pearson correlation coefficient?

(g) What effect on the correlation coefficient would you expect to observe if the range of values of the heart rate was greater than 125–225 beats/min?

10.7 The following summarizes the results of a study (based on Chiappe *et al.*, 1999) to assess the potential values of free serum osteocalcin or bone Gla protein (BGP) to reflect changes of bone turnover in Thoroughbred horses. Levels of osteocalcin were analysed in serum samples of 54 clinically normal animals aged between 8 and 36 months. Serum BGP was measured by an in-house-developed double antibody radioimmunoassay using bovine antigen. Differences between males and females were found to be significant in horses aged between 24 and 36 months, with higher values in females of 18.75 ± 5.00 ng/ml against 14.43 ± 10.47 ng/ml in the males. Correlation coefficients between age and serum BGP were $r = -0.598$ ($P < 0.001$) for males and $r = -0.807$ ($P < 0.001$) for females. A significant negative relationship could be established between these two parameters in males during the growth period. The regression equation between serum BGP (ng/ml) and age (months) for males was age $= 65.14 - 1.68$ BGP.

(a) Criticize the following statement with respect to its statistical content: 'Differences between males and females were found to be significant in horses aged between 24 and 36 months, with higher values in females of 18.75 ± 5.00 ng/ml against 14.43 ± 10.47 ng/ml in the males'. You should be able to list at least three mistakes or omissions.

(b) Criticize the regression equation quoted in the last sentence before (a).

(c) Explain what -1.68 is in the regression equation, and interpret its meaning.

(d) According to the estimated regression, a horse that has BGP $= 0$ ng/ml will be aged 65.14 months. This does not make any sense because a horse will never have BGP $= 0$ ng/ml – comment.

11 Further regression analyses

11.1 Learning objectives

By the end of this chapter you should be able to:

- Explain the difference between a univariable and a multivariable regression model.
- Explain the reasons for performing a multiple linear regression analysis.
- Describe how to choose which explanatory variables to include in a multiple regression model and how to code these variables if they are categorical.
- Explain how to centre and scale an explanatory variable and what is achieved by doing so.
- Explain when and how to include an interaction term in a multiple regression analysis.
- Conduct a valid multiple linear regression analysis, given the appropriate computer software.
- Test the assumptions underlying a multiple linear regression analysis.
- Explain the principles of maximum likelihood estimation.
- Identify a generalized linear model.
- Explain the circumstances in which a multivariable logistic regression analysis is indicated.
- Interpret the output from a logistic regression analysis.
- Explain the circumstances in which a Poisson regression analysis is indicated.
- Interpret the output from a Poisson regression analysis.
- Distinguish between various regression methods for analysing clustered data.

11.2 Introduction

In the last chapter we introduced you to the concepts involved in univariable (i.e. simple) linear regression where a numerical outcome variable is linearly related to a numerical explanatory variable. The regression equation describing the relationship defines a particular mathematical model which, as we explained in Chapter 10, is a simplified representation of a real-world situation or process that occurs in the population. This simple univariable model can be extended in a number of ways. For example, we may include more than one explanatory variable, either numerical or categorical, in the model. Strictly, it is then a multivariable regression model although it is more commonly referred to as a multiple regression model. Furthermore, we may have an outcome variable that is not numerical.

Such models often conform to the unified framework of a generalized linear model (GLM). In this chapter, we introduce you to the concepts underlying this type of model and to maximum likelihood estimation, which is the process generally used to estimate the parameters of the GLM. This is a growing area of statistics created not necessarily by more complex study designs, but by the ready availability of computer software which makes tackling such analyses within the scope of many more people. What follows is an introduction to the common models, and an indication of how they can be analysed. There are many issues that need to be considered in these

Statistics for Veterinary and Animal Science, Third Edition. Aviva Petrie and Paul Watson.
© 2013 John Wiley & Sons, Ltd. Published 2013 by John Wiley & Sons, Ltd.

analyses, and you should therefore consider seeking expert statistical advice if you are to embark on them yourself.

11.3 Multiple (multivariable) linear regression

11.3.1 Multiple linear regression equation

(a) Explanation

Section 10.4 was concerned with the linear relationship of a dependent variable, y, and a *single* independent variable, x. Very often we are interested in investigating the *simultaneous* effect of a *number of factors* on a response variable when we believe these factors may be interrelated. For example, Pearson and Ouassat (1996) found that, by using several variables rather than just one variable, they could get an improved estimate of the body weight of donkeys (see Section 11.3.5). We can extend the simple (univariable) linear regression equation, and form a **multiple linear regression equation** (since there is more than one explanatory variable in the equation, this is a type of **multivariable regression analysis**) to accommodate this situation. If there are k *independent*, *predictor* or *explanatory* variables, sometimes called *covariates*, $x_1, x_2, x_3, \ldots x_k$, which we believe may have an effect on a numerical *dependent* or *response* variable, y, the true regression model may be expressed as

$$Y_{\text{pop}} = \alpha + \beta_1 x_1 + \beta_2 x_2 + \beta_3 x_3 + \ldots + \beta_k x_k$$

where x_i is the ith predictor variable ($i = 1, 2, 3, \ldots, k$) measured on each individual; Y_{pop} is the predicted, fitted, expected or mean value of y in the population for the set of covariates; α is a constant term representing the mean value of y when all the explanatory variables are zero; and $\beta_1, \beta_2, \beta_3, \ldots, \beta_k$ are the **partial regression coefficients**, often simply called **regression coefficients**, corresponding to the k explanatory variables.

Then β_1 *represents the mean change in y for a unit change in x_1, when the other explanatory variables, $x_2, x_3, \ldots, x_k$, are held constant, i.e. after controlling for these variables.* A similar interpretation is afforded the other partial regression coefficients. The partial regression coefficients are obtained by the method of least squares, i.e. minimizing the sum of the squared residuals (a residual being the difference between an observed and a fitted value of y), as in univariable regression. The regression coefficients are estimated in the sample by $b_1, b_2, b_3, \ldots, b_k$, respectively, and α is estimated by a. The estimated regression line is thus

$$Y = a + b_1 x_1 + b_2 x_2 + b_3 x_3 + \ldots + b_k x_k$$

where Y is the estimated mean value of y.

We do not feel that it is necessary to give the formulae for estimating the coefficients or their standard errors since, invariably, you will use the computer to perform a multiple regression analysis. We outline the procedures involved, noting the similarity to simple linear regression and laying emphasis on the underlying concepts. You can obtain details of the analysis, and of the modifications to multiple regression, in more advanced texts such as Allen (1997), Draper and Smith (1998) and Kleinbaum *et al.* (2008).

(b) Uses

The main reasons for performing a multiple regression analysis are:

- To determine which explanatory variables are important predictors of the outcome variable, and the extent to which they influence the outcome variable.
- To be able to study the relationship between the outcome variable and each of the explanatory variables whilst controlling for the effect of the other explanatory variables in the equation.
- To predict the value of the outcome variable from the explanatory variables, using the optimal equation which relates y to the x values.

As we pointed out in Section 8.5.3, we can use multiple regression methodology instead of analysis of variance (ANOVA) techniques to compare means in different groups. If there are various categorical factors of interest, each of them is incorporated into the regression model as an explanatory variable, using the appropriate coding. For example, in the simple situation where we have 'treatment' as the only factor of interest, instead of performing a one-way ANOVA (see Section 8.6) to compare the mean response on two different treatments, A and B, we take 'treatment' as the explanatory variable in a regression model. We assign a code to 'treatment', so that its value for animals on treatment A, say, is 0 and its value for animals on treatment B is 1. The 'treatment' regression coefficient is interpreted as the difference in the mean responses between treatments A and B. If it is significantly different from zero, the mean response on A is significantly different from that on B. If it is positive, the mean response on B is greater than that on A (because of the way in which the treatment variable is coded); if it is negative, then the reverse is true. This concept can be extended so that a number of categorical factors are included in a multiple regression model.

Sometimes we use multiple linear regression as a form of **analysis of covariance** (ANCOVA), an extension of ANOVA, when we wish to evaluate the effect of different treatments, say, on a response variable if we believe it is necessary to take into account the effect of one or more explanatory variables (covariates) on response. In addition to adjusting for the effect of covariates which may not be balanced in the treatment groups, ANCOVA increases the precision (and, thereby, the power) of comparisons between groups by accounting for variation in important variables that affect outcome. In ANCOVA, we assume there is no group × covariate interaction (see Section 11.3.1(d)), so the slope of the regression line for a covariate is the same for each treatment. If our focus is in comparing two treatments, A and B, we interpret the 'treatment' coefficient in the multiple regression model as the difference between the mean responses on A and B, after adjusting for the covariates in the model.

(c) Categorical explanatory variables

It is straightforward to include numerical explanatory variables into our model, but we can also perform a multiple regression analysis when one

or more of our explanatory variables is categorical. We tackle the problem by assigning codes to the variable so we are able to distinguish its different categories. In particular, we need to assign two codes to the variable if we have a **binary** explanatory variable. For example, we could assign the codes 0 and 1 to the variable representing 'sex', so that a male takes the value '0' and a female takes the value '1'.

In the situation when a nominal categorical explanatory variable has more than **two** categories, we proceed by creating what are called **dummy** or **indicator variables**, but the approach is not straightforward. Within regression analysis, some computer software has the capability to respond to instructions and create dummy variables. However, if you need to create the dummies yourself, you proceed in the following way. Consider the variable 'treatment' which is a nominal variable comprising three treatments, A, B and C, where C is a control treatment. In order to incorporate 'treatment' into the regression model, you have to create two dummies, i.e. *the number of dummies is one less than the number of categories for that variable*. You choose one of the categories to be the reference category (let us say it is the control treatment, C) and the other categories will be compared with this reference category. For a given individual in the sample, the binary dummy variable that compares A with C is assigned the value 1 if the individual receives A and 0 otherwise; similarly, the binary dummy variable that compares B with C is assigned the value 1 if the individual receives B and 0 otherwise. By default, the individuals receiving C can be identified since they have the value 0 for both of the two binary variables. Then the regression coefficient for the dummy variable that compares A with C represents the difference in the mean values of y between A and C, after adjusting for the other explanatory variables in the model. The use of dummy variables is illustrated in the example described in Section 11.5.3.

If the categorical explanatory variable has more than two categories and is measured on an **ordinal scale**, we can create a series of dummy variables for it, treating the variable as if it were a nominal variable. However, if we want to take the ordering of the categories of the ordinal variable into account, we can assign values to the categories to represent their relative positions on an appropriate scale (typically we assume a linear scale and assign the successive digits, 1, 2, 3, . . . , to the categories) and then treat the variable as a numerical variable.

(d) Modifications

Centring and scaling

In some situations, we can improve the interpretation of the coefficients in a multiple regression equation by **centring** or **scaling** one or more of the explanatory variables. Both of these procedures can be adopted in simple linear regression (see Chapter 10) as well as in multiple linear regression analysis.

We explained in Section 11.3.1(a) that the coefficient for an explanatory variable, x_1, in a multiple regression equation represents the mean change in y for a unit change in x_1 after adjusting for the other explanatory variables (x_2, x_3, . . . , x_k). We also explained that the constant term is the mean value of y when all the explanatory variables are zero, but this is often a value which one or more of the explanatory variables cannot take. Suppose, for example, we are using a multiple regression equation to predict a Shetland pony's body weight (y) in kg from its gender (x_1, coded as 0 for males and 1 for females) and height from the withers (x_2) in cm. The regression coefficient for gender then represents the mean change in body weight for a unit change in gender (i.e. for females compared to males), for a given, but unspecified, value of height. In addition, the intercept is the mean value of weight for male (gender = 0) Shetland ponies of height zero. Clearly, this is nonsensical since the height of a Shetland pony cannot be zero. In fact, let us suppose that in our sample, the range of heights is from 75 to 97 cm, with a mean height of 86 cm. If we subtract the mean height of the sample from the height of each Shetland pony, the mean height of the transformed variable is zero. If we repeat the multiple regression analysis but use our modified value for height, the intercept represents the mean weight of male Shetland ponies at the mean height of the sample, and this is a much more meaningful interpretation. This process

of subtracting a mean (or some other value) from each observed value of an explanatory variable is called **centring**. If chosen carefully, it ensures that the interpretation of the constant term is both meaningful and relevant to the specific research question of interest and, in addition, may go some way to alleviate the problems of multicollinearity (see Section 11.3.2(b)). Note that centring an explanatory variable does not affect the magnitude of the estimated regression coefficient or its standard error, the significance of the regression coefficient or the fit of the regression model. It only affects the estimated intercept of the model.

Scaling an explanatory variable implies dividing or multiplying the value of that variable by a suitable constant to provide a more meaningful interpretation of the regression coefficient. This might be useful if, for example, the height of the Shetland ponies were measured in hands (as in the UK) rather than in centimetres (as in Europe). The coefficient for height in the multiple regression coefficient would represent the mean change in weight (kg) for a 1 hand change in height (after adjusting for gender): this would not be relevant in Europe. If, however, we were to scale height by multiplying it by 10.2, the unit of measurement for the rescaled variable would be centimetres and the interpretation of the regression coefficient for height would be more meaningful in Europe. Sometimes, we use scaling to place numerical explanatory variables on a common scale, achieved by dividing each variable by its standard deviation. If we were to do this for the height of the Shetland ponies, then its coefficient would represent the average change in weight for a 1 standard deviation increase in height, after adjusting for gender. Note that scaling an explanatory variable does not affect the estimated intercept, the significance of the regression coefficient or the fit of the regression model but it does affect the estimated regression coefficient and its standard error.

Interactions

You should note that it is possible to include **interaction** (also called **effect modification**) terms in the multiple regression equation. An interaction (see Section 5.9.1) occurs between two explanatory variables when the effect on the response variable of one of the explanatory variables is not the same for different values of the other explanatory variable.

Consider again the situation where we are using a multiple regression equation to predict a Shetland pony's body weight (y) in kg from its gender (x_1) and height (x_2) in cm. It may be that the slope of the line describing the relationship between body weight and height is different for males and females, i.e. there is an interaction between gender and height. We include an interaction term in the model by creating a new variable which is the product of the two explanatory variables, (x_1x_2), and examine its coefficient in the same way as we would that of any explanatory variable. In this example, gender is a binary variable and height is a numerical variable. The coefficient of the interaction term then represents the difference in the slopes for males and females of the relationship between body weight and height. If the coefficient for the interaction term is not statistically significant, the main effects (e.g. gender and height) are then believed sufficient for the model. If the coefficient for the interaction term is statistically significant, the main effects should not be evaluated in the model containing the interaction, but each should be investigated for the different categories of the other main effect in the interaction term, e.g. the effect of height should be investigated separately for males and females.

We could, instead, categorize height into a binary variable – short (say, < 86 cm) and tall (say, ≥ 86 cm) – and then the interaction would imply that the difference in the mean body weight for short and tall Shetland ponies is not the same for males and females, with the relevant interaction coefficient representing the difference between males and females of this difference in mean body weight for short and tall animals.

If one of the two categorical variables of interest is nominal, with more than two categories, and the other variable is binary, we have to create as many interaction terms as there are dummy variables for the nominal variable in the regression model: each interaction term is the product of one dummy variable and the binary variable. If, on the other hand, both variables are numeri-

cal, the interpretation of an interaction term in a regression analysis is more complex, and it may be advisable in these circumstances to produce an interaction term by creating a binary variable from one of the numerical variables.

Polynomial regression

Sometimes, you may find that you have a non-linear (i.e. curved) relationship between y and x, e.g. quadratic or cubic, in which case a **polynomial** regression may be appropriate. Polynomial regression for the single explanatory variable, x, can be thought of as a special form of multiple regression, and can be analysed as such. Each explanatory variable in the multiple regression equation is replaced by successively higher powers of x. For example, the estimated cubic equation is of the form

$$Y = a + b_1x + b_2x^2 + b_3x^3$$

11.3.2 Appropriateness of the model

(a) Assumptions underlying multiple regression

The assumptions underlying multiple linear regression are similar to those in simple linear regression (see Section 10.4.3).

- A linear relationship is stipulated between the response variable (which is a numerical random variable) and each of the explanatory variables (which may or may not be numerical and are measured without error).
- The residuals are independent – each individual is represented once in the sample.
- The residuals are Normally distributed with zero mean and constant variance.

We should produce appropriate plots of the residuals to verify the assumptions. These are similar to those illustrated in Figure 10.8. In particular:

- Separate plots of the residuals against each of the explanatory variables will verify the linearity assumption, providing no trend is apparent.

- A histogram or Normal plot of the residuals can verify the Normality assumption.
- A plot of the residuals against the fitted values of y will verify the constant variance assumption, providing there is no funnel effect.

As in simple regression, we can identify outliers and influential points in multiple regression by appraising residual plots and examining, for each individual, the values of the residual, leverage and Cook's distance (see Section 10.4.3). Note, however, that if there are k explanatory variables in the regression equation and n individuals in the study, a leverage of $2(k + 1)/n$ is regarded as high (this is equivalent to a leverage of $4/n$ if there is only one explanatory variable).

(b) Relationships between explanatory variables

We expect some of the explanatory variables in a multiple regression to be related to one another. If this were not so, the multivariable analysis would be redundant; we could equally well perform a simple univariable linear regression analysis between the response variable and each explanatory variable, and we would obtain the same regression coefficients as in the multiple regression incorporating all the variables. We can determine which numerical explanatory variables are associated by calculating the correlation coefficient between every pair of explanatory variables. You should be aware that extremely highly correlated variables often result in **collinearity** (also called **multicollinearity**) in the multiple regression analysis. Collinearity may be identified in a number of ways, for example, by observing if numerical variables have correlation coefficients that are close to the limits of ±1, whether the coefficients from univariable regression analyses are substantially different after fitting a multivariable model, or if the **variance inflation factor** (VIF_i) is greater than 10 (Kleinbaum *et al.*, 2008), where $\text{VIF}_i = 1/(1 - R_i^2)$ and R_i^2 is equal to the proportion of variance explained by the regression of the variable x_i on the remaining explanatory variables in a regression model. If collinearity exists between variables, the standard errors of their coefficients are extremely large, leading to test statistics which are very small so that their associated coefficients in the model are not statistically significant. However, even if the individual regression coefficients are non-significant in the multiple regression equation, they may have a statistically significant joint effect on the response of interest. You will find details of how to deal with collinearity in more advanced texts, for example Chatterjee and Hadi (2006). Note, however, that dropping relevant variables from the model or using automatic selection procedures (see Section 11.3.4) and/or centring (see Section 11.3.1(d)) may alleviate the problem.

11.3.3 Understanding the computer output in a multiple regression analysis

We can use the output from a multiple regression analysis to provide useful information that relates to the goodness-of-fit and to the coefficients of the model as a way of determining which, if any, of the covariates are important predictors of outcome. In particular:

1. We can assess how well the model fits the data by appraising the proportion of the total variability that is explained by the relationship of y on the x values. This proportion is denoted by R^2; its square root is called the **multiple correlation coefficient**. We cannot use R^2 to compare the fit of different models as its value will be greater for models that include a larger number of explanatory variables. To overcome this difficulty, an **adjusted R^2** is often calculated which affords a direct comparison of values to assess goodness-of-fit in models that contain different numbers of explanatory variables.

2. The computer output for a multiple regression analysis contains an **analysis of variance** table which separates the total variation of y into its two sources: that which is explained and that which is unexplained by the regression. The **F-test** in the table enables us to test the null hypothesis that *all* the partial regression coefficients are zero. If the result of the test is

significant, we conclude that at least one of the explanatory variables is associated with the response variable.

3. Then we can determine which of the explanatory variables has a partial regression coefficient that is significantly different from zero by performing a *t*-test on each coefficient. Each test statistic is the estimated regression coefficient divided by its standard error, and has a *t*-distribution on $n - k - 1$ degrees of freedom, where k is the number of explanatory variables in the model. Computer output lists each estimated regression coefficient, usually with its standard error or a confidence interval, together with the test statistic and its *P*-value.

11.3.4 Choosing the explanatory variables to include in the model

Just because a computer program is available to perform a multiple regression analysis, this does *not* give you carte blanche to include, indiscriminately, a disproportionately large number of explanatory variables in the model. As a rule of thumb, remember that the sample size should *not* be less than 10 times the number of explanatory variables. So, if you have 100 observations, you should include no more than 10 explanatory variables in the model. In any case, you should start by considering *only those explanatory variables that you know are likely, from clinical or biological reasoning, to have some relationship with the response variable.*

The next stage, if there are still very many potential variables to include in the model, is to eliminate those covariates that are clearly not associated with the outcome variable.

- If the covariate is binary, you could perform a two-sample *t*-test comparing the mean outcomes in the two groups defined by the two categories of the binary variable, probably using a less stringent significance level (e.g. taking $P < 0.10$ rather than the conventional $P < 0.05$ to determine significance). You then include that variable in the multiple regression analysis as a covariate only if the means are found to be significantly different.

- If the covariate is numerical, you could perform a univariable linear regression analysis in which the dependent variable is regressed on that covariate. You would include that covariate in the multiple regression analysis only if the slope (or, equivalently, the correlation coefficient) was significantly different from zero (probably at the 10% level).

It is also possible to use **automatic selection procedures** to reduce the number of covariates in the model; these procedures produce a multiple regression equation with the 'best' combination of covariates. (Note: automatic selection procedures can also be used in other multivariable regression models, such as logistic and Poisson regression – see Sections 11.4 and 11.5, respectively.) Such techniques are particularly useful when you are interested in using the model for predictive purposes, and/or when some of the explanatory variables are very highly correlated. There is no single definition of 'best' but, usually, those variables are selected which optimize the amount of explained variation in y, so that it will not be significantly greater for a different selection.

- In **forward step-up selection**, we start with the single explanatory variable that contributes the most to the explained variation in y, and include more variables in the equation, progressively, until the addition of an extra variable does not significantly improve the situation.

- In **backward step-down selection**, we start with all the variables, and take them away sequentially, starting with the variable that contributes the least, until the deletion of a variable significantly reduces the amount of explained variation in y.

- **Stepwise selection** is essentially step-up selection, but it permits the elimination of variables at each step according to defined statistical criteria specified by the computer package.

- In **all subsets selection**, we investigate all the possible combinations of variables and choose that one which is optimal in some sense, perhaps with the greatest adjusted R^2.

Unfortunately, you may find that the optimal combination of variables differs when using the various automatic selection procedures or that a slight change in the data produces a different set of variables defining the optimal model! In addition, you might find that the estimated coefficients of the *s* (say) variables in the final automatic selection model do not correspond to those that would be obtained when using these *s* variables directly to determine a multiple regression equation. This is because, unless missing data are imputed (see Section 5.9.4), the automatic procedures exclude any individuals that do not have complete information on all the variables, and this sample size may be smaller than that of the model which is obtained by including only those individuals who have no missing observations on these *s* variables. You should also be aware that some coefficients may be spuriously significant because of the multiple testing process that compares one model with another within a particular automatic procedure, an integral part of the automatic selection process (see Section 8.6.3). You might consider using a more stringent significance level (say, 0.01 instead of the conventional 0.05) to overcome this problem. At the end of the day, however, it is your responsibility to judge, in the context of *your* investigation, the *appropriate* combination of covariates to best explain your phenomenon and, if possible, you should attempt to validate the model on a different data set.

11.3.5 Example

In Section 10.4.2, we discussed an example of simple linear regression using a single explanatory variable, girth measurement, to estimate body weight in sheep. Another example of the problem of estimating body weight, this time using a multivariable regression approach in Moroccan working donkeys, is the subject of a study by Pearson and Ouassat (1996). Here they were concerned to avoid overloading the draft donkeys, and needed to be able to estimate body weight since weighing machines were a rarity! They chose a number of variables (the donkey's girth at the level of the heart (cm), girth at the umbilicus (cm), length from the olecranon to the tuber ischii (cm), height at the withers (cm), and the donkey's age (years) and sex (male = 0, female = 1)) to help them predict its body weight (kg). The variables were measured in a random sample of 400 adult donkeys. Many of these variables were interrelated but collinearity was absent since there was no extremely high correlation coefficient between any two explanatory variables. We performed a multiple linear regression analysis on a subset of these data (excluding pregnant females) using body weight as the outcome variable, and all other variables as the explanatory variables. The results from a computer analysis are shown in Display 11.1.

We can regard the model as a good fit since the adjusted R^2 is 0.857, i.e. 86% of the variation in body weight is explained by its linear relationship with the explanatory variables. Apart from independence of the observations (which is not in doubt), the assumptions underlying the regression model can be assessed by studying the residuals. The plots of the residuals against the three predictor variables (heart girth, umbilical girth and length) in Figure 11.1 show that the linearity assumption is satisfactory for these three variables. The plots for the other independent variables are omitted for brevity, but they all accommodate the linearity assumption. We can see from Figure 11.1 that the residuals are approximately Normally distributed, and, from the plot of the residuals against the predicted values, that they have constant variance and are centred around a mean of approximately zero.

The *F*-test in the ANOVA implies $P < 0.001$, indicating that at least one of the six partial regression coefficients is significantly different from zero.

In fact, as shown in the table of coefficients (in Display 11.1), four variables (heart girth, length, umbilical girth and sex) have partial regression coefficients which are significantly different from zero. We interpret these coefficients as follows: a donkey's body weight increases on average by 1.770 kg as its heart girth increases by 1 cm, adjusting for the other variables in the equation. Similarly, the body weight of a female donkey is 2.293 kg less, on average, than that of a male, after adjusting for the other variables, etc.

Display 11.1 SPSS computer output from the multiple linear regression analysis of the donkey data (six explanatory variables) discussed in Section 11.3.5.

Model summary

Model	R	R square	Adjusted R square	Std error of the estimate
1	0.927*	0.859	0.857	9.3812

*Predictors: (Const), UMBGIRTH, SEX, AGE, LENGTH, HEIGHT, HEARTGIR.

ANOVA*

Model	Sum of Squares	df	Mean Square	F	Sig.
1 Regression	203987.4	6	33997.899	386.305	0.000†‡
Residual	33354.959	379	88.008		
Total	237342.4	385			

*Dependent variable: BODYWT.
†Predictors: (Const), UMBGIRTH, SEX, AGE, LENGTH, HEIGHT, HEARTGIR.
‡Indicates $P < 0.001$.

Coefficients*

Model	Coefficients B	Std error	t	Sig.	95% confidence interval for B Lower bound	Upper bound
1 (Constant)	−216.3	7.667	−28.217	0.000‡	−231.403	−201.254
AGE	0.262	0.184	1.422	0.156	−0.100	0.623
HEARTGIR	1.770	0.115	15.390	0.000‡	1.544	1.996
HEIGHT	0.157	0.110	1.433	0.153	−0.058	0.373
LENGTH	0.893	0.117	7.605	0.000‡	0.662	1.123
SEX	−2.293	1.015	−2.260	0.024	−4.289	−0.298
UMBGIRTH	0.380	0.067	5.668	0.000‡	0.248	0.512

*Dependent variable: BODYWT.
‡Indicates $P < 0.001$.

As there is no evidence that the height and age of the donkey are useful predictors of body weight, the multiple regression analysis was repeated using only the four variables that had significant coefficients. The assumptions underlying this model were checked and found to be satisfactory. This second regression analysis (adjusted $R^2 = 0.856$) gives the following estimated multiple regression equation:

$$Bodywt = -216.4 + 1.840 Heartgir + 0.999 Length - 2.917 Sex + 0.396 Umbgirth$$

which can be used to predict a Moroccan donkey's body weight.

11.4 Multiple logistic regression: a binary response variable

11.4.1 Rationale

We can use a modification of the multiple regression equation to analyse data when we have a **binary outcome** of interest. For example, we may

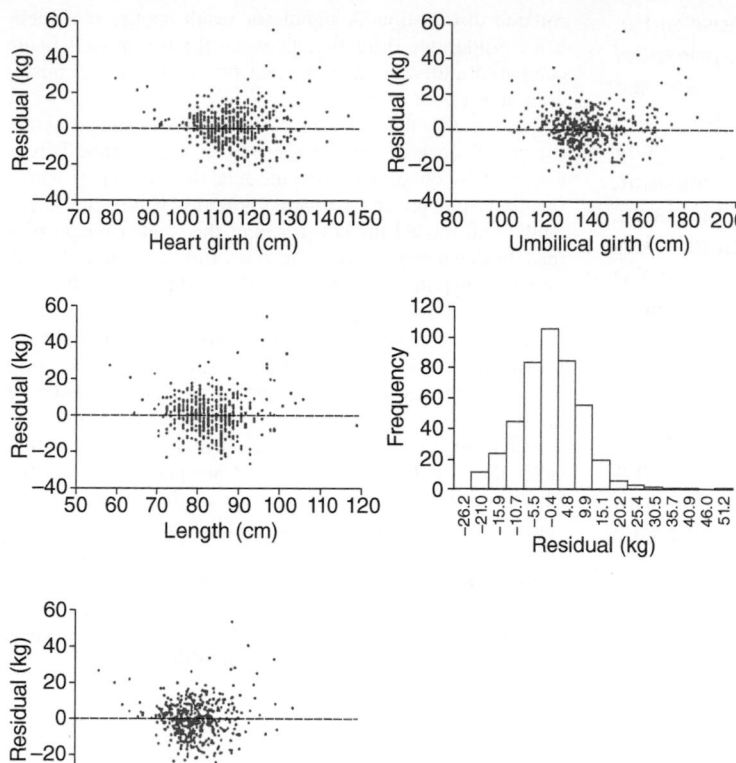

Figure 11.1 Diagrams for checking the assumptions underlying the multiple regression analysis of the Moroccan donkey data. In the histogram the *x*-axis labels relate to the midpoints of the intervals (from a subset of data from Pearson and Ouassat, 1996, with permission from the authors).

wish to relate a number of explanatory variables to an outcome such as the presence or absence of an abnormality. We can create a dummy variable for the outcome by coding 'presence' as one, say, and 'absence' as zero. However, we cannot use this as the dependent variable in a multiple regression equation because we would be unable to interpret any predicted values of it that are not exactly equal to zero or one. In order to overcome this problem, we use, as the dependent variable in our estimated regression equation, the *probability*, *p*, that an individual experiences a particular outcome (the larger of the coded outcomes, the value '1' in the abnormality example). Then, in order to linearize the relationship between the predicted value of the dependent variable and the covariates, we transform this dependent variable by taking the *logistic* or *logit*

transformation (see Section 13.2.2) of *p*, where logit(*p*) is equal to the logarithm to base *e* of the *odds* of the outcome, i.e. it is $log_e [p/(1 - p)]$. This leads to a **multiple** or **multivariable linear logistic regression** equation, often simply called a **logistic regression** equation.

11.4.2 Interpreting the coefficients

Each explanatory variable has a coefficient in the logistic equation that can be tested (the null hypothesis is that the true coefficient is zero) to determine whether that variable contributes significantly to an animal's chance of an abnormality, after adjusting for the possible confounding effects of the other variables. Because of the logistic transformation, the coefficients are interpreted in a different way from those in the multiple regression equation. The *exponential* of each logistic coefficient is the *odds ratio* (see Section 5.2.3) of a particular outcome for a unit increase in the explanatory variable, keeping the values of the other variables constant. For example, if we have an explanatory variable, x_1, indicating which treatment an animal has received ($x_1 = 0$ for treatment A, and $x_1 = 1$ for treatment B), the exponential of its coefficient in the logistic regression equation, e^{b_1}, is the estimated odds of the presence of the abnormality on treatment B compared with that on treatment A, after adjusting for the other variables in the equation. An odds ratio of unity indicates that the odds of the abnormality is the same for both treatments. The other coefficients in the logistic equation may be interpreted in a similar fashion. The odds ratio is often taken as an estimate of the relative risk, which is somewhat easier to interpret. However, the two are only similar if the outcome of interest is rare. You can obtain details of logistic regression analysis in a number of texts such as those by Hilbe (2009), Kleinbaum and Klein (2010) or Menard (2001).

11.4.3 Maximum likelihood estimation

We cannot use the method of least squares (see Section 10.4.1), as we do in simple and multiple linear regression analysis, to estimate the coefficients in the multiple logistic regression equation. Instead, the computer estimates these logistic coefficients by an iterative method called **maximum likelihood**. By way of explaining what this means, the **likelihood** of a model with particular values for the coefficients of the covariates is the probability of obtaining the observed results for that model. If we use a method of estimating the model coefficients which is based on maximum likelihood, we choose from all possible models with the same covariates that model which has the greatest chance of obtaining the observed results.

The *goodness-of-fit* of a model estimated by maximum likelihood is not assessed by considering the adjusted R^2 (see Section 11.3.3), as in simple and multiple linear regression. Instead, we use the **likelihood ratio statistic** (**LRS**), also called the **deviance** or **−2 log likelihood**. This compares the likelihood of two models – the model under consideration and the *saturated* model (i.e. the model that explains the data perfectly, having as many variables as individuals in the data set). The ratio of the two likelihoods approximately follows a Chi-squared distribution. A significant result implies that there is a considerable difference between the two models being compared and, consequently, that the model under consideration is a poor fit.

We can also use the likelihood ratio statistic to assess the significance of one or a group of coefficients. This is achieved by comparing two models, the smaller of which (i.e. that with fewer covariates) is *nested* within the larger model that has all the covariates of the smaller model plus the additional covariate(s) which is (are) being investigated. The null hypothesis is that all the additional coefficients are zero, a significant result implying that at least one of them is significantly different from zero. If, as a special case, the smaller model has no covariates (i.e. it has only a constant term) and the larger model comprises all the covariates of interest, the null hypothesis is that all these covariates have zero coefficients (e.g. Table 11.2). This latter test is often called the **model Chi-square** or the **Chi-square for covariates**. The alternative way of assessing the significance of a *single* coefficient in a multivariable regression model in which the coefficients are estimated by maximum likelihood is to use the **Wald test**. The test statistic of the Wald test, equal to the ratio of the estimated coefficient to its standard error, approximately follows the Normal distribution (its square approximates the Chi-squared distribution). □

11.4.4 Example

Hoeben *et al.* (1997) assessed 1000 Caesarian sections in standing cows performed under field conditions by veterinarians from the University of Ghent with a view to determining the factors that induce complications. This was in order to take some precautions to minimize the negative consequences, such as death of the cow or calf, placental retention, infection of the wound, etc. The most important complications are recumbency of the animal during the operation, difficulties with exteriorization of the pregnant uterine horn, and increased contractility of the uterus.

Initially, a simple univariable analysis was performed to evaluate the effects of each of a number of variables on the occurrence of each of the three main complications. For each binary variable, the relative risk was estimated as the proportion of animals developing the complication if the factor was present divided by that if it was absent, and its significance from unity determined. Significant variables ($P < 0.05$) included experience of the surgeon, type of cow (dairy or beef), parity, use of the sedative xylazine (yes/no), quantity of sedative (ml), attempt to extract the calf (yes/ no), use of epidural anaesthesia (yes/no), contractility of the uterus (relaxed/contracted), etc. For each of the three main complications, a multiple logistic regression analysis was then performed using only those variables that were shown to be significant in the univariable analysis.

In Table 11.1 we show the variables that had significant coefficients in the logistic regression analysis connected with recumbency of the animals during Caesarian section, after adjusting for the other prognostic variables. This table contains, for each variable, an estimate of the β coefficient in the logistic regression equation, with its standard error and P-value which results from the Wald test of the null hypothesis that the coefficient is zero. The estimated odds ratio of 1.95 for sedation implies that the odds of recumbency during the operation was 1.95 times greater if the animal was sedated than if it was not, after adjusting for the other variables. The confidence interval relating to sedation tells us that we can be 95% certain that the true odds ratio lies between 1.33 and 2.87. Note that this interval excludes unity; this is to be expected since we know that the coefficient is significant ($P = 0.001$).

From Table 11.1 we can see that there was approximately a twofold increase in the odds of recumbency of the animal during Caesarian section if the cow was sedated, or if the obstetrician met with difficulties when attempting to exteriorize the pregnant uterine horn. The odds of recumbency was approximately halved if the animal was a beef cow rather than a dairy cow, or if the cow was multiparous.

Similar analyses showed that attempting to extract the calf was the only factor that significantly increased uterine contractility. The experience of the surgeon, the parity, the increased uterine contractility, the position of the calf, and the presence of adhesions were associated with difficult exteriorization of the pregnant horn.

11.4.5 Checking the logistic regression model

- We usually check for outliers and influential points (see Section 10.4.3(d)) in logistic regression by drawing appropriate diagrams and looking for points that appear to be apart from the main body of the data. For example, we may plot the standardized residuals (the residuals divided by their standard errors) against each of the explanatory variables. If one or more points are disparate, we can perform a sensitivity analysis: the point(s) will be influential if the estimates of the regression coefficients are substantially different when the analysis is performed with and without the points.
- If we find that the deviance (see Section 11.4.3) divided by the degrees of freedom ($df = n - k - 1$ where n = number of individuals and k = number of explanatory variables) is substantially greater than one, we have **extra-Binomial variation**.

Table 11.1 Results of the logistic regression analysis for the recumbency of cows during Caesarian section (from Hoeben *et al.*, 1997, with permission from Taylor & Francis Ltd).

Variable, x_i	Numerical value of x_i	b_i	SE(b_i)	P-value	Estimated odds ratio	95% CI for odds ratio
Type of animal	Dairy = 0, Beef = 1	−0.6599	0.2087	0.002	0.52	0.34–0.78
Parity	Heifer = 0, Mult. cow = 1	−0.6708	0.2106	0.002	0.51	0.24–0.77
Sedation	No = 0, Yes = 1	0.6683	0.1972	0.001	1.95	1.33–2.87
Exteriorization of uterus	Easy = 0, Difficult = 1	0.7049	0.2153	0.001	2.02	1.33–3.09

CI, confidence interval; SE, standard error.

This occurs when the independence assumption is violated, perhaps because we have clustered data (see Section 11.6) or because an important explanatory variable has not been included in the model or because of the presence of one or more outliers. Then the standard errors of the regression coefficients will be underestimated, leading to increased Type I error rates (see Section 6.4).

- If we find that an estimated regression coefficient has an unexpectedly large standard error, we should investigate the possibility of collinearity (see Section 11.3.2(b)) when two or more of the explanatory variables are very highly correlated. An alternative explanation might be because a categorical explanatory variable has no individuals in one or more of its categories, i.e. a zero cell count. This problem can be overcome by combining one or more categories of this variable.

11.4.6 Applications of logistic regression

(a) Linear logistic regression analysis

We use multivariable linear logistic regression analysis when we have a binary outcome (e.g. success/failure) and wish to relate one or more covariates to it as a way of explaining the relationship between the variables, determining the covariates that are important predictors of outcome and/or predicting the outcome of interest. The logistic regression analysis provides an estimate of the odds ratio for each covariate, after controlling for the other covariates in the model. Odds ratios have a number of advantages over relative risks (see, for example, Kirkwood and Sterne, 2003) and, consequently, logistic regression analysis is usually the method of choice when analysing binary outcomes.

It is the only appropriate form of regression analysis for an *unmatched* case–control study (see Section 5.2.3(b)) when relative risks cannot be estimated directly. In such a study, the cases (often coded as one) and the controls (often coded as zero) define the binary outcome. The exponential of the estimated coefficient relating to a particular covariate in the model then represents the estimated odds of being a case (i.e. having disease) compared with that of being a control (i.e. being disease-free) as the covariate increases by one unit, after adjusting for the other covariates in the model. Linear logistic regression analysis can also be used if we want to investigate the factors that influence the incidence of disease in a longitudinal study, provided all the individuals in the study have the same length of follow-up. If the follow-up period is *not* the same for every individual, then the data

should be analysed using *survival analysis* (see Section 14.6) or *Poisson regression analysis* (see Section 11.5). We can also use logistic regression analysis when we have a binary outcome in a cross-sectional study (see Section 5.2.2).

(b) Conditional logistic regression analysis

There is a special form of logistic regression analysis, called **conditional logistic regression analysis**, which affords the analysis of a binary variable when the individuals are *matched*, as in a matched case–control study (see Section 5.2.3(b)). Conditional logistic regression analysis takes the matching into account and controls for confounding variables (although a factor which is used to match the cases and controls cannot be included as a covariate in the model). Any analysis that ignores the matching of individuals is inefficient and not to be recommended. Further details may be obtained from, for example, Kleinbaum and Klein (2010).

(c) Multinomial and ordinal logistic regression analysis

Logistic regression analysis can be extended to deal with the situation in which the categorical outcome variable is not binary but has more than two categories (i.e. it is **polycotomous**). In particular, we use **multinomial logistic regression analysis** when the categorical outcome variable is measured on a *nominal* scale (see Section 1.6), i.e. the distinct categories that define the variable are unordered (for example, Agresti (2010) used this approach to analyse data from a study of alligator length on primary food preference, in which the preferences were fish, invertebrates and other).

We use **ordinal logistic regression analysis** when the categorical outcome variable is measured on an *ordinal* scale (see Section 1.6), i.e. the categories of the variable have some intrinsic order but the intervals between the categories are not clearly defined or consistent (e.g. the disease stages I, II and III). Details on multinomial and ordinal logistic regression may be obtained from texts such as Agresti (2010) or Kleinbaum and Klein (2010).

As an illustration, Overton *et al.* (2003) used ordinal logistic regression analysis in a randomized, placebo-controlled, masked clinical trial to examine the prophylactic effect of 4 mg of estradiol cypronate (ECP) administered within 24–36 hours of calving on the three grades of severity of post-parturient metritis in primiparous dairy cows at high risk of metritis. Metritis was diagnosed by rectal palpation and the presence of a flaccid, fluid-filled uterus with vulval discharge and foetid odour and was categorized as absent, mild or severe. Explanatory variables in the regression analysis were treatment (ECP or placebo) and the calendar quarter of the year that the cow calved in, as well as some additional covariates which were found not to be significant. This analysis produced an estimated odds ratio of one for treatment (90% CI 0.5 to 1.8), after adjusting for the effect of year quarter of calving and some other covariates. This implies that the odds of a treated cow being in the same category of metritis (absent, mild or severe) or higher was equal to that of a control cow. The authors concluded that prophylactic administration of ECP did not reduce the severity of metritis.

Because these polycotomous regression methods are not straightforward, we often prefer to adopt a simple approach to the analysis of these data. If we dichotomize the nominal or ordinal variable (i.e. we create two categories from it by combining categories appropriately or by choosing a sensible cut-off point, if relevant), we can perform a logistic regression analysis on the data since the outcome is now binary. We have to decide how the data are to be dichotomized at the outset, before we have collected the data, as we may obtain biased results if we choose the point for dichotomy by looking at the data.

11.5 Poisson regression

11.5.1 Rationale

When we are interested in assessing the impact of certain factors on the occurrence of an event (such as disease or death) in a longitudinal study *in which the individuals are studied for varying lengths of time*, it is *inappropriate* to use logistic regression analysis. This is because we must take into account not only whether or not the event occurs in an individual but also the length of time that each individual is exposed to the risk of the event (the risk period). Two ways of achieving this are by using the Cox proportional hazards regression (see Section 14.6.2) or **Poisson regression analysis**.

The Poisson distribution (see Section 3.4.3) is the probability distribution of the number of events in a fixed time interval when these events occur randomly and independently in time (or space) at a constant rate. Poisson regression analysis is concerned with investigating the effect of various factors on the **rate** of occurrence of an event when this rate is constant over the time period of interest. If the time of follow-up is measured in years, the rate of an event is generally expressed as a rate per individual per year and is equal to the number of events occurring divided by the total number of years of follow-up for all individuals. If the individual is an animal, the latter is commonly called the animal-years of follow-up. A rate differs from a risk in that a rate takes the length of time that an individual is studied into account whereas a risk does not.

In the Poisson regression equation, we relate the predicted value of the *rate* of occurrence of the event to a linear function of the explanatory variables. However, to overcome mathematical difficulties, we use the logarithmic transformation (to base e) of the rate in the equation. This is analogous to logistic regression analysis, where we relate the predicted value of the *probability* or *odds* of the event to a linear function of the explanatory variables, and take the logit transformation of p to overcome mathematical difficulties. The coefficients of the Poisson regression model are usually estimated using the method of maximum likelihood (see Section

11.4.3). Since the response variable in Poisson regression is a rate, the exponential of an estimated coefficient in the Poisson model represents an estimated relative rate (often called an **incidence rate ratio**, **IRR**). If the associated covariate is binary (e.g. it is coded as 1 if the factor is present, and 0 otherwise), the incidence rate ratio is the rate of the event (say, disease) in those with the factor compared with the rate in those without the factor, after adjusting for all other covariates in the model. If the covariate is numerical, then the incidence rate ratio represents the ratio of the two rates for a unit increase in the covariate. If the incidence rate ratio is equal to one, then these rates are equal. A test of significance of the null hypothesis that the incidence rate ratio is equal to one is equivalent to a test of the null hypothesis that the associated coefficient in the model is equal to zero. The Wald test (see Section 11.4.3) is usually used to test the significance of each coefficient, as in logistic regression. You can generally find the results of such tests of the coefficients in the computer output of a Poisson regression analysis. We can assess the adequacy of the model using −2 log likelihood (or deviance), as for logistic regression (see Section 11.4.3). **Extra-Poisson variation** (analogous to extra-Binomial variation, see Section 11.4.5) occurs when the residual variance is greater than would be expected from a Poisson model: it results in underestimation of the standard errors leading to spuriously significant coefficients as well as confidence intervals that are too narrow. A value of the deviance divided by the degrees of freedom that is substantially greater than one is indicative of extra-Poisson variation.

11.5.2 Generalized linear models

The logistic transformation of the proportion (equivalent to the logarithmic transformation of the odds) used in logistic regression and the logarithmic transformation of the rate or count used in Poisson regression are examples of different **link functions**. A link function links the covariates of a regression model to a dependent variable (e.g. a proportion or rate) that has a known underlying probability distribution in such a way that the relationship between the predicted or mean value of the dependent variable and the set of covariates is linear. Note that no transformation is involved in multiple linear regression; the link function is then called the **identity link**. These models are particular forms of a **generalized linear model** (GLM); all generalized linear models conform to this unified framework. In particular, the probability distribution of the dependent variable associated with the outcome of interest is Normal in multiple regression where the outcome is continuous; it is Binomial in logistic regression where the outcome is binary; it is Poisson in Poisson regression where the outcome is a count.

The method of maximum likelihood (see Section 11.4.3) is usually used to estimate the parameters of a generalized linear model (although in multiple linear regression analysis, with the identity link, the method of least squares is generally adopted). We can use the likelihood ratio test to evaluate the significance from zero of one or a group of coefficients in a generalized linear model by comparing the deviances of two models, with the smaller model containing all the covariates of the full model apart from the covariate(s) under test. As an alternative procedure, we can use the Wald test to test the significance of just a single coefficient. We describe both of these tests in Section 11.4.3.

11.5.3 Example of Poisson regression

Equine grass sickness (EGS, equine dysautonomia) is a debilitating and often fatal neurodegenerative disease of horses which almost exclusively affects grazing horses. Newton *et al.* (2004) performed an epidemiological study with a view to identifying the risk factors associated with the recurrence of EGS on previously affected premises, and thereby possibly gaining insights into the pathogenesis of the disease. They collected data on disease history and risk factors from 305

premises, 100 of which were recurrent, by postal questionnaire from cases with EGS in the 6 years starting at the beginning of January 1997. The outcome of interest was the number of recurrent EGS incidents per 100 horses per premises per year, the overall median rate being estimated as 2.1 incidents/100 horses/premises/year. The authors performed a Poisson regression analysis because the nature of the data was events (i.e. recurrent EGS incidents) over time (risk period). In order to reduce the number of variables in the regression model they started by performing a series of univariable analyses, using each of the potential risk factors, one by one, as the single explanatory variable in a Poisson model (see Section 11.5.1). Those variables that were associated significantly ($P < 0.275$) with recurrence of disease in the univariable analyses were then incorporated into a stepwise multivariable Poisson regression analysis, together with interaction terms. Table 11.2 summarizes the results of the final multivariable model, which incorporated a set of dummy variables (see Section 11.3.1(c)) to replace each categorical covariate with more than two categories. The reference cat-

Table 11.2   Summary of Poisson regression analysis results showing significant covariates in the model (from Newton *et al.*, 2004, with permission from Wiley Blackwell).

Variable	Category	Coefficient	SE	IRR	95% CI for IRR Lower	95% CI for IRR Upper	LRS* or Wald *P*-value
Intercept		−2.57	0.28				
No. of horses on premises	1–5			Referent			<0.0001*
	6–10	0.08	0.37	1.08	0.52	2.22	0.838
	11–15	1.06	0.32	2.90	1.55	5.42	0.001
	16–20	2.46	0.35	11.7	5.91	23.1	<0.001
	21–40	1.27	0.30	3.56	1.98	6.40	<0.001
	40+	1.97	0.31	7.18	3.92	13.2	<0.001
Presence of horses age <2 years	No			Referent			<0.0001*
	Yes	0.53	0.24	1.70	1.06	2.71	0.027
Soil type	Clay			Referent			<0.0001*
	Sand	0.36	0.20	1.43	0.98	2.10	0.067
	Chalk	−1.48	0.61	0.23	0.07	0.76	0.016
	Loam	0.74	0.21	2.11	1.40	3.16	<0.001
	Other	−0.98	0.44	0.36	0.16	0.90	0.027
Method of faeces removal	Not removed			Referent			<0.0001*
	By hand	−1.71	0.49	0.18	0.07	0.48	0.001
	Mechanically	1.02	0.47	2.76	1.10	6.94	0.031
Pasture cut?	Not cut			Referent			<0.0001*
	Cut	−2.15	0.32	0.12	0.06	0.22	<0.001
Other domestic animals on pasture?	None			Referent			<0.0001*
	Ruminants	−2.22	0.41	0.11	0.05	0.24	0.001
	Birds/fowls	−0.09	0.30	0.91	0.50	1.65	0.780
	Other	−2.37	1.03	0.09	0.01	0.70	0.021

CI, confidence interval; IRR, incidence rate ratio; LRS, likelihood ratio statistic; SE, standard error.

egory for each of these sets of binary dummy variables is called the 'referent'. The *P*-value that tests the significance of a specific category when compared with the reference category was determined by the Wald test (see Section 11.4.3): the likelihood ratio statistic (see Section 11.4.3) was used to test the significance of the whole set of dummies for a particular covariate.

There was a significantly increased rate of recurrence of EGS with higher number of horses, presence of younger animals, study farms and livery/riding establishments, loam and sand soils, rearing of domestic birds and mechanical droppings removal. For example, the rate of recurrence was estimated to be 1.70 times greater in those premises that had horses aged <2 years than those that did not; it was estimated to increase by 176% if faeces were removed mechanically compared with when they were not removed (in each case, adjusting for the other variables in the model). The rate of recurrence decreased significantly with chalk soil, co-grazing ruminants, grass cutting on pastures and removal of droppings by hand. For example, if ruminants were on the pasture, the rate of recurrence was estimated to decrease by 89% (i.e. the IRR = 0.11) compared with when there were no other domestic animals on the pasture, after adjusting for the other variables in the model. In addition, several significant interactions were identified.

11.6 Regression methods for clustered data

11.6.1 What are clustered data?

When our observations can be grouped in such a way that the observations within a group or cluster are not independent, we have **clustered** data, sometimes called **repeated measures** data. The data are arranged hierarchically in that individual observations (called *level 1* units) are nested or hierarchical within a cluster (*level 2* unit); for example, litters from a sow, cattle in a farm, herds in a region, legs in a cat or a longitudinal data set in which observations are recorded at successive times (the level 1 units) for each animal (the level 2 unit) (Figure 11.2). The statistical analysis of these data

must take into account the fact that the observations within a cluster are correlated and, therefore, are not independent of each other (e.g. different litters from one sow are more likely to exhibit similar characteristics than litters that come from different sows). The standard errors of the estimates of interest are usually too small if we ignore the dependencies in the data, and consequently we may obtain confidence intervals that are too narrow and spuriously significant results when testing hypotheses relating to these estimates.

There are various valid strategies that we can adopt for the analysis of clustered data. In Section 14.5, we describe a simple non-regression approach to the analysis and discuss some inappropriate analyses. We can also use a procedure, such as one of the following, which relies on the specification of a *regression model* (for simplicity, we assume in this section that the outcome is numerical):

1. Regard the cluster (rather than the level 1 unit) as the unit of investigation and replace the set of responses within each cluster by an appropriate **summary measure** (e.g. in the sow example it may be the mean litter size). We then use this summary measure as the outcome or dependent variable in a univariable or multivariable regression analysis. The covariate(s) in this regression model must relate to the clusters, so, in the litters from a sow example, a covariate might be sow weight. Alternatively, if the trial is a **cluster randomized trial** in which we randomly allocate clusters of individuals to different treatments, the covariate may be a binary variable representing treatment group. Although this method of *aggregating the data* by using a summary measure has the advantage of simplicity, it does not make use of all the information provided in the sample and does not allow covariates relating to the level 1 units to be incorporated into the model.

2. Take clustering into account by calculating **robust standard errors** of the parameter estimates. These standard errors are 'robust' to violations of the assumptions relating to the probability model, such as lack of independence. Robust standard errors are calculated using the observed distribution of the response variable instead of relying on the specification of a full probability model for it, in contrast to the likelihood approach to estimation. This is a relatively simple approach that allows level 1 unit covariates

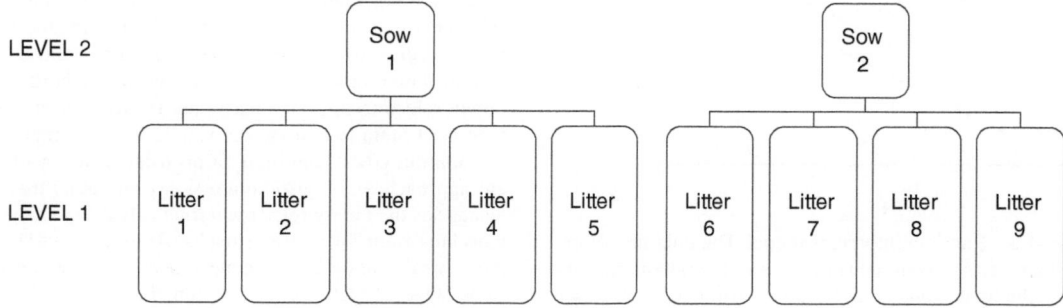

Figure 11.2 Diagrammatic illustration of a two-level hierarchical structure.

to be included in the model but suffers the disadvantage that the estimates of the coefficients in the model are not adjusted for clustering.

3. Use a **random effects regression model** (often called a **multilevel model**, usually abbreviated to MLM) which includes the two sources of random variation in the data: (i) the variation between the level 1 units *within* each cluster; and (ii) the variation *between* cluster means, representing what is termed the random effect (hence the name for the model). These sources of variation give rise to two sets of *residuals*, each of which is generally assumed to follow a Normal distribution if the outcome variable is numerical.

There are different forms of random effects models, one of the simplest being the **random intercepts model** with a single covariate. This assumes that, for a given cluster, there is a linear relationship between the numerical outcome variable, y, and the covariate, x, when x and y are measured on each level 1 unit in that cluster. Furthermore, if the regression line of y on x is determined for every cluster, then all these regression lines have the same slope but different intercepts which vary randomly about the intercept of the mean regression line (Figure 11.3).

This model can be extended by, for example, including more than one covariate, allowing both the intercepts and slopes to vary randomly (leading to a *random slopes model*), introducing additional levels into the hierarchical structure (e.g. a four-level structure with piglets in litters in sows in farms), or using it with Poisson regression if the outcome is a count.

4. Use the **generalized estimating equation** (**GEE**) approach (also called **population-averaged** or **marginal** approaches) to estimation which does not assume a particular probability distribution for the between-cluster residuals (as assumed in a random effects model). Without the distributional assumptions, it is impossible to calculate the likelihood of the observations, and so we cannot use the maximum likelihood method to estimate the parameters. In order to use the *quasi-likelihood* method of GEE, we essentially use the mean value per group as the outcome, and have to specify a 'working' correlation matrix (providing what we believe is a realistic description of the correlation of the outcomes within the clusters) instead of relying on the probability model to identify the correlation matrix. The GEE approach produces estimates of the parameters and their standard errors that are adjusted for clustering, and allows both level 1 and cluster level covariates to be included in the model. However, as clustering is of no intrinsic interest in a GEE analysis, we cannot obtain an estimate of the variation between clusters and thereby assess the importance of clustering in our data.

You can find further details of regression methods for clustered data in, for example, Burton *et al.* (1998), Diggle *et al.* (2002), Dohoo *et al.* (2010), Graubard and Korn (1994), Rabe-Hesketh and Skrondal (2012), Raudenbush and Bryk (2002) and Snijders and Bosker (2012). However, we recommend, if you find you have recourse to one of these approaches, that you seek help from a professional statistician to guide you.

11.6.2 Example

Milk leakage in dairy cows, a symptom of impaired teat sphincter function, is related to an increased risk of mastitis in heifers and cows, and causes hygiene problems. Klaas *et al.* (2005) conducted a longitudinal observational study to assess whether variables such as teat shape (short and thin, short and thick, normal, conical or thick), condition of teat orifice (protrusion, white ring, rough callosity or normal) and peak milk flow rate (defined as the maximum milk flow within eight measurements (over 22.4 s) and expressed in kg/min) were risk factors for milk leakage. Milk leakage was recorded for each mammary quarter as a binary variable (milk leakage = 1, no milk leakage = 0). Data were collected from 1600 primiparous and multiparous cows that were maintained in loose housing in 15 German dairy farms.

Although the data set conforms to a three-level hierarchical structure of quarters within cows within herds, we adopted the procedure justified by Klaas *et al.* and reduced it to a two-level hierarchical structure of cows within herds by randomly selecting one mammary quarter from each cow. We then used Stata to analyse the results from a sample of 579 primiparous cows from these farms using a variety of different approaches to logistic regression analysis, all using milk leakage as the binary response variable. In every analysis, the most important risk factor in first lactation cows was DevPMF, the cow's deviation from the mean peak milk flow within the same stage of lactation and within the same parity across herds. However, cows having canal protrusions were also at significantly greater risk of milk leakage than those having

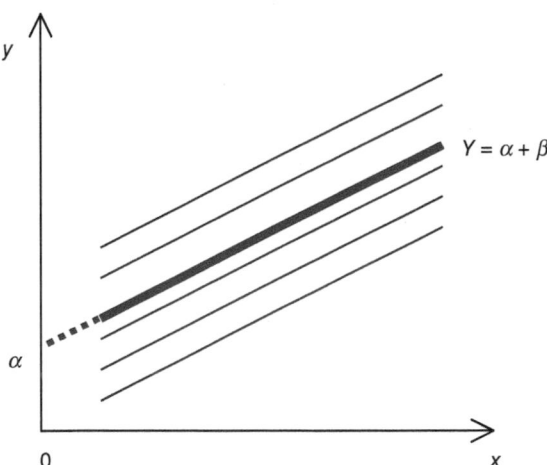

Figure 11.3 Random intercepts model. The bold line represents the mean regression line ($Y = \alpha + \beta x$) for all the clusters. Each of the lighter lines, one for each cluster, has a slope = β but they have different intercepts which vary randomly around the mean intercept = α.

Table 11.3 Summary of Stata results for the explanatory variable, deviation from peak milk flow (DevPMF), from different types of logistic regression analysis in which the binary response variable is milk leakage (Yes = 1, No = 0).

Logistic	Estimated OR	Std error	z	$P > |z|$	95% conf. interval for OR	
NC	1.760195	0.3203571	3.11	0.002	1.232086	2.514665
RoSE	1.760195	0.3563095	2.79	0.005	1.183737	2.617377
RaEf	1.690621	0.3166406	2.80	0.005	1.171178	2.44045
GEE	1.683941	0.3361768	2.61	0.009	1.138664	2.490337

Types of logistic regression analysis: NC, no account of clustering; RoSE, robust standard errors; RaEf, random effects; GEE, generalized estimating equations, robust standard errors, exchangeable correlation structure.
OR, odds ratio; $P > |z|$, P-value; z, Wald test statistic.

normal teat orifices and all other orifice characteristics. No other factors significantly influenced milk leakage.

Table 11.3 shows extracts of Stata output relating only to the explanatory variable, DevPMF, from different approaches to logistic regression analysis. In each case, DevPMF was a significant risk factor for milk leakage, with the odds of the cow having milk leakage nearly doubling as the deviation from the mean peak flow increased by 1 kg/min, after adjusting for the other factors in the model. However, the estimates of the odds ratios and their standard errors for DevPMF varied according to the type of analysis performed. As expected, the smallest P-value was obtained from the ordinary logistic regression analysis which ignored clustering. The estimated odds ratio from this analysis was the same as that from the logistic regression analysis which used robust standard errors, but ignoring clustering resulted in a standard error that was underestimated. The logistic regression analyses that used either a random effects approach or generalized estimating equations affected the magnitude of both the odds ratios and their standard errors when compared with the analysis that ignored clustering. The random effects analysis indicated that the variation in milk leakage due to the differences between herds, after adjusting for the other risk factors, accounted for 8.6% of the total variation. This was not statistically significant ($P = 0.09$), so it is not surprising that the logistic analysis that ignored clustering produced essentially similar results to the analyses that took clustering into account. Furthermore, the small and non-significant herd effect indicates that the impact of management or other herd-level factors on the occurrence of milk leakage is virtually negligible for practical purposes. ☐

Exercises

The statements in questions 11.1–11.5 are either TRUE or FALSE. Questions 11.3c–e, 11.4 and 11.5 relate to advanced sections in smaller type.

11.1 Multiple regression analysis:
(a) Requires all the independent variables to be Normally distributed.
(b) Requires the residuals to be Normally distributed.
(c) Can be used to determine whether the mean responses of animals on two treatments are significantly different.
(d) Can be performed with any number of independent variables.
(e) Is preferable to logistic regression analysis if the dependent variable has a binary response.

11.2 A partial regression coefficient in a multiple regression equation:
(a) Always lies between −1 and 1.
(b) Measures the degree of the relationship between its associated independent variable and the dependent variable, adjusting for the other independent variables.
(c) Measures the average change in the dependent variable for a unit increase in the associated independent variable, adjusting for the other independent variables.
(d) Describes the proportion of the variation in the dependent variable explained by its relationship with the associated independent variable.
(e) Is independent of the units of measurement.

11.3
(a) Logistic regression is an appropriate form of regression analysis when we have a binary explanatory variable and a numerical dependent variable.
(b) The coefficient attached to a particular explanatory variable in a logistic regression analysis is interpreted as an estimated odds ratio.
(c) The coefficients in a logistic regression model are estimated usually by maximum likelihood.

(d) The Wald test can be used to test the null hypothesis that a particular logistic coefficient is zero or, equivalently, that the relevant odds ratio is one.

(e) Conditional logistic regression analysis is used when the outcome variable has more than two categories.

11.4

(a) Poisson regression is only suitable for the analysis of fish data.

(b) Poisson regression is suitable for investigating the effect of various factors on the rate of occurrence of an event.

(c) Poisson regression is suitable when the individuals in the study are followed for varying lengths of time.

(d) The exponential of the coefficients of a Poisson regression model represents the ratio of the odds of the event as the relevant explanatory variable increases by 1 unit.

(e) The method of least squares is used to estimate the coefficients in a Poisson regression model.

11.5

(a) When we use regression methods to analyse clustered data, the standard errors of the estimates of the effects of interest are usually too small if the dependencies in the data are ignored.

(b) When we have clustered data, the level 1 unit represents the cluster that contains a number of level 2 units.

(c) The use of generalized estimating equations in the estimation of the coefficients of a multilevel regression model requires that the between-cluster residuals are Normally distributed.

(d) The two sources of variation in a random effects regression model for clustered data are the variation between the cluster means and the variation between the units within a cluster.

(e) The random intercepts model with a single explanatory variable for clustered data assumes that the regression lines for each cluster have different slopes and different intercepts that vary randomly about the mean slope and mean intercept, respectively.

11.6 Consider the following abstract describing the results of a study on the effects of cat ownership in children (from Fasce *et al.*, 2005, reproduced with permission from Elsevier):

BACKGROUND: Studies on the role of cat ownership in the development of allergy have led to conflicting results, probably owing to heterogeneity of the populations evaluated.

OBJECTIVE: To evaluate the possible effect of cat ownership on the frequency of sensitization and asthma or rhinitis in children living in Liguria, Italy, who attended a pediatric clinic for respiratory symptoms.

METHODS: We enrolled 269 consecutive school-aged children in 12 months. Sensitization to aeroallergens by skin prick testing and the presence of respiratory symptoms (i.e. asthma and rhinitis) were evaluated. To analyze the role of different independent variables in association with respiratory symptoms and sensitization, a multiple logistic regression analysis was performed.

RESULTS: Of 269 children, 81 were exposed to cats at home in the first 2 years of life ('early' cat owners), 65 after the first 2 years of life ('late' cat owners), and 123 never ('never' cat owners). Early cat ownership was significantly associated with a lower risk of cat sensitization compared with never cat ownership (adjusted odds ratio [OR], 0.32; 95% confidence interval [CI], 0.14–0.74; $P = 0.01$). Early cat ownership was also associated with a significantly lower risk of allergic rhinitis than late cat ownership (OR, 0.43; 95% CI, 0.22–0.85) or never cat ownership (OR, 0.51; 95% CI, 0.28–0.92). No differences in the frequency of asthma were found among the three groups ($P = 0.74$).

CONCLUSIONS: Cat ownership in early childhood can play an important role in preventing sensitization to cats and in lowering the frequency of allergic rhinitis, at least in children with the characteristics of the population studied.

(a) Why did the authors not have a single variable in each logistic regression to represent the level of cat ownership (none, early and late)? What did they use instead?

(b) Interpret the adjusted odds ratios of 0.32 and 0.51.

(c) Why do the authors refer to the odds ratios as adjusted odds ratios?

(d) The authors do not provide P-values for the odds ratios of 0.43 and 0.51. Provide the relevant P-values and explain how you obtained them.

(e) What hypothesis test would the authors have performed to compare the frequency of asthma in the three groups?

12 Non-parametric statistical methods

12.1 Learning objectives

By the end of this chapter you should be able to:

- List the different approaches to adopt if the assumptions of the parametric test are not satisfied.
- Describe the differences between parametric and non-parametric tests.
- Recognize when it is advisable to apply a non-parametric test to a data set.
- Identify a data set to which the sign test is suited and conduct the test.
- Identify a data set to which the Wilcoxon signed rank test is suited and conduct the test.
- Identify a data set to which the Wilcoxon rank sum (Mann–Whitney U) test is suited and conduct the test.
- Identify data sets to which the Kruskal–Wallis and Friedman ANOVAs are suited and interpret the results of such analyses.
- Calculate the Spearman's rank correlation coefficient and test the hypothesis that its true value is zero.

12.2 Parametric and non-parametric tests

12.2.1 Difference between parametric and non-parametric tests

The hypothesis tests that we discussed in earlier chapters for means and for regression and correlation coefficients are **parametric tests** in that each makes certain assumptions about the underlying form of the distribution of the observations. For example, in the two-sample t-test (see Section 7.4) we assume the data are Normally distributed. Animal research often results in data sets that are less than perfect either in terms of numbers of observations, or the distribution of the data. Hence the assumptions of the tests may not be satisfied. The alternative type of test is a **non-parametric test**, which does not make any distributional assumptions about the data. For this reason, they are often called **distribution-free tests**. The analyses in non-parametric tests

Statistics for Veterinary and Animal Science, Third Edition. Aviva Petrie and Paul Watson.
© 2013 John Wiley & Sons, Ltd. Published 2013 by John Wiley & Sons, Ltd.

are usually based on the **ranks** of the data, i.e. on the successive numbers assigned to the observations when they are arranged in increasing (or decreasing) order, rather than on the raw data. An extensive discussion of non-parametric methods may be found in, for example, Siegel and Castellan (1988) or Sprent and Smeeton (2007).

12.2.2 What if assumptions of the parametric test are not satisfied?

If the assumptions of the parametric test are *not* satisfied, then we have a number of choices. We can:

(a) Ignore the fact that the assumptions are not satisfied and proceed with the analysis. This approach may lead to an incorrect analysis in which the results of the test are distorted by its failure to adhere to the underlying assumptions. In particular, the *P*-value may not be the one that we believe we have evaluated. Some tests are **robust** against violations of certain assumptions (e.g. the Normality assumptions in the two-sample and paired *t*-tests – see Sections 7.4.2 and 7.5.2) so that the *P*-value is hardly affected if the assumptions are not satisfied (e.g. if the data depart from Normality).

(b) Take a particular **transformation** of every data value, and perform the analysis on the transformed observations. So, if the variable of interest is *x*, then we take a transformation of *x* to create a new variable, t_x, which is some function of *x*, for example, its logarithm, reciprocal or square root (see Section 13.2). There are a number of reasons for transforming data, the most common being:
 • To achieve a Normal distribution of t_x when the distribution of *x* is skewed.
 • To linearize a relationship; it is much easier to analyse data and investigate a relationship when that relationship can be described by a straight line.
 • To stabilize variance; equal variance is assumed in the two-sample *t*-test (see Section 7.4.2) and in analysis of variance

Box 12.1 Parametric analyses and some non-parametric equivalents.

Parametric analysis	Non-parametric analysis
One-sample *t*-test	Sign test
Paired *t*-test	Sign test, Wilcoxon signed rank test
Two-sample *t*-test	Wilcoxon rank sum test, Mann–Whitney *U* test
One-way ANOVA	Kruskal–Wallis one-way ANOVA
Two-way ANOVA	Friedman two-way ANOVA
Pearson correlation coefficient	Spearman rank correlation coefficient

(ANOVA – see Section 8.6.1), and statistical analyses often assume that the residuals (see Section 10.4.3) have constant variance in different circumstances.

(c) Perform an alternative **non-parametric test**, which does not make distributional assumptions. The non-parametric analyses that we discuss in this chapter are shown, against their equivalent parametric procedures, in Box 12.1. You should be aware that a non-parametric test may not produce an identical *P*-value to its parametric equivalent, and the exact formulation of the null hypothesis may not be the same. The most usual approach is to use the parametric test, provided its underlying assumptions are satisfied.

12.2.3 Advantages and disadvantages of using non-parametric tests

A non-parametric test can be used in the situation when the parametric equivalent is not appropriate for one or more of the following reasons:

 • The sample size is very small, comprising perhaps only five or six observations, and it is, therefore, difficult to establish that the data have a particular distributional form.
 • The distributional assumptions underlying the parametric test of interest are not satisfied.
 • The data are measured on ordinal or nominal scales.

However, if all the assumptions of the parametric test are satisfied, then the non-parametric test is less efficient because of the loss of information incurred by replacing the observations by their ranks. We can measure this loss of efficiency formally by evaluating the **power-efficiency** of the test: this is the extent (measured as a percentage) to which the sample size of the non-parametric test needs to be increased to make it as powerful as the parametric test for a fixed significance level. The power of a test, you will remember (see Section 6.4.2), is the chance of detecting as significant a real treatment difference, and this is proportional to the sample size. So, for example, if the power-efficiency of a test is 90%, this implies that the ratio of the sample size of the non-parametric test to that of the parametric test needs to be 10:9 if the two tests are to be equally powerful, provided all the assumptions underlying the parametric test are met. The power-efficiency of all the non-parametric tests discussed in this chapter is about 95%, with the exceptions of the sign test (falling eventually to 63% for very large sample sizes), the test for Spearman's rank correlation coefficient (91%) and the Friedman two-way analysis of variance (64–87%, depending on the number of groups). Details may be obtained from Siegel and Castellan (1988).

You should also be aware that non-parametric tests tend to be geared towards significance tests rather than to estimation. Although significance tests form an important part of statistical analysis, estimation of the effects of interest provide the necessary understanding of the biological processes involved. As the parametric counterparts of non-parametric tests usually incorporate parameter estimates in their calculation, parametric tests are preferred in many situations.

12.3 Sign test

12.3.1 Introduction

If we are concerned about the assumption of Normality, the sign test can be used as an alternative to the one-sample *t*-test or the paired *t*-test. We would use the one-sample *t*-test if we wanted to test the null hypothesis that the mean value of a numerical variable equals a specific value (see Section 7.3). Similarly, we can use the **sign test** to investigate whether the population from which our sample is taken has a specified median; we determine whether significantly more of the values are greater (or less) than this median.

We can also use the sign test when we want to establish whether the measurements of a single variable, measured on an ordinal (so they can be ranked) or numerical scale, are similar in two groups of paired observations. The pairing may be achieved by matching the animals in a pair with respect to any variables that may be likely to influence the response, or each pair may represent the same animal on different occasions (see Section 5.8.4).

For example, in investigating a test diet which it is believed may promote rapid growth in rats, each of a pair of age/sex-matched litter mates could be assigned to either the test diet or a control diet. The difference in weights (control versus test) between the litter mates after a prescribed time, say 60 days, could be used to determine whether the test diet is effective. In particular, we can use the *signs* of the differences for this purpose.

12.3.2 Rationale

- *One-sample test.* If the median of a sample of observations is approximately equal to the value for the population median specified under the null hypothesis, then we would expect to find an equal number of observations both above and below this specified value. Expressed another way, we would expect half the observations in our sample to be greater than the specified value. This means that we test the hypothesis, framed in terms of the population, that half the observations are greater than the specified median. We are investigating a binary response (above or below a given value); we can therefore use the Binomial distribution (see Section 3.4.2), and the Normal approximation to it (see Section 3.6.1), to test this hypothesis.

- *Paired test.* We start by evaluating the difference, in a defined direction, in the responses for each pair. If, overall, the responses in the two groups are similar, we would expect there to be the same number of positive and negative differences in the pairs. This means that we would expect about half of the differences to be positive if the null hypothesis – that there is no difference in the responses in the two groups – were true. Expressed another way, we test the null hypothesis that the true proportion of positive differences in the population, π, is 0.5. Because we have reduced the two-sample situation to a one-sample situation in which we are investigating a binary response variable (the difference, which can be either positive or negative), again we can use the Normal approximation to the Binomial distribution (see Section 3.6.1).

12.3.3 Assumptions

We assume that the variable under investigation is measured on an ordinal or numerical scale, and that for the paired analysis the observations in the two groups are matched (see Section 5.8.4 for types of pair).

12.3.4 Approach

We explain the approach in relation to the paired situation, but the same principles apply to the single-sample situation.

1. Specify the **null hypothesis**, H_0, that the true proportion of positive differences is 0.5. The alternative hypothesis is that this proportion is not equal to 0.5.
2. **Collect** the data and, if relevant, **display** them in the same way as for the paired *t*-test (see Section 7.5.3).
3. For a computer analysis, choose the *sign test* and proceed to Step 4. Otherwise, **count** the numbers of positive and negative differences (ignore zero differences) and note the smaller number, k. (In a one-sample test we would count the numbers of observations above and below the specified median and note the

smaller.) Suppose there are n non-zero differences; all tied pairs are excluded from the analysis.

If $n \leq 20$, proceed to Step 4.

If $n > 20$, calculate the **test statistic**. It approximately follows the Standard Normal distribution and is given by

$$Test_{12} = \frac{|p - 0.5| - 1/(2n)}{\sqrt{0.5^2/n}}$$

where $p = k/n$ is the observed proportion of positive (or negative) pairs out of n untied pairs; and $1/(2n)$ is a continuity correction that makes an allowance for using the continuous Normal distribution as an approximation to the discrete Binomial distribution.

4. Determine the **P-value** from the computer output, or:
   If $n \leq 20$ and $k \leq 9$, refer k and n to Table A.8. Otherwise, refer $Test_{12}$ to the table of the Standard Normal distribution (see Table A.1).
5. Use the *P*-value to judge whether the data are inconsistent with the null hypothesis. Then **decide** whether or not to reject the null hypothesis. Usually, we reject H_0 if $P < 0.05$.

12.3.5 Example

It was claimed at a regional veterinary meeting that the mean time for a consultation was 12 minutes. A young graduate challenged this statement on the grounds that with such a skewed population (a few cases take considerably more than 12 minutes), the median would be a better estimate to quote. Further discussion led to a general agreement that the median consultation time was also around 12 minutes. The young graduate, being sceptical, decided to test his own practice and conducted a time-and-motion study during morning surgery for 1 week. A total of 43 cases were seen; the results are summarized in Table 12.1.

In order to determine whether the results are inconsistent with a median value of 12, we perform the sign test.

1. The null hypothesis is that the true median duration of a consultation is 12 minutes, or,

Table 12.1 Duration of consultation times.

Duration of consultation	No. of cases
Less than 12 min	22
12 min	6
More than 12 min	15
Total	43

equivalently, that the true proportion of consultations of duration greater than 12 minutes is 0.5. The alternative hypothesis is that this proportion is not equal to 0.5.

2. There is no useful way in which to display these data diagrammatically.
3. There were 15 consultations with duration greater than 12 minutes and 22 consultations with duration less than 12 minutes out of 37 consultations whose duration was not exactly 12 minutes.
4. Thus $k = 15$ (the smaller number) and $n = 37$. This gives $Test_{12} = \{|15/37 - 0.5| - 1/74\}/\sqrt{0.5^2/37}$ $= 0.986$ which, when referred to Table A.1, gives $P = 0.32$.
5. Hence the data are not inconsistent with the null hypothesis that the true median duration is 12 minutes, and there is no evidence to reject it.

12.4 Wilcoxon signed rank test

We can also use the **Wilcoxon signed rank test** as a non-parametric alternative to the paired *t*-test.

12.4.1 Assumptions

We assume that the variable under investigation is measured on an ordinal or numerical scale, and that the observations in the two groups are paired (see Section 5.8.4 for types of pairs).

12.4.2 Approach

1. Specify the **null hypothesis**, H_0, that the samples come from populations with identical distributions and the same median, or from the same population. Generally, the alternative hypothesis is that they do not.
2. **Collect** the data and **display** them in the same way as for the paired *t*-test (see Section 7.5.3).
3. Either select the *Wilcoxon signed rank test* on the computer and proceed to Step 4, or:
   (a) Find the difference between each pair of observations, and indicate whether that difference is positive or negative.
   (b) Ignoring the signs of the differences, **rank** them in order of magnitude. This means that we have to assign successive numbers (the ranks), starting at unity, to the differences. The smallest difference (once we have ignored its sign) is given the rank 1, the next smallest difference gets the rank 2, etc. We ignore zero differences, and reduce the sample size accordingly, from n' to n, say. If two or more absolute differences (i.e. when we ignore their sign) have the same value, then these tied differences get the mean of the ranks they would have received had they not been tied.
   (c) Affix to each rank the sign of its corresponding difference.
   (d) Find the **sum of the ranks** that have a positive sign, T_+, or the sum of the ranks that have a negative sign, T_-, usually, whichever is the smaller. Let us assume here that $T_+ < T_-$.
   If $n \le 25$, proceed to Step 4.
   If $n > 25$, calculate the **test statistic**

$$Test_{13} = \frac{T_+ - n(n+1)/4}{\sqrt{n(n+1)(2n+1)/24}}$$

   which approximately follows the Standard Normal distribution. If there are a large number of ties, then a correction factor should be applied to the denominator. Details may be obtained from Siegel and Castellan (1988).
4. Determine the **P-value**. You may find this in your computer output. Alternatively:
   If $n \le 25$, refer T_+ to Table A.9.
   If $n > 25$, refer $Test_{13}$ to the table of the Standard Normal distribution (see Table A.1).
5. Use the information to determine whether the data are inconsistent with the null hypothesis.

Litter mate pair	Weight on test diet (g)	Weight on control diet (g)	Difference (control − test) (g)	Rank of difference
1	243	265	+22	15
2	161	165	+4	5.5
3	318	361	+43	16
4	270	270	0	–
5	214	235	+21	14
6	97	83	−14	11
7	189	170	−19	13
8	151	158	+7	9.5
9	143	143	0	–
10	117	121	+4	5.5
11	177	174	−3	3.5
12	204	211	+7	9.5
13	190	192	+2	1.5
14	134	131	−3	3.5
15	154	160	+6	8
16	273	291	+18	12
17	126	131	+5	7
18	188	190	+2	1.5

Table 12.2 Weights of litter mate rats on two different diets.

Then **decide** whether or not to reject the null hypothesis. Usually, we reject H_0 if $P < 0.05$.

6. Your computer output may provide a **confidence interval** for the difference in the medians. We refer you to Altman *et al.* (2000) for details of the calculation. Usually it is sufficient to provide the *difference in the sample medians*, together with the interquartile range (see Section 2.6.2) or the range of values that encloses 95% (or 90%) of the observations, to give an indication of the magnitude of the effect of interest. Alternatively, you could show the *median of the differences* in the sample, together with an appropriate range of the differences.

12.4.3 Example

A novel diet for laboratory rats was tested to see if it had any potential to promote rapid growth. Several different strains were included in this preliminary trial, and weanling litter mate rats, of the same sex, were used as the test unit. Eighteen pairs of litter mates were used; each rat in a pair was randomly allocated to the test or control diet, the second rat then receiving the other diet. At 60 days of age, the rats were weighed; these weights are shown in Table 12.2.

In order to investigate whether the test diet is effective, we go through the hypothesis testing procedure:

1. We are testing the null hypothesis that the rats' weight is unaffected by the novel diet, against the two-sided alternative that it is affected by the diet.
2. It is difficult to discern any obvious benefit of the diet from Figure 12.1, which displays the data. The differences in the weights are skewed to the right (you should sketch them to check this), indicating that a non-parametric test is advocated.
3. Proceeding by hand, we rank the absolute differences (ignoring the two zero differences), as shown in Table 12.2. There are only four negative differences, whilst there are 12 positive differences. We therefore find the sum of the ranks of the negative differences = 11 + 13 + 3.5 + 3.5 = 31.
4. Referring this sum to Table A.9, we find that $0.05 < P < 0.10$. In fact, the exact P-value from a computer analysis is $P = 0.06$.

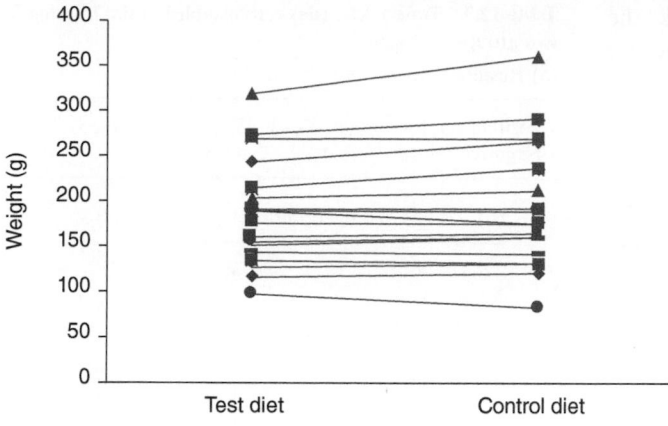

Figure 12.1 Dot diagram showing the weights of litter mate rats on two different diets.

5. There is insufficient evidence to reject the null hypothesis. We have reason to doubt the claim that the novel diet is effective in promoting an increase in growth.

6. The median rat weight (with 25th and 75th percentiles) after 60 days is 183 g (141, 221 g) on the novel diet and 175 g (140, 243 g) on the control diet. The median of the differences in weight is 4.0 g (−0.75, 9.75 g).

12.4.4 Choosing between the sign test and the Wilcoxon signed rank test

The sign test is less powerful than the Wilcoxon signed rank test because it uses only the information about the *direction* of the differences; it ignores their *magnitude*.

Performing the sign test on the rats' weight example of Section 12.4.3, we refer 4 (the number of negative differences, which is smaller than 12, the number of positive differences) to Table A.8. We find that $P = 0.076$, again having insufficient evidence to reject the null hypothesis.

12.5 Wilcoxon rank sum test

12.5.1 Introduction

We can use the **Wilcoxon rank sum test** or the **Mann–Whitney U test** as an alternative to the two-sample t-test if we are concerned that the underlying assumptions of the t-test (Normality and constant variance – see Section 7.4.2) are not satisfied. The two tests produce the same P-value. We shall explain the mechanics of the Wilcoxon rank sum test because its calculations are marginally simpler.

12.5.2 Assumptions

We assume that the variable under investigation is measured on an ordinal or numerical scale. The observations in the two independent samples are representative of the populations of interest.

12.5.3 Approach

1. Specify the **null hypothesis, H_0**, that the two samples could have been obtained from populations that have similar distributions with the same median, or from the same population. Generally, the alternative hypothesis is that they have not been obtained from such populations.

2. **Collect** the data and **display** them in the same way as for the two-sample t-test (see Section 7.4.3).

3. Using the computer, select the *Wilcoxon rank sum test* and proceed to Step 4, or follow the sequence below:

   (a) Suppose there are n_1 observations in the first sample and n_2 observations in the second sample, and $n_1 < n_2$. Rank the observations in the two samples together (i.e. assign successive numbers from 1 to $n_1 + n_2$ to the observations after they have been arranged in increasing order of magnitude). If two or more observations have the same value, then these tied values get the mean of the ranks they would have received had they not been tied.

(b) Find the **sum of the ranks** of one sample (usually the smaller sample), T_1.
If $n_1 \leq 10$ and $n_2 \leq 15$, proceed to Step 4. Otherwise, calculate the **test statistic**

$$Test_{14} = \frac{T_1 - n_1(n_1 + n_2 + 1)/2}{\sqrt{n_1 n_2 (n_1 + n_2 + 1)/12}}$$

which approximately follows the Standard Normal distribution. If there are a large number of ties, the denominator should be modified (Armitage *et al.*, 2002). Most computer packages adjust for tied ranks.

4. Determine the **P-value** from the computer output, or:
If $n_1 \leq 10$ and $n_2 \leq 15$, refer T_1 to Table A.10.
If $n > 10$, refer $Test_{14}$ to the table of the Standard Normal distribution (see Table A.1).

5. Use the *P*-value to determine whether the data are inconsistent with the null hypothesis. Then **decide** whether or not to reject the null hypothesis. Usually, we reject H_0 if $P < 0.05$.

6. Your computer output may provide a **confidence interval** for the true difference in the medians. The relevant formulae are given in Altman *et al.* (2000). Alternatively, you can provide an estimate of the median, together with the range (e.g. the interquartile range or that enclosing the central 95% of the observations) in each sample.

12.5.4 Example

Seventeen puppies were toilet-trained from weaning at 6 weeks of age by either positive reinforcement (praise and encouragement when defecating outdoors) or negative reinforcement (chastisement when defecating indoors). The

Table 12.3 Time taken (days) to establish toilet training in two groups of dogs.

(a) Results as they were obtained (time in days)

Positive reinforcement: 43, 41, 48, 44, 51, 48, 47, 35
Negative reinforcement: 42, 47, 57, 53, 74, 59, 65, 54, 46

(b) Results arranged in order (time in days)

Positive reinforcement	Negative reinforcement	Rank
35		1
41		2
	42	3
43		4
44		5
	46	6
	47	7.5
47		7.5
48		9.5
48		9.5
51		11
	53	12
	54	13
	57	14
	59	15
	65	16
	74	17

time taken for establishment of the habit (seven consecutive days without defecating indoors) was recorded in days. The results are shown in Table 12.3a. Are the two regimens equally effective?

1. The null hypothesis is that the two samples could have been selected from populations with the same median training time or from the same population. The alternative hypothesis is that they are from populations with different median training times.

2. The data are plotted in Figure 12.2; the sample sizes are small, and it would seem that the negative reinforcement training times are skewed to the right. Therefore, a non-parametric test is advocated.

3. The training times of the two samples are ranked together, as shown in Table 12.3b. There are eight observations in the sample with positive reinforcement and nine in the

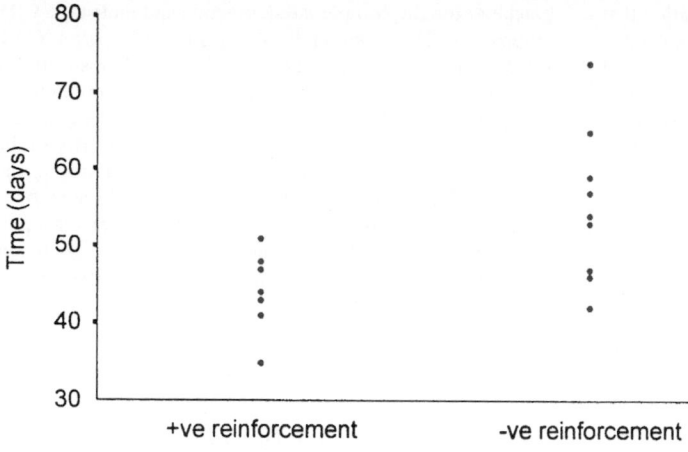

Figure 12.2 Dot diagram showing the time taken for puppies to become toilet-trained with positive or negative reinforcement.

sample with negative reinforcement. Hence we take T_1 to be the sum of the ranks of the sample with positive reinforcement = 1 + 2 + 4 + 5 + 7.5 + 9.5 + 9.5 + 11 = 49.5.

4. We refer 49.5 to Table A.10 with $n_1 = 8$ and $n_2 = 9$, and find that $P < 0.05$ since 49.5 lies outside the limits of 51–93, but $P > 0.01$ since the relevant tabulated limits are 45–99 (in fact, a computer analysis shows that $P = 0.03$).

5. The data are not consistent with the null hypothesis that the samples could have been selected from populations with the same median training time, and we have evidence to reject it. Hence we can conclude that there is evidence indicating that positive reinforcement is better than negative reinforcement.

6. The median training time (with the interquartile range) for the sample with positive reinforcement was 45.5 days (41.5, 48.0 days), and for that with negative reinforcement was 54.0 days (46.5, 62.0 days).

12.6 Non-parametric analyses of variance

12.6.1 Introduction

In this section we indicate the approach used in two particular forms of non-parametric ANOVA – the **Kruskal–Wallis** and the **Friedman ANOVA**. It is unlikely that you will ever have to perform these analyses by hand, so we omit the details of the calculations. You will find them in Siegel and Castellan (1988). In both analyses, we assume the data are measured on an ordinal or a numerical scale.

12.6.2 Kruskal–Wallis one-way ANOVA

(a) Procedure

In Section 8.6 we discussed the one-way ANOVA in some detail. You will recall that this may be regarded as an extension to the two-sample t-test if the means of more than two independent groups of observations are to be compared. However, if either or both of the assumptions underlying the parametric ANOVA (namely, Normality and constant variance – see Section 8.6.1) are not satisfied, perhaps because the data are measured on an ordinal scale, then we may prefer to analyse the data using the equivalent non-parametric **Kruskal–Wallis one-way ANOVA**. It tests the null hypothesis that the $k \geq 3$ independent samples are selected from identical populations with the same median or from the same population.

The appropriate test statistic is determined by replacing the observations in the samples by their ranks. This means that all the observations in the k samples are combined and are arranged in order of magnitude. The smallest observation receives the rank 1, the next smallest rank 2, etc. The test statistic is based on the sum of the ranks in each sample. It approximately follows the Chi-squared distribution with $k - 1$ degrees of freedom.

If the result of the Kruskal–Wallis test is significant, we reject the null hypothesis that all the samples are selected from identical populations with the same median. We infer that at least one of the samples comes from a population that is different from the others. We can then use the Wilcoxon rank sum test (see Section 12.5) to determine which pairs of groups differ. However, because of the potential for testing many combinations of groups (if we have k groups, we could make $k(k-1)/2$ comparisons), we are likely to find spurious significant results unless we adjust for multiple comparisons (see Section 8.6.3).

(b) Example

Barber and Elliott (1998) investigated the aetiopathogenesis of renal secondary hyperparathyroidism (RHPTH) in a prospective study of 80 cats with chronic renal failure (CRF) using routine plasma biochemistry and assays of parathyroid hormone (PTH). The presence of RHPTH can only be diagnosed by the demonstration of elevated plasma PTH concentrations. A knowledge of the prevalence and aetiopathogenesis of RHPTH in naturally occurring feline CRF is imperative before the institution of correct treatment modalities to reduce RHPTH.

Cats presenting as first opinion cases over a 3-year period and diagnosed with CRF were categorized subjectively into three groups (compensated, uraemic and end-stage), according to the severity of clinical signs. Plasma concentrations were determined from blood samples by immunoradiometric assay. Their distributions in the three CRF groups are shown in Figure 12.3. Note that here we have the common situation in which we perform a hypothesis test, in this case comparing the results of cats in three groups, which is not based on random allocation.

Because these distributions are skewed to the right, a Kruskal–Wallis one-way ANOVA is used to compare the medians. The sample medians (25th and 75th percentiles in

brackets) for the compensated, uraemic and end-stage CRF groups are 25.1 pg/ml (12.6, 40.0 pg/ml), 86.7 pg/ml (35.1, 176.2 pg/ml) and 301.2 pg/ml (148.7, 447.8 pg/ml), respectively. The null hypothesis is that the samples come from identical populations with the same median. The result of the Kruskal–Wallis test is that $P < 0.001$, indicating that at least two of the medians differ. Wilcoxon rank sum tests, incorporating the Bonferroni correction (i.e. multiplying each P-value by 3 because there are three two-sample tests) between each pair of groups shows that the median PTH is significantly greater in the end-stage CRF group than in the other two groups ($P < 0.001$) and that the median PTH is significantly greater in the uraemic CRF group than in the compensated group ($P < 0.003$).

12.6.3 Friedman two-way ANOVA

(a) Procedure

In Section 8.5.3 we gave an indication of the manner in which relatively complicated forms of designed experiments can be analysed by ANOVA. In particular, we mentioned the one-way repeated measures ANOVA (often confusingly called a randomized block or, sometimes, a two-way ANOVA) which may be regarded as an extension to the paired t-test when more than two groups of dependent observations are to be compared. The non-parametric equivalent, called the **Friedman two-way ANOVA**, may be performed when the underlying assumptions (Normality, constant variance) of the parametric ANOVA are not satisfied. It tests the null hypothesis that the $k \geq 3$ matched or dependent samples are selected from the same population or from populations with the same median.

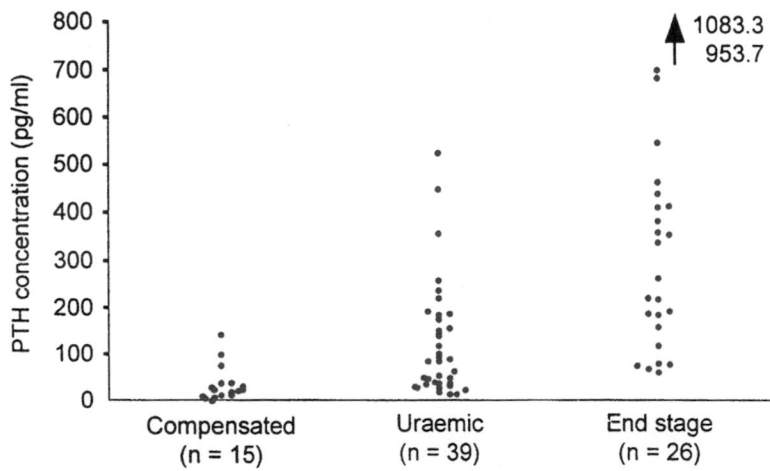

Figure 12.3 Dot diagram showing the distributions of plasma parathyroid hormone (PTH) concentration (pg/ml) in cats in three stages of chronic renal failure (from Barber and Elliott, 1998, redrawn with permission from Wiley-Blackwell).

The observed data are arranged in a two-way table, with the columns, say, representing the k samples (e.g. treatments) and each of the r rows representing a different individual (if each individual has an observation in each of the k samples) or matched individuals. The test statistic is determined by ranking the observations separately in each of the r rows. Thus, the observations in each row are replaced by the ranks $1, 2, \ldots, k$ according to their positions in the ordered set within that row. The test statistic is based on the sum of the ranks in each sample (column), and approximately follows a Chi-squared distribution with $k - 1$ degrees of freedom.

A significant test result implies that the k samples are not selected from populations with the same median. We can establish where the differences lie by performing the Wilcoxon signed rank test on pairs of samples, remembering, of course, to adjust for multiple comparisons (see Section 8.6.3).

(b) Example

Ketoprofen, a non-steroidal anti-inflammatory drug, was administered to horses rectally in three different bases to measure its bioavailability (%) by this route. One gram of drug was distributed in a fatty suppository suspension (A), as a polyethylene glycol solution (B) and as an aqueous suspension (C). Each of the six horses in the study received ketoprofen in the three different bases, with the order in which they received the 'treatments' being randomized. There was a wash-out period of 1 week between the administrations of the treatments. We show the results (derived from summary data presented by Corveleyn *et al.*, 1996) in Table 12.4. We can see that the variances in the treatment groups are quite different. Furthermore, it is difficult to establish Normality of the data since there are only six values in each treatment group. Hence we advocate a non-parametric analysis. The Friedman two-way ANOVA is appropriate because the samples are dependent, with each horse receiving all three treatments.

The null hypothesis is that the three repeated measures come from the same population or populations with the same medians. This null hypothesis implies that the bioavailabilities are the same in the three different treatment groups. The alternative hypothesis is that the three repeated measures do not come from populations with the same medians. A Friedman computer analysis gives $P = 0.31$. Thus, there is insufficient evidence to allow us to reject the null hypothesis; it appears that the formulation base makes little difference to the bioavailability. We show the summary measures, including the medians, for each base formulation in Table 12.4. □

12.7 Spearman's rank correlation coefficient

12.7.1 Introduction

The Pearson product moment correlation coefficient provides a measure of the strength of the linear association between two variables (see Section 10.3). Often we are interested in testing the null hypothesis that the true correlation coefficient in the population is zero, in which case there is no linear association between the two variables. In order to test this hypothesis, we assume that at least one of the two variables is Normally distributed. If we wish to calculate a confidence interval for the correlation coefficient, we assume that both of the variables are Normally distributed (see Section 10.3.2(a)). If we are concerned about these assumptions, we can calculate the **Spearman rank correlation coefficient** as a non-parametric equivalent to the Pearson correlation coefficient. You may also come across **Kendall's** τ (Greek letter tau) which is another non-parametric correlation coefficient.

12.7.2 Calculation

To calculate the Spearman rank correlation coefficient:

- We start by replacing the observations on each of the two variables, x and y, by their ranks. If our sample consists of a series of n pairs of x and y values, $\{(x_1, y_1), (x_2, y_2), (x_3, y_3), \ldots$

Table 12.4 Bioavailability (%) of ketoprofen administered in three bases, A, B and C (based on summary data from Corveleyn *et al.*, 1996, with permission from Wiley Blackwell).

	Bases		
Horses	A	B	C
1	22.5	28.2	37.5
2	11.5	43.8	25.1
3	16.7	36.8	28.9
4	32.1	48.6	33.3
5	36.7	2.1	40.0
6	27.5	12.9	22.9
Median (%)	25.0	32.5	31.1
Mean (%)	24.5	28.7	31.3
Variance (%²)	89.89	329.41	46.58
SD (%)	9.48	18.15	6.82
Range (%)	11.5–36.7	2.1–48.6	22.9–40.0

(x_n, y_n)}, we replace the $(x_1, x_2, x_3, \ldots, x_n)$ by the ranks from 1 to n according to the values of x in the ordered set (the smallest x gets rank 1, the largest x gets rank n), and we replace the $(y_1, y_2, y_3, \ldots, y_n)$ by the ranks from 1 to n according to the values of y in the ordered set. Tied values get the mean of the ranks they would have received had they not been tied.

- The sample value of the Spearman rank correlation coefficient, r_s, is then equivalent to the Pearson product moment correlation coefficient calculated using the ranks instead of the observations themselves. This is the easiest approach to calculating the Spearman rank correlation coefficient if not using computer software.

- Alternatively, we can calculate the Spearman rank correlation coefficient using the formula

$$r_s = 1 - \frac{6\sum d^2}{n^3 - n}$$

where each d is the difference between the ranks for a pair. This formula should be modified if there are tied values in a data set, although the effect is slight if there are few ties. Siegel and Castellan (1988) give details.

12.7.3 Interpretation

The Spearman rank correlation coefficient provides a measure of the association (not necessarily linear) between two variables, but does not imply causality. Similarly to the Pearson product moment correlation coefficient, its limits are −1 and +1. If it takes the value +1, then the individuals have the same *ranks* for both variables; if it takes the value −1, then the *rank* order of one variable is the reverse of that of the other variable. If the Spearman rank correlation coefficient is zero, the two variables are not associated.

12.7.4 Hypothesis testing and calculation of confidence intervals

In order to test the null hypothesis that the two variables, x and y, are not associated (i.e. the true correlation coefficient in the population, ρ_s, is zero), we follow the procedure for testing the Pearson correlation coefficient (see Section 10.3.2(b)). If we have 15 or fewer pairs of observations, we should assess significance using Table A.7. When the number of pairs is greater than 15, we can use, as an approximation, Table A.6 or $Test_{10}$ (replacing r by r_s), to assess significance, as for the Pearson correlation coefficient.

We calculate the confidence interval for ρ_s in the same way as for the Pearson correlation coefficient, replacing r by r_s (see Section 10.3.2(b)).

12.7.5 Example

At a recent dog show, two judges were asked to inspect the entrants, and give them a score out of 10 (including half marks) for conformation to the ideal breed type: the higher the score, the better the entrant. In this particular class, there were 12 entrants. Unfortunately, judge B misunderstood the instructions, and ranked the dogs in order (rank 1 being the best in the class) instead of assigning a score. The results are shown in Table 12.5a. We want to know if the two judges are assessing the dogs similarly, even though the scales of measurement are different. One way of evaluating this is by providing a measure of association between the two types of assessment, i.e. by calculating a correlation coefficient.

The Spearman rank correlation coefficient is preferred to the Pearson correlation coefficient since one of the two assessments was recorded on a ranking scale. We rank the scores for judge A and determine the differences between the two sets of ranks, as shown in Table 12.5b. Then the Spearman rank correlation is the Pearson correlation coefficient between the judges' ranks. This is estimated as 0.864. The alternative approach is to estimate it as

$$r_s = 1 - \frac{6\sum d^2}{n^3 - n} = 1 - \frac{6(38.5)}{1728 - 12} = 0.865$$

The small discrepancy between the two estimates is a consequence of there being three dogs tied at the same rank in the scores assigned by judge A.

Table 12.5 Two judges' assessments of 12 dogs.

(a) Scores given by judge A and ranks given by judge B.

Dog	1	2	3	4	5	6	7	8	9	10	11	12
Judge A	7.0	5.5	8.5	8.0	7.0	3.0	7.5	9.0	7.5	9.5	6.0	7.5
Judge B	6	11	4	2	5	12	7	3	8	1	10	9

(b) Ranks accorded to the scores of judge A with the ranks of judge B (in each case rank 1 is the best dog).

Dog	1	2	3	4	5	6	7	8	9	10	11	12
Judge A	8.5	11	3	4	8.5	12	6	2	6	1	10	6
Judge B	6	11	4	2	5	12	7	3	8	1	10	9
Diff. d	2.5	0	−1	2	3.5	0	−1	−1	−2	0	0	−3

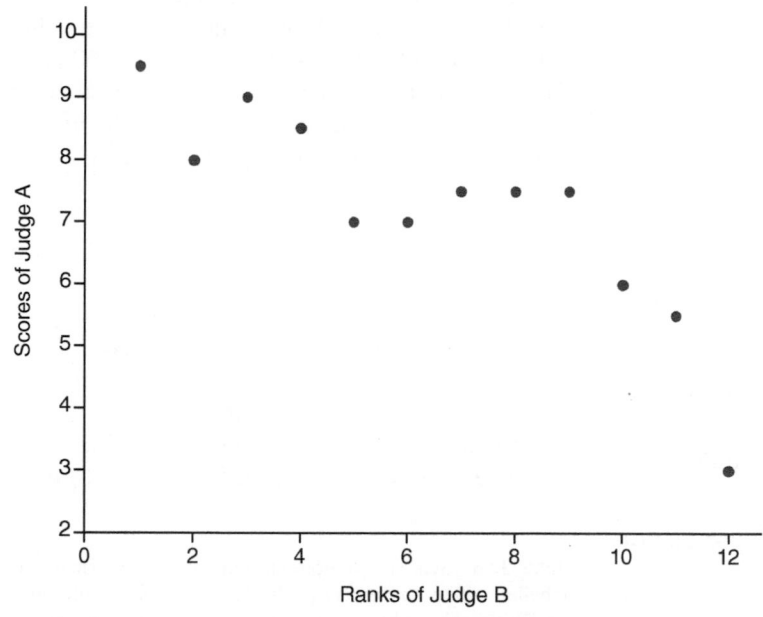

Figure 12.4 Scatter diagram of two judges' assessments of 12 dogs.

We can then assess the significance of the true correlation coefficient in the population by adopting the following procedure:

1. The null hypothesis is that the true Spearman correlation coefficient is zero. The alternative hypothesis is that it is not.
2. The data have been collected and are displayed in a scatter diagram, see Figure 12.4.
3. We refer $r_s = 0.865$ to Table A.7 with a sample size of 12.
4. Since 0.865 is greater than the tabulated value of 0.8182, $P < 0.002$.
5. We have evidence to reject the null hypothesis. This indicates that there is a significant association between the two judges' assessments of the dogs.
6. The 95% confidence interval for the true correlation coefficient is

$$\frac{e^{2z_1} - 1}{e^{2z_1} + 1} \quad \text{to} \quad \frac{e^{2z_2} - 1}{e^{2z_2} + 1}$$

where $z = 0.5\log_e\{(1 + r_s)/(1 - r_s)\} = 1.3129$,

$$z_1 = z - 1.96/\sqrt{(n-3)} = 0.6596, \text{ and}$$

$$z_2 = z + 1.96/\sqrt{(n-3)} = 1.9662.$$

Hence the confidence interval is from

$$\frac{2.7404}{4.4704} \quad \text{to} \quad \frac{50.0293}{52.0293}$$

i.e. from 0.58 to 0.96. This is a very wide confidence interval, as we would expect from a small sample, the lower limit of 0.58 suggesting that we may have some concerns about just how similar the two judges are in their assessments of the dogs.

Exercises

The statements in questions 12.1 and 12.2 are either TRUE or FALSE.

12.1 Non-parametric tests are preferred to parametric tests when:
(a) The data are measured on an ordinal scale.
(b) The sample size is large.
(c) A more powerful test is required.
(d) It is difficult to establish the distribution of the data.
(e) The emphasis is on estimation rather than significance testing.

12.2 The Spearman rank correlation coefficient:
(a) Takes values from −1 to +1.
(b) Measures the degree of association between two variables.
(c) Measures the degree of linear association between two variables.
(d) Requires that at least one of the variables be measured on a ranking scale.
(e) Is preferable to the Pearson correlation coefficient if the sample size is small.

12.3 In a preliminary investigation into the consequences of a treatment that altered growth hormone secretion, plasma insulin concentrations were measured in rabbits randomly assigned to the treatment or control group. There were five rabbits in each group. The rabbits' insulin levels (IU/dl) were measured before and after 6 weeks of treatment, and the difference in the before and after concentration found for each rabbit. Which of the following tests is appropriate for comparing the treatment and control groups?
(a) The sign test.
(b) The Wilcoxon signed rank test.
(c) The Wilcoxon rank sum test.
(d) The paired *t*-test.
(e) The two-sample *t*-test.

12.4 Two methods were used to test the degree of fluorescence of spermatozoa treated with a fluorophore. The subjective method was an ordinal score (0 = no fluorescence, 1 = slight, 2 = clear, 3 = strong fluorescence) and the value for each sample was the mean score for 60 cells. The fluorimeter measurements were on a scale reflecting light intensity emitted by cells in suspension when irradiated by ultraviolet light and detected by a photo-multiplier cell. The results are shown in Table 12.6.
(a) Examine the relationship between the two scores by plotting the data.
(b) Explain why it is more appropriate to calculate Spearman's rank correlation coefficient rather than Pearson's correlation coefficient as a measure of association.
(c) Estimate Spearman's rank correlation coefficient, and test the null hypothesis that its

Table 12.6 Scores of fluorescence intensity of spermatozoa labelled with a fluorescent probe. The scores are made on an arbitrary scale by eye and by means of a fluorimeter.

Sample	Subjective score	Fluorimeter score
1	2.000	0.944
2	2.833	1.048
3	2.667	1.040
4	2.667	1.007
5	1.667	0.845
6	2.500	1.000
7	2.333	1.001
8	2.833	0.990
9	1.008	0.746
10	1.500	0.811
11	1.657	0.862
12	2.000	0.883

value in the population is zero. What do you conclude?

12.5 A dog breeder wanted to establish whether large litter size is inherited. He randomly selected a bitch pup from each of nine large litters (litter size ≥ 5) and from 10 small litters (litter size ≤ 4). When each of these bitches reached adulthood, he counted the size of their second litters. The second litter sizes are shown below:

Bitches from large litters had litter sizes: 3, 7, 5, 6, 4, 6, 5, 7, 5

Bitches from small litters had litter sizes: 2, 3, 6, 4, 3, 4, 3, 5, 4, 5

Is there evidence to indicate that litter size is inherited?

12.6 Obesity is a problem in dogs kept as pets in the Western world. A novel weight control diet has been developed to address this problem. To test the diet, a veterinary surgeon investigates 18 successive obese dogs who present at her surgery, and she measures the dogs' weights (kg) at the time of presentation and after 8 weeks on the weight control diet. The data are shown in Table 12.7. Use an appropriate hypothesis testing procedure to determine whether the novel diet is effective at promoting weight loss. Comment on the limitation of this design and the implication this has for your conclusion.

12.7 This exercise follows on from Exercise 12.6, which you should attempt first. In assessing the effect of a special novel diet on weight in obese dogs, a veterinary surgeon randomly allocates 36 obese dogs who present at her surgery to two 'treatment' groups; either they are prescribed the special diet or they receive their standard diet administered by the owners in restricted quantities according to body weight and size. She records the dogs' weights at the time of presentation and 8 weeks after being put on the diet regimens. The results for the novel diet group are shown in Table 12.7. The results for the control group on the standard diet are shown in Table 12.8. What conclusions can you draw about the effectiveness of the novel diet in promoting weight loss?

12.8 In a study of gluten-sensitivity in Irish setter dogs, O. Garden (personal communication) has examined the activity of the enzyme, aminopeptidase N, in cultured explants of the small intestine of affected dogs. We show in Table 12.9 some results of an experiment in which matched explants from six dogs were studied in medium alone (negative control), under stimulation by a gluten digest (3 mg/ml) and in the positive control, phytohaemagglutinin (PHA). The entries in the table are the percentages of total enzyme activity present in the medium after culture (a measure of cell damage).

(a) How would you analyse the data set, using a non-parametric approach, to determine whether the percentage enzyme activity released is affected by the treatments? State

Table 12.7 Dogs' weights before and after a weight control diet.

Dog	Weight before (kg)	Weight after (kg)	Dog	Weight before (kg)	Weight after (kg)
1	26.5	24.3	10	12.1	11.7
2	16.5	16.1	11	17.4	17.7
3	36.1	31.8	12	21.1	20.4
4	28.0	27.0	13	19.2	19.0
5	23.5	21.4	14	13.1	13.4
6	8.3	9.7	15	16.0	15.4
7	17.7	18.9	16	29.1	27.3
8	15.8	15.1	17	13.1	12.6
9	14.3	14.3	18	19.0	18.8

Table 12.8 Dogs' weights before and after receiving the standard diet for 8 weeks.

Dog	Weight before (kg)	Weight after (kg)	Dog	Weight before (kg)	Weight after (kg)
19	26.0	22.9	28	20.3	19.7
20	21.9	21.3	29	8.7	9.9
21	19.7	16.8	30	18.8	17.2
22	7.5	8.5	31	14.7	14.0
23	15.6	12.7	32	12.7	12.9
24	25.5	27.3	33	16.0	16.9
25	11.4	14.4	34	13.5	11.8
26	16.1	17.0	35	15.4	14.7
27	20.4	21.0	36	13.5	13.3

Table 12.9 Percentage of total aminopeptidase released into the culture medium by duodenal explants stimulated by gluten and phytohaemagglutinin (PHA) (data adapted from O. Garden).

Dog	Medium	Gluten (3 mg/ml)	PHA
Bonnie	11.8	8.4	13.0
Bertie	10.8	8.9	9.1
Billie	17.3	10.3	13.5
Bonker	21.9	9.4	17.5
Barton	12.0	8.1	8.4
Barker	17.0	3.5	8.1
Median (%)	14.50	8.65	11.05
Range (%)	10.8–21.9	3.5–10.3	8.1–17.5

your null hypothesis clearly, and explain why you believe a non-parametric approach is suitable.

(b) If you have access to a computer, analyse the data. You should find that the appropriate non-parametric analysis, using all the data, gives $P = 0.006$. What are your conclusions?

12.9 A study was undertaken to investigate the relationship between aqueous vascular endothelial growth factor (VEGF) level and anterior segment ischaemia in rabbits (Tanaka *et al.*, 1998). Both long posterior ciliary arteries were occluded in six rabbits selected randomly from a sample of 11 rabbits to produce anterior segment ischaemia. The aqueous VEGF levels were measured in these rabbits and in the remaining five control rabbits on days 1 and 14 after entry into the study. The results were compared using appropriate Wilcoxon tests. The aqueous VEGF level was higher on average in rabbits with anterior segment ischaemia than in controls on both days (day 1, $P = 0.03$; day 14, $P = 0.04$), while the levels at day 14 were lower on average than those at day 1 ($P = 0.06$) in the rabbits with anterior segment ischaemia.

(a) Why was it sensible to perform non-parametric tests in this study?
(b) What other reasons could there be for performing non-parametric tests?
(c) Two different types of Wilcoxon test were performed in this study. What were they; when was each used?
(d) What are the null hypotheses for the test with a P-value of 0.03, and for the test with a P-value of 0.06?
(e) On the basis of the three P-values provided, what do you conclude about the comparisons?
(f) Which summary measures should be reported if you want to assess the importance of the findings of each of the three tests?

13 Further aspects of design and analysis

13.1 Learning objectives

By the end of this chapter you should be able to:

- Explain the purposes of data transformation.
- Choose an appropriate transformation where necessary, and demonstrate its effect.
- Explain why sample size is an important design consideration.
- List the factors that influence sample size determination.
- Use Altman's nomogram to determine optimal sample sizes for numerical and binary data.
- Explain the terms sequential analysis and interim analysis.
- Explain the principles underlying a meta-analysis.
- Describe the conditions to be fulfilled for random sampling.
- Elaborate the different ways of selecting a sample.

13.2 Transformations

By now you will be aware that not all data sets fulfil the inherent distributional assumptions of the required statistical procedure. Rather than turn immediately to a non-parametric analysis (see Chapter 12), we often consider transforming the data in order to be able to apply the statistical procedure. A **transformation** is a mathematical manipulation applied to each data point. The aim of the transformation is to produce a data set that satisfies the requirements of the proposed analysis.

The most common reasons for transforming data are to attempt to Normalize data, to linearize a relationship and/or to stabilize variance. So, if the variable of interest is x, then we take a transformation of each individual x-value to create a new variable, t_x, which is some function of x, e.g. its logarithm, reciprocal or square root. We give some examples of common transformations in the following sections.

13.2.1 Normalizing data

Many hypothesis tests and estimation procedures assume a Normal distribution of the variable of interest. There are various transformations that we can take in order to achieve a more nearly *Normal distribution* of t_x when the distribution of x is skewed. Two of the more common are:

1. **Log transformation** (Figure 13.1a and b). $t_x = \log x$ is a transformation that makes the distribution of x more nearly Normal if it is skewed to the right, in which case x is said to have a *Lognormal distribution* (see Section 3.5.3(f)). The logarithm is usually taken either to base 10 (as is common in many branches of medical science) or to base e (the Napierian

Statistics for Veterinary and Animal Science, Third Edition. Aviva Petrie and Paul Watson.
© 2013 John Wiley & Sons, Ltd. Published 2013 by John Wiley & Sons, Ltd.

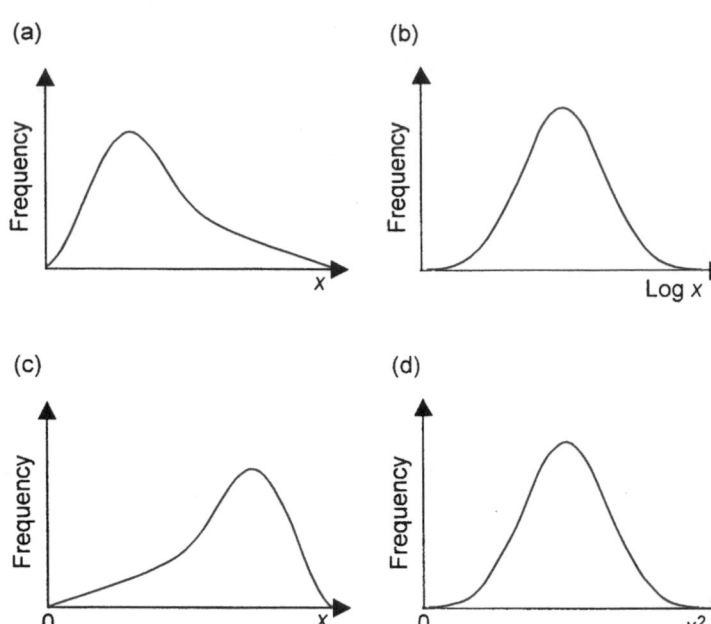

Figure 13.1   Normalizing transformations.

logarithm, written ln x, which is often more convenient in mathematics). Always remember that logarithms can be taken only of positive numbers.

2. **Square transformation** (Figure 13.1c and d). $t_x = x^2$ makes a left skewed distribution of x closer to a Normal distribution.

13.2.2 Linearizing a relationship

It is much easier to analyse data and investigate a relationship between two variables when that relationship can be described by a straight line. The most common transformations that may help to **linearize** a relationship are:

1. **Log transformation** (Figure 13.2a and b). If there is an exponential relationship between y and another variable x, say, such that the slope of the curve (when y is plotted against x) increases for increasing values of x, then a logarithmic transformation of y, $t_y = \log y$, often produces a linear relationship between t_y and x.

2. **Square transformation** (Figure 13.2c and d). $t_x = x^2$ often linearizes a relationship with a consistently decreasing slope.

3. **Logit transformation** (Figure 13.2e and f). Proportions (or percentages) often have a tendency to be grouped towards the lower or upper ends of the scale. If p is a proportion that has a sigmoid relationship with another variable, x, the *logit* or *logistic* transformation, $t_p = \ln\{p/(1 - p)\}$, produces a linear relationship between t_p and x.

4. **Arcsine transformation.** Another transformation of a proportion, p, which linearizes a sigmoid relationship is the *angular, inverse sine* or *arcsine* transformation, $t_p = \sin^{-1}\sqrt{p}$. This transformation can be used for percentages provided they are converted to proportions by dividing by 100.

13.2.3 Stabilizing the variance

Equal variance is assumed in the two-sample t-test (see Section 7.4.2) and in the analysis of variance (ANOVA) (see Section 8.6.1), and

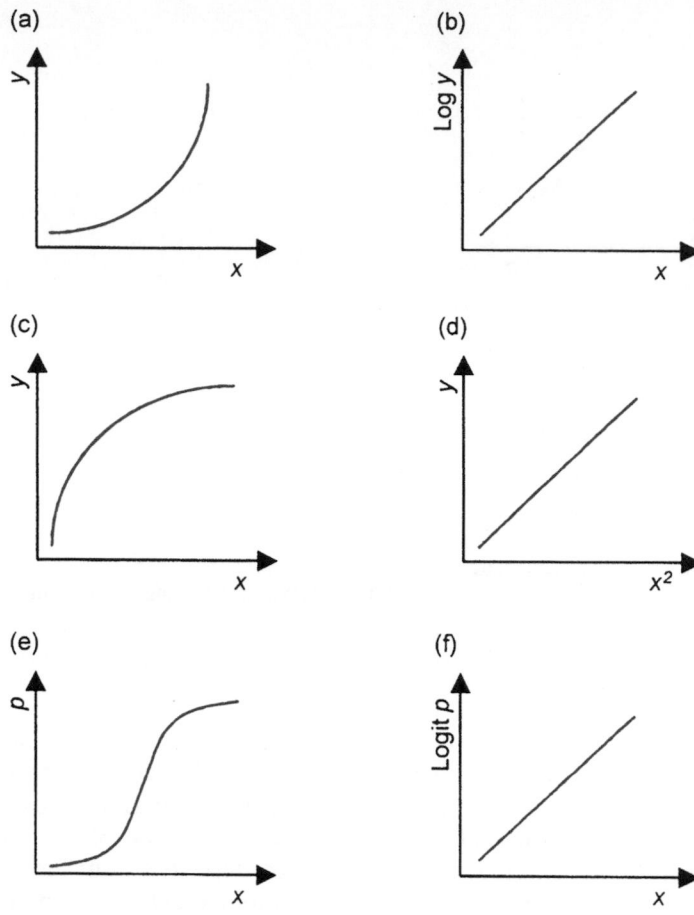

Figure 13.2 Linearizing transformations.

statistical analyses often assume that the residuals (see Section 10.4.3) have constant variance in different circumstances. The most common transformations that help to **stabilize variance** are:

1. **Log, reciprocal and square root transformations** (Figure 13.3a and b). If the variability of x tends to increase with increasing mean values of x (e.g. for groups defined by z), different transformations may be applied:
   - When the standard deviations of different samples are proportional to their means, then the logarithmic transformation, $t_x = \log x$, may stabilize the variance.
   - When the variability is particularly marked for increasing values of x (e.g. if the standard deviation is proportional to the square of the mean), then the reciprocal transfor-

mation, $t_x = 1/x$, may stabilize the variance. The reciprocal transformation is often applied to survival times.
   - When the variances of different samples are proportional to their means, then the square root transformation, $t_x = \sqrt{x}$, is used. This transformation is appropriate when observations are in the form of counts that follow the Poisson distribution (see Section 3.4.3).

2. **Square transformation** (Figure 13.3c and d). $t_x = x^2$, is often used when the variability of the observations decreases with increasing values of x.

3. **Arcsine transformation.** The angular transformation of the proportion, $t_p = \sin^{-1}\sqrt{p}$, described under linearizing transformations, also has the important function of stabilizing variance.

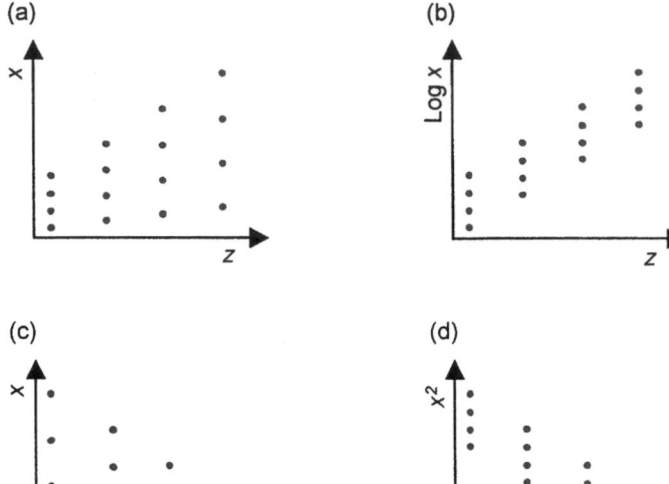

Figure 13.3 Variance stabilizing transformations.

13.3 Sample size

13.3.1 Importance of sample size

One of the most frequently asked questions of a statistician, and one of the hardest to answer, is 'How large a sample do I need if I am to conduct a particular experiment?' We usually design an experiment (see Section 5.4) to investigate the effect of a novel treatment (e.g. drug therapy or feeding regimen) or, perhaps, an intervention (e.g. a surgical procedure or a changed management routine). Usually, we wish to gauge whether it is superior to existing treatments or the absence of treatment, and obtain some estimate of its effect.

Clearly, we should aim to have a sample size large enough to have a good chance of detecting any clinically important treatment differences as statistically significant, and yet not so large as to be wasteful of animals thereby creating ethical difficulties (see Section 15.3) and squandering resources. An inadequate sample size can lead to biologically or clinically meaningful treatment differences that are overlooked, and parameter estimates that lack precision.

Fortunately, statistical techniques exist for determining the optimal sample size in different circumstances for both experimental and observational studies. The downside, however, is that these calculations usually depend on our having some idea of the results we expect at the end of the study before we have conducted it! An added difficulty is that a statistical approach to the sample size problem may produce numbers that are not commensurate with the available resources, such as cost, time and the accessibility of animals. At the end of the day, it must be a combination of practical, ethical and statistical considerations that govern the final decision of the choice of sample size.

13.3.2 Methods for determining the optimal sample size

The standard statistical approach to determining the optimal sample size of an experiment relies on the direct relationship between its **power** and sample size. Power, you will remember (see Section 6.4.2), is the chance of detecting as statistically significant a true treatment effect of a given magnitude. The greater the sample size, the greater the power.

We can use statistical formulae, tables or a diagram (Altman's nomogram) to determine the numbers of animals we require in an experiment of a particular design if we are to have a prescribed power (typically at least 80%) of detecting a real treatment effect. All these procedures are based on the same theory and therefore require the same input (specification of the power, significance level, the effect of interest in the populations being compared, and the variability of the observations), details of which we provide in Section 13.3.3. It is a matter of personal preference as to which approach you use. One option is *Altman's nomogram* because of the ease with which we can determine the sample size of a study under slightly varying conditions (e.g. with different power specifications, at a different level of significance, etc.). Also, it is simple to reverse the procedure and determine the power of a study of a given sample size. However, for small samples (< 100), it tends to overestimate the power.

Alternatively, you may have access to the appropriate computer software (e.g. nQuery Advisor 7.0 from Statistical Solutions Ltd or IBM SPSS Samplepower 3.0 or the freely available PS: Power and Sample Size Calculation software available at http://biostat.mc.vanderbilt. edu/wiki/Main/PowerSampleSize (accessed 16 October 2012)) which deals with both simple and complex designs including regression and survival analysis, and ANOVA. Computer programs speed up the process of sample size estimation, thus allowing us to produce, without any effort, power curves that show how the power varies as, for example, the sample size changes. However, bear in mind the fact that these computer programs require the same input as the other procedures, and it is acquiring this information which creates the real difficulties in sample size estimation.

You can find more on sample size estimation in Machin *et al.* (2009), which includes relevant software, and a full discussion in Cohen (1988). Altman (1980) introduces the nomogram, more details of which can be obtained in Altman (1991).

13.3.3 Nomogram

We can use **Altman's nomogram** to determine the optimal sample size for the comparison of two independent groups of animals (numerical or categorical data) or of paired observations (numerical data) (see Altman 1980, 1991). The calculations are for equally sized groups, but can be modified for unequal sample sizes and they can also be adjusted to allow for losses to follow-up (see Section 13.3.4).

The nomogram in Figure 13.4 shows the relation between the total study size (N), the power, the level of significance (two-tailed) and what is termed the '**standardized difference**'. The formula for the standardized difference is specific to the particular comparison; essentially, it is the difference of interest divided by its standard deviation (details in the following subsections). By drawing a straight line that joins a specified power and standardized difference, for a given level of significance, we can evaluate the required sample size. We can then easily appraise how variations in the power or the components of the standardized difference affect the sample size, or *vice versa*.

(a) Comparison of two independent groups – numerical data

Suppose we wish to determine the sample size of our proposed study if we are interested in comparing the means of a numerical variable using two independent groups. This is achieved by the two-sample *t*-test (see Section 7.4) provided the variable is Normally distributed and each group has the same variance. In order to use the nomogram, we have to specify:

1. The power of the test (usually this should be at least 80%).
2. The two-sided significance level (usually 0.05 but sometimes 0.01 or some other value).
3. The biologically or clinically relevant difference (δ); this treatment effect (see Section 6.3.1) is the difference in the means that we believe is important and which we would not want to overlook. It constitutes the smallest difference in means that represents a clinically

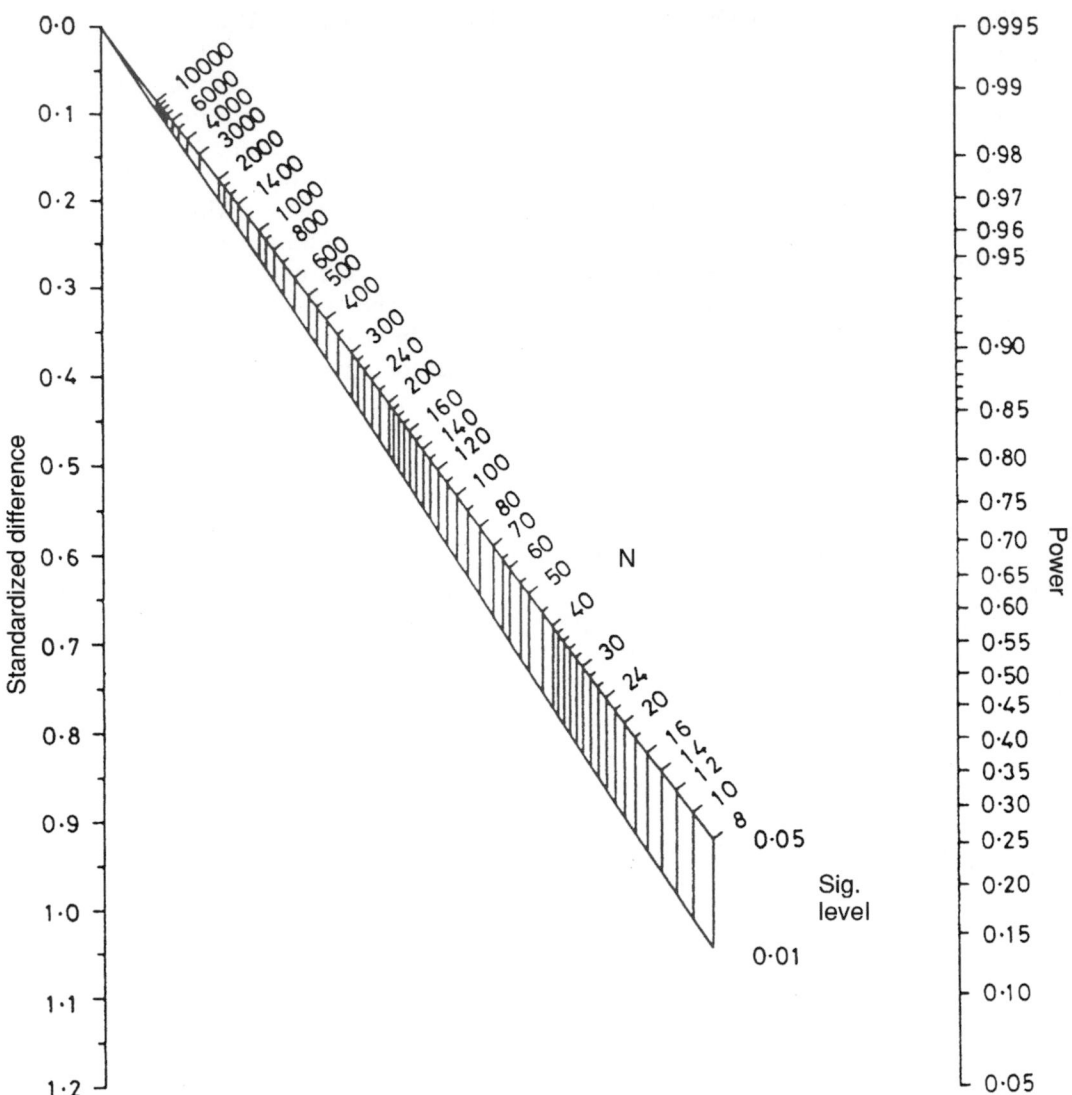

Figure 13.4 Nomogram for sample size determination (from Altman, 1980, reproduced with permission from BMJ Publishing Group Ltd).

meaningful effect and is not necessarily the difference that is expected.

4. The standard deviation of the observations in each group (σ); here we are assuming constant variance, as in the two-sample *t*-test. This is where the real problem lies – we require an estimate of the standard deviation *before* we have collected the data. We can obtain this

estimate either from a previous study that we may have performed which is similar to that which is proposed, from published papers or after we have conducted a pilot study (see Sections 5.9.6 and 13.3.5).

Then the standardized difference = δ/σ, and N = the total number of observations.

Example

Published information suggests that the mean standard lactation (305 days) for Holstein cows in the UK is about 8000 kg and the standard deviation of milk yield is about 1425 kg. Suppose we want to compare the mean milk yields of Holstein cows in Devon with those in Cheshire. We want to know how many animals to sample from each of the two counties if we require an 85% chance of detecting a difference in mean milk yield of 250 kg (this is the minimum difference we would consider of importance to our investigation) at the 5% level of significance.

Thus, δ = 250 kg, σ = 1425 kg, and the standardized difference is 250/1425 = 0.175. If we mark 0.18 on the standardized difference axis, and 0.85 on the power axis of the nomogram, a line that joins these two points cuts the 0.05 significance level axis at N = 1000. Hence, each of the two random samples should comprise 500 cows.

Example

We want to measure the growth of weaner pigs under different growing conditions. We intend to choose matched pairs of weaners from pig litters and assign each weaner pig randomly to one of the two 'condition' groups; the second weaner pig in the pair will then be assigned to the other group. We want to know how many weaner pigs to select in order to have an 80% chance of detecting a mean difference in body weight of 25 g per day (such a difference or a greater one would be considered biologically important) at the 5% level of significance. We believe, from a pilot study, that the standard deviation of the differences is about 45 g per day.

The standardized difference = 2 × 25/45 = 1.11. If we mark 1.11 on the standardized difference axis of the nomogram, and 0.80 on the power axis, a line that joins these two points cuts the 0.05 significance level axis at approximately N = 24. Hence, we require about 24 pairs of weaners.

(b) Comparison of two paired groups – numerical data

Suppose we wish to determine the sample size of our proposed study if we are interested in comparing the measurements of a numerical variable in two paired groups of observations. This is achieved by the paired t-test (see Section 7.5) provided the differences of the pairs are approximately Normally distributed. In order to use the nomogram, we have to specify:

1. The power of the test (usually this should be at least 80%).
2. The two-sided significance level (usually 0.05 but sometimes 0.01 or some other value).
3. The biologically or clinically relevant difference (δ).
4. The standard deviation of the *differences* (σ_d); this is likely to be very difficult to estimate and will probably have to be obtained from a pilot study.

Then the standardized difference = $2\delta/\sigma_d$.

(c) Comparison of two independent groups – categorical data

Suppose we wish to determine the sample size of our proposed study if we are interested in comparing proportions in two independent groups of individuals; for example, those possessing a certain attribute, such as a disease, or having a particular outcome, such as death. This can be achieved by the Chi-squared test (see Section 9.4). In order to use the nomogram, we have to specify:

1. The power of the test (usually this should be at least 80%).
2. The two-sided significance level (usually 0.05 but sometimes 0.01 or some other value).
3. The clinically important difference in the two proportions, $p_1 - p_2$. So, if we know the proportion, p_1, that we expect in one group, we take the proportion, p_2, in the other group to be that which makes $p_1 - p_2$ represent a clinically relevant difference.

Then the standardized difference equals

$$\frac{p_1 - p_2}{\sqrt{\overline{p}(1 - \overline{p})}}$$

where

$$\overline{p} = \frac{p_1 + p_2}{2}$$

Example

Toxocara canis is a dog parasite that can cause blindness in children. We want to know whether the prevalence of *T. canis* infestation is different in puppies compared with adult dogs (based on Ramirez-Barrios *et al.*, 2004). We expect the prevalence in puppies to be about 20% and would be interested in detecting a difference of 15%, i.e. if we found that the prevalence in the adult dog was below 5%, we should regard this difference in prevalence to be biologically important for control measures. We need to know how many adults and puppies to sample if we are to have a 90% chance of detecting this 15% difference at the 5% level of significance.

The mean prevalence

$$\overline{p} = \frac{0.20 + 0.05}{2} = 0.125$$

and the standardized difference equals

$$\frac{0.20 - 0.05}{\sqrt{0.125(1 - 0.125)}} = 0.45$$

Connecting 0.45 on the standardized difference axis of the nomogram to a power of 0.90, we find that we will require about 210 animals in total if we are to achieve significance at the 5% level. Hence our study should comprise about 105 puppies and 105 adult dogs.

13.3.4 Adjustments

- If we believe that there may be withdrawals or dropouts during the course of the study, we will have to increase our sample size estimate to allow for these **losses to follow-up**. This is likely to occur in a longitudinal observational study when animals are studied for a long time or, perhaps, in a clinical trial of a novel treatment. If we expect r% of our animals to be losses to follow-up, we modify the unadjusted estimated optimal sample size, obtained using the methods described in Section 13.3.3, by multiplying it by $100 \div (100 - r)$. Consider, for example, the cross-over study in Section 7.5.4 that used the paired t-test to compare the effect on serum glucose of two diets in insulin-dependent diabetic dogs. These dogs each received one diet for 8 months before being switched to the other diet for a further 8 months. Suppose the investigators had expected a 5% attrition rate and had estimated that they needed 10 dogs using the approach described in Section 13.3.3(b). Then the adjusted sample size would be $1000 \div (95) = 10.5$: rounding this up results in a requirement for 11 dogs.

- We showed in Section 13.3.3 how we can use the nomogram to estimate the optimal sample size if we were intending to use a two-sample t-test to compare two means and a Chi-squared test to compare two proportions. In both instances we assumed that the requirement was for equal numbers in the two comparison groups. Sometimes, however, we may want **groups of different sizes**, perhaps because the availability of the novel treatment in a clinical trial is restricted or because the disease is rare in a case–control study (see Section 5.2.3(b)). Suppose we wish to have k times as many animals in one group as in the other. Then the adjusted overall sample size is equal to $N(1 + k)^2/(4k)$, where N is the unadjusted overall sample size obtained using the methods described in Section 13.3.3. As an example, consider the study to compare the prevalence of *Toxocara canis* infestation in puppies and adults dogs (see Section 13.3.3(c)). On the premise that a Chi-squared test would be used to compare the two proportions with *T. canis* infestation, we estimated the overall optimal sample size to be 210, comprising 105 puppies and 105 adult dogs. If the investigators had wanted twice as many puppies as adult dogs, they would need to recruit $210(1 + 2)^2/8 = 237$ (rounded up from 236.25) dogs in total. This would imply that they should have $237/3 = 79$ adult dogs and 158 puppies in their study. The overall optimal sample size is greater in this example with unequal sample sizes than with equal sample sizes, and this is generally the case, provided all the factors relevant to the estimation of sample size remain unaltered.

13.3.5 Internal pilot study

We indicated in Section 13.3.3(a) that, when determining sample size, we might have to rely on a pilot study to provide a value for the expected standard deviation of the observations in each group. A pilot study is generally regarded as a preliminary investigation that is distinct from the main study. However, when animals are in short supply, perhaps because they are rare or costly, or when the measurements on them are laborious and/or expensive, we can use an **internal pilot study** which incorporates the results from the pilot study into the main study. In this process, explored by Birkett and Day (1994), we estimate the overall sample size using the information currently available and then conduct a pilot study whose size is pre-specified and often determined by practical considerations. We use the measurements obtained from this pilot study to provide appropriate estimates of interest (e.g. of the standard deviation) which we then employ to re-evaluate the optimal sample size. The results from the animals used in this internal pilot study are treated as belonging to the main body of the data rather than distinct from it. To ensure that the conclusions from the study are valid:

- All details of this process must be documented in the protocol.
- The calculations of the optimal sample size at the second stage of this procedure must be based on the effect of interest (e.g. the smallest difference in means that constitutes a mean-

ingful clinical effect) that was specified at the design stage of the trial and used in the initial sample size calculations; it is *not* the effect of interest observed in the pilot study.
- The final sample size can never be less than that determined from the initial calculations: the latter can only be increased if a revision is advocated.

13.4 Sequential and interim analysis

The designs that we have considered so far have been **fixed sample size plans**; we make a decision about the approximate sample size in advance of performing the experiment. In certain circumstances, we can avoid choosing our sample size at the start of the investigation, and design the trial in such a way that the data are analysed as they are collected. We call this kind of trial, in which we have continuous monitoring of the treatment differences, a **sequential trial**. Generally, **sequential analysis** is performed on pairs of observations, one member of each pair being allocated at random to one of the two treatments; the other member of the pair receives the other treatment. We analyse the results from the pairs as they accumulate; we stop the trial when the evidence for one treatment is overwhelming or when we believe that it is unlikely that any difference will emerge. The stopping rules (determining when to 'stop') are defined by specifications of the null and the alternative hypotheses and of the significance level and power of the test. You may obtain full details in Armitage (1975).

Sequential trials tend, on average, to require smaller sample sizes than the equivalent fixed sample size plans. However, they are only amenable to the study of conditions in which the response to treatment can be evaluated soon after its administration. They are limited to trials in which there is only one response variable of predominant importance.

Sometimes we wish to design our trial as a fixed sample size study, but would like to have the option of terminating the trial before the end by performing a *predetermined* number of **interim analyses**. We must decide in advance when any intermediate analyses are to be carried out, and *not* be tempted to interrupt the investigation at whim. Then, if we find treatment differences that are convincingly large, we can stop the trial early, thereby ensuring:

- In the clinical setting, that the maximum number of animals receive the better treatment.
- In the experimental setting, that only a minimum number of animals are subjected to any adverse conditions.

Such a trial is also called a **group sequential design** (the data are analysed after the results of groups of animals become available, rather than after each pair as in the continuous sequential design) and is based on the idea of **repeated significance tests**. The significance test at each of the interim analyses uses the same form of test statistic as at the final stage, and not the stopping rules of sequential analysis. Multiple significance tests have the effect of increasing the chance of finding a significant difference when the treatments really are the same (see Section 8.6.3). In effect, we will increase the significance level at the final stage after repeated significance tests unless we make appropriate adjustments. For example, if we have five repeated tests, each at the 5% level, the *overall* significance level becomes 14%, i.e. in effect we reject H_0 if $P < 0.14$. In order to keep this overall significance level at, say, 0.05, we must choose a more stringent *nominal* significance level for each of the repeated tests (an appropriate value less than 0.05). In particular, for our example of five repeated tests, the nominal level is 0.016. You can obtain further discussion of the method and the required nominal significance levels for varying numbers of interim analyses in Pocock (1983). □

13.5 Meta-analysis

13.5.1 Introduction

We may find that the results of a study are not statistically significant because its sample size is small and, hence, its power is low, even though there is a clinically important treatment difference. One way of improving the power of an investigation and increasing the precision of the estimates of treatment effects, without undertaking a much larger study, is to combine the results from similar trials in an appropriate manner. This is achieved by performing what is termed a **meta-analysis** or **overview** which provides a statistical summary of the numerical outcomes of the separate studies. A meta-analysis is a quantitative example of a **systematic review** that examines the literature in a rigorous and clearly defined manner; this contrasts with a traditional review which is often not very systematic and mixes together opinions and evidence.

A meta-analysis plays an important role in evidence-based veterinary medicine (see Sections 16.3–16.6) as it often provides the most comprehensive material, already well assimilated and critically appraised, from which to draw conclusions concerning the optimal treatment for a given condition. Although meta-analyses are becoming increasingly popular in medicine, and

are gaining favour in veterinary and animal science, they are not without their critics. Several **problems** can arise; for example:

- It may be difficult to decide exactly which studies should be included (e.g. must they be randomized? Should poor quality trials be excluded?).
- The conclusions may be affected by **publication bias** (the tendency for journals to give substantially more space to papers in which the treatment effects are statistically significant) so that many trials with non-significant results are excluded from the meta-analysis.
- The data summarized may not be homogeneous (e.g. because of methodological or clinical differences: this is called **clinical heterogeneity**) and the studies may differ in their quality.

However, if handled correctly (see Stroup *et al.*, 2000), a meta-analysis will improve the reliability and accuracy of recommendations.

You can obtain further discussion of meta-analysis in, for example, Borenstein *et al.* (2009), Egger *et al.* (2001), Freemantle *et al.* (1999), Sutton *et al.* (2000) and Whitehead (2002). In addition, the **Cochrane Collaboration**, an international non-profit and independent organization, produces and disseminates systematic reviews of healthcare interventions and promotes the search for evidence in the form of clinical trials and other studies of interventions. Although the systematic reviews currently in its library relate only to human investigations, its website (www.cochrane.org, accessed 20 October 2012) provides useful information relating to workshops, discussion lists and aspects of training. Review Manager (RevMan Version 5.1. Copenhagen: The Nordic Cochrane Centre, The Cochrane Collaboration, 2011) is the Cochrane Collaboration's freely downloadable software which can be used to help reviewers be systematic and explicit when performing a meta-analysis.

In promoting good practice, we refer you to the PRISMA statement (see Section 17.7), aimed at helping authors report systematic reviews and meta-analyses to assess the benefits and harms of a healthcare intervention.

13.5.2 The process

(a) Effect of interest in a single study

A quantitative summary of a study is usually provided by the **effect of interest**. For example, in a clinical trial comparing a novel treatment with a control treatment, as judged by a numerical response (e.g. weight gain), the effect of interest is commonly the difference in the mean responses. Alternatively, if we have a binary response (e.g. presence or absence of disease) or are investigating the results of a case–control study, the effect of interest is generally the odds ratio, equal to the odds of disease in the treated group (or those with the factor) divided by the odds of disease in the control group (or those without the factor) – see Section 5.2.3(b). The treatment has no effect if the means are equal or the odds ratio is one (or, equivalently, if the logarithm of the odds ratio is zero).

(b) Combining the effects of interest from different studies

The aim of a meta-analysis is to combine the estimates of the effect of interest from k (say) single studies under review to obtain one overall estimate of the effect of interest. However, it is really only sensible to obtain an overall estimate if the estimates from the separate studies are similar (i.e. they are *statistically homogeneous* rather than *heterogeneous*). There are two commonly used approaches to investigating statistical homogeneity, and both are usually employed in a meta-analysis.

- We calculate the I^2 **statistic**, which can be viewed as a measure of inconsistency of the findings across the studies and represents the proportion of the total variation that is due to heterogeneity. It takes values from 0% when there is no observed heterogeneity to 100%, with larger values showing increasing heterogeneity. Higgins *et al.* (2003) suggest that values of the order of 25%, 50% and 75% might be considered as low, moderate and high, respectively. The I^2 statistic has the advantages that

it is independent of the scale of measurement of the observations and of the choice of effect of interest (e.g. relative risk, odds ratio or difference in means) and is not directly affected by the number of studies in the analysis. It can therefore be compared in meta-analyses with different types of outcome data and with different numbers of studies.

- We perform a **hypothesis test of homogeneity** (i.e. the null hypothesis is that there no difference in the true effects of interest in the k studies) by calculating Cochran's Q test statistic which approximately follows a Chi-squared distribution. A *significant result* implies heterogeneity. A *non-significant result* does not indicate that the estimates are similar, only that there is no evidence to show that they are different, i.e. a non-significant result does not necessarily imply homogeneity. It may be that there are only a small number of studies in the meta-analysis, in which case the power (see Section 6.4.2) of the test will be low.

If we are confident that there is no statistical heterogeneity, we generally use a **fixed effects** approach to estimation. We then assume that the separate studies are the only ones of interest and that the underlying effects from the different studies are all equal to each other and, in turn, to the overall effect. When there is evidence of statistical heterogeneity, it is customary to use a **random effects** approach to estimating the overall effect (although we should carefully investigate the reasons for this statistical heterogeneity before proceeding, and decide whether or not it is sensible to derive an overall estimate). In the random effects approach, we regard the separate studies as a random sample of studies from a population of studies. Thus we expect the estimated effects from the different studies to exhibit variability and to have a mean equal to the true mean effect in the population. However, if we are concerned about the heterogeneity and believe that a single overall measure of effect would be inappropriate, instead of performing a random effects analysis, we could stratify the studies into homogenous *subgroups* (i.e. where there is no evidence of heterogeneity within each subgroup) and perform a separate, usually fixed effects, meta-analysis in each stratum. We must take care when interpreting *P*-values in these subgroup analyses: lack of significance may be due to low power (see Section 6.4.2) whilst, at the other extreme, spuriously significant results may be a consequence of multiple testing (see Section 8.6.3).

Whether we assume a random or a fixed effects approach to estimating the overall effect of interest has algebraic repercussions. The estimate is usually determined as a **weighted mean** of the *k* separate estimates. Thus, if the *i*th study effect of interest is estimated by E_i where $i = 1, 2, \ldots, k$, and each study has a weight, w_i, then the weighted mean is given by:

$$\bar{E}_w = \frac{\sum w_i E_i}{\sum w_i}$$

and the variance of this weighted mean is estimated by $\mathrm{Var}(\bar{E}_w) = 1/\sum w_i$ so that its standard error is $\sqrt{\mathrm{Var}(\bar{E}_w)}$.

The weight, w_i, for the *i*th study ($i = 1, 2, \ldots, k$) typically reflects the precision of the estimate, and is generally taken as the inverse of the associated estimated variance. In this way, studies with greater precision are given more weight. Since larger studies provide augmented information and therefore have more precise estimates, we occasionally take the study sample sizes as the weights for the different studies instead of the inverse of the variances.

However, the weight, w_i, is affected by the extent to which there is statistical heterogeneity. In the *fixed effects* approach (with no evidence of statistical heterogeneity), we consider the variance of the estimated effect for the *i*th study to be the only variance that is relevant to that study, and so this variance is the only component of w_i. In contrast, in the *random effects* approach (with statistical heterogeneity), we include in the w_i both the variance of the estimated effect for that study as well as some measure of the variability of the estimates between studies. The weight for the *i*th study in a random effects analysis is therefore less and the standard error of the overall estimate greater than that of the comparable fixed effects analysis. Consequently, the confidence interval for the overall effect of interest for the random effects model is wider if there is statistical heterogeneity.

(c) Testing the overall effect of interest

Once we have obtained an estimate for the overall effect of interest, we generally want to use it to assess whether there is a 'treatment' effect. (Is one treatment better than the other? Is the presence of a factor associated with disease?) The null hypothesis in a fixed effects analysis is that the true effect of interest is zero in every study (e.g. the true treatment means are equal so that their difference is zero, or the true odds ratio is one so that its logarithm is zero). The null hypothesis in a random effects model is that the true mean effect is zero. We can calculate a test statistic that approximately follows the Chi-squared distribution to test this hypothesis. A significant result suggests that there is evidence of a treatment effect. We have not provided formulae in this book either for the homogeneity test or for this test of the effect of interest as you will invariably perform a meta-analysis using computer software, and will not need the details. You can obtain the formulae in many texts such as those suggested in Section 13.5.1.

(d) Displaying the results

We generally display the results from the separate studies in a diagram called a **forest plot** (Figure 13.5). This is usually drawn with the horizontal axis indicating the different values for the effect of interest. A vertical line is drawn through the value that represents 'no effect' (e.g. it is zero for a difference in means or for a log odds ratio). The studies are identified at the side of the plot, and for every study the estimated effect of interest with its associated confidence interval is marked appropriately; the overall estimate with its confidence interval is also included, usually at the bottom of the plot. Sometimes, the area of the symbol for an estimated effect reflects the size of that study; the larger the area, the bigger the study. From the forest plot, we can get a visual impression of the extent to which the estimates differ, and decide, subjectively, whether or

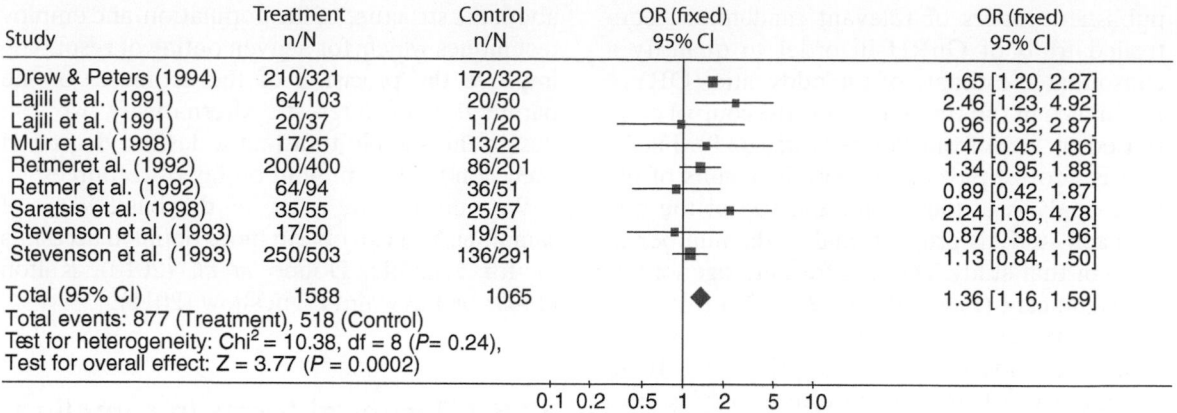

Figure 13.5 Forest plot of the estimated odds ratio (OR) of pregnancy in cows treated with gonadotrophin-releasing hormone (GnRH) and control cows, with 95% confidence intervals (CI) (derived from Review Manager (RevMan) [Computer program]. Version 5.1. Copenhagen: The Nordic Cochrane Centre, The Cochrane Collaboration, 2011).

not there is statistical heterogeneity by looking at the overlap, or absence of it, of the confidence intervals. Furthermore, we have evidence that an effect, either from a single study or from all studies combined, is statistically significant if its confidence interval does not cross the 'no effect' line.

Another plot that is commonly used in meta-analysis is a **funnel plot**, which may allow us to assess whether publication bias is present. Publication bias occurs when there is selective publication of studies on the basis of the magnitude and direction of their findings. It occurs in the meta-analysis when there is a tendency to favour studies with statistically significant results as those manuscripts are more likely to be submitted to journals and published. In such circumstances the missing studies are systematically different from those that are included (see Section 5.9.4). Usually, for a given sample size, they will have smaller effects of interest (e.g. difference in means) or, *vice versa*, for a given effect of interest, they will be smaller studies. Traditionally the funnel plot is a scatter diagram in which the effect of interest is plotted on the horizontal axis and some measure of the sample size is plotted on the vertical axis. The latter may be the actual sample size or may be, for example, the standard error of the effect of interest, as smaller studies tend to have larger standard errors. If the

standard error is used, the scale on the vertical axis is reversed, going from high values at the bottom to low values at the top. In the absence of publication bias, the studies in the funnel plot are distributed symmetrically about the average effect of interest, exhibiting an inverted funnel (hence the nomenclature) demonstrating increasing spread of studies as the sample size decreases, with few studies at the top where the sample size is large and widely dispersed studies at the bottom. If publication bias is present, there is likely to be symmetry at the top but asymmetry at the bottom of the funnel, with an absence of studies in the area where the small studies with non-significant results or negative findings would have been. This would be on the left-hand side of the plot if the effect of interest was, for example, the difference in two means, with zero representing no effect of treatment and positive values to the right representing a treatment effect.

13.5.3 Example

Although a number of studies have used gonadotrophin-releasing hormone (GnRH) between 11 and 14 days after first insemination to improve pregnancy rates in cows, the results have not been consistent. We show the results of a meta-analysis on nine studies from six published papers of relevant randomized controlled trials of GnRH in order to quantify a consolidated estimate of the odds ratio (OR) of pregnancy in the treated versus the control cows (based on data from Peters *et al.*, 2000). Figure 13.5 is a forest plot that shows the results of the meta-analysis of these data; the size of the box for each study is proportional to the number of cows in that study. The test for heterogeneity is not significant ($P = 0.24$) and $I^2 = 23\%$ (low heterogeneity) and so it is reasonable to use the estimated odds ratio of 1.36 (95% CI 1.16 to 1.59), derived from a fixed effect analysis, as a combined estimate of the effect of interest. Thus, it can be seen that there is a significant improvement in the pregnancy rate of cows on treatment with GnRH ($P = 0.0002$); the odds of a cow becoming pregnant is increased by 36% if the cow is treated.

13.6 Methods of sampling

13.6.1 Introduction

When we are interested in certain features of a population, it is usually impractical to appraise the complete population because of the constraints of time, finance or labour. Instead, we conduct a **sample survey** in which we study only a portion of the population. A sample survey is a particular type of observational study (see Section 5.2.1); it is usually concerned with estimating the parameters in the population from which it is selected. These should be **unbiased** (free from bias) and **precise**. If an estimate is free from bias, then the mean of its sampling distribution is equal to the value of the parameter in the population (see Section 4.4.3). The precision of an estimate is measured by its standard error, a more precise estimate having a smaller standard error.

We can attempt to eliminate selection bias if we use a mechanism based on chance to select a **random sample** of individuals (see Section 1.9.2), each individual having the same probability of selection. Random sampling is sometimes called **probability sampling**. Then we build on the initial premise of random selection, using information about the structure of the population, and employ techniques which, for a given outlay of resources, improve the precision of the estimates of the parameters of interest. Alternatively, we can design the sample to attain a desired degree of precision for a minimum outlay of resources.

We only outline some of the basic ideas of sampling. You can obtain more detailed accounts in, for example, Dohoo *et al.* (2010), Kalton (1983) or Levy and Lemeshow (2011).

13.6.2 Technical terms in sampling

An **element** is a single object or individual on which a measurement can be taken. The **population** from which we take our **sample** comprises an aggregate of **sampling units**. These are non-overlapping collections of elements, i.e. every element in the population belongs to only one unit. If each sampling unit contains only one element, then the sampling unit and the element are identical. The **frame** is a list of sampling units.

13.6.3 More common sampling designs

You may find Figure 13.6 helpful in conceptualizing the following descriptions of the more common sampling designs.

(a) **Simple random sampling** is the basic sampling design. The sampling units are chosen in such a way that:
   - The selection of one unit has no influence on the chance of any other being selected, i.e. they are *independent*.
   - Each possible sample of *n* units from the population of *N* units has an equal chance of being selected. This implies that every member of the population has an equal chance of being included in the sample.

   As an example, consider a trout farm in which scientists want to sample the trout from a pond for heavy metal contamination. A random sample is taken of sufficient size to be representative of the population. For

(a) Random sampling

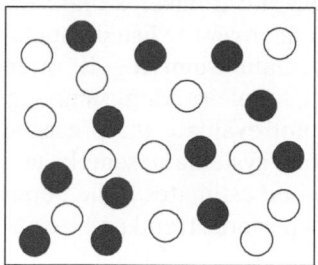

(b) Stratified sampling
(some units of all strata)

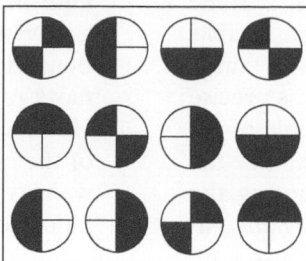

(c) Cluster sampling
(all units of selected clusters)

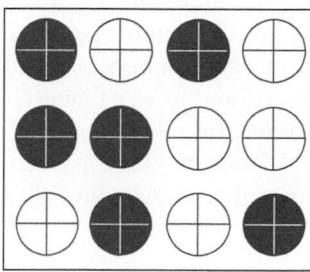

(d) Systematic sampling
(each unit in same relative position)

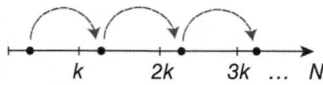

Figure 13.6 Diagrammatic illustration of different sampling techniques.

example, for a stock of 8000 fish we might take a random sample of 2%, i.e. 160 fish.

(b) In **stratified sampling**, we divide the population into various subpopulations called strata. We select a simple random sample of units from each stratum, and compute parameter estimates from each stratum. We combine these estimates appropriately, using a weighted technique, to provide the required estimates of the parameters of interest. For example, in a wildlife population study in a particular location, the strata may be hedgerow, open field and woodland. These different habitats are likely to influence parameters such as population density, plumage and development rate. The sites would be identified and a simple random sample of animals taken from each. The estimates of each parameter of interest would be obtained from the three habitats and then combined to obtain an overall population estimate for this location.

Stratified sampling usually results in more precise estimates for a given cost than simple random sampling. For maximum precision, we construct the strata so that the strata means are as different as possible, and the units within each stratum are as alike as possible. Stratified sampling is the method most commonly employed in wildlife population surveys.

(c) In **cluster sampling**, we divide the population into clusters of units. We select a simple random sample of clusters from the population of clusters, and observe all the units in the selected clusters. As an example, suppose a veterinary practitioner wants to investigate the incidence of calving problems in his practice area. He could define the cattle farms on his books as the clusters, and note all the incidents of dystokia over the period of the study in a random selection of these farms.

Cluster sampling is cheaper and more practical than simple or stratified random sampling if the clusters represent a geographically compact set of units. We may have to resort to cluster sampling if a frame that lists all population units is unavailable. However, the parameter estimates obtained from a cluster sample tend to be less precise than those of a simple random sample of the same number of units. We can maximize the precision of the estimates by choosing the clusters so that cluster means are as alike as possible, and the units within each cluster are as diverse as possible. Furthermore, we will obtain more precise estimates from a large number of small clusters than a small number of large clusters.

Although cluster sampling bears a superficial resemblance to stratified sampling in that a cluster, like a stratum, is a grouping of the units in the population, the two techniques are quite different. In stratified sampling, every stratum is represented in the final sample, and we select units at random from each sample; in cluster sampling, we select a random sample of clusters from a population of clusters in the same way as we select individual units from a population of units in simple random sampling. In cluster sampling we observe every unit in the selected clusters.

(d) We can extend cluster sampling by introducing one or more stages to the basic technique to obtain a **multi-stage sample**. For example, in two-stage sampling, we start by dividing the population into clusters. At the first stage, we select a random sample of clusters from the population of clusters. At the second stage, we select a random sample of units from the selected clusters rather than enumerating every unit in the selected clusters.

(e) In **systematic sampling**, we randomly select one unit from the first k units in the frame, and then every kth unit thereafter. In the strict sense, a systematic sample is not a true random sample because only the first unit is selected at random. Once the first unit has been selected, the remaining units are predetermined in that every one occupies the same relative position in each group of k

units. A systematic sample is appealing because it is relatively easy to assemble the units in the sample and it ensures that they are evenly distributed over the listed population. Hence systematic sampling is often more precise than simple random sampling. However, we cannot evaluate the precision of the estimates in a systematic sample, and we may obtain biased estimates if the population consists of a periodic trend and k coincides with the period or a multiple of it.

Multi-stage and systematic sampling have less use in veterinary and animal science than in human investigations. Systematic sampling depends on being able to list all the individuals. Unlike humans with their voting registers, National Insurance or Social Security numbers, animals are usually more dispersed and less regimented. However, the tagging of individuals accompanying the need to trace all food animals for veterinary disease control measures is now providing opportunities for systematic sampling.

You may be interested to note the relationship of systematic sampling to both stratified and cluster sampling. The systematic sample is almost equivalent to a stratified sample if we regard each stratum as a group of k consecutive units in the frame. Our sample comprises a single unit from each 'stratum', although only the first unit is selected at random. The systematic sample is equivalent to a cluster sample if we define the ith cluster ($i = 1, 2, 3, \ldots, k$) as that containing the ith unit in every group of k consecutive units in the frame. Then there exist k possible clusters to choose from, and in a systematic sample we are selecting a simple random sample of one cluster from this population of k clusters. □

13.6.4 Sampling from wildlife populations

It is important to be able to estimate the size of many wildlife populations for the study of growth, evolution and maintenance. There are a number of ways in which the estimate can be obtained.

(a) Capture–tag–recapture

The **capture–tag–recapture** method can be split into two types of sampling procedure: direct sampling and inverse sampling.

1. **Direct sampling:**
   (a) We take a random sample of size t from the wildlife population, tag each animal sampled, and return these animals to the population.
   (b) At some later date, we take a second random sample, this time of a predetermined size, n, from the population, and observe the number tagged, s.

   For example, suppose we want to estimate the pigeon population in Trafalgar Square. We take a random sample of $t = 500$ pigeons and ring (tag) them before release. A week later, we take another sample of $n = 200$ pigeons and note that $s = 29$ are ringed.

2. **Inverse sampling:**
   (a) We take a random sample of size t from the wildlife population, tag each animal sampled, and return these animals to the population.
   (b) At some later date, we select animals from the population, using random sampling, and observe whether or not the animals captured are tagged. We continue sampling until we observe exactly s (a predetermined number) tagged animals. Let us suppose that we need to select n animals in this second sample to obtain s tagged animals.

   As an illustration, suppose we start by taking a random sample of $t = 500$ pigeons and ring them before release. We decide that we are going to capture $s = 25$ ringed pigeons 1 week later. At that time we find that we have captured $n = 173$ pigeons of which $s = 25$ are ringed.

   For both direct and inverse sampling

   $$\text{Estimated population size} = \frac{t}{s/n}$$

where the denominator represents the proportion of tagged animals in the second sample, estimating the proportion of tagged animals in the population.

In our example, we estimate the pigeon population in Trafalgar Square to be

$$\text{Direct sampling,} \frac{t}{s/n} = \frac{500}{29/200} \approx 3448 \text{ pigeons}$$

$$\text{Inverse sampling,} \frac{t}{s/n} = \frac{500}{25/173} \approx 3460 \text{ pigeons}$$

However, the variance of the estimate is different in each case. The estimated variances of the estimated population size for direct and inverse sampling are, respectively,

$$\frac{t^2 n(n-s)}{s^3} \text{ and } \frac{t^2 n(n-s)}{s^2(s+1)}$$

In our pigeon example, the standard errors of our estimates (i.e. the square roots of the variances) are approximately 592 and 628 for the direct and inverse methods, respectively. If the size of the second sample, n, is small compared with the overall population size, then inverse sampling provides a more precise estimate of the population size than direct sampling. However, if we know very little about the size of the population, then it is difficult to gauge the most appropriate t, which, if too great, could make n very large; in these circumstances, direct sampling is the preferred choice. Details of choosing sample sizes for direct and inverse sampling may be obtained from Mendenhall *et al.* (1971).

An explanation and further discussion of the methods of estimating wildlife population sizes is given by Greenwood and Robinson (2006). They explain how to estimate total population size by simultaneously tagging and recapturing animals by using traps of two different sorts in a closed population. The estimate is obtained by assessing, at the endpoint of the study, the relative numbers of animals caught in one type of trap from which they cannot escape, and from the other type in which the animals are tagged before they are allowed to escape.

Unfortunately, the methods, which rely on tagging and recapturing the animals, assume that all animals in the population have the same probability of recapture. This is often not the case, so that the population estimates may be inaccurate, and their calculated standard errors wildly off the mark. Sometimes, more reliable information can be obtained by estimating birth and survival rates having followed the fortunes of a group of marked animals.

Several other references provide useful help in exploring this subject further, avoiding some of the pitfalls awaiting the novice: Buckland *et al.* (1993), Peres (1999), Southwood (1966), Thompson *et al.* (1998) and Witmer (2005).

(b) Bootstrapping

Another approach to estimating population numbers, if the relevant sampling distribution is unknown, is based on a simulation process called **bootstrapping** (see Section 4.8). Suppose it is of interest to estimate the population numbers of a particular species in a given area. The underlying sampling process that precedes the bootstrapping estimation procedure is often cluster sampling, the clusters being equivalent sized areas derived from an appropriate map. (More details of territory mapping techniques are given in Bibby *et al.*, 1992.) The entire population in a random selection of areas is then counted within a short period, often by recruiting volunteer labour.

For example, in a national survey of corn buntings (Donald and Evans, 1995), tetrads (2×2 km) were selected at random from areas that had previously been recorded as having the birds. Populations were calculated separately for 11 different regions representing Scotland, England and Wales to reduce geographical bias, and a national estimate of corn buntings obtained. Having obtained a random sample (in this case, of mapped areas), a bootstrapping technique can be used to refine the estimation process. A set of simple random subsamples (often 999 subsamples, as recommended by Manly, 2007), each of the same size as the original sample, is created from it by sampling with replacement (see Section 4.8). A single estimate of the population size is determined from each subsample and, using the relevant percentiles of the sampling distribution of these estimates, it is possible to obtain a confidence interval for the population size of corn buntings.

(c) Distance sampling

A variant sampling procedure is that of **distance sampling** from a transect line. A transect line is drawn and the number and frequency of species recorded by an observer along the transect. The method is based on the proposition that the detection of randomly distributed subjects declines with distance from the transect line; an increasing number of subjects will be undetected with increasing distance from the line. Distance sampling methods model the decline in detectability with distance for a given species, and arrive at an estimate of population based on the data. More details can be found in the volume by Bibby *et al.* (1992).

Childs *et al.* (1998) used both a capture–tag method and a distance sampling technique to make estimates of rural dog populations in the Philippines. They concluded that distance sampling was a simple and satisfactory method for estimating dog population density.   □

Exercises

The statements in questions 13.1–13.4 are either TRUE or FALSE.

13.1   The logarithmic transformation:
(a) Normalizes data that are skewed to the left.
(b) Linearizes an exponential relationship.
(c) Stabilizes variance when the variability of the data increases as the magnitude of the observations increases.
(d) Is particularly useful for transforming proportions.
(e) Is applied when the sample size is small.

13.2   You will need more animals to find a significant difference between two treatments in a clinical trial if (all other factors remaining constant):
(a) You increase the power of the test.
(b) You decrease the significance level from 0.05 to 0.01.
(c) You have been informed that the clinically important treatment difference is greater than you believed it to be.
(d) The response of interest is numerical, and you have underestimated the standard deviation of the observations in each group.
(e) The standardized difference is increased.

13.3
(a) Sequential analysis is particularly appropriate when the response to treatment is prolonged.

(b) The nominal significance level in a group sequential design is always less than the overall significance level.
(c) Random allocation of animals to treatment groups is ensured by random sampling.
(d) A stratified sample is more precise than a simple random sample of the same size if it is designed so that the units within a stratum are as alike as possible, and the strata means are as different as possible.
(e) A cluster sample is more precise than a simple random sample of the same size if it is designed so that the units within a cluster are as alike as possible, and the cluster means are as different as possible.

13.4   A meta-analysis:
(a) Is a statistical analysis of transformed data.
(b) Is a particular type of systematic review.
(c) Uses a random effects approach to estimating an overall effect of interest if the separate estimates from the different studies are heterogeneous.
(d) Has results that are clinically heterogeneous if each of the separate studies are focusing on different clinical endpoints of interest.
(e) Can use a forest plot to determine if the data in each study are Normally distributed.

13.5   The Indian water buffalo, like domestic cattle, suffers from gut parasite infestations, some of which cause severe anaemia. We want, therefore, to be able to detect a change in haemoglobin (Hb) content in buffalo blood. We know that the Hb content of buffalo blood has a mean value of 11.1 g/dl with a standard deviation (SD) of 0.96 g/dl (Jain *et al.*, 1982). In an investigation comparing the effects of infestation with those in a control group, we want an 80% chance of detecting a mean change of, say, 1 g/dl. Will this be a one- or two-tailed test? How many animals would be needed to detect a change of this magnitude, assuming equal numbers in the two groups:
(a) At a significance level of 0.05 with a power of 80%?
(b) At a significance level of 0.05 with a power of 90%?
(c) At a significance level of 0.01 with a power of 80%?

(d) If the standard deviation was 1.3 g/dl, at a significance level of 0.05 with a power of 80%?

(e) At a significance level of 0.05 with a power of 80% if, instead of equal numbers, we want twice as many controls as water buffalos with the infestation?

13.6 We want to compare two different exercise regimens for horses on a treadmill as judged by the plasma lactate concentration at the end of the exercise period. We will conduct a randomized cross-over trial (each horse undergoes both exercise regimens in a randomized order) on a group of randomly selected animals with two different cantering speeds for a period of 7 minutes. A difference in plasma lactate of 1 mmol/l is considered an important difference. From a previous pilot trial, we know that the SD of the differences in plasma lactate concentration under the two regimens is likely to be around 1.7 mmol/l. Use Altman's nomogram to answer the following:

(a) How many horses will we need to test in order to have a probability of 0.85 of detecting, at a 1% significance level, a difference in mean plasma lactate concentrations of 1.0 mmol/l between these exercise regimens?

(b) We actually have 20 horses available. What is the power of the test if the significance level remains at 1%?

(c) Now what is the effect on power of changing the significance level to 5%?

13.7 A study is to be conducted on the effectiveness of attenuated canine parvovirus vaccine (A-CPV) to protect 6-week-old puppies. It is anticipated that maternally derived passive immunity would interfere with the establishment of an adequate immunity (titres greater than 1:80 in a haemagglutination-inhibition (HI) test) 1–2 weeks after vaccination. Puppies will be divided into seronegative (<1:10 HI titre) and seropositive (>1:20 HI titre) groups before vaccination. We anticipate that, in the seronegative group, a successful vaccination programme will produce a high percentage (i.e. >90%) of protected animals (>1:80 HI titre). If we find that vaccination in the seropositive group produces less than 50% protection, this will be considered a serious limitation. How many puppies will be required if we want a power of 90% of detecting this difference in percentages protected at the 5% level of significance?

13.8 Investigators were interested in comparing two systems of management of pigs to reach slaughter weight. The mean number of days for the pigs to reach slaughter weight using the old system of management was 165 days and the investigators were hoping that the new system of management would require fewer days on average for the pigs to reach slaughter weight. The following statement was made about the choice of optimal sample size for a randomized controlled trial to compare the two systems. 'Using a two-tailed two-sample *t*-test, approximately 32 pigs are required for each system in order to have a power of 80% to detect, at the 5% level of significance, a difference in means of 5 days for the bacon pigs to reach slaughter weight, if the standard deviation of the observations is likely to be about 7 days in each group.'

(a) Explain what is meant by a significance level of 5%.

(b) Explain what is meant by a power of 80%.

(c) How do the significance level and the power of the test relate to the Type I and Type II errors?

(d) If all other factors remained unchanged, would the required sample size increase or decrease if the significance level was increased to 10%?

(e) If all other factors remained unchanged, would the required sample size increase or decrease if the power of the test were increased to 90%?

(f) If all other factors remained unchanged, would the required sample size increase or decrease if the difference in means to be detected was increased to 7 days?

14 Additional techniques

14.1 Learning objectives

By the end of this chapter you should be able to:

- Define the terms 'sensitivity', 'specificity' and 'predictive value' as used in diagnostic tests.
- Evaluate the performance of a diagnostic or screening test.
- Interpret a receiver operating characteristic (ROC) curve and explain how it can be useful in evaluating a diagnostic test.
- Explain what is meant by a Bayesian analysis and how it differs from the frequentist approach.
- Distinguish between uninformative and informative priors and explain the terms 'posterior probability' and 'likelihood' in the context of Bayesian analysis.
- Apply Bayesian reasoning in evaluating a diagnostic test.
- Investigate both repeatability and method agreement in paired numerical data. Explain why the Pearson correlation coefficient is an inappropriate measure of agreement and why the paired *t*-test does not give full information about agreement for pairs of numerical data.
- Investigate agreement in categorical data using Cohen's kappa.
- Explain what is meant by a time series, and state the issues that are relevant for analysis.
- Identify the appropriate analyses for repeated measures data.

- Recognize when a survival analysis should be performed.
- Interpret the results of Kaplan–Meier and Cox proportional hazards survival analyses.
- Explain the terms 'competing risks' and 'frailty' in the context of survival analysis.
- Explain the difference between univariate, univariable, multivariable and multivariate analysis.
- Outline different multivariate methods.

14.2 Diagnostic tests

14.2.1 Introduction

We can often use the result of a test to **diagnose** or exclude a disease in a sick animal or as a **screening** device in a population of apparently healthy animals. The **screening test** procedure is usually the first step in a process that involves further investigation on each animal which has an initially positive test result. However, screening for disease is only worthwhile if the disease is serious, and if diagnosing it and treating the animal at the pre-symptomatic stage positively affects its long-term outcome. For simplicity, we shall explain the statistical theory underlying these tests in terms of diagnosis.

Each animal either has the disease (is **positive**) or is disease-free (is **negative**). If the **diagnostic test** is based on a numerical variable, then we

Statistics for Veterinary and Animal Science, Third Edition. Aviva Petrie and Paul Watson.
© 2013 John Wiley & Sons, Ltd. Published 2013 by John Wiley & Sons, Ltd.

may decide that the animal is likely to have the disease if the numerical measurement for that animal exceeds or is below a certain range of values. Typically, this range will be the limits of a reference range (see Section 2.7). For example, we may use plasma thyroxin (T4) measurements in the diagnosis of hypothyroidism in dogs. A dog could be diagnosed as having an underactive thyroid gland if its plasma thyroxin measurement is less than 15 nmol/l, the lower limit of the reference range. Alternatively, our diagnostic test may be based on a categorical response, such as the presence or absence of some symptom or sign. In either situation, we must be able to evaluate the performance of this diagnostic test. We want to know:

- How effective the test is at identifying animals with the disease (**sensitivity**).
- How effective the test is at identifying animals without the disease (**specificity**).
- How likely it is that the test will give a correct diagnosis, whether the animal is diseased or disease-free (**predictive value**).

The sensitivity and specificity are characteristics of the test that provide measures of its **accuracy** whereas the predictive value gives an indication of the usefulness of the test.

14.2.2 Characteristics of the test: sensitivity and specificity

The true or 'gold standard' diagnosis may be made using information from a variety of sources such as clinical examination, laboratory or postmortem results or an expert's opinion. Table 14.1 shows the observed frequencies obtained from the gold standard test (true results) and the diagnostic test when each is applied to n animals. From this table, we can see that the **prevalence** of the disease in the sample is $(a + c)/n$, the proportion of animals in the study with the disease. We use the following measures to assess the effectiveness of the test.

- **Sensitivity** = $a/(a + c)$ is the proportion of true (gold standard) positives identified by the test

Table 14.1 Table of observed frequencies.

Test result	True diagnosis		Total
	Positive (diseased)	Negative (healthy)	
Positive	a	b	$a + b$
Negative	c	d	$c + d$
Total	$a + c$	$b + d$	$n = a + b + c + d$

as positive. It gives an indication of the ability of the test to correctly identify those animals with the disease.

- **Specificity** = $d/(b + d)$ is the proportion of true (gold standard) negatives identified by the test as negative. It gives an indication of the ability of the test to correctly identify those animals without the disease.

Because we are using sample data to provide estimates of the relevant measures, we should accompany the estimates of the prevalence and the sensitivity and specificity by their standard errors and/or associated confidence intervals. Each measure is a proportion (although it is often multiplied by 100 and expressed as a percentage), and we explained how to calculate the standard error of, and a confidence interval for, a proportion in Sections 4.6.2 and 4.7, respectively.

Generally, the sensitivity and specificity of the test are not affected by the prevalence of the disease. They are used to assess the performance of the diagnostic test and provide measures of its accuracy in relation to the 'gold standard' diagnosis. However, *verification bias* may arise if the gold standard is not a true reflection of the real disease state of the animal, in which case the sensitivity and specificity may be related to prevalence. We explain how to estimate the sensitivity and specificity of a test when there is no true gold standard in Section 14.2.5. Verification bias may also arise if the selection of animals to receive the gold standard test is influenced by the result of the diagnostic test under investigation. For example, the animal may not receive an invasive gold standard test if the diagnostic test result is negative.

Ideally, we should like a test that has both a high sensitivity and a high specificity but these two measures are dependent, so that as one increases, the other tends to decrease. The relative importance of the sensitivity and specificity of a test depends on the particular disease that is being tested and the implications of the animal either having or not having the disease.

- If we are concerned with identifying animals with the disease so that we can treat them, then we should use a test that has a high sensitivity, e.g. the glucose tolerance test in dogs to diagnose diabetes mellitus.
- If our concern is with excluding diseased animals and identifying those that are disease-free, then we require a test with a high specificity, e.g. tuberculin testing in cattle.

If our test is based on a numerical variable, we can alter the sensitivity and the specificity of a diagnostic test by raising or lowering the cut-off value for the variable, where this cut-off determines whether the test result is positive or negative. So, for example, in our hypothyroid example in dogs where a low T4 level is taken as indicative of the existence of a pathological state, e.g. an underactive gland, we can increase the sensitivity and decrease the specificity if we raise the critical cut-off to a value above 15 nmol/l, the lower limit of 'normal'.

14.2.3 Using the ROC to assess a diagnostic test and to determine the optimal cut-off

Sometimes a **receiver operating characteristic (ROC) curve** is plotted as a means of determining the best cut-off for a diagnostic test based on a numerical variable, and for comparing two or more tests for a given condition. The ROC curve plots the sensitivity (the true positive rate, TPR) against 1 minus the specificity (the false positive rate, FPR) for different cut-off values (Figure 14.1). A 'good' test is one that has a high true positive rate and a low false positive rate and

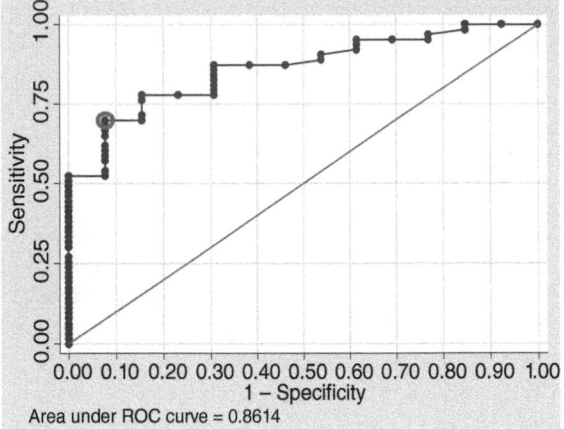

Area under ROC curve = 0.8614

Figure 14.1   Receiver operating characteristic (ROC) curve determined using different cut-off values of phosphate to diagnose renal secondary hyperparathyroidism (RHPTH) in cats (the enlarged circle indicates a phosphate value of 1.86 mmol/l). See Section 14.2.11.

whose value, therefore, lies close to the top left-hand corner of the ROC curve.

In addition, we can use the **area under the ROC curve (AUROC)** to describe the overall ability of the diagnostic test to distinguish between animals with and without the disease. This area, sometimes designated by the term '*c* statistic', represents the probability that a randomly chosen diseased animal has a higher predicted probability of having the disease than a randomly chosen disease-free animal. Expressed another way, if the AUROC is equal to 0.7, say, this means that, on 70% of occasions, a randomly chosen diseased animal will have a higher predicted probability of having the disease than a disease-free animal. A test that is perfect at discriminating between animals with and without the disease has an AUROC = 1, and a test that performs no better than chance has an AUROC = 0.5. The AUROC is particularly useful when we wish to compare the diagnostic accuracy of two or more diagnostic tests that are used for the same condition. The test with the greater AUROC is better at distinguishing between the two disease outcomes.

Further details may be found in Greiner *et al.* (2000), Jekel *et al.* (1996), Zweig and Campbell (1993) and similar texts.

14.2.4 Using logistic regression to determine the optimal cut-off

Logistic regression analysis (see Section 11.4) is a modification of multiple regression (see Section 11.3), utilized when we have a binary outcome of interest, e.g. disease or no disease. We may use it instead of the ROC curve to determine the optimal cut-off for a diagnostic test based on a numerical variable. In this situation, the outcome variable is the dichotomous result of the gold standard test (coded as 1 for a diseased animal and 0 for a disease-free animal) and the explanatory variables or covariates, in addition to the numerical measurement from the diagnostic test, are those variables that are thought to influence the disease outcome. Comprehensive statistical software (such as SPSS and Stata) uses the logistic regression model to estimate the sensitivities and specificities of the diagnostic test for various cut-offs. We can plot a ROC curve from these values and choose the optimal cut-off as the most extreme point in the top left-hand corner of the curve. Another approach is to simply choose a cut-off that provides what we regard as the optimal combination of sensitivity and specificity for the particular scenario of interest. Alternatively, we can plot the predicted probability of the disease (this may be obtained from the logistic regression analysis) against the associated cut-off and choose the cut-off that corresponds to the probability of interest (typically 0.50).

14.2.5 Estimating the sensitivity and specificity with no gold standard

We may be in a situation where we have a sample of animals that can be used to assess a new diagnostic test for a particular condition, but there is no gold standard test available to enable us to estimate the sensitivity and specificity of the new diagnostic test. However, we may be able to compare the results of the new test with some other standard test which, although good, does not detect the disease status of the animals perfectly. If the sensitivity (Sen_s) and specificity (Sp_s)

of this standard test are known, then it is possible to estimate the sensitivity (Sen_{new}) and specificity (Sp_{new}) of the new test by employing the following formulae (using the notation of Table 14.1):

$$\text{Sensitivity}_{new} = \frac{(a+b)Sp_s - b}{nSp_s - (b+d)}$$

$$\text{Specificity}_{new} = \frac{(c+d)Sen_s - c}{nSen_s - (a+c)}$$

Standard error formulae for these estimates may be found in Gart and Buck (1996). Further details of this and other approaches to estimating the sensitivity and the specificity of a new test using a standard or reference test instead of a gold standard test may be found in, for example, Enoe *et al.* (2000).

14.2.6 Using logistic regression to estimate the sensitivity and specificity

When we wish to estimate the sensitivity and specificity of a test if we believe that these measures will be affected by various characteristics of the population (e.g. males and females, different age categories, disease stages), it is tempting to approach the problem by performing subgroup analysis, i.e. by estimating the measures using the formulae in Section 14.2.2 for each subgroup or category of the factors of interest. However, it is usually impractical to use this technique because of the problem of small sample sizes after stratification. A preferred approach is to undertake a logistic regression analysis (see Section 11.4) in which the outcome variable relates to the dichotomous result of the diagnostic test (taking the value 1 or 0 if the disease is present or absent, respectively). One of the covariates is the disease status as determined by the gold standard; it takes the value 1 if the disease is present and 0 if it is absent. The other covariates are those factors that might affect the sensitivity and specificity of the test, for example, the gender of the animal or its age. In this way, we are able to estimate the sensitivity and specificity of the diagnostic test for a particular set of covariate values.

If the logistic regression equation is estimated by

$$\text{logit}\,(p) = \log_e(p/(1-p))$$
$$= a + b_1x_1 + b_2x_2 + b_3x_3, \ldots, + b_kx_k$$
$$= a + \Sigma b_ix_i$$

where x_1 is the binary result from the gold standard test and p is the estimated value of the probability that an animal with a particular set of covariate values of $x_2, x_3, \ldots, x_k$ is presumed to have the disease by the diagnostic test, then we estimate sensitivity and specificity as

$$\text{Sensitivity} = 1/(1 + \exp(-a - \Sigma b_ix_i))$$
$$\text{where } x_1 = 1$$

$$\text{Specificity} = 1 - 1/(1 + \exp(-a - \Sigma b_ix_i))$$
$$\text{where } x_1 = 0$$

Full details, including the formulae for confidence intervals, may be obtained from Coughlin *et al.* (1992). See also Sections 14.2.4 and 14.2.9 for further use of logistic regression for diagnostic tests.

14.2.7 Usefulness of the test: positive and negative predictive values

We use the sensitivity and specificity to assess the accuracy of the test and determine the optimal test for a given condition. However, these two measures do not help us decide how likely it is that a particular animal has the condition if it tests positive or does not have the condition if it tests negative. The positive and negative predictive values (PPV and NPV, respectively) are useful in this regard. Using the notation of Table 14.1, these are estimated as:

- **Positive predictive value** (PPV) = $a/(a + b)$, the proportion of animals with a positive test result that really are positive.
- **Negative predictive value** (NPV) = $d/(c + d)$, the proportion of animals with a negative test result that really are negative.

As with the sensitivity and specificity, we should accompany the estimates of the PPV and NPV by their standard errors and/or associated confidence intervals. However, unlike the sensitivity and specificity, the PPV and NPV are affected by the prevalence of the disease. As the prevalence of the disease is raised, we have more animals with the disease in the population, and we have greater confidence that a positive test result is correct; the positive predictive value of the test is increased and the negative predictive value is decreased. The reverse is true as the prevalence of the disease is lowered. *We should therefore not compare predictive values of tests that have been evaluated in populations in which the prevalence of the disease is different.*

14.2.8 Estimating the PPV and NPV with no gold standard: the likelihood ratio

The positive predictive value (PPV) of a test evaluates the chance that an animal has the disease if its test result is positive. In the statistical technique described in Section 14.2.2 and illustrated in Table 14.1, the estimation of the PPV relies on information being available on a sample of animals, all of which have been categorized as disease positive or negative both by the test and by the gold standard. Unfortunately, we cannot produce this information when attempting to diagnose the condition of an individual animal when only a single test result and no gold standard result is available for that animal. An alternative way of deciding how likely it is that a particular animal has the disease if it tests positive is to give consideration to the relevant **likelihood ratio**, a concept we introduced in Section 11.4.3. We can use the likelihood ratio to assess how good a diagnostic test is and to compare the usefulness of different tests for a given condition.

The **likelihood ratio of a positive test result** (**LR₊**) describes how much more likely the animal is to have a positive test result if it has the disease than if it is disease-free (i.e. it is the ratio of the likelihoods of having and not having the disease).

So, for example, if the $LR_+ = 5$, a positive test result is five times more likely to occur in an animal that has the disease than in one that does not have it. If the $LR_+ = 1$, then a positive test result is equally likely in diseased and disease-free animals, and the test is useless. A high likelihood ratio (e.g. $LR_+ > 10$) indicates that the test can be used to *rule in* the disease, whilst a low likelihood ratio (e.g. $LR_+ < 0.1$) can *rule out* the disease. (Note that it is also possible to calculate the likelihood ratio of a negative test result (LR_-) which describes how much more likely the animal is to have a negative test result if it has the disease than if it is disease-free.)

We may use the following formulae to calculate the likelihood ratios of positive and negative test results. In each case, we assume that sensitivity and specificity are expressed as probabilities taking values from 0 to 1 (if they are expressed in percentage terms, we should replace the '1' in the denominator and numerator, as appropriate, by 100).

$$LR_+ = \frac{\text{Sensitivity}}{1 - \text{Specificity}}$$

$$LR_- = \frac{1 - \text{Sensitivity}}{\text{Specificity}}$$

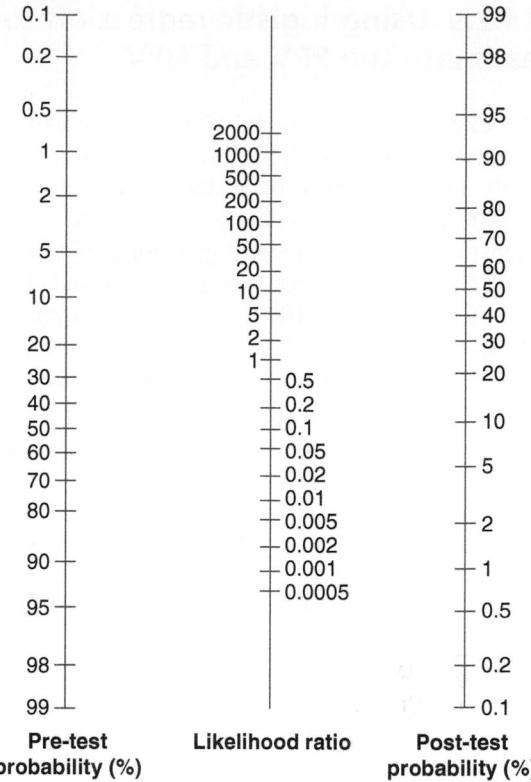

Figure 14.2 Fagan's nomogram (from Fagan, 1975, reproduced with permission from the Massachusetts Medical Society).

Commonly, we use the likelihood ratio, which provides information about the performance of the diagnostic test, together with any prior information that the clinician has regarding the possibility that the animal is diseased (the **pre-test probability**) to estimate the chance that the animal has the disease (the **post-test probability**) if it tests positive. This process of using the current evidence (e.g. the test result) to revise and update the researcher's initial estimate of the probability of the event of interest (e.g. the presence of disease) is described as **Bayesian** (see Section 14.3 for more details). Using conventional Bayesian terminology, the pre-test and post-test probabilities are the **prior** and **posterior probabilities**, respectively.

Although it is possible to evaluate the post-test probability from the pre-test probability using formulae, we recommend using **Fagan's nomogram** (Figure 14.2) for simplicity. Suppose

that an animal tests positive for the disease of interest. How likely is it that the animal actually has the disease? In the absence of any additional information, we usually take the prevalence of the disease in the relevant geographical area as the pre-test probability. With knowledge of the sensitivity and specificity of the diagnostic test, we can evaluate the likelihood ratio of a positive test result using the formula provided. We then connect the pre-test probability (expressed as a percentage) on the left-hand axis of the nomogram to the likelihood ratio and extend the line to the point at which it cuts the right-hand axis, and this gives us the post-test probability that the animal has the disease. With this knowledge, the clinician can decide on the appropriate therapeutic action for the animal in his/her care. We illustrate the use of Fagan's nomogram in the example in Section 14.2.11.

14.2.9 Using logistic regression to estimate the PPV and NPV

We explained in Section 14.2.6 how we can use a logistic regression model to estimate the sensitivity and specificity of a diagnostic test, after adjusting for factors likely to influence these measures. In that logistic regression analysis, we took the diagnostic test result (coded as 1 if the disease is present and 0 otherwise) as the outcome variable and the gold standard result as one of the covariates, the other covariates being those factors that were likely to affect the outcome. If, alternatively, we wish to use a logistic regression model to estimate the PPV and NPV of a diagnostic test, we use a similar approach but take the gold standard result (coded as 1 if the disease is present and 0 otherwise) as our outcome variable and the diagnostic test result as an explanatory variable, together with any other covariates of interest. We then use the formulae in Section 14.2.6 for the estimated sensitivity and specificity to estimate the PPV and NPV, respectively (Coughlin *et al.*, 1992).

14.2.10 Using two (or more) diagnostic tests

One of the main uses of a diagnostic test is to provide good probabilistic evidence that a particular animal has (or does not have) the disease of interest. That is, we are particularly interested in the positive predictive value of the test: we want to know how likely it is that the animal actually has the disease if it has a positive diagnostic test result. Clearly, a high PPV is a reflection of a useful test. For a given population, if we increase the specificity of the test, this will increase the PPV in a given population because *b* in Table 14.1 will decrease. We may achieve this, for example, by choosing a higher cut-off value to designate disease, if higher values of the variable of interest are more indicative of disease.

An alternative approach to strengthening the evidence that an animal has the disease is to test each animal using two (or more) diagnostic tests and combine the findings in one of two ways.

- We perform the tests **sequentially**, most usefully when we are interested in arriving at a diagnosis without necessarily performing both tests (or all the tests if there are multiple tests) on every animal. This may be recommended if one test is a cheaper, quicker, more practical and/or less invasive test than the other. Then we use the cheaper or less invasive test, which should have high sensitivity but low specificity, on all the animals, and we use the second, more expensive or more invasive test, which should have equally high sensitivity but also high specificity, only on those animals that tested positive to the first test. We regard an animal as testing positive for the disease if *both* tests have positive results.

- A similar interpretation is elicited from the results for **series** testing. In this situation, we administer both tests to *all* animals and we regard an animal as testing positive for the disease only if we obtain a positive test result from *both* tests. An example of series testing is described by Muma *et al.* (2007). The investigators conducted a cross-sectional study to investigate the risk factors of *Brucella* seropositivity in cattle herds reared in livestock–wildlife interface areas of the Blue Lagoon and Lochinvar National Parks in Zambia between August 2003 and September 2004. Sera were collected from cattle aged ≥2 years from 124 herds. Data on husbandry practices, grazing strategies and herd structure were also collected. Sera were screened for anti-*Brucella* antibodies using the Rose Bengal test (RBT) as a presumptive test and a competitive enzyme-linked immunosorbent assay (c-ELISA) as a confirmatory test. A herd was classified as *Brucella* seropositive if at least one animal tested positive on both RBT and c-ELISA in series testing.

- A third approach is to use **parallel** testing when we administer both tests to all animals but then regard an animal as having a positive outcome if *at least one test* has a positive result.

If, on the other hand, we wish to provide good probabilistic evidence that an animal is *free* of the disease, we will be interested in increasing the negative predictive value which can be accommodated by increasing the sensitivity of

Table 14.2 Results (observed frequencies) of the diagnostic test for renal secondary hyperparathyroidism (RHPTH) in cats with chronic renal failure (data from Barber and Elliott, 1998, with permission from Wiley-Blackwell).

Diagnostic test	'True diagnosis'		Total
	RHPTH (PTH >25.5 pg/ml)	No RHPTH (PTH ≤25.5 pg/ml)	
RHPTH (phosphate >1.86 mmol/l)	43	1	44
No RHPTH (phosphate ≤1.86 mmol/l)	20	12	32
Total	63	13	76

Sensitivity = 43/63 = 0.68 (95% CI 0.57 to 0.80) or 68%.
Specificity = 12/13 = 0.92 (95% CI approximately* 0.78 to 1.00) or 92%.
PPV = 43/44 = 0.98 (95% CI approximately* 0.93 to 1.00) or 98%.
NPV = 12/32 = 0.38 (95% CI 0.21 to 0.54) or 38%.
Observed prevalence = 63/76 = 0.83 (95% CI 0.74 to 0.91) or 83%.
*Note that these confidence intervals are only approximate because the Normal approximation to the Binomial distribution does not hold well with such small numbers. A better estimate can be made following a method given by Wilson (1927).
NPV, negative predictive value; PPV, positive predictive value; PTH, parathyroid hormone.

the test and thereby reducing c in Table 14.1. We might achieve this, for example, by choosing a lower cut-off point to designate disease, if higher values of the variable of interest are more indicative of disease.

14.2.11 Example

Barber and Elliott (1998) investigated the aetiopathogenesis of renal secondary hyperparathyroidism (RHPTH) in cats with chronic renal failure (CRF). We used this example in Section 12.6.2 to illustrate the Kruskal–Wallis test, which compared the distributions of plasma parathyroid hormone (PTH) concentrations in the cats in three stages of CRF. We showed that, on average, the PTH concentrations were significantly higher in those groups of cats with a greater degree of renal dysfunction.

Assay of PTH is, at the moment, expensive and not widely available. Barber and Elliott therefore investigated the use of more routine biochemical measurements to act as markers for the presence of RHPTH. In particular, they found that use of plasma phosphate concentrations was the most efficient diagnostic test for RHPTH in feline CRF. As the 'gold standard', they used the upper limit of the reference range of PTH in an

age-matched control group as the cut-off point for determining whether or not the cat suffered from RHPTH (a cat was thus defined as having RHPTH if its PTH >25.5 pg/ml). Similarly, they used the upper limit of the reference range of phosphate (i.e. phosphate >1.86 mmol/l) as the cut-off for the diagnostic test. Table 14.2 shows the results they obtained in 76 cats with CRF. (It could be argued that the use of the upper limit of the reference range of PTH is not the true gold standard for the diagnosis of RHPTH in these cats. If so, the estimated values of the sensitivity and specificity displayed in Table 14.2 might have been affected by verification bias. Had the sensitivity and specificity of the test based on a PTH > 25.5 pg/ml been available, it would have been preferable to use the formulae in Section 14.2.6 to estimate the sensitivity and specificity of the diagnostic test based on a phosphate value of greater than 1.86 mmol/l.)

If the sensitivity and specificity are expressed as percentages, the ROC curve created by plotting the sensitivity against 100 minus the specificity for each of a number of different cut-off points of the raw phosphate values to identify cats with RHPTH is shown in Figure 14.1. The area under the curve (AUROC) = 0.86 (95% CI 0.77 to 0.95) which suggests that phosphate is reasonably good at identifying cats with RHPTH.

The circle on the ROC curve, which lies towards the top left-hand corner of the graph, suggests an optimal cut-off of phosphate. It is of interest to note that this cut-off corresponds to the cut-off chosen by the investigators as the upper limit of the reference range of phosphate, i.e. phosphate 1.86 mmol/l. It gives a sensitivity of 68% and a specificity of 92%.

Although the diagnostic test based on plasma phosphate >1.86 mmol/l is well able to identify those CRF cats without RHPTH (specificity = 92%, 95% CI 77.8% to 100%), its ability to detect RHPTH in CRF cats who have this complication is low (sensitivity = 68%, 95% CI 56.8% to 79.7%). However, the PPV value of the test is very high (98%, 95% CI 93.3% to 100%), indicating that if a CRF cat has a positive test result, it almost certainly does have RHPTH. Note that the prevalence of RHPTH is high (83%, 95% CI 74.4% to 91.4%) in this group of CRF cats, so we would expect the PPV to be high as well.

In addition, the likelihood ratio of a positive test result is equal to (sensitivity)/(100 − specificity) = (68)/(100 − 92) = 8.5. This means that a cat is 8.5 times more likely to test positive if it is diseased than if it is disease-free, and is an indication that the test is helpful in diagnosing cats with RHPTH if the test result is positive. Furthermore, if we use the prevalence of 83% as the pre-test probability, and connect this value on Fagan's nomogram to a likelihood of 8.5, we obtain a post-test probability of about 97% when we extend the line to the right-hand axis. As expected, this corresponds well to the PPV of 98%.

Although this diagnostic test has poor sensitivity, plasma phosphate concentrations proved to have superior efficiency compared with other variables that were investigated. It could certainly be used as a filter for instituting dietary phosphate restriction in CRF cats. Monthly monitoring of phosphate would then be used to establish whether phosphate concentration can be stabilized within or above the normal range. The cats in the latter group, those with persistently high phosphate concentrations, are likely to have RHPTH which could then be confirmed by analysis of hormone levels.

14.3 Bayesian analysis

14.3.1 The process

The **Bayesian approach to statistical inference** involves the use of external evidence (e.g. subjective judgement based on signs and symptoms, prevalence of the condition, trials of similar interventions, pilot studies) to supplement the information obtained from the sample (i.e. the data derived from the current study) to draw a conclusion about the hypothesis of interest, the latter often being framed in terms of one or more population parameters.

The Bayesian approach is based on a theorem devised in 1763 by Thomas Bayes, a nonconformist minister from Tunbridge Wells. Before we conduct a study such as a clinical trial comparing the effects of two treatments, we may be able to quantify our belief in probabilistic terms in the hypothesis of interest (e.g. the null hypothesis, H_0, that the two treatment means are equal). This is called the **prior probability** and we shall denote it by $Pr(H_0)$. The evidence we obtain from the results of the current study is expressed as a **likelihood** which describes how likely it is that we would obtain the observed results if the hypothesis were true (see Section 11.4.3). The likelihood is a conditional probability (see Section 3.2.4) and may be written as $Pr(\text{data}|H_0)$. In a dynamic process, **Bayes' theorem** uses the likelihood, which quantifies the new information, to update the prior probability into a **posterior probability**, the belief that we now have about the hypothesis *after* conducting the study, i.e. it is the conditional probability $Pr(H_0|\text{data})$.

More specifically, Bayes' theorem states that the posterior probability is proportional to the product of the prior probability and the likelihood, that is

$$Pr(H_0|\text{data}) \propto Pr(H_0) \times Pr(\text{data}|H_0)$$

In fact,

$$Pr(H_0|\text{data}) = \frac{Pr(H_0) \times Pr(\text{data}|H_0)}{Pr(\text{data})}$$

where the denominator is a normalizing factor that makes the total probability equal to one when all possible hypotheses are considered.

14.3.2 Choice of prior

Clearly, the choice of prior probability plays a crucial role in a Bayesian analysis. There are different types of prior that encompass the spectrum of information they contain:

- An **uninformative prior** does not influence the posterior probability as it provides no relevant information. For example, this would occur if all possible values for the parameter under test (e.g. the difference in two means) are believed to be equally likely before the sample data are collected. Sometimes an uninformative prior is virtually indistinguishable from a *vague* or *diffuse prior* when the sample data swamp the prior information so that the posterior and likelihood are virtually equal.
- At the other extreme is an **informative prior** that provides such strong information (for example, if it suggests that there is only one possible value for the parameter under test) that the likelihood does not influence the posterior and the posterior is identical to the prior. More usually, the informative prior will be *substantial*, providing considerable empirical or theoretical relevant information about the unknown parameter with the consequence that the posterior departs substantially from the likelihood.

In addition, there are different ways in which the prior can be chosen:

- A *reference prior* represents minimal prior information and is usually used as a baseline against which the other priors can be compared.
- A *clinical prior* expresses the opinions of well-informed specialists or is derived from reputable published material.
- A *sceptical prior* is pessimistic in nature, reflecting the worst possible outcome (e.g. that the difference between two means is zero, indicating that there is no treatment effect).
- An *enthusiastic prior*, in contrast, is optimistic in nature, reflecting the best plausible outcome.

There is considerable scepticism (especially amongst non-Bayesians) on the subjectivity associated with the choice of prior and its consequence on the interpretation of the findings. One solution is to use an uninformative prior which is regarded as less subjective than a prior based on clinical judgment. Alternatively, a *sensitivity analysis* may be performed to assess how robust the conclusions are to changes in the prior distribution. Using this approach, the interpretation of the results from the posteriors derived from a number of different priors obtained from varying sources are compared. If the conclusions are consistent (e.g. the novel treatment is always found to be significantly superior to the existing treatment), then the choice of prior is not influential and should not be regarded as problematic.

A more difficult situation arises when there is limited information extraneous to the sample data so that it is hard or impossible to specify an appropriate prior. In these circumstances it may be possible to perform an *empirical Bayesian analysis*, with observed data being used to estimate the prior, instead of a full Bayesian analysis. Further details may be obtained from Louis (1991).

14.3.3 Comparing the Bayesian and frequentist philosophies

The approach to statistical hypothesis testing we have presented elsewhere in this book is based on the **classical** or **frequentist** theory originally espoused in the late 1920s and early 1930s by two statisticians called Jerzy Neyman and Egon Pearson.

- In contrast to the Bayesian philosophy, the only relevant information used for statistical inference in the frequentist approach is that obtained from the evidence provided by the sample data from the current investigation, i.e. the frequentist approach uses only the sample data to make inferences about the true but unknown value of the parameter of interest (e.g. the difference in means). This contrasts with the Bayesian approach which uses the sample data to update the prior information to make inferences about the parameter.

- Furthermore, whereas the Bayesian interpretation of a probability is *subjective*, reflecting a personal degree of belief in an outcome, the *frequentist* probability (see Section 3.2.2) associated with the classical approach to inference is (or should be!) interpreted as the percentage or proportion of times that the event of interest would occur if the experiment were repeated many times, independently and under essentially the same circumstances. Thus, strictly, the 95% confidence interval for a mean is the interval that would contain the population mean on 95% of occasions if the experiment were to be repeated many times. The 95% confidence interval for the true value of a parameter used in the frequentist approach is replaced by the 95% *credible interval* in the Bayesian approach: this interval has a 95% chance of containing the true parameter (i.e. this is the interpretation commonly, but falsely, attributed to the frequentist 95% confidence interval).

- Bayesian theory assumes that the parameter of interest (e.g. that defining the hypothesis under test) is a random variable with a probability distribution, so that it is possible to evaluate the probability that the parameter has a particular value. Initially, this probability is the prior probability, but, using the sample data, it is modified to become the posterior probability. Consequently, the Bayesian approach allows us to calculate the probability that a particular hypothesis is true, as opposed to the frequentist approach in which we regard the parameter as having a fixed value (i.e. that defined in the null hypothesis), and which evaluates the less useful *P*-value, the probability of obtaining the observed (or more extreme) sample results if the null hypothesis is true.

- The results of a Bayesian and a frequentist analysis are very similar if the prior is uninformative because the influence of the prior is minimal or non-existent compared with that of the data. However, if the prior is informative, the two approaches can give very different results and it is this discrepancy that fuels the controversy between the proponents of the two methodologies.

14.3.4 Applications

Bayesian analysis has substantially increased in popularity since the advent of powerful computers and specialist software, as the process of estimating the posterior distributions usually relies on simulation methods that are extremely computer intensive. Free software, WinBUGS (hosted by the MRC Biostatistics Unit, Cambridge, UK) is described by Lunn *et al.* (2000) and is available at www.mrc-bsu.cam.ac.uk/bugs/ (accessed 23 October 2012). We may apply the Bayesian approach to many areas of veterinary and animal science, such as diagnosis, prognosis, clinical trials, survival analysis, meta-analysis and diagnostic and screening tests.

The example in Section 14.2.11 illustrates a Bayesian approach to diagnostic testing. A relatively simple diagnostic test for assessing whether a cat suffering from renal failure had renal secondary hyperparathyroidism (RHPTH) was to determine whether its plasma phosphate concentration was greater than 1.86 mmol/l. The sensitivity and specificity of the test were found to be 68% and 92%, respectively. Here the prevalence of RHPTH (83%) in cats with chronic renal failure was taken as the prior probability of having RHPTH (this was called the pre-test probability). The likelihood of a positive test result describes how likely it is that a cat tests positive if it has RHPTH compared with when it does not have RHPTH. This likelihood can be calculated as the sensitivity of the diagnostic test divided by (100 − specificity) and was equal to 8.5. Instead of laboriously working through the formula for Bayes' theorem (as shown at the end of this subsection), Fagan's nomogram was used to determine the posterior or post-test probability of a cat having RHPTH. By connecting the pre-test probability of 83% to the likelihood of 8.5, and extending the line, we found that the post-test or posterior probability of RHPTH was about 97%. That is, the initial belief that a cat which tested positive for RHPTH actually had RHPTH was updated by the test result from 83% to about 97%.

As a point of possible interest, we show how to evaluate the posterior probability of a cat having RHPTH from first principles. We can express Bayes' theorem in terms of odds (see Section 5.2.3(b)) in the following way:

Posterior odds of RHPTH = prior odds $\times$ LR$_+$

where, if the probability takes a value from 0 to 1:

Prior odds = prior probability/(1 – prior probability)
LR$_+$ = likelihood ratio of a positive test result

We then convert the posterior odds into the posterior probability using the following formula

Posterior probability

   = posterior odds/(1 + posterior odds)

Hence in the cat example:

Prior odds = 0.83/(1 – 0.83) = 0.83/0.17 = 4.88
Posterior odds = 4.88 $\times$ LR$_+$ = 4.88 $\times$ 8.5 = 41.48

and

Posterior probability = 41.48/42.48 = 0.976.

This result is virtually identical to that obtained from Fagan's nomogram (and differs only because of rounding errors and the inaccuracies relating to lack of precision of the nomogram).

You can obtain further details about Bayesian analysis from texts such as Bernardo and Smith (2000), Gelman *et al.* (2013) or Spiegelhalter *et al.* (2004) or from the paper by Bland and Altman (1998).

14.4 Measuring agreement

14.4.1 Introduction

Often we find ourselves wanting to question the reliability of our observations. To do this we need to measure the degree of closeness of results between observers or different methods or repeated observations, and this presents us with questions of how this is best assessed statistically. Typically, we are interested in assessing the similarity or agreement between two, three or more observations obtained on a numerical or categorical variable.

- **Repeatability** evaluates the extent to which a given observer obtains the same results when s/he takes successive measurements on an item (e.g. animal) in identical circumstances (i.e. using the same measuring instrument and procedure under the same conditions in the same location within a short period of time).
- A related problem is when we wish to investigate **reproducibility**, sometimes called **method agreement**. Do two 'methods' of measurement (using the same scale) agree with one another? These 'methods' may be, for example, different observers using the same technique or a single observer using different techniques.

Repeatability and reproducibility are both aspects of the *reliability* of measurements. For simplicity, in Sections 14.4.2 and 14.4.3, we assume that we have *pairs* of measurements and we wish to assess the agreement between the members of a pair. To this end, we need to consider both the systematic and random effects that can arise. A *systematic* effect implies that there is a tendency for the differences in the paired results to go in one direction (e.g. to be positive if the variable of interest is numerical). A *random* effect implies that sometimes the differences go in one direction and sometimes they go in the opposite direction, but they tend to balance out on average. By using all the available evidence from our analysis, including possible measures and/or indices to quantify the magnitude of the agreement, we can decide whether the agreement is acceptable in the context of the study. We explain the approach comparing two methods to assess reproducibility for numerical (see Section 14.4.2) and categorical (see Section 14.4.3) data. The approach is essentially similar if we wish to compare two successive measurements in a set of such pairs to assess repeatability. *Remember, however, that it is necessary to establish that a method is repeatable before comparing two methods for reproducibility.*

For further reading on the methods of assessing agreement, we suggest a review by Watson and Petrie (2010) and the book by Lin *et al.* (2012) which blends the theory with applications and provides many examples. In addition, Bland and Altman (2007) describe methods of agreement for analysing clustered numerical data, i.e. when there are multiple observations per individual.

14.4.2 Repeatability and reproducibility of numerical measurements

In this section, we assume that we are assessing reproducibility by comparing two methods of measuring a numerical variable. Bland and Altman (1986) give a detailed discussion of the problem; they explain how the approach can be modified when more than two measurements are to be compared, e.g. when three or more methods are to be compared or when each observer takes more than two repeated measurements on the same item.

(a) Correct analysis of repeatability and reproducibility

(i) Checking for a systematic effect

We calculate the difference between each pair of measurements. If the mean of these differences ($\bar{d}$) is not significantly different from zero (this can be investigated by the paired t-test – see Section 7.5), then there is evidence that the methods agree *on average*. All we can say in this situation is that the differences are evenly scattered above and below zero. The differences could be large (indicating that there is substantial disagreement between the two methods) or they could be small (indicating good method agreement). A non-significant result, therefore, does not imply good method agreement. It implies only that there is no systematic difference between the observations in a pair (if one method is assumed to be the gold standard providing the 'true' measurement, the absence of a systematic effect implies that there is no *bias* – see Section 4.4.3).

(ii) Bland and Altman approach and measures of agreement

In order to assess how well the measurements in a pair agree, we determine the limits within which most (typically, 95%) of the differences are expected to lie. These are called the **limits of agreement**. Provided the differences approximately follow a Normal distribution, we estimate the limits to be $\bar{d} \pm 2s_{diff}$, where $\bar{d}$ is the sample mean of the differences, and s_{diff} is the estimated standard deviation of the differences. Based on clinical judgement of the particular problem at hand, we can decide whether the limits of agreement are acceptable and, therefore, whether we are prepared to conclude that the methods have good agreement.

Clearly, we require these limits of agreement to be the same for all the measurements in a given data set, whatever the magnitude of the measurement. This implies that the variability of the differences should be similar for large and small values of the measurement. In order to check whether this is so, and that there is no systematic effect, we use the **Bland and Altman** approach and plot the difference between the two measurements in a pair against their mean (see Figure 14.3). If there is no evidence of a systematic effect, we should see the points scattered evenly above and below the line corresponding to a zero difference. If the variability of the differences is constant, there should be no funnel or cone effect as the mean of the two measurements increases. If the variability of the differences is not constant, we should take a transformation of the data (see Section 13.2) and repeat the process. Note that it is easier to spot outliers (see Section 5.9.3) in this plot than in the plot of one measurement in a pair against the other. If we find an outlier, we should check it to determine if there is any obvious reason for its presence.

We can utilize the standard deviation of the differences, s_{diff}, as a **measure of agreement**. This may be useful if we wish to compare the repeatabilities of different methods when the scale of measurement is the same for all the methods: the smaller the measure of agreement, the greater is the repeatability. Commonly, we multiply the standard deviation of the differences by 2 (an approximation to 1.96) to obtain the **British Standards Institution reproducibility** or **repeatability coefficient** (British Standards Institution, 1975) which gives an indication of the maximum difference likely to occur between two measurements in a pair. We expect approximately 95% of the absolute differences (i.e. ignoring their sign) to be less than this repeatability/reproducibility coefficient. Expressed another way, the coefficient is the value below which the difference between paired results may be expected to lie with 95% certainty. You may find that, instead of the standard deviation of the differences, s_{diff}, being used in the reproducibility/repeatability coefficient, the quantity $\sqrt{\sum d^2/n}$ is employed instead. This is derived from

$$s_{\text{diff}} = \sqrt{\left\{\sum\left(d-\bar{d}\right)^2\right\}/(n-1)}$$

when $\bar{d} = 0$ and $(n-1)$ is replaced by n. Note that if there is no systematic effect, we would expect the mean of the differences to be zero, and if the sample size is reasonably large, $n-1$ is virtually the same as n.

Just to confuse the issue, Dahlberg's formula (Dahlberg, 1926), $\sqrt{s_{diff}^2/2}$, is sometimes called the **standard error of measurement**. It is used in studies of repeatability to provide an estimate of the standard deviation of the *individual measurements*, s_w, rather than that of the *differences*. If there are many, rather than just two, repeated measurements on a given individual, the standard error of measurement is equal to the square root of the residual or within-group variance in the one-way analysis of variance (see Section 8.6) in which, here, the different individuals represent the groups. It may be of interest to note that the British Standards Institution repeatability coefficient can also be calculated as 2.83 times the standard error of measurement (i.e. the coefficient is $2\sqrt{s_{diff}^2} = 2\sqrt{2s_w^2} = 2.83s_w$).

(iii) Indices of agreement

An index of repeatability or reproducibility that is sometimes used is called the **coefficient of reliability**. It takes a value ranging from zero (when there is no agreement between the observations in a pair) to one (when there is perfect agreement). Often the coefficient is multiplied by 100 and expressed as a percentage. It is numerically equal to a form of the **intraclass correlation coefficient (ICC)** and represents the proportion of

the total variability in the observations that is due to the differences *between* (as opposed to within) the pairs.

If there is no evidence of a systematic difference between the observations in a pair, the estimated ICC is most easily computed in the following way. Suppose we have n pairs of measurements on a single variable which are to be compared. Let us call the first and second members of the ith pair, x_i and X_i, respectively, where $i = 1, 2, \ldots, n$. We create a set of $2n$ pairs by adding to the original set of n pairs another set of n pairs. This second set is obtained by switching the members of a pair in the first set, so what was x_i becomes X_i and *vice versa* for $i = 1, 2, \ldots, n$. The coefficient of reliability is then estimated by the Pearson correlation coefficient between the $2n$ pairs of measurements. This approach is illustrated in the example in Section 14.4.2(b) which examines the reproducibility of two different laboratory methods (a spectrophotometer and a haemocytometer) for evaluating sperm counts of sheep.

If a systematic difference between the measurements in a pair is to be taken into account, the difference between and the sum of the observations in each of the n pairs is determined, and then the ICC is estimated as

$$s_{sum}^2 - s_{diff}^2 \, s_{sum}^2 + s_{diff}^2 + \frac{2\left(n\bar{d}^2 - s_{diff}^2\right)}{n}$$

where,

s^2_{sum} is the estimated variance of the n sums;
s^2_{diff} is the estimated variance of the n differences;
and $\bar{d}$ is the sample mean of the differences.

Another index that we can use to assess agreement is **Lin's concordance correlation coefficient** (Lin, 1989, 2000) which is very similar to the ICC. If we were to plot one measurement in a pair against the other, we might be tempted to calculate the Pearson correlation coefficient to assess the agreement between the pairs of observations. The problem with this approach, however, is that it only gives an indication of *precision* (i.e. the random variation describing the tightness of the points about the best-fitting straight line) but it ignores *accuracy* (i.e. the systematic effect describing the closeness of the points to the line of perfect agreement, the 45° line through the origin). Lin's concordance correlation coefficient is a comprehensive index that can be used to assess agreement because both accuracy and precision are incorporated into it.

If we have n pairs of measurements, x_i and X_i ($i = 1, 2, 3, \ldots, n$), Lin's coefficient can be estimated as

$$r_c = \frac{2rs_x s_X s_x}{s_x^2 + s_X^2 + (\bar{x} - \bar{X})^2}$$

where

r is the estimated Pearson correlation coefficient between the n pairs of results; and
$\bar{x}$ and $\bar{X}$ are the sample means of x and X, respectively.

$$s_x^2 = \frac{\sum(x_i - \bar{x})^2}{n}$$

$$= \frac{n-1}{n} \text{ times the estimated variance of } x$$

$$s_X^2 = \frac{\sum(X_i - \bar{X})^2}{n}$$

$$= \frac{n-1}{n} \text{ times the estimated variance of } X$$

As with the ICC, perfect agreement is achieved when Lin's concordance correlation coefficient equals one, and there is no agreement when it is zero. McBride (2005) proposed the following categories to assess the strength of agreement for values of Lin's concordance correlation coefficient when the variable of interest is continuous:

- 'Poor' if $r_c < 0.90$.
- 'Moderate' if $0.90 \leq r_c \leq 0.95$.
- 'Substantial' if $0.95 < r_c \leq 0.99$.
- 'Almost perfect' if $r_c > 0.99$.

(b) Example of measuring agreement for a numerical variable

We have two ways of evaluating sperm counts in the laboratory: we can count them directly using a haemocytometer (a time-consuming procedure but regarded as the gold standard) or we can count them indirectly using the calibration curve of optical density using a spectrophotometer. From time to time, however, we have to check that the instrument is giving the correct count. Table 14.3 shows the pairs of counts of sperm concentration in 22 samples of ram ejaculates using the two methods. When we calculate the difference in counts between each member of a pair and produce a dot plot of them, we find that these differences are approximately Normally distributed. A paired t-test produces a test statistic of 0.42 ($df = 21$) which gives $P = 0.68$, indicating that there is no evidence of a systematic difference between the two methods of measurement. Figure 14.3 is a Bland and Altman diagram showing the difference in the paired counts plotted against their mean. From Figure 14.3 we can see that the points are evenly scattered above and below the line corresponding

Spectrophotometer	Haemocytometer	Spectrophotometer	Haemocytometer
0.82	1.01	1.73	1.52
2.34	2.46	3.11	3.37
2.34	2.20	3.76	3.60
4.13	4.29	1.12	1.09
4.03	3.82	3.28	3.41
4.70	4.59	3.25	3.16
4.78	4.66	1.28	1.41
5.00	4.75	3.82	3.77
5.04	4.97	3.48	3.49
5.17	5.24	1.43	1.23
5.27	5.35	3.14	3.33

Table 14.3 Sperm counts ($\times 10^9$/ml) of 22 sheep ejaculates using two methods of counting.

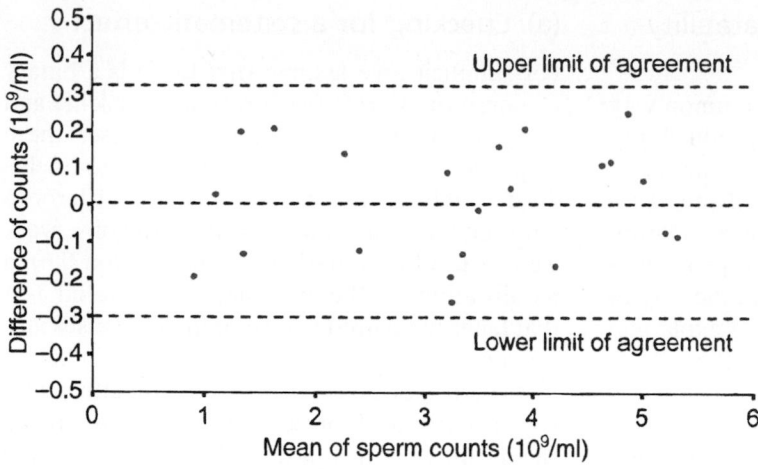

Figure 14.3 Difference between the counts of sperm concentration using a spectrophotometer and a haemocytometer (S – H) plotted against their mean (S + H)/2 in an investigation of method agreement.

to no difference. Furthermore, the scatter of the points is random with no funnel effect, indicating that the size of the discrepancy between the two methods of counting is not related to the magnitude of the count. Thus it is reasonable to calculate the limits of agreement for the two methods. These are approximately equal to $\bar{d} \pm 2s_{diff}$, where the mean of the differences, $\bar{d} = 0.0136 \, (10^9/\text{ml})$, and the standard deviation of the differences, $s_{diff} = 0.1543 \, (10^9/\text{ml})$. Hence the limits are approximately equal to $0.0136 \pm 0.3104 = (-0.295, 0.322) \, 10^9/\text{ml}$. These limits are shown as dashed lines in Figure 14.3: we expect 95% of differences to lie within these limits. Expressed another way, we expect 95% of the absolute differences to be less than the reproducibility coefficient, $2s_{diff} = 0.31$ (i.e. 0.3086 corrected to two decimal places) $10^9/\text{ml}$. For these methods, this is satisfactory agreement; we conclude that we can use the spectrophotometer with reasonable confidence.

In addition, since there is no evidence of a systematic effect, we can estimate the ICC by creating a sample of 44 pairs of observations by adding to the original sample of 22 pairs, a set of 22 pairs of observations in which the values in each pair from the original sample are interchanged. For example, for the first three pairs of readings in the original set, we have the values (0.82, 1.01), (2.34, 2.46) and (2.34, 2.20) $10^9/\text{ml}$ so

that, in the second set, these readings become (1.01, 0.82), (2.46, 2.34) and (2.20, 2.34) $10^9/\text{ml}$. We find that the estimated Pearson correlation coefficient calculated using all 44 pairs of observations created in this way (i.e. the coefficient of reliability) is 0.994, i.e. from this intraclass correlation coefficient we believe that 99.4% of the variability in the observations is due to the differences between the pairs and only 0.6% is due to the differences within a pair. This suggests extremely high reliability.

Another approach is to estimate Lin's concordance correlation coefficient using the formula provided in Section 14.4.2(a). The estimated correlation coefficient between the 22 pairs of counts is 0.994. The sample means of the sperm counts from the spectrophotometer and the haemocytometer are $3.3191 \left(\text{SD} = \sqrt{2.001} \right) 10^9/\text{ml}$ and $3.3055 \left(\text{SD} = \sqrt{1.956} \right) 10^9/\text{ml}$, respectively. Thus, using the suffix 's' for spectrophotometer and 'h' for haemocytometer and noting that $21/22 = 0.9545$, we find that $s_s^2 = 0.9545 \times 2.001 = 1.910 \, (10^9/\text{ml})^2$ and $s_h^2 = 0.9545 \times 1.956 = 1.867 \, (10^9/\text{ml})^2$ so that $s_s = 1.382 \, 10^9/\text{ml}$ and $s_h = 1.366 \, 10^9/\text{ml}$. Hence the estimated value of Lin's concordance correlation coefficient is 0.994. This is identical to the ICC and, according to the categorization of the values specified in Section 14.4.2(a), it represents almost perfect agreement between the two methods.

(c) Erroneous analysis of repeatability and method agreement

Unfortunately, you will find that a common way of investigating repeatability and reproducibility for numerical data is by performing a paired *t*-test (see Section 7.5) on the pairs of measurements and by calculating the Pearson correlation coefficient (see Section 10.3.1) to provide a measure of the agreement. This is *not* the way to proceed for the reasons that we have explained in Section 14.4.2(a) and summarize in the following bullet points.

- The paired *t*-test tests the null hypothesis that the mean of the differences is zero. If the differences are large (indicating that there is poor agreement between the two methods) but evenly scattered around zero, we will obtain a non-significant result. We can conclude only that there is no evidence of a *systematic difference* (see Section 4.4.3), not that the methods have good agreement.
- The Pearson correlation coefficient gives an indication of how close the observations in the scatter diagram (plotting the measurements of one method against the other) are to a straight line. To assess agreement we also need to know how close the points are to the line of perfect agreement, i.e. the 45° line through the origin.

14.4.3 Kappa measure of agreement for a categorical variable

We may be interested in assessing repeatability or reproducibility when the variable of interest is categorical. For example, we may wish to assess the reproducibility of two observers after each observer has classified each of a number of animals into one of several categories, say when judging at dog and cat shows or at agricultural shows. As in Section 14.4.2, we limit our explanation to assessing reproducibility when we have pairs of results (in this section, the responses are obtained from two observers): the statistical techniques can also be applied to the evaluation of repeatability.

(a) Checking for a systematic effect

For simplicity, we assume that there is a binary response of interest (e.g. present or absent) and that each of the two observers assesses these responses on the same *n* units (e.g. animals). To determine if there is a *systematic* difference between the results obtained from the observers, we can use McNemar's test (see Section 9.6), a modification of the ordinary Chi-squared test that takes the paired nature of the responses into account. A statistically significant result indicates that there is evidence of a systematic effect with the proportion of 'present' responses, say, being significantly greater in one observer than in the other. Note that when there are more than two categories of response, we can use an extension of McNemar's test such as Cochran's Q test or the McNemar–Bowker test of symmetry to assess whether there is a systematic effect. Tests such as these are available in many computer software packages but they are rather cumbersome to perform by hand (details of Cochran's test may be found in Siegel and Castellan (1988) and details of the McNemar–Bowker test may be found in Krampe and Kuhnt (2007)).

(b) Cohen's kappa coefficient

The most usual measure of agreement is **Cohen's kappa coefficient**, written κ. It assesses overall observer agreement by relating the actual agreement obtained with that which would have been attained had the categorization been made at random, i.e. it compares the actual agreement with chance agreement, and may be interpreted as the chance corrected proportional agreement.

Unfortunately, there are a number of difficulties associated with using kappa.

- There are no objective criteria for judging kappa. Its maximum value of one represents perfect agreement. A value of zero indicates that the agreement is the same as chance agreement. A negative value, which rarely occurs, indicates that the agreement between the observers is less than chance agreement. Landis and Koch (1977) provide a reasonable approach to interpreting kappa; very approximately, they regard the agreement as:

- 'Poor' if $\kappa \leq 0.20$.
- 'Fair' if $0.21 \leq \kappa \leq 0.40$.
- 'Moderate' if $0.41 \leq \kappa \leq 0.60$.
- 'Substantial' if $0.61 \leq \kappa \leq 0.80$.
- 'Good' if κ exceeds 0.80.

• The value of kappa depends on the proportion of individuals in each category. Thus different kappa values should not be compared in studies in which these proportions differ.

• Kappa depends on the number of categories that are used in its calculation, with its value being greater if there are fewer categories.

In order to calculate kappa, we arrange the data in a square two-way contingency table of frequencies (see Section 9.4.2 and Table 14.4). The rows represent the categories of response of one observer, and the columns represent the same categories of response of the second observer. Perfect agreement is obtained when both of the observers believe an animal belongs to the same category; the frequency with which this occurs is shown in the diagonal cells of the table. For each of the observed frequencies along this diagonal, we calculate the corresponding frequency we would expect if there were chance agreement. The calculations are similar to those for the Chi-squared statistic (see Section 9.5.3), i.e. each expected frequency is the product of the relevant marginal totals divided by the overall

total. The observed frequencies along the diagonal are added and their sum is divided by the total observed frequency to obtain a proportion (p_o) which represents the 'observed agreement'. 'Chance agreement' (p_c) is the sum of the expected frequencies along the diagonal, divided by the total observed frequency. Then

$$\kappa = \frac{\text{Observed agreement} - \text{Chance agreement}}{\text{Maximum agreement} - \text{Chance agreement}}$$

where maximum agreement = 1. The approximate 95% confidence interval for kappa is given by $[\kappa \pm 1.96 \times \text{SE}(k)]$ where, approximately,

$$\text{SE}(\kappa) = \frac{p_o(1 - p_o)}{n(1 - p_c)^2}$$

(Note: the correct formula for $\text{SE}(\kappa)$ is complex; details may be obtained from Fleiss *et al.*, 2003.)

This unweighted kappa coefficient considers only perfect agreement of the observers, as demonstrated by the frequencies along the diagonal of the contingency table. It has the disadvantage that it takes no account of the *extent* to which the observers disagree. This is relevant if the categories are *ordered* so that observers differing by one category show less disagreement than if they differ by two categories, etc. Then, the greater the discrepancy, the greater the distance of the cell from the diagonal in the contingency table. In these circumstances, we should calculate

Table 14.4 Table of observed frequencies of body condition scores accorded to 160 pigs by a pigman and a trainee (expected frequencies are in brackets).

		Experienced pigman					
	Score	1	2	3	4	5	Total
Trainee	1	**4 (0.400)**	3	1	0	0	8
	2	4	**7 (1.463)**	5	2	0	18
	3	0	2	**15 (7.813)**	7	1	25
	4	0	1	16	**36 (29.656)**	12	65
	5	0	0	13	28	**3 (4.400)**	44
	Total	8	13	50	73	16	160

a **weighted kappa coefficient**; this is determined by assigning weights to the frequencies representing disagreements according to the magnitude of the disagreement. In fact, the weighted kappa is very similar to the intraclass correlation coefficient or, equivalently, the index of reliability (see Section 14.4.2(a)).

You can obtain full details of the calculations of the weighted kappa, together with formulae for its standard error from which confidence intervals can be derived, in Cohen (1960) and Cohen (1968).

(c) Example of the kappa measure of agreement

Scoring of body condition is routinely used in pig management. Generally, the score is on a subjective scale ranging from 1 to 5 (1 is very poor condition, 5 implies a pig with excellent fat and muscle). To be consistent, the scoring system must be learned. Table 14.4 gives body condition scores of 160 pigs by two independent scorers. The first scorer is an experienced pigman, and the second is a trainee.

The McNemar–Bowker test gives a Chi-squared value of 23.0 with 7 degrees of freedom and $P = 0.002$, suggesting that there is a systematic difference in the scoring between the trainee and the experienced pigman: the trainee tends to give higher body condition scores than the experienced pigman.

$$\text{Observed agreement} = \frac{4+7+15+36+3}{160}$$
$$= 0.406$$

Chance agreement
$$= \frac{0.400+1.463+7.813+29.656+4.400}{160}$$
$$= 0.273$$

Hence, $\kappa = \dfrac{0.406 - 0.273}{1 - 0.273} = 0.183$

and, using the approximate formula,

$$\text{SE}(\kappa) = \frac{0.406(1-0.406)}{160(1-0.273)^2} = 0.0534$$

So the approximate 95% confidence interval for kappa is given by $0.183 \pm 1.96 \times 0.0534$, i.e. from 0.078 to 0.288. (Note, using the correct formula, the estimated $\text{SE}(\kappa) = 0.051$ and the 95% confidence interval is from 0.082 to 0.284.)

We can see that with a kappa of only 0.18 (or possibly as low as 0.078), the agreement between the assessors is poor, although the upper limit of the confidence interval suggests that it could be classified as fair. In fact, when the extent to which the scorers disagree is taken into account, the weighted kappa, using linear weights, is estimated as 0.384, which may also be considered fair. However we classify the measure, though, it is clear that the trainee requires more experience and help!

14.5 Measurements at successive points in time

14.5.1 Time series

A **time series** is a sequence of observations made at many successive time points. Generally these observations are recorded on groups of animals or other phenomena of interest at each of the time points. Typical examples in agriculture are the average number of eggs per hen in a poultry farm in successive months, or the national herd or flock population in successive years. Sometimes, however, a time series is generated by recording observations on a single animal over many successive time points, e.g. the milk yield of a dairy cow throughout lactation. The *order* in which the observations are made is of particular relevance in a time series. Usually the successive observations are *dependent*, so that the expected value of an observation at one time point cannot be regarded in isolation because it is likely to be related to the magnitude of the observation at the previous time point. This is known as an **autoregressive series**.

The aim of a statistical analysis of a time series is to describe it by constructing the appropriate mathematical model that explains both the systematic and the random, or unsystematic, variation. The systematic variation may comprise a trend or long-term movement, oscillations about the trend and/or a seasonal effect. From this model we may gain some insight into the causal mechanisms that generated the time series, and may be able to predict future observations.

Although it may seem appropriate to analyse a time series by regressing the variable of interest against time (see Section 10.4), this approach is rarely feasible. It is very unusual to find that a simple linear model is an adequate description of the time series. Furthermore, the fact that successive observations are dependent implies that these observations have deviations about any long-term trend which are associated.

This so-called **serial correlation** violates the independence assumption underlying regression analysis. Therefore, special techniques have been devised to analyse time series. The details of this analysis are beyond the scope of this book, and we refer you to Chatfield (2003) or Diggle (1990) for further information. □

14.5.2 Analysis of repeated measurements

(a) Correct analysis

Suppose we are interested in analysing the results of a *within-animal study* in which measurements of a numerical variable are taken on each of a number of animals at more than one time. Another type of within-animal study occurs when data are collected at one time point but we obtain more than one observation on each animal, for example on different body parts such as the two forelegs of a cow, both ears of a rabbit or teeth in the mouth of a horse. Such within-animal studies embody what is called **clustered** data, with the results within each cluster (e.g. animal) being correlated, a feature which must not be ignored in the analysis. For simplicity, we shall provide explanations in this section in terms of measurements taken serially in time, although our explanations can be applied equally to any form of clustered data. Typically, we may wish to compare such data in two or more groups of animals. Although we could regard the serial measurements on any one animal as a time series, we do not use time series analysis (see Section 14.5.1) to evaluate the results because the series are generally too short, and because of the difficulty of combining the series from different animals.

There are a number of ways of analysing the data. We can choose from one of the following:

- Perform a **repeated measures analysis of variance** (see Section 8.5.3) using the appropriate computer software, provided the design is completely balanced.
- Perform a suitable **regression analysis** by using, for example, a **random effects model** (also called a **multilevel, hierarchical, mixed, cluster-specific** or **cross-sectional time series model**)

or **generalized estimating equations (GEE)** or by **aggregating the data** in a sensible manner (e.g. by calculating the mean value of the outcome variable for each animal so that its multiple responses are reduced to a single measurement which is then used as the value of the dependent variable in the regression). We discussed these regression methods in Section 11.6.

- Use a (non-regression) approach based on **summary measures**. The analysis is simpler to perform and the results easier to interpret than the alternative elaborate analyses, such as repeated measures ANOVA or multilevel modelling, which often rely on relatively complex software. The summary measures approach therefore has much to recommend it (Everitt, 1995).

The **summary measures approach** reduces the serial responses for each animal to a single statistic which describes some important aspect of that animal's response curve. For example, the summary measure might be:

- The maximum (or minimum) value.
- The time to maximum (or minimum) response.
- The time to reach a particular value.
- The difference between the initial and the final responses.
- The slope of the line.
- The area under the curve.
- The overall mean.

The summary measure should have some clear clinical or biological relevance and it should be chosen before the data are collected. The summary measure for each animal is then used in the analysis as if it is the raw data.

So, for example, suppose we wish to compare serial measurements over time in two groups of animals, with each group receiving a different treatment. We may decide that we are interested in determining whether the average time to reach the peak response is the same using both treatments. We find the time to reach the peak response in each animal, and perform a significance test (e.g. a two-sample *t*-test (see Section 7.4) or a Wilcoxon rank sum test (see Section

12.5)) on the times to peak response in the two groups to determine whether there is a treatment effect.

The statistical analysis is incomplete without a **graphical representation** of the data. However, it is often difficult to know how to provide this in an informative way. Avoid the temptation to draw the average curve for a group (i.e. by joining the mean responses for a group at successive time points) as it may not describe a typical curve for an animal. You should start by producing a separate graph of the responses against time for each animal. Then, perhaps, you could arrange them in some order or in a panel or grid with separate panels for each group. If the sample size is large, you could classify the curves in a meaningful way, and plot representative examples. Be sure that your examples are truly *representative* and not simply the best! It may also be helpful to plot the chosen summary measures, such as histograms for each measure or a scatter plot of any two summary measures (e.g. the maximum value for each animal against the time that the maximum occurred).

(b) Incorrect analysis

Repeated measures data are frequently analysed inappropriately. The most usual approach when two groups are being compared is to apply separate two-sample tests (e.g. the two-sample *t*-test or the Wilcoxon rank sum test) at each time point. The main criticism of this approach is that:

- No account is taken of the fact that measurements at different time points are from the same animal, i.e. the within-animal changes are ignored.
- Successive observations on an animal are likely to be correlated, so that the results of significance tests at adjacent time points are not independent, which leads to difficulties in interpretation.
- A group may comprise a different set of animals at various time points if the missing observations do not come from the same animals at these time points.
- Spuriously significant results may arise because of multiple testing (see Section 13.4).

The most usual approach to the graphical display of the data is to draw the average curve for each group, often with error bars for each mean. As we point out in Section 14.5.2(a), this is generally inappropriate because the average curve may have quite a different shape from that of the individual curves, and individual variation will be obscured. One possibility is to represent all the individual curves in the background (e.g. in pastel colours) together with the average curve in bold.

(c) Example

In a study of the effect of thawing rate on the motility and survival of cryopreserved dog semen, the motility of the spermatozoa from individual dogs was recorded over a 4-hour period. The semen from six of the dogs (chosen randomly from the 12) was thawed at 39°C, and the remaining semen samples were thawed at 70°C. The mean curves in Figure 14.4a show the general trend but obscure the very real differences between dogs, which are shown in Figure 14.4b and c. To address the problem of repeated measures data, the times for spermatozoa to reach a motility of 75% and 25% of the original values were measured from the plotted curves for each dog, and these summary measures were used for the statistical analysis to investigate differences in the two groups.

The times to reach a motility of 75% were 80.2, 53.5, 75.7, 57.8, 56.2 and 55.8 minutes (median = 57.0 min) for the sperm of the six dog semen straws thawed at 39°C, and 107.2, 63.0, 92.7, 97.0, 76.3 and 80.5 minutes (median = 86.6 min) for the sperm of the six dog semen straws thawed at 70°C. A Wilcoxon rank sum test (see Section 12.5) comparing the two distributions from which these samples were selected gives $P = 0.02$, which is statistically significant, indicating that there is a tendency for the time to reach a motility of 75% to be greater in the sperm thawed at 70°C than in the sperm thawed at 39°C.

Furthermore, the times to reach a motility of 25% were 167.5, 124.3, 158.2, 170.2, 112.5 and 140.3 minutes (median = 149.3 min) for the sperm of the six dogs thawed at 39°C, and 190.6, 160.0, 182.0, 195.0, 148.5 and 186.0 minutes (median =

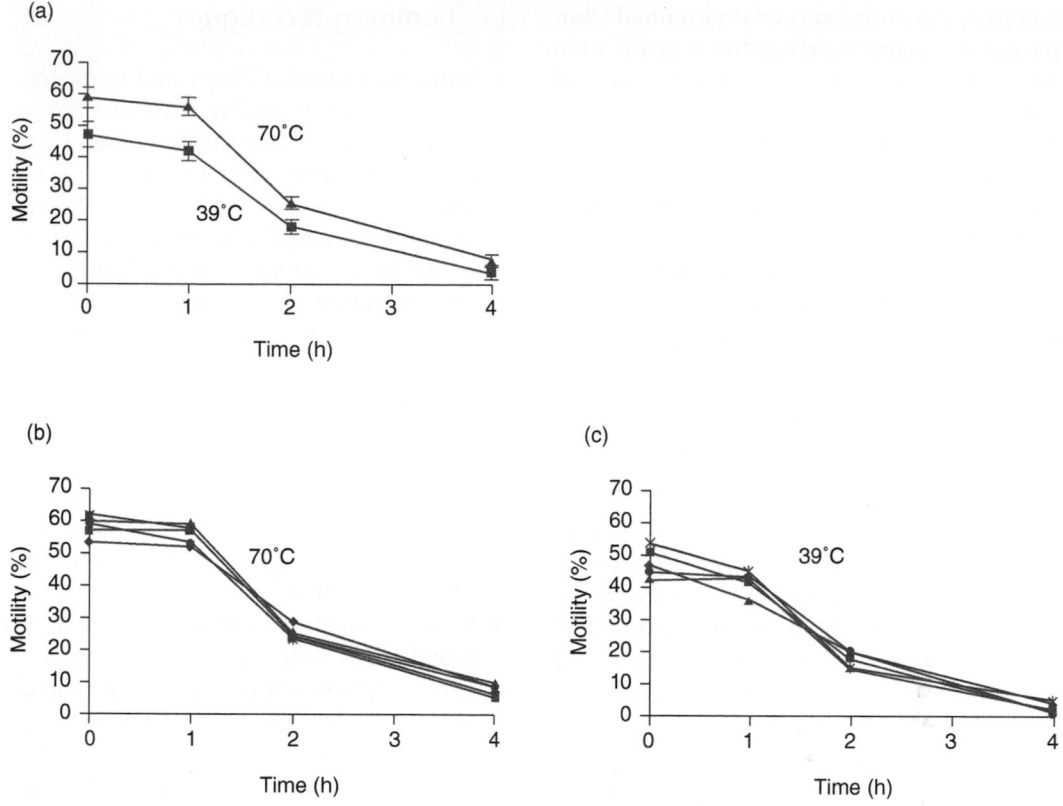

Figure 14.4   Repeated measures data showing the effect of thawing rate on the motility of dog semen. (a) Mean curves for thawing at 70°C and 39°C (mean ± SD at hourly intervals). (b) Individual curves for thawing at 70°C. (c) Individual curves for thawing at 39°C (data from England, 1992, with permission from the author).

184.0 min) for the sperm of the six dogs thawed at 70°C. A Wilcoxon rank sum test comparing the two distributions from which these samples were selected gives $P = 0.04$, which is statistically significant, indicating that there is a tendency for the time to reach a motility of 25% to be greater in the sperm thawed at 70°C than in the sperm thawed at 39°C. Thus, it was concluded that rapid thawing at 70°C was preferable for recovering viable spermatozoa.

14.6 Survival analysis

14.6.1 Introduction

Another form of statistical analysis that focuses on time is known as **survival analysis**. Here we are concerned with the time (the **survival time**) it takes for some critical event (the **failure**), such as death, to occur in an individual after a particular starting point, such as the initiation of treatment. The most common situation is when the failure can occur at most once in any individual (although in Section 14.6.2(b) we briefly describe frailty models that allow for the situation where the failure can occur more than once in an individual). Examples of the 'individual' are an animal, a machine component in industrial reliability or a tooth filling; examples of the 'failure' are death, remission or recurrence. For purposes of discussion, we shall assume that the individual is an animal in a clinical trial, that the animal is being treated for a particular condition, and that the failure is death as a result of the condition. We may be interested in:

- Estimating the probability that an animal from a particular group survives for a given time period, say 6 months (the 6-month survival rate).
- Estimating the median survival time for a given group of animals.
- Comparing the survival experience in two groups of animals receiving different treatments.
- Assessing the impact of one or more factors on survival, whilst controlling for the effect of other factors.

The analysis of survival times warrants special techniques because of **censored data**; these arise when some of the animals never experience the failure during the course of the study. Either they are alive at the end of the study period, or they are lost to follow-up (such animals are called **withdrawals**) or they die during the study period from some cause unrelated to the condition of interest. It is important to note that it is assumed in the analysis that we have **uninformative** or **non-informative censoring**: this implies that the probability that an animal is censored is not related to the probability that the animal will experience the failure. If we have **informative censoring** (say, when animals are removed from the study because their condition is deteriorating or, conversely, because their condition has improved substantially) then any bias that is introduced because of it has to be adjusted for in the analysis. Furthermore, the animals may be observed for varying lengths of time because they have been recruited into the study at different times and there is a single time point at which the study period ends, when **administrative censoring** occurs.

The mathematical theory underlying survival analysis is relatively complex. We omit details of the calculations and refer you to, for example, Collet (2003), Kleinbaum and Klein (2005), Machin and Cheung (2006) or Smith (2002).

14.6.2 Approaches

There are various approaches to the analysis of survival data, some of which are illustrated in the example in Section 14.6.3.

(a) Common techniques

- When the survival times and censored times are *grouped into intervals*, we can analyse survival data using the **Berkson–Gage** approach which bases the calculations on the methods involved in actuarial life tables. We can estimate the chance that an individual will survive a particular length of time from a relevant starting point (e.g. diagnosis of condition or surgical operation). The Berkson–Gage method suffers from a number of disadvantages: (i) the choice of interval is arbitrary; (ii) it involves a loss of information if exact survival times are known; and (iii) it generally assumes that individuals lost to follow-up are censored at the midpoint of the interval and makes adjustments to the calculations to account for this.
- If the survival and censored times are known exactly, it is better to use the **Kaplan–Meier** approach to survival analysis. The calculations are similar to those of the life table, but the time 'interval' is chosen to correspond to the smallest unit used to record the time at which an event occurred (e.g. if survival time is recorded in days, each time interval is a day). However, unlike the Berkson–Gage approach, it assumes that losses to follow-up at a given time survive longer than deaths at that time, and so these censored data are included in the calculations without the need for adjustments. The Kaplan–Meier analysis provides estimates of the probabilities of surviving from the starting point to particular time points, e.g. the probability of surviving 20 days. A **Kaplan–Meier survival curve** is obtained (see Figure 14.5) when we plot the survival probability against the time from the starting point. Conventionally, the survival curve is drawn in steps (this is because the curve should be horizontal when there is no event (e.g. death)), and the **median survival time**, corresponding to a survival probability of 0.5, may be read from it. This median survival time provides a reasonable summary of survival; the mean survival time should *not* be calculated when there are censored data and/or animals are followed for different lengths of time.

We often compare survival curves in two (or more) groups by using the non-parametric **logrank test** which utilizes all the information in each curve but does not make assumptions about the shape of the curve. It tests the null hypothesis that the survival experience is the same in the two groups. The test statistic, following a Chi-squared distribution, compares the observed number of deaths at each time at which there is a death with the numbers expected if the null hypothesis were true. Using the logrank test is preferable to the much more restricted comparison of survival rates at a specific time (say, 6 months).

- If we wish to investigate the effect on survival of several variables at the same time, as a way of assessing which factors affect survival and, perhaps, estimating the probability of survival to a particular time in different circumstances, we can use the **Cox proportional hazards regression model**. This is more appropriate than performing a multiple logistic regression analysis (see Section 11.4) because the Cox regression analysis, unlike logistic regression analysis, makes allowances for censored data and the fact that animals are generally followed for different lengths of time, as well as utilizing the time that an animal spends in the study even if it does not experience the failure.

The dependent variable in a Cox regression analysis is called the **hazard**, the probability of dying/failing at a particular time, conditional on the animal surviving up to that time. It can be thought of as an instantaneous death rate. There is no requirement in a Cox regression analysis for the death rate to be constant over the time period of interest, as in a Poisson regression (see Section 11.5), but there is an assumption of **proportional hazards**. This means that the ratio of the hazards in two groups that are to be compared (e.g. the ratio of the hazards in the treatment and control groups) remains constant over time. If this assumption is satisfied, the survival curves for the two groups will move apart progressively over time or, alternatively, the lines will be roughly parallel in a log–log plot (i.e. when we plot $\log_e(-\log_e(\text{survival probability}))$ versus $\log_e(\text{time})$). Another approach is to incorpo-

rate into the model an interaction between the covariate and $\log_e(\text{time})$ and ensure that it is not statistically significant. If there is concern about the proportional hazards assumption, a separate Cox regression analysis may be performed for each of a number of successive time intervals within which the proportional hazards assumption is satisfied or, if appropriate, for different strata of the population.

The proportional hazards regression model links the *logarithm* of the hazard at a particular time to a linear function of the k explanatory variables (i.e. of the form $\beta_1 x_1 + \beta_2 x_2 + \beta_3 x_3 + \ldots + \beta_k x_k$) and an arbitrary baseline hazard (the latter is the hazard when all the explanatory variables take their baseline values; it is of no inherent interest). It is a *semiparametric* model in that no distribution is assumed for the survival times although, as explained in the previous paragraph, it does make an assumption about the hazard ratio. The coefficients, β_1, $\beta_2, \ldots, \beta_k$, are estimated using a form of maximum likelihood estimation (see Section 11.4.3). The exponential of a particular coefficient (for example, $\exp(\beta_1)$) represents a relative hazard, the ratio of the two hazards when the value of x_1 is increased by 1 unit, after adjusting for the other explanatory variables in the model. If this exponential is equal to one, there is no increased or decreased risk of reaching the endpoint (typically, death) when the explanatory variable increases by 1 unit. Comprehensive computer output of a Cox regression analysis will contain estimates of the coefficients, the associated confidence intervals and Wald or likelihood ratio significance tests, with P-values (each resulting from the test of the null hypothesis that the relevant coefficient is equal to zero or, equivalently, that its exponential is equal to one). We show some typical computer output in Display 14.1 relating to the example in Section 14.6.3.

The Cox model assumes that the covariates are measured at a single time point for each individual at the beginning of the study. A **time-dependent covariate** is a variable that changes over time during the course of the study, and such covariates may also be included in a Cox analysis. However, caution should be

Display 14.1 Stata output of Cox survival analysis of uraemic cats' data with diet (standard = 1; low phosphorus, low protein = 2) and creatinine (mild = 1; moderate = 2) as covariates.

```
No. of subjects   =          50          Number of obs.  =        50
No. of failures   =          42
Time at risk      =       27597
                                          LR chi2(2)      =     15.97
Log likelihood    =  -128.33447           Prob > chi2     =    0.0003
```

_t	Haz. ratio	Std. err.	z	P > |z|	[95% conf. interval]	
Diet	0.3345698	0.1138069	-3.22	0.001	0.1717684	0.6516741
Creatine	2.711757	0.8927078	3.03	0.002	1.422447	5.169702

adopted as they have a great potential for bias and they do not lead to prediction for the individual survival experience as does the usual Cox model with fixed covariate values (Fisher and Lin, 1999).

- Sometimes, we assume a **particular distributional form for the survival function** (i.e. the survival curve obtained when we plot the survival probability against time), such as the exponential, gamma or Weibull distributions, and use our data to estimate the parameters that define the model. Using this parametric approach, we can compare survival curves in two or more groups, each assuming the same distributional form, by comparing their estimated parameters.

(b) Additional techniques and issues

- It may be that survival analysis is required when there is some natural or artificial clustering of individuals and the observations within a cluster are not independent (for example, the characteristics of mice in a litter, or when failure is remission and an animal can go into remission more than once so that there are recurrent failures for each animal). We discuss the problems of clustered data in Section 11.6 where we briefly describe some of the special methods that are required to accommodate the dependencies in the data. One of these methods is the use of a random effects regression model in which the random effect represents the variability between the clusters. The **frailty model** is a random effects proportional hazards model, used when analysing survival

in clustered data where failure times are not independent. The frailty is the unknown tendency for an individual to fail, and in frailty models, the common value of the frailty is shared by the individuals in a cluster. In the proportional hazards model, the frailty factor, representing the frailty in a cluster, is random with a specified distribution for which there are a number of choices. Full details of the analysis may be obtained, for example, in Duchateau and Janssen (2010).

- Let us suppose that death from a specific cause (e.g. lamb mortality from birth to weaning due to dam-related problems such as dystocia and starvation (Southey *et al.*, 2004)) is the failure or event of interest in a particular study. It may be that the lambs die from some other disease (e.g. pneumonia) in which case they cannot experience the event of interest. These events are termed **competing risks** in that the one event precludes the occurrence of the event of interest. In the Southey study the investigators examined the mortality records from birth to weaning of 8301 lambs from a composite population at the US Meat Animal Research Center. The data were analysed using a competing risks model in which specific causes of mortality were grouped into dam-related (e.g. dystocia and starvation), pneumonia, disease excluding pneumonia, and other categories, so different hazards of mortality could be assigned to different causes. Although the authors found that the influence of type of birth and age of dam on mortality were generally consistent across the categories (indicating that the effect of these factors on mortality was not dependent on the cause of mortality), the effect of sex varied with the cause of mortality. Thus, ignoring the cause of the event could hide important genetic differences.

Death from a cause other than that related to the event of interest is one common form of competing risk but there are other types of events, such as undergoing some treatment, that are also competing risks in that they modify the probability of the occurrence of the event of interest. Special methods are used to analyse survival data with competing risks. Further details of the approaches may be found in, for example, Putter *et al.* (2007).

14.6.3 Example

The outcome achieved by dietary control of uraemia in domestic cats was investigated by

Elliott *et al.* (2000). They studied 50 cats from the day of diagnosis, at which time the cats were divided into two diet groups created by animal and/or owner compliance. Twenty-nine cats accepted a restricted phosphorus and protein diet and 21 cats continued to receive their standard diet. Figure 14.5 shows the Kaplan–Meier survival curves that depict the survival experience of these two groups of uraemic cats in the days following diagnosis. The tick marks indicate the censored data: these cats were still alive at the last follow-up at the times indicated. Also shown are the numbers at risk in each group at intervals of 250 days.

The **median survival time** from diagnosis for the control group on the standard diet was 367 days (95% CI 194 to 541 days), and for the test group receiving the low phosphorus and low protein diet it was 677 days (95% CI 503 to 851 days). In each case, the median is the value on

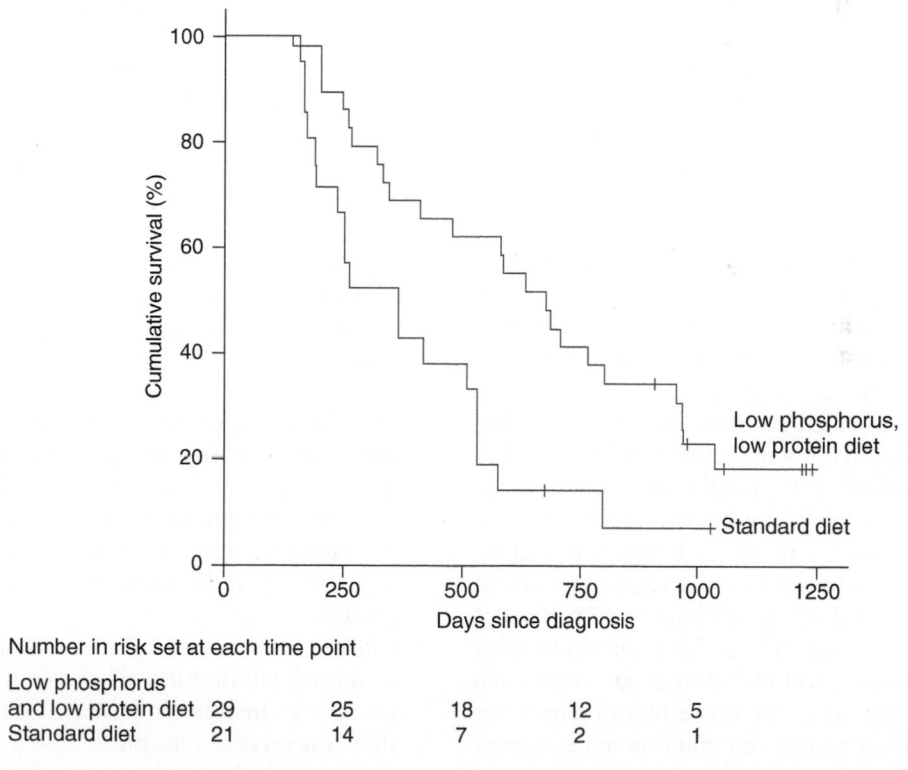

Number in risk set at each time point

Low phosphorus and low protein diet	29	25	18	12	5
Standard diet	21	14	7	2	1

Figure 14.5 Kaplan–Meier curves showing the survival probability, expressed as a percentage, of cats following diagnosis with uraemia, stratified by diet. The tick marks indicate cats lost to follow-up at the time indicated (based on data in Elliott *et al.*, 2000, with permission from Wiley-Blackwell).

the horizontal axis that corresponds to a 50% survival on the vertical axis. These two groups were compared with a **logrank test**, giving a Chi-squared test statistic of 7.65 on 1 degree of freedom and a highly significant result ($P = 0.006$); thus the survival experience of the cats on the restricted diet was significantly better than those on the standard diet.

A **Cox proportional hazards survival analysis** was performed to investigate whether the effect of diet on survival could be explained by differences in the cats' initial blood creatinine concentrations at the time of diagnosis (after clinical stabilizing by fluid therapy, if necessary). The mild creatinine group was defined as having creatinine concentrations between 177 and $250\,\mu$mol/l and the moderately severe group had creatinine concentrations $>250\,\mu$mol/l. Stata computer output relating to a Cox regression analysis that used both diet and creatinine as binary covariates is shown in Display 14.1. The model Chi-square (see Section 11.4.3) of 15.97 on 2 degrees of freedom with $P < 0.001$ indicates that at least one of the two coefficients in the model is significantly different from zero. The estimated hazard ratio is provided for each covariate, together with a Wald test statistic (indicated by 'z') and a P-value (indicated by $P > |z|$) which results from the test of the hypothesis that the relevant coefficient in the model is zero (or equivalently that its hazard ratio is one).

We can conclude that each of the covariates has a hazard ratio that is significantly different from one, after adjusting for the other covariate. Thus both diet and creatinine level are independently and significantly associated with survival. A cat is estimated to be nearly three times more likely (but, with 95% confidence, it could be five times more likely) to die if it has a moderate rather than a mild creatinine level, and its risk of dying is reduced by an estimated 67% (but it could be as much as 83%) if it is put on the low phosphorus/low protein diet at diagnosis, in each case after adjusting for the effect of the other covariate. Thus we can see that this analysis gives some very helpful guidelines for prognosis and treatment of this condition.

14.7 Multivariate analysis

We have already introduced you to *multiple regression* (see Section 11.3), *multiple logistic regression* (see Section 11.4), *Poisson regression* (see Section 11.5) and *regression methods for clustered data* such as *multilevel modelling* (see Section 11.6) where, in each case, we look at the effect of a number of explanatory variables on a single response variable. A similar model building approach, *log-linear analysis*, can be used to investigate associations in multiway contingency tables derived from a number of categorical variables (i.e. each individual is categorized with respect to several categorical variables). In all these regression-type analyses, there is only a single dependent or response variable and so, strictly, these methods are termed **univariate**; generally, these models incorporate more than one explanatory variable, in which case they are **multivariable** models.

The procedures gathered under the general heading '**multivariate analysis**' are traditionally directed at situations in which there are several response variables, and we wish to examine the variation in these variables simultaneously. Multivariate techniques are increasingly used, especially now that computer techniques can take the drudgery out of the calculations. As with all statistical procedures, you should aim to understand what the computer is doing, and how, before embarking on multivariate analyses.

Some of the more common multivariate analyses are:

- *Discriminant analysis* – given the existence of different groupings of the population, it uses the information from a sample of individuals, in which each individual is known to belong to a particular group, to devise a rule for allocating further individuals to the appropriate groups.
- *Cluster analysis* – determines whether there is a natural subdivision of the individuals into groups or clusters on the basis of the observations on several variables.
- *Factor analysis* – defines a model (with distributional and other assumptions) in which the

k original variables are replaced by another set of $j < k$ variables (called factors), each of which is a linear combination of the original variables together with a residual. In order to present the most economical model, j is chosen to be as small as possible.

- *Principal component analysis* – replaces the k original variables by another set of k variables (the principal components), each of which is a linear combination of the original variables. The first few principal components often account for most of the variability of the original data, so that the remaining principal components can be discarded and thereby reduce the dimensionality of the data.
- *Multidimensional scaling* – concerned with expressing the main content of the data in fewer dimensions with as little distortion as possible. It is based on the distances between the points, and is closely related to principal component analysis.
- *Canonical correlation* – concerned with investigating the interdependence between two sets of variables, $(y_1, y_2, y_3, \ldots, y_p)$ and $(x_1, x_2, x_3, \ldots, x_m)$.
- *Multivariate analysis of variance (MANOVA)* – an extension of the univariate ANOVA for multiple dependent variables. So, for example, in the one-way MANOVA, we test the null hypothesis that the vector of population means is the same for all the independent groups.

We suggest, if you require to utilize these multivariate analytical methods, you refer to books such as those by Dugard *et al.* (2010), Everitt and Dunn (2001) or Krzanowski (2000) before embarking on the analysis. The methods are sometimes difficult to understand, and need careful assessment to avoid misuse. It may also be advisable to seek advice from a professional statistician to ensure you are applying the methods appropriately.

Exercises

The statements in questions 14.1–14.6 are either TRUE or FALSE.

14.1 The sensitivity of a screening test for a particular disease is 0.99. This means that:
(a) The proportion of animals correctly identified by the test as having the disease is 0.99.
(b) The proportion of animals with the disease, out of those which tested positive, is 0.99.
(c) The specificity of the test is 0.01.
(d) The test is particularly useful for identifying animals with a disease that is treatable.
(e) The prevalence of the disease in the population must be high.

14.2 The most appropriate way to investigate the agreement between two observers when each has measured a numerical response on each of 20 animals is to:
(a) Calculate Cohen's kappa.
(b) Perform a paired t-test.
(c) Calculate the correlation coefficient, and test its significance from zero.
(d) Calculate two times the standard deviation of the differences, and use this as a measure of agreement.
(e) Estimate the standard deviation of the individual measurements, s_w, and use this as a measure of agreement.

14.3 Suppose 16 animals are randomly allocated to one of two treatments, and there are eight animals in each treatment group. We take a single measurement of a numerical variable at six successive time points on each animal. An appropriate analysis that investigates the treatment effect may be:
(a) A time series analysis.
(b) A repeated measures ANOVA.
(c) A two-sample t-test, comparing the observations in the two groups, at each time point.
(d) A two-sample t-test, comparing the changes from baseline in the two groups, at each time point.
(e) A two-sample t-test, comparing the differences between the initial and final responses in the two groups.

14.4 A Cox regression analysis:
(a) Is used to analyse survival data when individuals in the study are followed for varying lengths of time.

(b) Can only be used when there are censored data.
(c) Assumes that the relative hazard for a particular variable is constant at all times.
(d) Uses the logrank test to compare two survival curves.
(e) Relies on the assumption that the explanatory variables in the model are Normally distributed.

14.5　Using a single-detector computed tomography (CT) examination, sixteen 6-month-old male minipigs were scanned under general anaesthesia and two radiologists assessed the Hounsfield unit (HU) value of subcutaneous abdominal fat in each minipig by drawing the region of interest manually at the T13 level. The HU is the numerical information relating to density contained in each voxel (volume unit) of a three-dimensional CT image. The HU values from one radiologist were plotted against those from the second radiologist in a scatter diagram. The Pearson correlation coefficient was estimated as 0.95 and Lin's concordance correlation coefficient was estimated as 0.70 (based on Chang *et al.*, 2011).

(a) The Pearson correlation coefficient of 0.95 indicates that there was almost perfect agreement between the HU values obtained by the two radiologists.
(b) It would have been preferable to calculate the kappa measure of agreement instead of either the Pearson correlation coefficient or Lin's concordance correlation coefficient.
(c) Lin's concordance correlation coefficient was substantially less than the Pearson correlation coefficient. This would suggest that there was a systematic difference between the two radiologists' measurements, with one tending to give a higher HU value than the other for each minipig.
(d) Lin's concordance correlation coefficient was substantially less than the Pearson correlation coefficient. This would suggest that there was poor precision.
(e) The difference between the two correlation coefficients could only arise if there was both poor precision and poor accuracy.

14.6　A receiver operating characteristic (ROC) curve for a diagnostic test:

(a) Is a plot of the sensitivity against the specificity.
(b) Is a plot of the sensitivity against one minus the specificity, when each is expressed as a proportion.
(c) Is a plot of the true positive rate against the true negative rate.
(d) With an AUROC of 0.5 indicates that the diagnostic test is better than chance at discriminating between subjects with and without the disease of interest.
(e) With an AUROC of 0.6 indicates that, on 60% of occasions, a randomly chosen diseased animal will have a higher predicted probability by the diagnostic test of having the disease than a disease-free animal.

14.7　Quantitative determination of the corticosteroid-induced isoenzyme of alkaline phosphatase (CAP) was evaluated as a diagnostic test for hyperadrenocorticism (HAC) in dogs (Solter *et al.*, 1993). A cut-off value of 90 U/l was selected for use for this assay as a diagnostic test for HAC, with values of CAP greater than this cut-off value being indicative of HAC. This cut-off value was used in Harrogate on 46 dogs with a combination of historical and clinical signs of HAC and on 92 date-matched healthy control dogs (i.e. there were two controls for every HAC dog). The results are shown in Table 14.5.

(a) Determine the sensitivity and specificity of the test.
(b) Do you think that this cut-off is reasonable?
(c) What is the effect on sensitivity and specificity of raising the cut-off of CAP to >500 U/l (when, in this sample of dogs, 37 HAC dogs and four healthy dogs had CAP >500 U/l)?
(d) When the CAP cut-off value of 90 U/l was used on all canine serum samples submitted

Table 14.5　Observed frequencies in two groups of dogs (based on results of Solter *et al.*, 1993).

	HAC dogs	Healthy dogs	Total
CAP >90 U/l	43	12	45
CAP ≤90 U/l	3	80	83
Total	46	92	138

to the laboratory over a 3-month period, the positive predictive value of the test was 21.4% and the negative predictive value was 100%. What do you infer from these results in terms of the usefulness of the CAP test as a screening test rather than a diagnostic test?

(e) Why do these predictive values not agree with what you would obtain if you were to calculate them using the information from Table 14.5?

14.8 Studies conducted in 98 mithuns (*Bos frontalis*) maintained at the National Research Centre, Nagaland, India, using the 'gold standard' enzyme-linked-immunosorbent assay, revealed that the seroprevalence of brucellosis in these cattle of Indian origin was 34% (Rajkhowa *et al.*, 2005). The sensitivity and specificity of the standard tube agglutination test were found to be approximately 61% and 99.9%, respectively. Using Fagan's nomogram, evaluate the chance that a mithun that tests positive for brucellosis using the standard tube agglutination test actually has brucellosis.

14.9 A sheep farmer has a problem with foot rot. He decides to score the degree of foot rot in each sheep in his flock and then to treat them; later he scores them again to see if there has been any improvement. He scores them as follows: 1 = no lameness, perfect feet; 2 = no lameness, but at least one misshapen claw requiring trimming; 3 = mild lameness involving infection and damage to one foot only; 4 = severe lameness, foot rot and injury in more than one foot. Table 14.6 shows the frequency of occurrence of the scores before and after treatment. Conduct a suitable analysis and present the result. Is it reasonable to presume that the treat-

Table 14.6 Observed frequencies of scores of foot condition in sheep.

Score after treatment	Score before treatment				
	1	2	3	4	Total
1	34	78	27	4	143
2	1	16	36	13	66
3	0	6	14	49	69
4	0	0	2	3	5
Total	35	100	79	69	283

Table 14.7 Measurement of plasma glucose concentrations (mmol/l).

	First reading	Second reading
Sample 1	3.665	3.751
Sample 2	4.297	4.297
Sample 3	3.639	3.545
Sample 4	3.146	3.171
Sample 5	3.331	3.342
Sample 6	3.060	3.026
Sample 7	3.089	3.129
Sample 8	3.299	3.193
Sample 9	2.983	2.992
Sample 10	2.761	2.813
Sample 11	2.975	2.881

ment has helped to alleviate the problem of foot rot?

14.10 When conducting any sort of assay measurement, it is common to put duplicate samples through the assay. In an assay of plasma glucose concentration (mmol/l) in sheep blood, the duplicate results, shown in Table 14.7, were used to assess the repeatability of the method. Conduct an appropriate analysis to assess the extent to which the results are repeatable.

15 Some specialized issues and procedures

15.1 Learning objectives

By the end of this chapter, you should be able to:

- Explain what ethical issues surround the use of animals in research.
- List the five 'freedoms' for animals in our care.
- Outline the three Russell and Burch approaches for limiting harm to animals in research.
- Describe the stages involved in preparing an application for animal research.
- Propound the contribution of spatial statistics to veterinary investigations.
- Outline the potential hazards in the use of spatial statistics.
- Outline the importance of veterinary surveillance in animal health monitoring and planning.
- Explain what is involved in veterinary surveillance.
- Elaborate the generally accepted understanding of molecular genetics.
- Briefly explain the basis of quantitative genetics.
- Outline the benefits of quantitative genetics.

15.2 Introduction

This chapter contains several apparently disparate topics in veterinary and animal science that are either relevant to the conduct of animal research, or have specialized data collection and display, or demand a range of newer statistical approaches. We have attempted to introduce the scientific basis for the statistical procedures without going into the details of the methods used since often these are beyond the scope of this book. In each case we give references so that you can, if desired, pursue these methods further.

15.3 Ethical and legal issues

15.3.1 Ethics and animal 'rights'

Ethics is essentially a branch of philosophy that investigates the moral value of human conduct and the rules and principles that ought to govern it. Often the terms morality and ethics are used indiscriminately but 'morality is concerned with what is right and what is wrong conduct whereas ethics is really concerned with why certain conduct is considered to be right or wrong' (Dolan, 1999).

Many argue that animals have rights but an alternative, and more ethically sustainable, position is that humans have duties and responsibilities towards animals in considering their use for man's benefit. Indeed, one of the more influential philosophers of our time, Peter Singer, has argued that animals do not need to be accorded rights; instead, he maintained that, to the extent that an animal can suffer pain, it should be given

Statistics for Veterinary and Animal Science, Third Edition. Aviva Petrie and Paul Watson.
© 2013 John Wiley & Sons, Ltd. Published 2013 by John Wiley & Sons, Ltd.

equivalent consideration to that of humans (Singer, 2005), although this is not a widely accepted view. Nonetheless, in discharging our responsibilities regarding animals, we should be clear about what this implies, both in legal and moral terms. The UK Farm Animal Welfare Council in 1979 defined explicitly, for animals in our care, the fundamental duty of protection we owed to animals used for human food production, summarized as the five freedoms:

- Freedom from thirst and hunger.
- Freedom from discomfort.
- Freedom from pain, injury and disease.
- Freedom from fear and distress.
- Freedom of normal behaviour by providing proper facilities and company.

These freedoms are now considered to be widely applicable to our diverse use of animals and provide a framework for the creation of an acceptable animal welfare system (see also Section 15.3.4).

When we think about the ethics of animal experimentation, our concern generally lies with the animals and their suffering. However, we should remember that animals, both domesticated and in the wild, have also benefited from human activity. Some of these benefits are:

- Shelter from the elements and protection from predators.
- Regular supply of food, usually of better quality than that which would be obtained in the wild.
- Superior strains produced by selective breeding providing resistance to disease or adverse climatic conditions.
- Improved health due to veterinary medicine.
- Preservation of species by laws of protection.

Clearly, the whole area of the ethics of animal investigation is fraught with controversy. There will always be those who completely oppose the use of animals in research whatever the potential benefits, and, on the other hand, those who believe these animals are essential for establishing important innovative procedures that benefit human or animal health and recreation. At the end of the day, we must strike a balance between the expected benefit to be accrued from the research and the likely suffering of the animal, i.e. we must give consideration to what might be termed the cost–benefit equation. We do this by ensuring that the principles of the three Rs (see Section 15.3.2) are upheld, all research on animals is carefully regulated (see Section 15.3.3) and that ethical dilemmas are given due consideration by indepth discussions by those on ethics committees (see Section 15.3.4). You can find a detailed discussion of the ethics of animal experimentation in Dolan (1999) and an overall guide to the legal obligations in the care of laboratory animals in Dolan (2000).

15.3.2 The three Rs

Wherever we contemplate experimental approaches using animals, issues of animal welfare and ethics are present. Even the seemingly innocuous question of a control group may present an ethical dilemma. For example, can we justify failing to treat a random selection of diseased animals in order to compare the effect of a treatment protocol? The answer we give will depend on the severity of the condition, the effectiveness of existing treatments and the degree of suffering involved. Perhaps, as we suggest in Section 5.5, it may be appropriate to compare a novel treatment with the best existing treatment, thereby offering the most effective available treatment to the control group. However, with a novel treatment it is possible that this treatment group itself is at risk, and we have every duty to ensure that the risk is minimal and assessed as far as it is in our power to do so.

In experimental situations, we have a moral duty (and in much of Europe and the USA, a legal duty) to apply the principles of the 'three Rs' (Box 15.1), originally proposed by Russell and Burch (1959). Specifically, we must demonstrate that we have considered:

- *Reduction* (minimizing the numbers of animals used, consistent with achieving the desired scientific objectives). Clearly, a real understanding of statistical methodology is at the heart of Reduction. The minimum number of animals

Box 15.1 The three Rs: a strategy for minimizing the use of animals in research (Russell and Burch, 1959).

- *Reduction*: minimizing the numbers of animals used, consistent with achieving the desired scientific objectives.
- *Refinement*: aiming to minimize pain, suffering or lasting harm to each individual animal.
- *Replacement*: involving, where appropriate, the use of lower organisms, tissue culture, or other cell culture techniques instead of conscious living vertebrates.

must be decided upon using stringent statistical procedures that involve power considerations (see Sections 6.4.2 and 13.3) and the use of efficient experimental designs as well as appropriate statistical analyses. This avoids both wasted trials owing to inadequate group sizes and using unnecessarily large numbers of animals.

- *Refinement* (aiming to minimize pain, suffering or lasting harm to each individual animal). Here we make use of sedation and anaesthesia, as appropriate, together with expert pain management by the use of analgesics; this may necessitate the presence of veterinarians in the research team.

- *Replacement* (could we use 'lower' organisms, tissue culture, etc., instead of conscious living vertebrates?). In this area, much has been achieved with the development of tissue culture techniques, although it should be recognized that this experimental setting can only reveal the response of isolated cells or tissues and not the integrated responses of the whole organism.

15.3.3 Legislation controlling animal investigation

(a) Historical note

Many have criticized the use of animals in experiments over the ages. Leonardo da Vinci (1452–1519), an alleged vegetarian, predicted that experimentation on animals would one day be judged as a crime. Dr Johnson, in the middle of the 18th century, wrote a number of articles on the plight of animals subjected to cruelty in the pursuit of medical knowledge, a concern which was emerging in English society at that time. In the late 18th century there was an official scrutiny of the treatment of animals, culminating in the licensing of slaughterhouses. Early in the 19th century, Martin's Act gave protection to some animals from cruelty and the RSPCA (Royal Society for the Prevention of Cruelty to Animals), a leading animal welfare charity, was formed in the UK. As the 19th century progressed, concern was voiced by many, including Disraeli, about the use of animals for research. Leading figures of the time, such as Darwin, Huxley and Jenner, signed a petition requesting legislative control of animal experimentation. Finally in 1876, the Cruelty to Animals Act was passed, limiting painful experiments on animals to take place only for specific purposes and under certain conditions, at the same time enforcing a licensing and inspection system for vivisection.

There have been many attempts to add more stringent controls in the UK since then but it was not until 1911 that the Protection of Animals Act was passed, and it was only in 1986 that the Animals (Scientific Procedures) Act (amended in 2012), regulating the use of laboratory animals in the UK, came into being. More recently, the Animal Welfare Act of 2006 outlawed the causing of 'unnecessary suffering' to animals, although specific exemptions apply to experiments licensed under the 1986 Act. This slow development of controls on animal use has also been witnessed in other countries and continents. For example, minimal restrictions on animal experimentation prevailed in the United States until 1966 when the first federal Laboratory Animal Welfare Act (now known as the Animal Welfare Act or AWA) was passed by Congress; this has been modified by various measures in 1970, 1976 and then again in 1985.

(b) Current allowable practices

In the UK, any invasive act of veterinary surgery, such as obtaining a blood sample or a tissue biopsy, is prohibited except when carried out for diagnostic purposes, and is limited to being performed under veterinary supervision, preventing exploitation of animals. Obtaining samples from healthy animals by a veterinary surgeon without causing any significant discomfort, pain, suffering, distress or lasting harm in order to support a diagnosis, or to provide information relating to animal husbandry or clinical management, is permissible, providing it is done with the informed consent of the owner. The main exceptions to this are under the Animals (Scientific Procedures) Act 1986, when particular biological scientists are licensed by the Home Office to perform specific procedures after completing adequate training. Even modifying the diet of an animal for experimental purposes is controlled under this Act and may not be carried out without a licence.

In fact, it is rather easier to obtain human volunteers for research than to assemble animals for a study. This is partly because the principle of informed consent is easier to apply, although the situation for animals is not dissimilar to the situation involving children too young to give their own informed consent, where the parent or guardian must give consent for a procedure to be performed.

15.3.4 Principles of animal welfare and ethics committees

In order to keep animal welfare in the forefront, we must devise protocols that minimize the inconvenience and discomfort to animals and provide safety for humans.

In medical establishments it is widely recognized that approval from an ethics committee is required to institute investigative studies carried out on human subjects. Similarly, studies of animals in the UK are subject to ethics committee approval. An ethics committee for animal investigations provides a forum for discussion about the concerns of animal welfare in relation to the proposed investigation on animals. Its particular format will vary according to the nature of the investigation and the institution at which the investigation will take place. An ethics committee often includes individuals from the administrative team of the institution, academics in the

field, social workers, clergy, academic ethicists and statisticians, as well as lay members of the public. The committee will meet at regular intervals and provide a serious appraisal of the cost–benefit equation, paying particular attention to the three Rs (see Section 15.3.2), and benefiting from the various views expressed in open discussion by its members. It serves to protect the rights of the animals whilst promoting the advancement of knowledge in a carefully controlled environment.

Under the Animals (Scientific Procedures) Act 1986, the experiments must be justified by the welfare benefit to the animal population at large or by the advantage to human medicine before they can be approved. Furthermore, welfare concerns must be addressed by reducing the numbers of animals used and by minimizing the discomfort to be applied (see Section 15.3.2). Furthermore, a veterinary surgeon is appointed to oversee the care of the experimental animals and must, if necessary on grounds of animal welfare, remove animals from the study.

15.4 Spatial statistics and geospatial information systems

15.4.1 What is spatial statistics?

We define **spatial statistics** as modifications, extensions and additions to statistical techniques that focus on the importance of locations or spatial arrangement. If data are spatially distributed, we give explicit consideration to the potential importance of their positional arrangement in the analysis. A **geographical** or **geospatial information system** (**GIS**) is a data handling system that merges statistical analysis, database technology and cartography. Its output includes the mapping of the data in a variety of meaningful ways to allow its geographical or locational context to be emphasized. It therefore enables us to capture, manage, manipulate, analyse and store location-referenced data.

The combination of spatial statistics and GIS allows us to handle the analysis of data involving two- or three-dimensional space, often linked with chronological data to consider time trends, and to present them in a readily comprehensible form. Thus it has applications in a wide variety of fields, not least any animal studies interested in locational information such as the geographical spread of disease, which is of fundamental interest in epidemiology. To deal with this, there are spatial versions of descriptive statistics, pattern analysis, regression analysis to assess relationships, and surface modelling for prediction.

Spatial autocorrelation occurs when there is a relationship between the values of a single variable that is due to the geographical areas in which these values occur; this implies that there is a dependency between the values of the variable in one location and in neighbouring areas. In other words, values from sites located closer together may have a greater similarity to one another than were they to be more widely separated. This dependency creates problems for statistical methods that make assumptions about the independence of residuals (a residual is the difference between an observed and a predicted value – see Section 10.4.3(b)), so particular statistical techniques should be employed. For example, a regression analysis that ignores spatial dependency may have biased parameter estimates and inappropriately low P-values, whereas a regression model that takes into account the possibility of spatial autocorrelation will not exhibit these flaws. Spatial autocorrelation analysis tests whether autocorrelation is present and, if it is, measures the degree of dependency and the nature of it among the observations in a geographic space. Such associations point to the influence of geography or location on the data which might otherwise appear random in nature when viewed by traditional statistics that ignore the spatial aspects.

15.4.2 Displaying the data

In the first steps in spatial analysis, we often need to display the data and then inspect them for any clues as to their meaning, for any errors and for possible models to test. With geographical data, for example, we might construct a map of the incidence of a disease and look for evidence of a non-random distribution, for example, clustering

or large-scale patterns. In Plate 15.1 we see evidence of the incidence of bovine tuberculosis increasing from a relatively restricted occurrence mainly in the southwest of England to a much more extensive coverage in the UK, even as far as Scotland, in a short 5-year period. The pattern suggests infection is by contact since it is seen in a non-random distribution developing mainly from the sites infected in 1997, but it may also imply the existence of persistent local reservoirs of infection.

As we hinted in Section 15.4.1, there are many situations where geographical aspects of data can add a further dimension to the data set and may provide us with clues to underlying patterns within the data. Such maps, apart from presenting useful information in a readily accessible format, can also provide indications as to the type of analysis that will be most instructive. It is particularly relevant in veterinary epidemiology where the spatiotemporal spread of contagious disease may help us identify particular causative conditions. Using the software available, it is relatively easy to create a map showing the locations of events recorded and then, using the power of GIS, to overlay this with, for example, topological features or vegetation cover or human population densities or road maps. This helps us to identify patterns of relationships between the data collected and other data features that may not otherwise be obvious.

15.4.3 Examples of spatial statistics in veterinary and animal science

We list in the bullet points that follow some of the applications of spatial statistics and GIS for veterinary and animal science, illustrating the sort of studies that benefit from these techniques.

- Bessell *et al.* (2010) used data collected in the 2001 foot-and-mouth disease (FMD) outbreak in Great Britain to study risk factors at farm level, and identified conditions that were associated with a high risk of transmitting FMD to other premises. This kind of work enabled the

Department for Environment, Food and Rural Affairs (Defra) in the UK to plan more targeted policies to combat the disease spread. Given that disease outbreaks are single discrete events often spatially and temporally distributed, spatial regression models using a Poisson distribution (see Section 3.4.3) are commonly employed to analyse disease outbreaks.

- Spatial autocorrelation was seen concerning Danish mink farms infected with plasmacytosis (Themudo *et al.*, 2011); the authors demonstrated the clustering of the disease persistently over a 10-year period in a particular region of Northern Jutland.
- Spatial statistics is used in studies of wild animal migration patterns, allowing us, for example, to identify repeating patterns year by year and their associations with climatic conditions (Clegg *et al.*, 2003; Holdo *et al.*, 2009). This is useful for wildlife land management, for monitoring sea fish stocks and for understanding how wildlife influences domestic animal disease control.
- Myers *et al.* (2008) used a topological overlay to study conditions leading to road deaths of elk and deer in Washington State, USA. The authors were able to show that deaths occurred in relation to traffic speed and density, but also were influenced by roadside ground cover and time of year (the latter relating to mating months and migration patterns).

15.4.4 What are the hazards of using these methods?

Spatial statistics is a fast-developing subject with a number of traps for the unwary. Some of the problems we may encounter are involved with the assumptions inherent in the statistical procedures being applied, while others are associated with inadvertent misunderstandings about the data. Potential sources of error are explained in the following bullet points.

- **Location.** Data are accorded specific point locations. In the case of animal data, this may be the registered address of the farm or the owner and not the actual location or the area where the animals in question are kept. In some cases, the latter may be some distance away from the registered address and may lead to inappropriate conclusions.
- **Sampling.** At the outset we need to consider data sampling. Given that an assumption of spatial statistics is that data may be influenced by location, we need to plan how many data are necessary to represent the evidence faithfully. Adjacent areas may be affected by local conditions which make them differ, so sampling must be frequent enough to represent such a local variation. We may need to employ sampling methods such as stratified or cluster sampling (see Chapter 13).
- **Clustering.** Data points may not be randomly distributed but clustered in small areas. If the sampling is not frequent enough nor ranges widely enough, this clustering may be missed and generalized conclusions may be inappropriately drawn from a small area displaying clustering. Unless we also take into account the distribution of the population density, we might be misled by concentrations of cases merely associated with clusters of the population.
- **Cartograms.** A way of emphasizing a particular non-random distribution is to show the incidence data in areas redrawn geometrically proportional in size to the item under consideration. Such maps or cartograms are said to have a demographic (isodemographic) base in contrast to those constructed according to the two-dimensional shape of the region, which have a geographic base. An example is shown in Plate 15.2. While such maps often have a dramatic impact, they have potential dangers similar to those that we saw with pictograms (see Section 2.5.1): in this instance we have difficulty in determining how to interpret the distortion of a particular area to assess its associated incidence data.
- **Length or distance.** This is a potential source of error depending on the units of measurement employed. Should we be interested in borders of an area (farm borders, town or county boundaries, etc.), the scale of the measurement unit used to determine the boundary can seriously distort the distance or area of interest. This is due, essentially, to the approximations

involved. For example, Mandelbrot (1967) showed that the measurement of the coastline of Great Britain could be seriously influenced by the units of distance used (Plate 15.3). In other circumstances, such as the distance between objects, it may be important to decide whether the straight line distance, 'as the crow flies', or, for example, the connecting road distance is the relevant data. Such details may have a profound effect on the conclusions to be drawn.

- **Modifiable areal unit problem (MAUP).** This gives rise to a potential source of error that can affect spatial studies which utilize aggregate data sources (Unwin, 1996). In practice it means that when data collected in relation to specific geographical point locations are amalgamated into areas for comparison, the choice of area boundaries can result in potentially misleading conclusions. The areas are not uniform in size and characteristics may be modified at whim. This is of particular importance to veterinary surveillance (see Section 15.5) since data are reported in relation to local areas delineated by, for example, a veterinary diagnostic laboratory, county or other area unit. Disease incidence in the UK is often reported in relation to county boundaries; the boundaries are arbitrary in relation to disease transmission and may be misleading in terms of the actual spread of the disease.
- **Ecological fallacy.** This occurs when we believe mistakenly that an association we observe between variables at the group or aggregate level (e.g. in a region) reflects the corresponding association at an individual level (e.g. individual animals in the region) in the same population. Such errors occur in part from spatial aggregation and the topic is closely related to the MAUP. Thus, when a piece of information in respect of a location is recorded (e.g. environmental temperature), the assumption is often made that all points in that locality share the same characteristics although this may be far from the truth. Tree cover, the proximity of buildings and other local features may all affect temperature or wind speeds or rainfall; care must be exercised in drawing conclusions.

15.4.5 Some useful references

This subject of spatial analysis is growing rapidly and there are a number of sources of information to further enhance knowledge. Freely available as a pdf on the internet at the time of publication of this book is a primer in spatial statistics by Câmera *et al.* (2008). A helpful introduction to the analysis of spatial data is to be found in a chapter by Pfeiffer (2009). Other suitable books include a veterinary primer by Pfeiffer *et al.* (2008) and a more advanced text by Ripley (2004). In addition, the veterinary literature now contains several good published reviews, such as those of Carpenter (2001) and Rinaldi *et al.* (2006).

15.4.6 Example

In a study by Chhetri *et al.* (2010), information about foot-and-mouth disease (FMD) outbreaks reported by Village Development Committees (VDCs) in 75 districts of Nepal was collected in order to quantify associations between hypothesized epidemiological factors and the spatial distribution of FMD. This study depended on the use of a spatial scan statistic to identify the spatial clustering of reports and a Bayesian mixed effects Poisson regression model to quantify the association between the number of reports and 25 potential risk factors. Plate 15.4a illustrates the three regional terrains, and Plate 15.4b shows the observed-to-expected ratios (O_i/E_i) of reported outbreaks as well as the numbers of VDCs per district. Two significant clusters of districts with a risk of VDC-reported cases of FMD higher than the background risk of the country were identified using the spatial scan statistic. One primary cluster located in the Kathmandu and Nuwakot districts (bold circle) had a relative risk (RR) of 7.6 of VDCs reporting FMD compared with the overall country background, and one secondary cluster located in the Mahottari and Saralahi districts (faint circle) had a RR = 2.7 (Plate 15.4b). Elevated risk was associated with large numbers of people, buffalo and animal health technicians.

15.5 Veterinary surveillance

15.5.1 What is veterinary surveillance?

According to the World Health Organization's International Health Regulations (WHO, 2005), '"surveillance" means the *systematic ongoing* collection, collation and analysis of data for public health purposes and the timely dissemination of public health information for assessment and public health response as necessary' [our italics]. This definition, of course, relates to the monitoring and control of human public health, and specifically involves information about disease outbreaks. The use of the term 'ongoing' in the definition enables us to distinguish surveillance from a survey, and by the inclusion of 'systematic' we imply that the data have a format that is predetermined by the collecting authority in response to the potential uses of the data set.

Veterinary surveillance (or animal disease surveillance) is thus the process of collecting information on animal diseases and infections in order to provide early indication of changing patterns of animal health which may affect productivity or pose a threat to human health. The main aim of veterinary surveillance is to inform decision-making for rapid and appropriate responses should disease patterns change.

15.5.2 Why is veterinary surveillance conducted?

A US government public health organization, the Centers for Disease Control and Prevention (www.CDC.gov, accessed 17 October 2012), has outlined the following purposes for disease surveillance, with particular reference to human diseases:

- To collect data to better understand the extent of health risk behaviours, preventive care practices and the burden of chronic diseases.
- To monitor the progress of prevention efforts.
- To help public health professionals and policy-makers make more timely and effective decisions.

Box 15.2   The purposes of veterinary surveillance

- To continuously collect data on agricultural, but also companion and wild, animal disease for the purpose of monitoring risks to animal enterprises and human health.
- To monitor animals and animal products in the human food supply chain that might pose a threat to the disease status of humans or animals.
- To monitor drug residues in animal products entering the human food chain.
- To collect reports of drug resistance to assess the threats to drug effectiveness.
- To inform governments and other agencies charged with responding to disease threats in order that appropriate, measured and targeted responses can be initiated in a timely manner.
- To analyse information to determine changes in risk that require targeted responses.

Veterinary surveillance, on the other hand, has a rather wider perspective in that we are concerned not only with the disease status of our food-producing animals, but also with wild and companion animal health since that may indicate transmissible infections or environmental toxicity that may affect humans (Box 15.2). We therefore obtain our information from a wide range of sources in order to encompass the potential hazards:

- Bacterial and viral diseases, prion diseases, poisonings and other welfare issues affecting agriculturally important species.
- Changes in animal husbandry practices that may affect disease incidence.
- Changes of animal movement controls that might allow new conditions to come to light, such as the introduction of an exotic disease or the emergence of a novel disease. (These controls are temporary UK government restrictions in place to limit animal movements, usually instituted in the light of a reported outbreak of a notifiable disease.)
- Pet disease – our pets live generally in close association with us, and their health can be an indicator of potential problems with contamination of the human food supply.
- Wildlife disease, which can be a sign of an infectious disease transmissible to agricultural

species, or evidence of toxic substances endangering farm animals and/or humans.

- Drug resistance, for example antibiotic resistance in bacteria.
- Drug residues in animal products – these are monitored to protect the human population against inadvertent exposure to drugs.
- The importation of meat products and live animals, which are monitored to identify potential sources of exotic diseases. For example, smuggling of 'bushmeat' (the meat of wild animals), often from West and Central Africa, is a growing concern to European governments because of the risk of inadvertent importation of African wild animal viruses which are known to have the potential to 'jump' species by mutation. A by-product of this monitoring is a contribution to the protection of endangered species.

Some surveillance is focused on a particular disease, e.g. bovine tuberculosis surveillance, and some surveillance is generic, e.g. general monitoring of patterns of disease outbreaks.

Veterinary disease surveillance has become an integral part of the strategies of the developed world to understand and control the spread of disease in animals and its transmission both within and beyond national borders. With the migration of people from one region to another caused by the promise of a better standard of living, as well as the mass movement of refugees under persecution, together with modern business and vacation travel, the risks of disease dissemination are vastly increased. For these reasons, data collection and monitoring of disease incidence together with its geographical locations, facilitated by the developments of computer recording of large bodies of information, have become a necessity. Veterinary disease surveillance covers all major animal diseases including zoonoses (any infectious diseases that can be transmitted naturally from animals, both wild and domestic, to humans) and hence public health issues; it impacts national and international trade in live animals and their products. It is generally conducted by governmental or national organizations, but requires input from animal owners, veterinarians and laboratory and animal scientists, aided by volunteer groups such as bird watchers and ramblers who may notice problems in wildlife or grazing farm animals.

15.5.3 How is veterinary surveillance conducted?

We commonly find veterinary epidemiologists at the centre of surveillance programmes, since their discipline is frequently based on disease surveillance on populations of animals. Obviously the collection of such a body of information would be of little use without the application of statistical methods to control and reduce the data to provide useful and accessible information. It is for this reason that we have included a section on surveillance in this book.

We gather surveillance data from reports emanating from veterinary diagnostic laboratories, post-mortems and clinical cases, and directly from veterinary surgeons and farmers. While the data are systematically collected, there is always a potential for bias. The value of the data is only as good as the quality of data provided; we must ensure that relevant data are collected, and that they are accurate and as complete as possible.

Much of the data collection, analysis and dissemination of the data are the responsibility of national government departments, such as, in England and Wales, the Department for Environment, Food and Rural Affairs (Defra); details can be explored on their website (http://archive.defra.gov.uk/foodfarm/farmanimal/diseases/vetsurveillance/, accessed 17 October 2012). In Scotland, the details are available from the Scottish government under the topic of veterinary surveillance at (www.scotland.gov.uk/Topics/farmingrural/Agriculture/animal-welfare/Diseases/, accessed 17 October 2012). Similar information pertaining to the USA is available through US Department of Agriculture (www.aphis.usda.gov/vs/nahss/, accessed 17 October 2012). In sophisticated data banks such as these, **performance indicators** are used to monitor the quality of the data. Performance indicators are specifically designed key measures of quality, sensitivity and quantity of a surveillance system: they evaluate whether the achievements of a national disease surveillance programme are fulfilling the purposes for which they were established.

15.5.4 How are veterinary surveillance data analysed?

We use mostly simple procedures to analyse surveillance information and this can be readily achieved, providing the facilities are in place to cope with a large amount of data. Usually, the routine analysis of veterinary surveillance data relies on presenting prevalence or incidence rates using graphs, histograms and maps. Of particular value is the illustration of these rates by the individual animal (or herd, farm or breed) and area or time, or both. Surveillance analysis has recourse to spatial statistics (see Section 15.4).

As an example, Plate 15.5 shows an indication of bovine tuberculosis-positive herds in the UK by county between July 2009 and June 2010 (the data are proportions of herds that had their official disease-free status withdrawn in the period). It demonstrates the use of GIS to display recorded data graphically and indicates the high prevalence, particularly in the southwest of England. There are, of course, many further variations on the use of descriptive statistics in this context. Although simple graphical illustrations are appealing and useful, more sophisticated statistical methods are also being used, such as time series analyses to model epidemics (Montgomery *et al.*, 2008) and small area analysis of clustering (Alexander and Boyle, 1996; Olsen *et al.*, 1996).

One of the important outcomes from surveillance data analyses is a risk estimate. Particular disease risk estimates can be used to identify hazards to surrounding flocks and herds or the human population, or may be used to rank priorities for resource allocation to control disease spread. For example, Yousey-Hindes *et al.* (2011) compared the risk to humans of a bite from foxes infected with raccoon variant rabies and rabid raccoons in New York State, and showed that rabid foxes were more likely than rabid raccoons to bite and that rabid grey foxes were more dangerous than rabid red foxes in this regard.

15.5.5 Uses of veterinary surveillance in the UK

The value of surveillance is dependent on a number of factors including the timing and validity of its output and the costs involved. It is generally considered to be essential to health management in agricultural animals. The following points provide some examples of the uses of veterinary surveillance in the UK.

- Good surveillance is imperative for the early detection of outbreaks of foot-and-mouth disease and for control measures to be implemented in a timely manner (e.g. Bessell *et al.*, 2010). Because outbreaks are infrequent (at the time of publication, the last major outbreak in the UK was in 2001, some 34 years after the previous one), practice is only refined slowly; nevertheless, models have now been developed to predict airborne dissemination based on Meteorological Office data about local weather patterns (Gloster *et al.*, 2005, 2010). This allows the targeting of inspections of premises around an early case to detect spreading of the condition. Other measures developed from surveillance data from earlier outbreaks include the extent of restricted movement zones and localized slaughter zones.
- The appearance of a new disease revealed by veterinary surveillance was bovine spongiform encephalopathy (BSE) (Wilesmith *et al.*, 1992). This disease is linked to variant Creutzfeldt–Jakob disease in humans, and caused a considerable scare when it was first described in the 1980s. Its progress throughout the UK was monitored and the management co-ordinated using surveillance information.
- The ongoing management of tuberculosis in cattle in the UK depends on accurate recording and standard procedures in the event of a positive skin test. The success of these procedures to limit the dissemination in the cattle population is monitored on an ongoing basis.
- The emergence of porcine respiratory and reproductive syndrome (PRRS) was first recognized through surveillance in North America in 1987 and in Europe in 1990. PRRS was considered by the Food and Agriculture

Organization in 2007 as the most economically important viral disease of intensive pig farms in Europe and North America. Similarly, another globally emergent epizootic disease of pigs, porcine post-weaning multisystemic wasting syndrome (PMWS) was first detected in UK in 1999.

- A cattle and sheep midge-borne disease, blue-tongue, has been found by surveillance to be spreading northwards in Europe since around the turn of the 21st century: it reached the UK in 2007.
- Veterinary surveillance is being used, at the time of writing, to monitor 'bleeding calf syndrome', also known as bovine neonatal pancytopenia (BNP), a newly emergent disease in calves. A link has recently been found between BNP and a now withdrawn vaccine, but this is not the only or main cause, which currently remains unknown.

15.5.6 Further reading in veterinary surveillance

There are few comprehensive books on veterinary surveillance at the time of writing but Brookmeyer and Stroup (2003), concerning surveillance with regard to human public health, explain many of the principles and methods that are also relevant to the veterinary field. The textbook by Sainsbury (1998) describes the factors having most implications for the health of animals kept for production purposes and covers much of the background to veterinary surveillance. For further reading, you might consult Dufour and Hendrikx (2009) or Salman (2003). In addition, good basic information, as well as data, can be found in the government websites listed in Section 15.5.3. The current practice of veterinary surveillance has been under review in Great Britain, and reports on the present state of coverage and desirable steps forward are available: see Animal Health and Veterinary Laboratories Agency (Defra), *The Surveillance Advisory Group Final Report April 2012* (http://vla.defra.gov.uk/ science/docs/sci_sag_final_report.pdf, accessed 17 October 2012) and *Review of Veterinary Surveillance: How information on animal disease is gath-ered, analysed and disseminated in Scotland. Final Report, November 2011* (www.scotland.gov. uk/Resource/Doc/362344/0122619.pdf, accessed 17 October 2012).

15.6 Molecular and quantitative genetics

15.6.1 Molecular genetics

In Mendelian terms a gene is a unit of inheritance, whereas in molecular terms it is a region of DNA (deoxyribonucleic acid) which is transcribed into mRNA (messenger ribonucleic acid) and this is then used to synthesize protein. **Molecular genetics** is concerned with studying the structure and functions of DNA at a molecular level. It employs the methods both of genetics and molecular biology to answer questions about the make-up of genes and the mechanism of gene replication, giving rise to an understanding of genetic mutations that can cause certain diseases, as well as discovering why traits (genetically determined phenotypes or characteristics of an organism) are passed on from one generation to another.

Modern molecular biology has generated a considerable armoury of research techniques to explore the genetic composition of an entire animal. The **genome** (the complete DNA of an organism) of each of several domestic animals has recently been established and other species are being added. New terms have been coined to encompass each of the functional stages of the cellular processes originating in the genome – **genomics** (the branch of molecular biology concerned with the structure, function, evolution and mapping of genomes), **transcriptomics** (an examination of the expression level of mRNA molecules in one or a population of cells), **proteomics** (the study of the proteome, the complete set of proteins expressed by an organism, tissue or cell) and **metabolomics** (the scientific study of chemical processes involving metabolites, small molecules produced or taking part in metabolism in a tissue or cell). Together with these developments is the ability to explore the activity of multiple genes simultaneously using array technology, which generates enormous data banks stored digitally for further exploration. With vast computing power so readily available, a new science, **bioinformatics** (the application of computer science and information technology to 'omic' information in the field of biology, agriculture and medicine), often referred to as **computational biology**, has grown up around these data banks to manage the exploration and harvesting of the information. These techniques, which are advancing steadily over time, are all employed in basic veterinary and animal science. In general, the statistical approaches build on the concepts introduced in this book – probability theory, distinguishing important changes from background variation, significance testing, regression analysis, Bayesian analyses, clustering procedures, maximum likelihood estimation, etc. For example, empirical DNA sequence analysis is often incomplete and contains errors; iterative procedures are used to find a match to the sequence in published data banks and to estimate the probability of the accuracy of the match. Algorithms to deal with iterative methodology and computer 'learning' from evidence within the data sets are frequently generated to answer new questions being asked.

For those who want to explore the statistics behind molecular genetics applications, we recommend Balding *et al.* (2007) and Laird and Lange (2011).

15.6.2 Quantitative genetics

It is generally accepted that both genetic and environmental factors give rise to continuous distributions of phenotypic characteristics, affecting the incidence of diseases or patterns of growth and carcass conformation. **Quantitative genetics** encompasses the scientific study and analysis of such phenomena, and refers to the study of genetic variation of complex traits (characteristics of an individual influenced by a multitude of genes and their interactions with the environment). Most often, quantitative genetic analysis is performed on traits showing a continuous range of values, such as live weight. However, traits displaying a discrete number of values (such as litter size) and even binary traits

(such as disease presence or absence) are all amenable to quantitative genetic analysis using maximum likelihood methods or Bayesian approaches (Xu *et al.*, 1998; Yi and Xu, 2000).

There is now an active branch of medicine concerned both with identifying diseases that appear to have a polygenic inheritance component, and with attempting to estimate the risks of those diseases in populations. Unlike the original genetic experiments of Gregor Mendel where the phenotype of certain characteristics of pea plants was either of one kind or another with no intermediate appearance, the traits studied by quantitative genetics are not controlled by a single gene with only two alleles, but are controlled by multiple genes. While each gene behaves according to Mendel's Laws, the sum of their actions, together with environmental influences, result in a full range of intermediate phenotypic appearances that behave as continuous variables with a Normal distribution in the population. The straightforward mathematical calculations based on discontinuous distributions of limited different types derived from Mendel's Laws no longer serve for the complexity of multiple gene interactions: instead, they are replaced by complicated statistical probability estimations.

Many common human diseases, such as Type II diabetes, fall into this category of having phenotypic appearances behaving as continuous variables. In veterinary medicine and in agriculture, as well as an interest in the genetics of disease susceptibility, we also explore the potential of these techniques to estimate the heritability of *desirable* traits such as growth rate, milk production and drought resistance, and carcass traits, like subcutaneous fat and lean meat percentage in pigs. Litter size or clutch size, which are characterized by discrete values, can also be considered since the influence of multiple genes can affect the likelihood of increased sizes. The probability of twinning in sheep and the susceptibility of developing a given disease are similarly amenable to quantitative genetics analysis. It is expected that new applications will be found in the future as more is understood of the inheritance of complex traits under the influence of multigene interactions both with one another and the environment.

While the details of the techniques used in quantitative genetic analysis are beyond the brief of an introductory statistical text, we should appreciate that it is a quantitative issue, and we use statistical analysis to look for markers that follow the phenotype characteristic in which we are interested. The methodology derives largely from concepts introduced in this book, such as the Normal distribution (see Section 3.5.3), correlation and simple regression (see Chapter 10) and more complex linear models (see Chapter 11) as well as the analysis of variance (see Sections 8.5 and 8.6), but takes them to a more advanced level.

Further information can be found in the texts by Falconer and McKay (1995) and Nicholas (2010). Quantitative genetics applications in veterinary science and animal breeding are explored in the book by Simm (2002). Saxton (2004) is a primer with good information on how to use SAS as a statistics package in this field. Sorensen and Gianola (2002) is a more advanced text designed for the biologist with some mathematical background, introducing more sophisticated methodology for the analysis of quantitative genetics data, but with sufficient detail for non-mathematicians to follow the derivation of the equations employed.

Exercises

The statements in questions 15.1–15.4 are either TRUE or FALSE.

15.1 An investigator using live animals has a duty:
(a) To focus on benefits of the new knowledge promised and not be diverted into consideration of possible harms to the animals.
(b) To leave all welfare aspects to the ethics committee.
(c) To minimize possible pain and suffering while still designing a meaningful experiment/trial.
(d) To focus exclusively on the welfare of the animals in the experiment.

(e) To design the experiment/trial to obtain the most information responsibly.

15.2 The benefit of spatial statistics in veterinary medicine and animal research is:
(a) To provide the only way to include data collected in different locations.
(b) To offer good spatial maps for output.
(c) To allow for the analysis of data pertaining to events in time.
(d) To aid our understanding of animal research in space and time.
(e) To explore the spatial aspects of data.

15.3 Veterinary surveillance is used:
(a) To check whether all animals coming into the country are free of disease.
(b) To monitor the spread of animal diseases important to the economy or public health.
(c) To audit the quality of veterinary practices.
(d) To control animal movements.
(e) To inspect slaughter houses before licensing.

15.4 Quantitative genetics:
(a) Is used to study traits that are determined by multiple genes and their interactions with the environment.
(b) Is concerned with studying the structure and function of genes at a molecular level.
(c) Builds on concepts of Mendelian genetics.
(d) Uses exclusively non-parametric analysis methods.
(e) Is the identification of the entire genome in a new species.

15.5 The distribution of Q fever (a zoonotic disease caused by *Coxiella burnetii*) was studied in the goat population throughout the Netherlands (Schimmer *et al.*, 2011). In the diagram (Plate 15.6), we show their observations regarding both serology and bulk milk testing of goats in the study.
(a) What conclusions can you draw about infection with Q fever from the distribution of the goat farms?
(b) What additional information is contained in the distribution of goat density?
(c) What hypotheses might you be able to test with this spatial information?

16 Evidence-based veterinary medicine

16.1 Learning objectives

By the end of this chapter, you should be able to:

- Explain the concept of evidence-based veterinary medicine.
- Describe the hierarchy of reliability of evidence and give reasons for the relative positions of types of evidence.
- List the stages involved in practising evidence-based veterinary medicine.
- Identify the aspects of a study design that avoid bias.
- From a report of a clinical trial, critically appraise the value of the evidence.
- Explain what is meant by the absolute risk reduction (ARR) and the relative risk reduction (RRR).
- Explain what is meant by the number needed to treat (NNT) and how to calculate the confidence interval for the NNT.
- Interpret the usefulness of the evidence in the clinical/professional setting.

16.2 Introduction

In our reflections in recent years on the application of statistics in the veterinary field, we have become aware that so-called **evidence-based veterinary medicine (EBVM)** is now a buzz-word throughout the veterinary profession. By this is meant the integration of the results of scientifically conducted studies into day-to-day clinical practice with the aim of improving clinical outcome. At first sight, this seems to be a statement of what veterinary practice has been all along. However, the real difference is that scientific 'literature' is now available to everyone who has access to the internet wherever s/he may be. Furthermore, a blueprint for the practice of EBVM, incorporating sound statistical principles in critical appraisal, has been formulated to make its processes more accessible to veterinary professionals. Like human medicine, veterinary science is developing an emphasis on the latest experimental evidence to guide clinical judgements. Moreover, for both performance and production in animals, there is also a growing awareness of the relevance of scientifically conducted studies to direct progress. We have gathered the consideration of these themes into this chapter to set the foregoing information in an effective context. We direct our thoughts particularly to the professional practitioner in all branches of animal or veterinary science. The following sections will give you a feel of what is encompassed by EBVM; for further exploration of these concepts we direct you to Cockcroft and Holmes (2003), Marr (2003) and Straus *et al*. (2011).

Statistics for Veterinary and Animal Science, Third Edition. Aviva Petrie and Paul Watson.
© 2013 John Wiley & Sons, Ltd. Published 2013 by John Wiley & Sons, Ltd.

Box 16.1 Evidence-based veterinary medicine: a definition

> The conscientious, explicit and judicious use of the best scientific evidence to inform clinical judgements with a view to improving clinical outcome at the level of the individual unit, i.e. animal or group of animals.

Useful websites include:

- www.cebm.net (accessed 24 October 2012).
- http://ktclearinghouse.ca/cebm (accessed 24 October 2012).
- www.vetmed.wsu.edu/courses-jmgay/EpiLinks.htm (accessed 24 October 2012).

16.3 What is evidence-based veterinary medicine?

We provide a formal definition of EBVM in Box 16.1: it is derived from the widely quoted definition for evidence-based medicine devised by Sackett (1996). EBVM implies the basing of clinical judgement not simply on clinical experience but also on the available relevant and valid scientific studies of the condition, its diagnosis and/or its treatment. In practice, this means the integration of individual clinical expertise, tempered by local knowledge and circumstances, with the best available external clinical evidence which is assessed in a methodological fashion using well-defined strategies. It involves a conscious choice to use this approach towards achieving best practice, it is conscientious in that it implies a scrupulous application, and it is explicit in that the practitioner is able to justify judiciously any clinical decisions made that rely on this external evidence.

Evidence comes with variable reliability so we are faced with the task of selecting and critically evaluating the best evidence. In human medicine, properly designed trials of sufficient size are readily organized, given the structure of health services around the world, and thus there is a large and growing body of good evidence on which to draw. In veterinary medicine, however, the most reliable types of evidence, systematic reviews or randomized controlled trials, are still quite rare so we must resort to less reliable, often

smaller, studies. We consider this in more detail in Section 16.5.2.

In veterinary practice, the outcome may have a wider definition than in human medicine, as we generally take into account economic issues as well as animal welfare; for example, our concern may be improved economic use of animal treatments and therefore better production efficiency. Cost–benefit analysis is clearly implicated at the level of the individual case in EBVM, more so than in human medicine. It involves addressing the client's values and providing reliable evidence on which informed decisions can be taken jointly.

16.4 Why has evidence-based veterinary medicine developed?

Following human medicine, veterinary medicine has now espoused the emphasis on scientific publications, in their widest sense, to guide clinical practice. Driven by the advent of the ready availability of electronic media for disseminating scientific observations, no longer can we, as practitioners, fall back on 'clinical opinion' as the sole guide to our practice. Today, more than ever before, we need to demonstrate that our decisions are based on current knowledge of the condition. This is not to say that 'clinical judgement' now has no place in clinical practice. Far from it: clinical judgement must use the best information to guide good practice. Decisions are to be *based on* the evidence, not *made by* the evidence.

This requires the development of a number of new skills for the veterinary and animal scientist in the 21st century. We cannot expect to carry in our heads all the knowledge needed for our practice; instead, we need to learn how to marshal the evidence available to us to guide our decision-making. Foremost amongst these skills is the ability to phrase the right questions to direct the search, and next, to search the databases, extract the relevant information efficiently, and then evaluate it appropriately. We, as practitioners, must recognize that in veterinary medicine, as in human medicine, the evidence-based approach is here to stay: it is increasingly becoming part of expectations in veterinary schools and in the profession at large.

Moreover, this activity is not limited to clinical veterinary practice, but also embraces animal science in its broader sense. The use of training regimens, feed supplements and nutritional additives, the relative values of husbandry practices, and the use of physiotherapy to aid recovery in equine subjects will all be influenced by this approach. Indeed, professional advisors, in whatever capacity, will be required to demonstrate that they are using the best available knowledge, not least in response to legal challenges when the legal profession will have at their disposal the same body of literature and information.

16.5 What is involved in practising evidence-based veterinary medicine?

Evidence-based veterinary medicine applies to several aspects of diagnosis, therapy, prognosis and prevention in clinical practice (Box 16.2). For example, a query may arise as to what is

Box 16.2 Clinical activities which are central to evidence-based veterinary medicine

- **Diagnosis**: this may involve the choice and interpretation of an appropriate diagnostic test, with an assessment of its reliability. Consideration of the possible causes of a disease, its likelihood and an evaluation of signs and symptoms will lead to a differential diagnosis about which clinical judgement, informed by the evidence, is exercised.
- **Treatment**: evidence relating to the efficacy of competing therapeutic regimens has to be evaluated with a view to offering the animal the therapy which will be of the greatest benefit, weighed against the potential harm inflicted and the costs involved. In contrast to human medicine, euthanasia will sometimes remain a potential course of action.
- **Prognosis**: consideration must be given to the likelihoods of the possible outcomes of the disease, the timing of these outcomes, and their effect on the animal, and its owner, in the presence and absence of treatment.
- **Prevention**: prophylactic measures, such as vaccination, may be taken after appraising the known risk factors associated with the disease, estimating the risk of the disease, and the efficacy, cost and side effects of the procedure.

Box 16.3 Evidence-based veterinary medicine: the process

1. Phrase the question(s).
2. Search available resources for all relevant information (i.e. the evidence).
3. Critically appraise the retrieved information for its validity and clinical applicability.
4. Make a clinical judgement by integrating the appraisal with clinical expertise and take action accordingly.
5. Review the process and evaluate its performance.

known of the relative importance of certain clinical signs in differential diagnosis, or what reliance can be placed on a particular diagnostic test. In the therapeutic area, which particular therapeutic approach has the best chance of success and the least chance of an adverse outcome? In prognosis, what is the likelihood of a successful outcome and at what cost, especially when, unlike in human medicine, the client has the option of euthanasia?

Broadly, the process can be broken down into five stages (Box 16.3) which are elaborated in Sections 16.5.1–16.5.5.

16.5.1 Phrasing the question

The first task is to ask the appropriate focused questions. In order to get clear answers and to avoid wasting time in searching, we must phrase appropriate questions that can be answered precisely, given the availability of the evidence. For example, what diagnostic tools are available and what is known about their reliability? In prognosis, what is the probability of a favourable outcome? Once questions have been phrased, specific answers can be sought from a variety of resources. Some guidelines for formulating appropriate questions are given on the Centre for Evidence-Based Medicine's web page (http://www.cebm.net/index.aspx?o=1036, accessed 24 October 2012). Here the use of the PICO structure is advocated, specifically:

- **P**: Patient or problem – what type of patients (animals) or problem do we have in mind? How would we describe a group of patients similar to ours?

- **I**: Intervention – what main treatment/intervention are we considering?
- **C**: Comparison – if necessary, what is the main alternative to compare with the intervention?
- **O**: Outcome – what can we hope to accomplish or what could this exposure really affect?

Once we have formed the question using the PICO structure, we can think about what type of question it is we are asking, and therefore what type of research (e.g. systematic review or randomized controlled trial) would provide the best answer. As an example, consider the following PICO questions that might be asked of a study to investigate the efficacy of a single oral dose of oxfendazole against *Fasciola hepatica* in naturally infected sheep (Gomez-Puerta *et al.*, 2012):

- Patient or problem: naturally infected sheep.
- Intervention: single oral dose of oxfendazole.
- Comparison: no treatment.
- Outcome: the number of eggs per gram of stools after 10 days.

Clearly a randomized controlled trial would be advocated in these circumstances. In fact, the authors found that in groups of 20 sheep, none of the treated group had *Fasciola* eggs in the faeces 10 days after treatment, while all the untreated (control) group had similar numbers of eggs as before. They concluded that a single dose of 30 mg/kg oxfendazole was highly effective.

16.5.2 Obtaining the information

Evidence comes with various degrees of reliability; in particular, in assessing the value of the evidence, we should remember to be extremely cautious about relying on the results contained in publications that have not been peer-reviewed. To select information on a scientific basis, we need to have in mind a hierarchy of value from the most helpful and reliable, to the least (see Table 16.1 for a summary).

The evidence of the greatest reliability is obtained from systematic reviews and meta-analyses (see Section 13.5) which rely on the combined evidence from available and valid studies to draw dependable conclusions. Next in the hierarchy we have experimental studies, generally clinical trials, which are randomized (to avoid assessment bias; see Section 5.6), controlled (so that there is an objective assessment of the treatment effect; see Section 5.5) and of sufficient size to give statistically sound results (see Section 13.3). Ideally these should be blinded trials (see Section 5.7) to control for subjective elements at the point of delivery or assessment and thus avoid bias. Smaller randomized controlled trials are less dependable because of lower statistical power yielding wide confidence intervals and greater doubt about the treatment effect. In clinical investigations, an experimental study which is relatively simple and easy but may be of limited value is one using historical controls (see Section 5.5.3); a novel treatment is applied to all new cases and the outcome compared with that of cases treated earlier by the more traditional approach. It lacks a contemporary control and is therefore less reliable and subject to bias.

There is still a considerable lack of dependable experimental studies of many aspects of veterinary clinical practice, but observational studies (see Section 5.2), provided they are properly structured to contain suitable controls, make a valuable contribution to the information base and form the next level of hierarchy. In terms of the strength of evidence, these are followed by case reports and then the views of an expert sought by referral; those with expertise in a particular field might be expected to have a superior knowledge of the specific subject and the published literature relating to it. With perhaps less reliability, we might consider the opinions of trusted colleagues; this allows for there to be a collective view derived from multiple experiences and reading. Lastly, there is the individual's own clinical expertise based on memories and impressions of past experience. While the latter used to be the sole basis of clinical judgement, no longer is it as useful because of the rate at which advances are being made in the veterinary field.

Today, personal access to the worldwide literature is available over the internet to the vast majority, accessed via search engines and databases, and generally downloadable free of charge or for a small fee. Devising the correct search

Table 16.1 Hierarchy of evidence.

Hierarchy of evidence	General description	Methodology	Description
Strongest	Overview	*Systematic review and meta-analysis*	*Systematic review*: a literature review focused on a single question that tries to identify, appraise, select and synthesize all high-quality research evidence relevant to that question *Meta-analysis*: a systematic review that uses quantitative methods to synthesize and summarize the results (see Section 13.5)
	Experimental study	*Randomized controlled trial*	Animals are randomly allocated into one or more experimental groups or a control group and followed over time for the variables/outcomes of interest (see Sections 5.3–5.9)
	Observational study	*Cohort study*	Groups (cohorts) of animals are selected on the basis of their exposure to a particular factor and followed prospectively to see if they incur a specific outcome (e.g. disease) (see Section 5.2.3(a))
		Case–control study	Animals that have the outcome of interest (cases) and those that do not have the same outcome (controls) are identified, and a retrospective analysis performed to see if there are differences between the groups in their exposure(s) of interest (see Section 5.2.3(b))
		Cross-sectional survey	A defined population is observed at a single point in time or time interval. Exposure and outcome are determined simultaneously
	Observation	*Case series and case report*	A report based on a single animal; sometimes collected together into a short series but there are no controls
	Opinion	*Expert opinion*	A view or consensus of views from one or more persons with a high degree of skill in or knowledge of the relevant subject
Weakest		*Anecdotal*	Based on casual observations or indications rather than rigorous or scientific analysis

terms and structuring the search is now a well-developed art; helpful restriction tools exist in some of the search websites to focus our search – for example in PubMed (www.ncbi.nlm.nih.gov/pubmed, accessed 24 October 2012), which provides free access to MEDLINE, a database of indexed citations and abstracts to medical, nursing, dental, veterinary, healthcare and pre-clinical sciences journal articles.

16.5.3 Evaluating the information: the role of statistics

Having located the body of knowledge on our subject, we must set about evaluating the retrieved information. It is in this part that an *understanding of statistics*, its terms and its procedures, is essential. We need to have a sound grasp of the principles of **design** and **analysis**, as applied in both experimental and observational studies, in order to be able to critically appraise the methods used and assess whether the information provided is valid and applicable to our problem. This book provides the background that is required to pursue this aspect of EBVM.

The information in the following bullet points provides a brief summary of the steps involved in appraising the information.

- We need to know that the study has been designed in such a way so as to avoid **bias** (see Section 5.4). In an experimental situation investigating a new therapy, this means that the study should incorporate a control, randomization and blinding (see Sections 5.6 and 5.7). For the evaluation of a diagnostic test, there should be an independent, blind comparison with a reference ('gold') standard of diagnosis (see Section 14.2).
- In order to further assess **validity**, we should check that the appropriate statistical procedures have been applied in the correct manner, and determine whether the subjects were sufficient in number and of a wide enough range to render the results of the study useful and generalizable to the population of interest. For a prognostic problem, we should ensure that the follow-up time for all animals was sufficiently long and complete.
- We have to **extract the most useful results**, in particular, those that relate to the primary aim(s) of the study. In clinical trials and epidemiological studies, these results should be expressed as estimated **effects of interest** (e.g. difference in means, difference in risks, odds ratio, relative risk, hazard ratio) with associated estimates of precision or, preferably, confidence intervals. If a confidence interval is wide, this will indicate poor precision and an unreliable estimate. For a diagnostic test (see Section 14.2), we need the **sensitivity** and **specificity** of the test (describing the performance of the test) and the **likelihood ratios** which can be calculated from them, as well as the **positive** and **negative predictive values** of the test (indicating the chances that the animal does or does not have the disease, given the test result). In

prognostic studies, the **median survival times**, **survival curves** and/or the **probabilities of survival to a particular time** may be of interest (see Section 14.6). In all situations, confidence intervals, where appropriate, should be provided.

- We must decide whether the results are **important clinically**. We can often achieve this by studying the **confidence intervals** of the outcomes of interest. For example, in a comparative study, we might ask: 'if the observed effect is equal to either the upper limit or the lower limit of the confidence interval, would the result be considered clinically important?' Another approach is to determine the **number of animals needed to treat** (**NNT**) with the novel treatment to prevent one adverse outcome: this is equal to the inverse of the **absolute risk reduction** (**ARR**; the difference in the risks of the adverse outcome between the control and treated groups – see Section 5.2.3). Sometimes it is also helpful to determine the **relative risk reduction** (**RRR**; the percentage reduction in risk of the adverse outcome in the treated group compared with the control group, i.e. it is the ARR divided by the risk in the control group). Bear in mind, though, that we can only put a relative risk (RR), RRR or ARR in context if we know the underlying risk in each group – a large relative risk may be clinically unimportant if the actual risk of the disease outcome is low. Appendix Table B.1 provides formulae for the confidence intervals for the ARR, RR and NNT, and an example that derives values for these indices is given at the end of this subsection. The **post-test probability** of disease is particularly useful when assessing the clinical usefulness of a diagnostic test. This is calculated from the pre-test probability (often simply an estimated prevalence of the disease in the population under investigation) and the likelihood ratio, and is closely allied to the positive and negative predictive values of the test (see Section 14.2).

Example of ARR, RRR and NNT

Bacterial overgrowth and translocation from the gut lumen to extraintestinal sites is a cause of concern after massive gut resection in human cancer patients. In order to assess whether the administration of *Bifidobacterium lactis* (BL), a probiotic bacterium, reduces the incidence of bacterial translocation in adult Wistar rats fed orally after 80% gut resection, Eizaguirre *et al.* (2002) found that the incidence of bacterial translocation in the RES group (those rats having 80% resection only) was 87% (34 of 39) whereas it was only 50% (nine of 18) in the RES-PRO rats (those with the same resection and daily administration of 7.8×10^8 colony-forming units BL). In these data, the relative risk (see Section 5.2.3(a)) of bacterial translocation is 0.57 (95% CI 0.36 to 0.92) so that the risk of bacterial translocation is reduced by 100% − 57% = 43% if a rat is treated with the probiotic; i.e. this is the relative risk reduction (RRR). The difference in the two incidences of bacterial translocation is the absolute risk reduction (ARR), equal to 37% (95% CI 11.8% to 62.5%; see point 6 of Section 9.4.3(c)). The results indicate that treatment with the probiotic significantly improves the incidence of bacterial translocation ($P = 0.006$ from Fisher's exact test). The number needed to treat (NNT) is the reciprocal of the ARR when the latter is expressed as a probability, i.e. NNT is $1/(0.37) = 2.7$. When this is rounded up, the NNT = 3. This implies that only three rats need to be treated with the probiotic after gut resection instead of just having resection in order for one of them to be free of bacterial translocation. The 95% confidence interval for the NNT is obtained by finding the reciprocal of the limits of the 95% confidence interval for the ARR, i.e. it is $1/(0.625) = 1.6$ to $8.5 = 1/(0.118)$. The study demonstrates the distinct advantage of the probiotic regimen following gut resection in controlling the bacterial translocation.

16.5.4 Applying the results and making a clinical judgement

In order to use the critically appraised external evidence in clinical practice, we should ensure that the results are applicable to the animal(s) in our care. Then we need to come to a clinical judgement, bringing to bear local and/or individual knowledge of the particular case in ques-

tion. Here the clinicians, with their particular experience of the background, can integrate the scientific understanding derived from the EBVM process, the local setting (e.g. prevalence of the disease condition locally) and the client's own values in order to arrive at a suitable course of action.

16.5.5 Reviewing the process

Lastly, there is a further stage – that of reflection on the process and its outcome to refine the skills. Have I conducted the EBVM process effectively and has it influenced my decision-making process for the better? In what areas do I need to improve? Have I learnt from the experience?

16.6 Integrating evidence-based veterinary medicine into clinical practice

It has been suggested that the introduction of the evidence base is causing as big a change in clinical practice as the Enlightenment. Whether that is an overstatement or not, it is sufficient to make the point that big changes in the practice of clinical medicine are afoot. The veterinary profession is being swept along by this change, and cannot stand against it. In the veterinary schools, EBVM is being taught as the best mode of practice, and more and more publications are providing the evidence base on which it is built.

16.7 Example

Box 16.4 contains an abstract adapted from a paper reporting the results of a randomized controlled trial to evaluate the clinical efficacy of pimobendan compared with ramipril in dogs with mild to moderate heart failure (HF) (Smith *et al.*, 2005). We use it in the process of demonstrating an EBVM approach (with particular emphasis on assessing the statistical information highlighted in Section 16.5.3) to establishing the

Box 16.4   Abstract showing the important aspects of the design, conduct and reporting of a clinical trial

- **Objectives**: to evaluate the clinical efficacy of pimobendan by comparing it with ramipril over a 6-month period in dogs with mild to moderate heart failure (HF) caused by myxomatous mitral valve disease (MMVD).
- **Methods**: this was a prospective, randomized, single-blind, parallel-group trial. Client-owned dogs ($n = 43$) with mild to moderate HF caused by MMVD were randomly assigned to one of two groups for 6 months of treatment: 22 dogs received 0.3 mg/kg pimobendan every 12 hours orally and 21 dogs received 0.125 mg/kg ramipril every 24 hours orally. The main outcome measure studied was adverse HF outcome, defined as failure to complete the trial as a direct consequence of HF.
- **Results**: treatment with pimobendan was well tolerated compared to treatment with ramipril. The characteristics of the two groups were similar at baseline in terms of the dogs' echocardiogram features, echocardiographic measurements, laboratory data and most clinical features but there was some evidence that pimobendan dogs may have had more advanced disease as the two groups exhibited substantial differences in mobility and demeanor scores at baseline. Four (18.2%) of the pimobendan dogs suffered an adverse HF outcome compared to 10 (47.6%) of the ramipril dogs (RR = 0.38; 95% CI 0.14 to 1.03; $P = 0.08$). The NNT was 4 (95% CI 1.8 to 37.3).
- **Clinical significance**: because dogs treated with ramipril may have had more advanced disease at baseline, these results should be interpreted cautiously but a low RR of 0.38 and NNT of 4 suggests that pimobendan warrants further investigation.

Adapted from Smith *et al.*, 2005, with permission from Wiley-Blackwell.

adverse HF outcome in each group is estimated and evaluated for significance: the RR is put into context since the estimated risk, as well as actual numbers with adverse effects, in each group is also provided. The NNT is determined. The statistical methods are appropriate although, since the pimobendan group had more advanced disease, it would be better to adjust for this in the analysis using a multivariable logistic regression approach (see Section 11.4).

- *Effect of interest*: this is the estimated relative risk, RR = 0.38 so the RRR = 1 − 0.38 = 0.62, i.e., the risk of an adverse HF outcome was reduced by 62% if the dog received pimobendan ($P = 0.08$).
- *Clinical importance*: the estimated 95% confidence interval for the RR is from 0.14 to 1.03. This is a wide confidence interval indicating poor precision and suggesting that the results may not be clinically important. The upper limit of the 95% confidence interval is 1.03, just exceeding 1 which is reflected by $P = 0.08$, a non-significant result. The NNT = 1/(0.476 − 0.182) = 3.4 implies that four dogs should be treated with pimobendan to prevent one of them suffering an adverse HF outcome. In view of these findings, and the fact that dogs treated with pimobendan may have had more advanced disease, it is correct to indicate that these results should be interpreted cautiously.

value of the novel treatment, pimobendan. In particular:

- *Bias*: the study was randomized to avoid allocation bias and blinded to avoid assessment bias.
- *Validity*: the authors checked that the two groups were comparable at baseline with respect to factors likely to influence response. Important factors were comparable apart from an indication that pimobendan dogs had more advanced disease. The relative risk (RR) of an

Exercises

The statements in questions 16.1 and 16.2 are either TRUE or FALSE.

16.1
(a) EBVM uses only published literature as evidence.
(b) EBVM is intended to protect veterinary professionals against litigation following errors of judgement.
(c) Randomized controlled experimental studies provide more reliable evidence than observational studies.
(d) EBVM is what has been practised all along.

(e) EBVM enables veterinary practitioners to draw on the best and most reliable evidence to guide their decision-making.

16.2 The number needed to treat (NNT) is:

(a) The number of animals treated with the novel treatment in an experimental study.

(b) The total number of animals on the novel and control treatment in an experimental study.

(c) The number of animals needed to be treated with the novel treatment compared with the control treatment to prevent one adverse outcome occurring.

(d) Equal to the inverse of the absolute risk reduction.

(e) Equal to the ratio of the risks of the outcome of interest in the treated and control groups.

16.3 Choose the most appropriate answer. If I am a veterinary practitioner, EBVM is intended to:

(a) Make sure I read the veterinary literature every week.

(b) Make me more aware of the literature available to improve my professional practice.

(c) Enable me to justify my clinical decisions based on the best possible information available.

(d) Enable me to apply the global clinical experience relevant to my case to my clinical decision-making.

(e) Share the responsibility for decision-making.

16.4 Which one of the following is *not* a component of a PICO question?

(a) *P*-value to determine significance of the finding.

(b) Intervention under consideration.

(c) Comparative intervention, if relevant.

(d) Outcome(s) of interest.

16.5 Which one of the following statements is *not* one of the steps of EBVM?

(a) Producing a clinically focused question.

(b) Searching available resources for the relevant information.

(c) Designing a clinical trial to answer a clinical question.

(d) Appraising the retrieved information for its validity and clinical judgement.

(e) Reviewing the process and evaluating its performance.

16.6 Read the following abstract with a view to evaluating the statistical information.

This investigator-blinded randomized controlled trial was designed to determine whether tacrolimus ointment (Protopic, Fujisawa Healthcare) decreased the severity of localized lesions of canine atopic dermatitis (AD). Twenty dogs with AD were enrolled if they exhibited lesions on both front metacarpi. Each foot was randomized to be treated with 0.1% tacrolimus or placebo (Vaseline) ointment twice daily for 6 weeks. Before, and every 2 weeks during the study, erythema, lichenification, oozing and excoriations each were graded on a 10-point scale (maximal total score: 40). The primary outcome measures were the percentage reduction from baseline of lesional scores and the number of subjects whose scores had decreased by 50% or greater at study end. Intention-to-treat analyses were used. At study onset, lesional scores were not significantly different between sites treated with tacrolimus or placebo. After 6 weeks, the percentage reduction from baseline scores was higher for tacrolimus-treated sites (median: 63%; 95% confidence interval: 39–67) than for placebo-treated feet (median: 3%; confidence interval: -2–13) (Wilcoxon test; $P = 0.0003$). When tacrolimus was applied, lesions decreased by 50% or greater in 15/20 dogs (75%); these dogs were those that completed the study. In contrast, this benchmark was not reached for any placebo-treated feet (Fisher's test; $P < 0.0001$). Adverse drug events consisted of minor irritation in some lesional areas treated with tacrolimus. Results of this trial suggest that the application of 0.1% tacrolimus ointment is useful for reducing the severity of localized skin lesions of canine AD.

From Bensignor and Olivry, 2005, reproduced with permission from Wiley-Blackwell.

(a) What attempts were made to eliminate bias?

(b) What statistical tests were employed and were they suitable?

(c) What do the *P*-values indicate?

(d) What is the main effect of interest?

(e) What can be understood from the confidence intervals of the responses?

(f) Do you agree with the conclusion?

17 Reporting guidelines

17.1 Learning objectives

By the end of this chapter, you should be able to:

- Expound the importance of reporting guidelines in veterinary research.
- Explain the function of the EQUATOR network.
- Describe the function of the CONSORT guidelines.
- Describe the aims of the REFLECT guidelines.
- Explain the benefit of the REFLECT guidelines.
- Describe the purpose of the ARRIVE guidelines.
- Explain in what circumstances you use the STARD, STROBE and PRISMA guidelines.

17.2 Introduction to reporting guidelines (EQUATOR network)

17.2.1 Introduction

The Declaration of Helsinki was developed in June, 1964, at the 18th World Medical Association (WMA) General Assembly, Helsinki, Finland. It was written as a statement of ethical principles for medical research involving human subjects but is relevant, then and now, to animal research.

The ethical principles of the Declaration of Helsinki included the following statement:

Authors, editors and publishers all have ethical obligations with regard to the publication of the results of research. Authors have a duty to make publicly available the results of their research on human subjects and are accountable for the completeness and accuracy of their reports. They should adhere to accepted guidelines for ethical reporting. Negative and inconclusive as well as positive results should be published or otherwise made publicly available. Sources of funding, institutional affiliations and conflicts of interest should be declared in the publication. Reports of research not in accordance with the principles of this Declaration should not be accepted for publication.

This serves at a starting point for scientists to ensure that they report their work in an accurate and open manner in such a way that it is, as far as possible, reproducible and verifiable.

If research is not reported in full or if the reporting is inadequate, it is difficult or impossible to assess the strengths and weaknesses of the research and thereby draw proper conclusions about the validity of the findings. To avoid this pitfall, it is essential that researchers have standardized and comprehensive guidelines of reporting to follow. The guidelines are not necessarily absolutely prescriptive but they can guide authors preparing manuscripts for publication, and those involved in peer review for quality assurance, to ensure completeness and transparency. They are also helpful for study planners and are a valuable aid to promoting good practice.

Statistics for Veterinary and Animal Science, Third Edition. Aviva Petrie and Paul Watson.
© 2013 John Wiley & Sons, Ltd. Published 2013 by John Wiley & Sons, Ltd.

If you are less familiar with writing scientific English, you may find the European Association of Science Editors (EASE) 2012 guidelines (*EASE Guidelines for Authors and Translators of Scientific Articles to be published in English*, available from www.ease.org.uk/publications/author-guidelines, accessed 24 October 2012) helpful in ensuring that your scientific communication is efficient. They provide simple advice that promotes the writing of complete, clear and concise scientific papers. For example, the guidelines include expressions that can be simplified or deleted, distinguishes between British and American spelling, and gives guidance on grammatical form and how to make acknowledgements and cite references.

17.2.2 EQUATOR Network

The EQUATOR Network (**E**nhancing the **QUA**lity and **T**ransparency **O**f health **R**esearch, www.equator-network.org, accessed 24 October 2012) is an international initiative that seeks to improve the reliability and value of medical research literature by promoting transparent and accurate reporting of research studies. The EQUATOR Network convened initially in Oxford, UK, in 2006. Its 27 participants from 10 countries, including journal editors, peer reviewers, researchers and funders, met with a view to providing standardized reporting guidelines that would facilitate a clear, comprehensive and transparent description of the procedures involved and the results obtained from a research study. It should be noted that these guidelines were not written as tools for assessing the methodological quality of a study. For the latter, we refer you to Whiting *et al.* (2003), a paper devoted to quality assessment in reported research.

A number of reporting guidelines (e.g. for randomized controlled trials, observational studies, diagnostic tests and systematic reviews and meta-analysis) fall under the auspices of the EQUATOR Network and many medical journals have embraced their recommendations. The veterinary journals are somewhat slower to adopt the same or similar guidelines but progress is being made in this field (More, 2010). To this end,

the REFLECT statement, a modification of the CONSORT statement for randomized controlled trials (RCTs) on human subjects, was drawn up in 2008 to provide reporting guidelines for livestock trials with production, health and food-safety outcomes. In addition, the ARRIVE guidelines are aimed specifically at research using laboratory animals. There is also some reporting guidance (as distinct from formalized guidelines) for animal studies on certain topics, such as systematic reviews, animal stroke modelling and prognostic studies in veterinary oncology. References with full details may be obtained at www.equator-network.org/resource-centre/library-of-health-research-reporting/reporting-guidelines-in-other-research-fields/ (accessed 24 October 2012).

Although at the time of writing, REFLECT and ARRIVE are the only formalized guidelines aimed specifically at animal research, we also present in this chapter the guidelines written for research on human subjects, as these guidelines are easily adapted for analogous research on animals. In particular, we present the following guidelines:

- REFLECT (a modification of CONSORT, for reporting of RCTs on humans, applicable to the reporting of livestock trials with production, health and food-safety outcomes).
- ARRIVE (research using laboratory animals).
- STARD (diagnostic accuracy studies).
- STROBE (observational studies in epidemiology).
- PRISMA (systematic reviews and meta-analysis) which replaced QUOROM.

The guidelines usually include the following:

- **A checklist**: this follows the format of an academic paper, namely, a title, abstract, introduction, methods, results, discussion and, finally, other information relating to funding and conflicts of interest. Each of these topics comprises a section in the checklist and these sections are divided into a number of subsections (items) indicating what should be included and how to report the information relevant to them.

- A **flow diagram**: this provides information about the flow of participants (or samples) through the study, with an indication of the numbers and information about when, why and how many participants were excluded or lost to follow-up during the course of the investigation.
- An **Explanation and Elaboration** document: this enhances the use, understanding and dissemination of the checklist by providing the meaning and rationale for each checklist item.

These guidelines are constantly evolving since they are subject to periodic updating as new evidence emerges. We present, in the sections which follow, the versions of the statements and flow charts that were current when this book went to print. We also provide website addresses so that it is possible to obtain the most up-to-date versions when required.

17.3 REFLECT statement (livestock and food safety RCTs)

17.3.1 CONSORT and its history

The first of the reporting guidelines, CONSORT (**CON**solidated **S**tandards **O**f **R**eporting **T**rials) was produced in 1998, after a merger in 1996 of proposals put forward by two independent groups of experts who met in Canada and the USA in 1993. It has since been updated (www.consort-statement.org (accessed 24 October 2012) and, for example, Schulz *et al.*, 2010). The CONSORT statement encompasses various initiatives to alleviate the problems arising from inadequate reporting of RCTs on humans. Its intention is to enable readers to understand the design, conduct, analysis and interpretation of the RCT and to assess its validity. Its checklist comprises what are believed to be the essential 25 items for assessing the reliability and relevance of the findings. Its flowchart (Figure 17.1) shows the passage

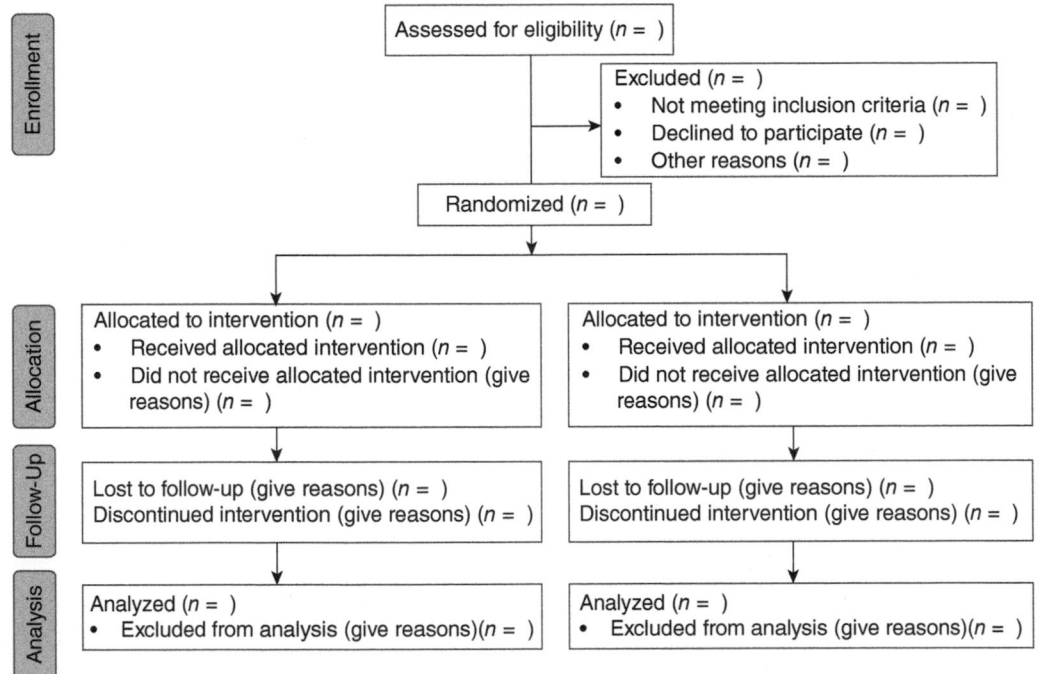

Figure 17.1   CONSORT flow diagram (the REFLECT guidelines for reporting randomized controlled trials in livestock and food safety are a modification of the CONSORT guidelines for reporting randomized controlled trials in humans; the CONSORT flow diagram may be used as a surrogate for REFLECT) (from Schultz *et al.*, 2010, reproduced with permission, under the terms of the Creative Commons Attribution License).

of participants through the four stages of a parallel group RCT, namely, enrolment, intervention allocation, follow-up and analysis. The diagram explicitly indicates the number of participants included in the primary data analysis in each intervention group. Inclusion of these numbers allows the reader to judge whether or not the authors have performed an intention-to-treat analysis (see Section 5.9.5).

17.3.2 REFLECT statement

In 2008, the CONSORT statement was adapted for animal research to produce the REFLECT Statement (**R**eporting guid**E**lines **F**or randomized contro**L**led trials for liv**E**sto**C**k and food safe**T**y: www.reflect-statement.org/ (accessed 24 October 2012) and O'Connor *et al.*, 2010), an evidence-based minimum set of items for reporting livestock trials with production, health and food-safety outcomes. It focuses on field trials and challenge studies with either therapeutic or preventive interventions. The REFLECT statement consists of a 22-item checklist (Table 17.1: bold print indicates modifications of the CONSORT statement on which is it based). Figure 17.1 shows the flow diagram for the CONSORT guidelines, which can be used with the REFLECT statement.

17.4 ARRIVE guidelines (research using laboratory animals)

17.4.1 Background

The **N**ational **C**entre for the **R**eplacement, **R**efinement and **R**eduction of Animals in Research (NC3Rs: www.nc3rs.org.uk, accessed 24 October 2012), established by the UK Government, is an independent scientific organization, and the largest funder of 3Rs research in the UK. In 2009, the NC3Rs carried out a systematic and detailed survey to assess the quality of reporting, experimental design and statistical analysis of published research using laboratory animals (Kilkenny *et al.*, 2009). The results demonstrated that many publications reporting publicly funded animal research

from the UK and USA lacked key information on how the study was designed, conducted and analysed, which could have limited their value in informing future scientific studies and policy. In particular, they showed that the hypothesis or objective of the study, the number of animals used, and characteristics of the animals (i.e. species/ strain, sex, and age/weight) were all included in only 59% of 271 randomly chosen articles. Furthermore, bias in animal selection and outcome assessment may well have been present in most of the papers as 87% of them did not report using randomization and 86% did not report blinding. The statistical methods used were only fully and properly described in 70% of the publications and 4% of the articles did not report the number of animals used anywhere in the methods or the results sections.

17.4.2 ARRIVE guidelines

In view of the findings summarized in Section 17.4.1, the NC3Rs produced the ARRIVE guidelines (**A**nimal **R**esearch: **R**eporting of *In Vivo* **E**xperiments: www.nc3rs.org.uk/ARRIVE (accessed 24 October 2012) and Kilkenny *et al.*, 2010) with the intention of improving the reporting of research using laboratory animals. Developed in consultation with the scientific community, including scientists, statisticians, journal editors and research funders, the guidelines consist of a 20-point checklist (Table 17.2), based on CONSORT, of the essential information that should be included in publications reporting animal research. ARRIVE has been endorsed by a number of leading scientific journals, along with the major funders of animal research in the UK.

17.5 STROBE statement (observational studies)

Observational research comprises several study designs and many topic areas. The STROBE statement (**ST**rengthening and **R**eporting of **OB**servational studies in **E**pidemiology: www.strobe-statement.org (accessed 24 October 2012) and, for example, von Elm *et al.*, 2008) provides guidelines for reporting cohort, case–control and cross-sectional studies, the three main analytical designs that are used in observational research. Checklists are available for the three study designs separately and for all three together (Table 17.3). The STROBE checklist is best used in conjunction with the Explanation and Elaboration article (freely available at, for example, www.plosmedicine.org (accessed 24 October 2012) where there are links to relevant papers, for example, Vandenbroucke *et al.*, 2007). The recommendations offered by STROBE are not intended to be prescriptions for designing or conducting studies, but they provide useful guidance in these areas. Its relevance to veterinary studies was reviewed by Boden and Parkin (2008).

17.6 STARD statement (diagnostic accuracy)

Diagnostic accuracy describes the extent to which a diagnostic test is able to differentiate between patients who do and do not have the disease outcome of interest (see Section 14.2). The STARD (**STA**ndards for the **R**eporting of **D**iagnostic accuracy studies: www.stard-statement.org, accessed 24 October 2012) guidelines were created in 2003 (Bossuyt *et al.*, 2003) with a view to improving the accuracy and completeness of reporting of studies of diagnostic accuracy. Using the guidelines should facilitate the assessment of both the internal (potential for bias) and external validity (generalizability) of the diagnostic study.

The STARD statement (Table 17.4) consists of a checklist of 25 items, similar to those of the CONSORT statement. The flow diagram (Figure 17.2) provides information about the method of recruitment of patients or samples, the order of test execution and the number of patients undergoing the diagnostic test under evaluation and the reference test to which it is compared.

17.7 PRISMA statement (systematic reviews and meta-analysis)

A systematic review uses systematic and explicit methods to identify, select and critically appraise research relevant to a clearly formulated question. Statistical methods (meta-analysis) may or may not be used to integrate and summarize the results of the included studies (see Section 13.5).

The aim of the PRISMA statement (**P**referred **R**eporting **I**tems for **S**ystematic reviews and **M**eta **A**nalysis: www.prisma-statement.org, accessed 24 October 2012) is to help authors report systematic reviews and meta-analyses to assess the benefits and harms of a healthcare intervention. It focuses on RCTs but can also be used as a basis for reporting other types of systematic reviews. It provides an updated and expanded version of the QUOROM statement (**QU**ality **O**f **R**eports **O**f **M**eta-analyses of randomised controlled trials) (Moher *et al.*, 1999) which it now supersedes.

The PRISMA statement consists of a 27-item checklist (Table 17.5) which has adopted the definitions of systematic review and meta-analysis used by the Cochrane Collaboration (see Section 13.5.1 and www.cochrane.org, accessed 24 October 2012). The statement and the flow diagram (Figure 17.3) are intended to be accompanied by the PRISMA Explanation and Elaboration document (Liberati *et al.*, 2009), freely available in, for example, the *British Medical Journal* (2009, vol. 339: b2700, doi: 10.1136/bmj. b2700).

Table 17.1 The REFLECT statement. For an Explanation and Elaboration of the REFLECT statement see also Sargeant *et al.* (2010) (from O'Connor *et al.*, 2010, reproduced with permission of the authors, under the Creative Commons Attribution License).

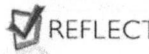 REFLECT **Checklist for REFLECT statement: Reporting guidelines for randomized controlled trials in livestock and food safety**. Bold text are modifications from the CONSORT statement description (Altman DG *et al.* Ann Intern Med 2001; 134(8):663–694).

Paper section and topic	Item	Descriptor of REFLECT statement item	Reported on Page #
TITLE AND ABSTRACT	1	How **study units** were allocated to interventions (e.g., 'random allocation,' 'randomized,' or 'randomly assigned'). **Clearly state whether the outcome was the result of natural exposure or was the result of a deliberate agent challenge.**	
INTRODUCTION Background	2	Scientific background and explanation of rationale.	
METHODS Participants	3	Eligibility criteria **for owner/managers and study units at each level of the organizational structure**, and the settings and locations where the data were collected.	
Interventions	4	Precise details of the interventions intended for each group, **the level at which the intervention was allocated**, and how and when interventions were actually administered.	
	4b	**Precise details of the agent and the challenge model, if a challenge study design was used.**	
Objectives	5	Specific objectives and hypotheses. **Clearly state primary and secondary objectives (if applicable).**	
Outcomes	6	Clearly defined primary and secondary outcome measures and the levels at which they were measured, and, when applicable, any methods used to enhance the quality of measurements (e.g., multiple observations, training of assessors).	
Sample size	7	How sample size was determined and, when applicable, explanation of any interim analyses and stopping rules. **Sample-size considerations should include sample-size determinations at each level of the organizational structure and the assumptions used to account for any non-independence among groups or individuals within a group.**	
Randomization-Sequence generation	8	Method used to generate the random allocation sequence **at the relevant level of the organizational structure**, including details of any restrictions (e.g., blocking, stratification).	
Randomization-Allocation concealment	9	Method used to implement the random allocation sequence **at the relevant level of the organizational structure**, (e.g., numbered containers ~~or central telephone~~), clarifying whether the sequence was concealed until interventions were assigned.	

Continued

Table 17.1 *Continued*

Paper section and topic	Item	Descriptor of REFLECT statement item	Reported on Page #
Randomization-Implementation	10	Who generated the allocation sequence, who enrolled **study units,** and who assigned **study units** to their groups **at the relevant level of the organizational structure**.	
Blinding (masking)	11	Whether or not ~~participants~~ those administering the interventions, **caregivers** and those assessing the outcomes were blinded to group assignment. If done, how the success of blinding was evaluated. **Provide justification for not using blinding if it was not used.**	
Statistical methods	12	Statistical methods used to compare groups for all outcome(s); Clearly state the level of statistical analysis **and methods used to account for the organizational structure, where applicable;** methods for additional analyses, such as subgroup analyses and adjusted analyses.	
RESULTS **Study flow**	13	Flow **of study units** through each stage **for each level of the organization structure of the study** (a diagram is strongly recommended). Specifically, for each group, report the numbers of **study units** randomly assigned, receiving intended treatment, completing the study protocol, and analyzed for the primary outcome. Describe protocol deviations from study as planned, together with reasons.	
Recruitment	14	Dates defining the periods of recruitment and follow-up.	
Baseline data	15	Baseline demographic and clinical characteristics of each group, **explicitly providing information for each relevant level of the organizational structure. Data should be reported in such a way that secondary analysis, such as risk assessment, is possible.**	
Numbers analyzed	16	Number **of study units** (denominator) in each group included in each analysis and whether the analysis was by 'intention-to-treat.' State the results in absolute numbers when feasible (e.g., 10/20, not 50%).	
Outcomes and estimation	17	For each primary and secondary outcome, a summary of results for each group, **accounting for each relevant level of the organizational structure**, and the estimated effect size and its precision (e.g., 95% confidence interval).	
Ancillary analyses	18	Address multiplicity by reporting any other analyses performed, including subgroup analyses and adjusted analyses, indicating those pre-specified and those exploratory.	
Adverse events	19	All important adverse events or side effects in each intervention group.	
DISCUSSION **Interpretation**	20	Interpretation of the results, taking into account study hypotheses, sources of potential bias or imprecision, and the dangers associated with multiplicity of analyses and outcomes. **Where relevant, a discussion of herd immunity should be included. If applicable, a discussion of the relevance of the disease challenge should be included.**	
Generalizability	21	Generalizability (external validity) of the trial findings.	
Overall evidence	22	General interpretation of the results in the context of current evidence.	

Table 17.2 The ARRIVE guidelines – a checklist of items that should be included in reporting of research using laboratory animals (from Kilkenny *et al.*, 2010, reproduced with permission under the terms of the Creative Commons Attribution License).

	Item	Recommendation
TITLE	1	Provide as accurate and concise a description of the content of the article as possible
ABSTRACT	2	Provide an accurate summary of the background, research objectives (including details of the species or strain of animal used), key methods, principal findings and conclusions of the study
INTRODUCTION		
Background	3	a. Include sufficient scientific background (including relevant references to previous work) to understand the motivation and context for the study, and explain the experimental approach and rationale b. Explain how and why the animal species and model being used can address the scientific objectives and, where appropriate, the study's relevance to human biology
Objectives	4	Clearly describe the primary and any secondary objectives of the study, or specific hypotheses being tested
METHODS		
Ethical statement	5	Indicate the nature of the ethical review permissions, relevant licences (e.g. Animal [Scientific Procedures] Act 1986), and national or institutional guidelines for the care and use of animals, that cover the research
Study design	6	For each experiment, give brief details of the study design, including: a. The number of experimental and control groups b. Any steps taken to minimize the effects of subjective bias when allocating animals to treatment (e.g. randomization procedure) and when assessing results (e.g. if done, describe who was blinded and when) c. The experimental unit (e.g. a single animal, group, or cage of animals). A time-line diagram or flow chart can be useful to illustrate how complex study designs were carried out
Experimental procedures	7	For each experiment and each experimental group, including controls, provide precise details of all procedures carried out. For example: a. How (e.g. drug formulation and dose, site and route of administration, anaesthesia and analgesia used [including monitoring], surgical procedure, method of euthanasia). Provide details of any specialist equipment used, including supplier(s) b. When (e.g. time of day) c. Where (e.g. home cage, laboratory, water maze) d. Why (e.g. rationale for choice of specific anaesthetic, route of administration, drug dose used)
Experimental animals	8	a. Provide details of the animals used, including species, strain, sex, developmental stage (e.g. mean or median age plus age range) and weight (e.g. mean or median weight plus weight range) b. Provide further relevant information such as the source of animals, international strain nomenclature, genetic modification status (e.g. knock-out or transgenic), genotype, health/immune status, drug- or test-naïve, previous procedures, etc.
Housing and husbandry	9	Provide details of: a. Housing (e.g. type of facility, e.g. specific pathogen-free (SPF); type of cage or housing; bedding material; number of cage companions; tank shape and material, etc. for fish) b. Husbandry conditions (e.g. breeding programme, light/dark cycle, temperature, quality of water, etc. for fish, type of food, access to food and water, environmental enrichment) c. Welfare-related assessments and interventions that were carried out before, during or after the experiment

Continued

Table 17.2 *Continued*

	Item	Recommendation
Sample size	10	a. Specify the total number of animals used in each experiment and the number of animals in each experimental group b. Explain how the number of animals was decided. Provide details of any sample size calculation used c. Indicate the number of independent replications of each experiment, if relevant
Allocating animals to experimental groups	11	a. Give full details of how animals were allocated to experimental groups, including randomization or matching if done b. Describe the order in which the animals in the different experimental groups were treated and assessed
Experimental outcomes	12	Clearly define the primary and secondary experimental outcomes assessed (e.g. cell death, molecular markers, behavioural changes)
Statistical methods	13	a. Provide details of the statistical methods used for each analysis b. Specify the unit of analysis for each dataset (e.g. single animal, group of animals, single neuron) c. Describe any methods used to assess whether the data met the assumptions of the statistical approach
RESULTS		
Baseline data	14	For each experimental group, report relevant characteristics and health status of animals (e.g. weight, microbiological status, and drug- or test-naïve) before treatment or testing (this information can often be tabulated)
Numbers analysed	15	a. Report the number of animals in each group included in each analysis. Report absolute numbers (e.g. 10/20, not 50%) b. If any animals or data were not included in the analysis, explain why
Outcomes and estimation	16	Report the results for each analysis carried out, with a measure of precision (e.g. standard error or confidence interval)
Adverse events	17	a. Give details of all important adverse events in each experimental group b. Describe any modifications to the experimental protocols made to reduce adverse events
DISCUSSION		
Interpretation/ scientific implications	18	a. Interpret the results, taking into account the study objectives and hypotheses, current theory and other relevant studies in the literature b. Comment on the study limitations including any potential sources of bias, any limitations of the animal model and the imprecision associated with the results c. Describe any implications of your experimental methods or findings for the replacement, refinement or reduction (the 3Rs) of the use of animals in research
Generalisability/ translation	19	Comment on whether, and how, the findings of this study are likely to translate to other species or systems, including any relevance to human biology
Funding	20	List all funding sources (including grant number) and the role of the funder(s) in the study

Table 17.3 The STROBE statement – checklist of items that should be included in reporting of observational studies (from von Elm *et al.*, 2008, reproduced with permission, under the terms of the Creative Commons Attribution License).

	Item no.	Recommendation
TITLE AND ABSTRACT	1	(*a*) Indicate the study's design with a commonly used term in the title or the abstract
		(*b*) Provide in the abstract an informative and balanced summary of what was done and what was found
INTRODUCTION		
Background/ rationale	2	Explain the scientific background and rationale for the investigation being reported
Objectives	3	State specific objectives, including any pre-specified hypotheses
METHODS		
Study design	4	Present key elements of study design early in the paper
Setting	5	Describe the setting, locations and relevant dates, including periods of recruitment, exposure, follow-up and data collection
Participants	6	(*a*) *Cohort study* – Give the eligibility criteria, and the sources and methods of selection of participants. Describe methods of follow-up *Case–control study* – Give the eligibility criteria, and the sources and methods of case ascertainment and control selection. Give the rationale for the choice of cases and controls *Cross-sectional study* – Give the eligibility criteria, and the sources and methods of selection of participants
		(*b*) *Cohort study* – For matched studies, give matching criteria and number of exposed and unexposed *Case–control study* – For matched studies, give matching criteria and the number of controls per case
Variables	7	Clearly define all outcomes, exposures, predictors, potential confounders and effect modifiers. Give diagnostic criteria, if applicable
Data sources/ measurement	8*	For each variable of interest, give sources of data and details of methods of assessment (measurement). Describe comparability of assessment methods if there is more than one group
Bias	9	Describe any efforts to address potential sources of bias
Study size	10	Explain how the study size was arrived at
Quantitative variables	11	Explain how quantitative variables were handled in the analyses. If applicable, describe which groupings were chosen and why
Statistical methods	12	(*a*) Describe all statistical methods, including those used to control for confounding
		(*b*) Describe any methods used to examine subgroups and interactions
		(*c*) Explain how missing data were addressed
		(*d*) *Cohort study* – If applicable, explain how loss to follow-up was addressed *Case–control study* – If applicable, explain how matching of cases and controls was addressed *Cross-sectional study* – If applicable, describe analytical methods taking account of sampling strategy
		(*e*) Describe any sensitivity analyses

Continued

Table 17.3   *Continued*

	Item no.	Recommendation
RESULTS		
Participants	13*	(a) Report numbers of individuals at each stage of study, e.g. numbers potentially eligible, examined for eligibility, confirmed eligible, included in the study, completing follow-up, and analysed
		(b) Give reasons for non-participation at each stage
		(c) Consider use of a flow diagram
Descriptive data	14*	(a) Give characteristics of study participants (e.g. demographic, clinical, social) and information on exposures and potential confounders
		(b) Indicate number of participants with missing data for each variable of interest
		(c) *Cohort study* – Summarize follow-up time (e.g. average and total amount)
Outcome data	15*	*Cohort study* – Report numbers of outcome events or summary measures over time
		Case–control study – Report numbers in each exposure category, or summary measures of exposure
		Cross-sectional study – Report numbers of outcome events or summary measures
Main results	16	(*a*) Give unadjusted estimates and, if applicable, confounder-adjusted estimates and their precision (e.g. 95% confidence interval). Make clear which confounders were adjusted for and why they were included
		(*b*) Report category boundaries when continuous variables were categorized
		(*c*) If relevant, consider translating estimates of relative risk into absolute risk for a meaningful time period
Other analyses	17	Report other analyses done, e.g. analyses of subgroups and interactions, and sensitivity analyses
DISCUSSION		
Key results	18	Summarize key results with reference to study objectives
Limitations	19	Discuss limitations of the study, taking into account sources of potential bias or imprecision. Discuss both direction and magnitude of any potential bias
Interpretation	20	Give a cautious overall interpretation of results considering objectives, limitations, multiplicity of analyses, results from similar studies and other relevant evidence
Generalizability	21	Discuss the generalizability (external validity) of the study results
OTHER INFORMATION		
Funding	22	Give the source of funding and the role of the funders for the present study and, if applicable, for the original study on which the present article is based

*Give information separately for cases and controls in case–control studies and, if applicable, for exposed and unexposed groups in cohort and cross-sectional studies.

Note: An Explanation and Elaboration article discusses each checklist item and gives methodological background and published examples of transparent reporting. The STROBE checklist is best used in conjunction with this article (freely available on the websites of *PLoS Medicine* at http://www.plosmedicine.org/, *Annals of Internal Medicine* at http://www.annals.org/, and *Epidemiology* at http://www.epidem.com/ (all accessed 24 October 2012)).

Table 17.4 The STARD checklist for reporting of studies of diagnostic accuracy (version January 2003) (from Bossuyt *et al.*, 2003a, reproduced with permission from BMJ Publishing Group Ltd). (See also http://www.stard-statement.org/, accessed 24 October 2012.)

Section and Topic	Item		On page
TITLE/ABSTRACT/ KEYWORDS	1	Identify the article as a study of diagnostic accuracy (recommend MeSH heading 'sensitivity and specificity')	
INTRODUCTION	2	State the research questions or study aims, such as estimating diagnostic accuracy or comparing accuracy between tests or across participant groups	
METHODS			
Participants	3	Describe the study population: The inclusion and exclusion criteria, setting and locations where data were collected	
	4	Describe participant recruitment: Was recruitment based on presenting symptoms, results from previous tests, or the fact that the participants had received the index tests or the reference standard?	
	5	Describe participant sampling: Was the study population a consecutive series of participants defined by the selection criteria in items 3 and 4? If not, specify how participants were further selected	
	6	Describe data collection: Was data collection planned before the index test and reference standard were performed (prospective study) or after (retrospective study)?	
Test methods	7	Describe the reference standard and its rationale	
	8	Describe technical specifications of material and methods involved including how and when measurements were taken, and/or cite references for index tests and reference standard	
	9	Describe definition of and rationale for the units, cut-offs and/or categories of the results of the index tests and the reference standard	
	10	Describe the number, training and expertise of the persons executing and reading the index tests and the reference standard	
	11	Describe whether or not the readers of the index tests and reference standard were blind (masked) to the results of the other test and describe any other clinical information available to the readers	
Statistical methods	12	Describe methods for calculating or comparing measures of diagnostic accuracy, and the statistical methods used to quantify uncertainty (e.g. 95% confidence intervals)	
	13	Describe methods for calculating test reproducibility, if done	

Continued

Table 17.4 *Continued*

Section and Topic	Item		On page
RESULTS			
Participants	14	Report when study was performed, including beginning and end dates of recruitment	
	15	Report clinical and demographic characteristics of the study population (at least information on age, gender, spectrum of presenting symptoms)	
	16	Report the number of participants satisfying the criteria for inclusion who did or did not undergo the index tests and/or the reference standard; describe why participants failed to undergo either test (a flow diagram is strongly recommended)	
Test results	17	Report time interval between the index tests and the reference standard, and any treatment administered in between	
	18	Report distribution of severity of disease (define criteria) in those with the target condition; other diagnoses in participants without the target condition	
	19	Report a cross-tabulation of the results of the index tests (including indeterminate and missing results) by the results of the reference standard; for continuous results, the distribution of the test results by the results of the reference standard	
	20	Report any adverse events from performing the index tests or the reference standard	
Estimates	21	Report estimates of diagnostic accuracy and measures of statistical uncertainty (e.g. 95% confidence intervals)	
	22	Report how indeterminate results, missing data and outliers of the index tests were handled	
	23	Report estimates of variability of diagnostic accuracy between subgroups of participants, readers or centres, if done	
	24	Report estimates of test reproducibility, if done	
DISCUSSION	25	Discuss the clinical applicability of the study findings	

Note: an Explanation and Elaboration article may be found at Bossuyt *et al.* (2003b) *Clin Chem* **49**: 7–18.

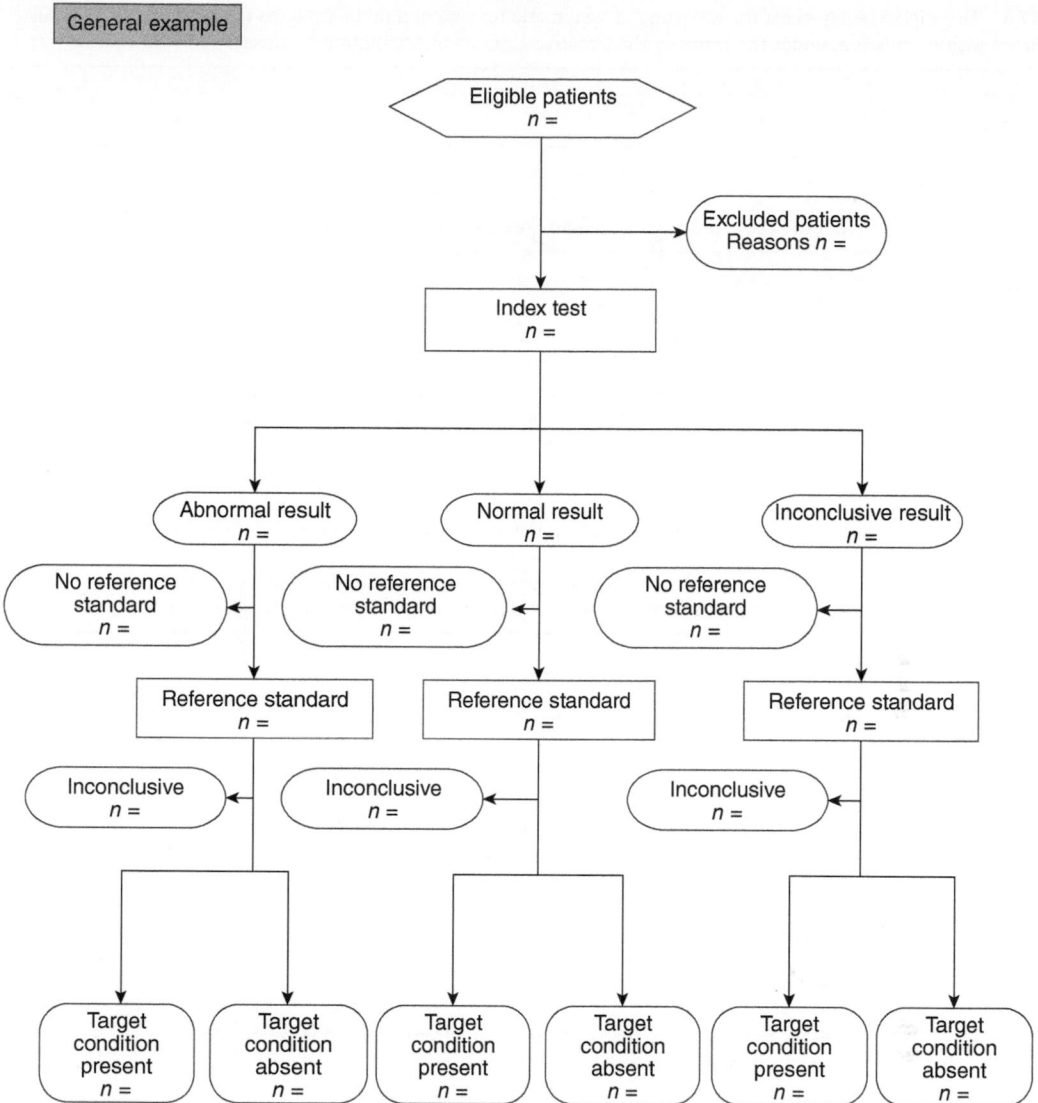

Figure 17.2 STARD flow diagram for reporting tests of diagnostic accuracy (from Bossuyt *et al.*, 2003a, reproduced with permission from BMJ Publishing Group Ltd).

Table 17.5 The PRISMA checklist for reporting of systematic reviews and meta-analyses (from Moher *et al.*, 2009, reproduced with permission, under the terms of the Creative Commons Attribution License).

Section/topic	#	Checklist item	Reported on page #
TITLE			
Title	1	Identify the report as a systematic review, meta-analysis, or both	
ABSTRACT			
Structured summary	2	Provide a structured summary including, as applicable: background; objectives; data sources; study eligibility criteria, participants, and interventions; study appraisal and synthesis methods; results; limitations; conclusions and implications of key findings; systematic review registration number	
INTRODUCTION			
Rationale	3	Describe the rationale for the review in the context of what is already known	
Objectives	4	Provide an explicit statement of questions being addressed with reference to participants, interventions, comparisons, outcomes, and study design (PICOS)	
METHODS			
Protocol and registration	5	Indicate if a review protocol exists, if and where it can be accessed (e.g. web address), and, if available, provide registration information including registration number	
Eligibility criteria	6	Specify study characteristics (e.g. PICOS, length of follow-up) and report characteristics (e.g. years considered, language, publication status) used as criteria for eligibility, giving rationale	
Information sources	7	Describe all information sources (e.g. databases with dates of coverage, contact with study authors to identify additional studies) in the search and date last searched	
Search	8	Present full electronic search strategy for at least one database, including any limits used, such that it could be repeated	
Study selection	9	State the process for selecting studies (i.e. screening, eligibility, included in systematic review, and, if applicable, included in the meta-analysis)	
Data collection process	10	Describe method of data extraction from reports (e.g. piloted forms, independently, in duplicate) and any processes for obtaining and confirming data from investigators	
Data items	11	List and define all variables for which data were sought (e.g. PICOS, funding sources) and any assumptions and simplifications made	
Risk of bias in individual studies	12	Describe methods used for assessing risk of bias of individual studies (including specification of whether this was done at the study or outcome level), and how this information is to be used in any data synthesis	
Summary measures	13	State the principal summary measures (e.g. risk ratio, difference in means)	

Table 17.5 *Continued*

Section/topic	#	Checklist item	Reported on page #
Synthesis of results	14	Describe the methods of handling data and combining results of studies, if done, including measures of consistency (e.g. I^2) for each meta-analysis	
Risk of bias across studies	15	Specify any assessment of risk of bias that may affect the cumulative evidence (e.g. publication bias, selective reporting within studies)	
Additional analyses	16	Describe methods of additional analyses (e.g. sensitivity or subgroup analyses, meta-regression), if done, indicating which were pre-specified	
RESULTS			
Study selection	17	Give numbers of studies screened, assessed for eligibility, and included in the review, with reasons for exclusions at each stage, ideally with a flow diagram	
Study characteristics	18	For each study, present characteristics for which data were extracted (e.g. study size, PICOS, follow-up period) and provide the citations	
Risk of bias within studies	19	Present data on risk of bias of each study and, if available, any outcome level assessment (see Item 12)	
Results of individual studies	20	For all outcomes considered (benefits or harms), present, for each study: (a) simple summary data for each intervention group, (b) effect estimates and confidence intervals, ideally with a forest plot	
Synthesis of results	21	Present the main results of the review. If meta-analyses are done, include for each, confidence intervals and measures of consistency	
Risk of bias across studies	22	Present results of any assessment of risk of bias across studies (see Item 15)	
Additional analysis	23	Give results of additional analyses, if done (e.g. sensitivity or subgroup analyses, meta-regression; see Item 16)	
DISCUSSION			
Summary of evidence	24	Summarize the main findings including the strength of evidence for each main outcome; consider their relevance to key groups (e.g. healthcare providers, users, and policy-makers)	
Limitations	25	Discuss limitations at study and outcome level (e.g. risk of bias), and at review level (e.g. incomplete retrieval of identified research, reporting bias)	
Conclusions	26	Provide a general interpretation of the results in the context of other evidence, and implications for future research	
FUNDING			
Funding	27	Describe sources of funding for the systematic review and other support (e.g. supply of data); role of funders for the systematic review	

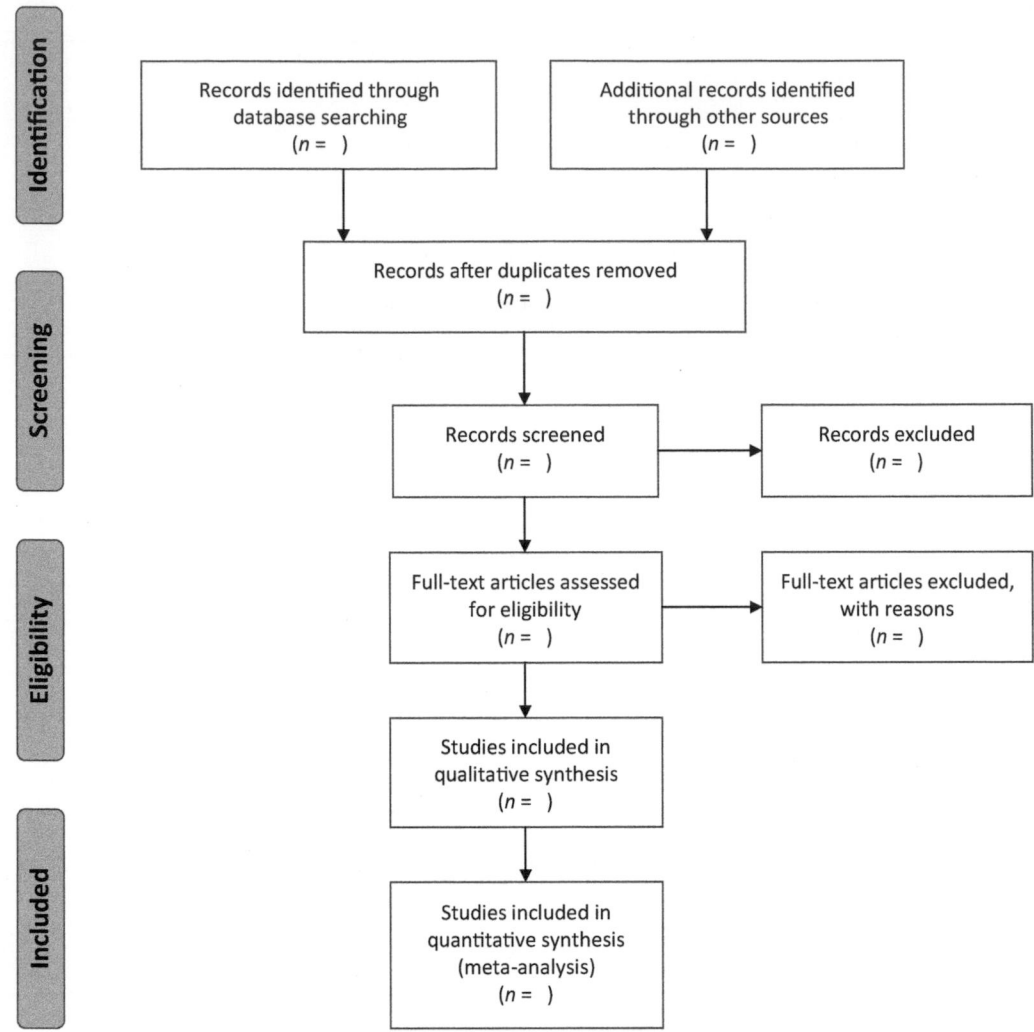

Figure 17.3 PRISMA flow diagram for reporting systematic reviews and meta-analyses (from Moher *et al.*, 2009, reproduced with permission, under the terms of the Creative Commons Attribution License).

18 Critical appraisal of reported studies

18.1 Learning objectives

By the end of this chapter you should be able to critically appraise a paper describing a randomized controlled trial or observational study. This means that when you have read the paper, to evaluate it you should be able to:

- Decide whether the title adequately describes the design and purpose of the study.
- Assess whether the rationale is explained.
- Evaluate whether the primary aim has been stated in relation to the outcome of interest and whether secondary objectives have been identified.
- Determine if the numbers of animals used are clearly specified.
- Decide whether all the methods are clearly described.
- Establish if the design is fully described and whether any steps have been taken to avoid bias.
- Determine if an appropriate power analysis has been performed to justify the numbers.
- Decide whether correct statistical methods have been used to analyse the data.
- Judge whether the descriptive data are comprehensive.
- Decide whether there is full information on the outcomes and effects of interest, including measures of precision.
- Assess whether all harms have been documented.

- Establish whether the conclusions drawn are correct and important.
- Decide whether all the limitations have been considered.
- Judge whether the generalizability of the findings is appropriate.

18.2 Introduction

It is our concern that the quality of reporting of animal research is generally poor and lags behind that of medical research (Kilkenny *et al.*, 2009). As we reach the conclusion of this book we want to leave you with a methodology to appraise the studies you read about. Its purpose is not simply to find holes in other people's work, but to enable you to evaluate a study constructively and critically. In so doing, you will be able to choose those studies that are of most use in informing your understanding of the subject, and you will sharpen your own critical faculties to design, conduct and report your own studies. Our approach is to provide a template for critical appraisal of published research involving animals (see Section 18.3). We have devised this template by drawing on those principles propounded by the CONSORT, STROBE and REFLECT statements and the ARRIVE guidelines (all discussed in Chapter 17) and have based it on the templates provided by Petrie and Sabin (2013). As illustrations of its applicability, we invite you to use our template to critically appraise the two

Statistics for Veterinary and Animal Science, Third Edition. Aviva Petrie and Paul Watson.
© 2013 John Wiley & Sons, Ltd. Published 2013 by John Wiley & Sons, Ltd.

publications provided in Sections 18.4 and 18.6. Our own appraisals of these two papers are to be found in Sections 18.5 and 18.7, respectively.

18.3 A template for critical appraisal of published research involving animals

(1) Title and abstract

(a) Is the type of study or study design mentioned in the title? For example, randomized controlled trial (RCT), cross-sectional or longitudinal study, prospective or retrospective survey, cohort or case–control study.

(b) Does the abstract summarize the study approach: its primary objective, its design, methods, results, conclusions and any limitations?

(2) Introduction

(a) Has the rationale for the study been set out logically and clearly? Is it based on the relevant existing scientific background? Has all the necessary information from previous studies and other pertinent evidence been included?

(b) Is the primary aim of the study indicated, has the outcome of interest been identified and, if appropriate, has a relevant hypothesis based on the outcome of interest been explicitly stated? Are any secondary objectives identified? If a cohort study, were there any modifications to the original study protocol following the publication of new evidence after the cohort study was initiated?

(3) Materials and methods

(a) Animals
(i) Is the number and choice of animals clearly stated?
  • If a clinical trial, how have the animals been selected? Are inclusion and exclusion criteria provided?
  • If a case–control study, is the rationale for the choice of cases and controls explained?
  • If a cohort study, is the method of follow-up described?
  • If a matched study, is full information provided on the matching criteria?
(ii) Was the study conducted using an appropriately wide range of animals?

(b) General methodology
(i) Are all methods clearly presented with sufficient information to carry them out, or a reference given to the original method in the literature?
(ii) Are details provided on the comparability of assessment methods if there is more than one group?

(c) Study design
Is the study design adequately described? Is there a description of the study setting and location and are relevant dates provided? Were the authors aware of any potential biases and what steps were taken to avoid them? For example, if a clinical trial, were the following considered?

(i) **Randomization.** Are full details of the randomization process provided, e.g. the type of randomization, the method used to generate the random allocation sequence and the unit of randomization (e.g. animal, farm)? Is the implementation of the randomization described (e.g. who enrolled the subjects and who assigned the participants to the treatments)?

(ii) **Blinding.** To what extent was the study blinded? If relevant, is a description provided of the similarity of the interventions?

(iii) Was the **allocation sequence concealed** from those assigning subjects to treatments and those responsible for care of the animals?

(iv) With the exception that they received different treatments, were the groups treated in a similar fashion?

(d) Variables
(i) Is consideration given to all important outcomes?
(ii) Are the primary and secondary outcomes precisely defined?

(iii) Were any changes made to outcomes after the start of the study?

(iv) Is there a clear description of treatments (in a clinical trial), exposures (observational study), predictors, potential confounders and effect modifiers?

(e) Sample size

(i) Is there a power statement to justify the overall sample size, and does it state the form of the statistical analysis on which it is based? Is the reader made aware of all the relevant factors that influence sample size for this power calculation?

(ii) If relevant, is there a reference to any pilot studies that informed the power analysis?

(iii) If relevant, is there a full explanation of any interim analysis, including any steps taken to reduce the Type I error rate?

(iv) If subgroup analyses have been described, are the subgroup sample sizes based on power calculations, and were any further steps taken to reduce the Type I error rate? Alternatively, is it acknowledged that these subgroups may lack sufficient power to detect an effect as statistically significant?

(f) Statistical methods

(i) Is the unit of investigation (e.g. single animal, cage of animals, farm) clearly identified?

(ii) Are the statistical methods employed for all data analyses identified?

(iii) Are the statistical methods appropriate, for example:
- Have the correct considerations of the nature of the data been made?
- Have underlying assumptions been verified?
- Have data dependencies (e.g. pairing) been taken into account in the analysis?
- If transformations have been taken of the data, have they been justified?

(iv) Is there a description of how numerical variables were handled in the analysis, including any choice of groupings?

(v) Is there a description of additional analyses, such as subgroup analyses? Were any additional analyses undertaken *specified a priori* or were they *post hoc* analyses?

(vi) Is there a description of how missing data have been dealt with in the analysis?

(vii) Is there a description of how losses to follow-up (cohort and clinical trial), matching (case–control) or sampling strategy (cross-sectional) have been dealt with?

(viii) If it was necessary to perform a sensitivity analysis to assess how robust or sensitive the results of the study were to the methods employed or assumptions made, is it fully described?

(ix) Have the *P*-value to determine statistical significance and the statistical software, with version number, used to analyse the data been reported?

(4) Results

(a) Animal numbers and dates

(i) If a RCT, is there a full explanation for each treatment group, of the numbers of participants who were randomly assigned, received the intended treatment, and were analysed for the primary outcome? Is this information presented in prose, or preferably, in a participant flow chart or table?

(ii) If an observational study, is there a report of the number of subjects included at each stage of the study (e.g. the numbers potentially eligible, examined for eligibility, included in the study, completed follow-up, included in the analysis), preferably in a participant flow chart.

(iii) If relevant, are numbers of and reasons for losses to follow-up and exclusions documented?

(iv) Are dates provided that define the periods of recruitment and follow-up?

(b) Baseline data

(i) Is there a table that shows the baseline demographic and clinical characteristics for each group if there is more than one group?

(ii) If there is more than one group, are the groups comparable?

(c) Descriptive data

(i)   Are the characteristics (e.g. at baseline in a cohort study or RCT) of study participants provided for each group (if there is more than one group)? In particular, are the sex, age, developmental stage and weight distributions of the animals summarized? Are the strains (rodents), lines, breeds and species (animals) reported? If relevant, is information provided on the source of the animals, genetic modification status, etc.?

(ii) If relevant, is information provided on housing (e.g. type of facility, number of cage or pen companions, fish-tank shape and material) and husbandry conditions (e.g. breeding programme, temperature, quality of water and air, type of food, etc.)?

(iii) Can the reader be satisfied that if groups are to be compared (e.g. case–control study, RCT), they are comparable?

(iv) Is there an indication of the number of participants with missing data for each variable of interest?

(v)   If a cohort study or an analysis of survival data, is the follow-up time summarized (e.g. average and total amount)?

(d) Numbers analysed

(i)   If an RCT, is there a specification of whether an 'intention-to-treat' (ITT) analysis was performed? Is a justification given for the choice of analysis (ITT or other) and is this appropriate?

(ii) If there were protocol deviations, was a sensitivity analysis performed (e.g. as per protocol analysis or an analysis with imputed data for missing observations)?

(e) Outcomes of interest

(i)   **Main outcome of interest.** Is there full information on outcomes? For example:

- If a clinical trial, is there an appropriate summary measure of the main outcome variable (i.e. that which relates to the primary aim of the study) for each group? For example, the rate/risk/odds of occurrence of the outcome (e.g. death) for a *binary* outcome variable, giving absolute numbers when feasible; or the mean (median) of a *numerical* outcome variable.
- If a cohort study, are the numbers of outcome events or summary measures over time provided?
- If a case–control study, are the numbers in each exposure category or summary measures of exposure provided?
- If a cross-sectional study, are the numbers of outcome events or summary measures provided?

(ii) **Magnitude of the effect of interest:**

- Is there an indication of the magnitude of the effect of interest? For example, a ratio such as the relative rate/risk/odds or a difference such as the absolute difference in risk if the outcome variable is *binary*; or a difference in means (medians) if the main outcome variable is *numerical.*
- If adjusting for confounding, are unadjusted estimates and confounder-adjusted estimates provided? If confounder-adjusted estimates are provided, is there a clear indication of which confounders were adjusted for in the analysis and why they were selected?

(iii) **Precision of the effect of interest.** Is there an indication of the precision of the effect of interest (e.g. a 95% confidence interval or standard error)?

(f) Additional analyses

Are the results of any additional (e.g. subgroup or sensitivity) analyses given, and are *post hoc* analyses distinguished from those that were pre-specified?

(g) Harms

If a clinical trial, are all important harms in each group documented?

(5) Discussion

(a) Deciding whether the results are important

(i)   Are the key findings summarized with reference to the study objectives?

(ii) Do the results make **biological sense**?

(iii) If a **confidence interval** for the effect of interest (e.g. the difference in means) has been provided:

- Would you regard the observed effect clinically important if the true value of the effect was equal to either the upper or lower limit of the confidence interval (irrespective of whether or not the result of the relevant hypothesis test is statistically significant)?
- If your answers do not differ markedly, do you conclude that the results are unambiguous and important?

(iv) If a clinical trial, is there an evaluation of the **number of subjects needed to treat** (NNT) with the experimental treatment rather than the control treatment in order to prevent one of them developing the 'bad' outcome?

(v) If feasible, have any estimates of relative 'risk' (e.g. relative risk odds ratio) been translated into absolute 'risks' for a meaningful time period?

(vi) If relevant, has a discussion of herd immunity been included?

(b) Limitations

Is there a discussion of all the study limitations, including any potential sources of bias and imprecision?

(c) Generalizability

Is there a discussion of the generalizability of the results (i.e. the extent to which the subjects are representative of the wider population) together with any acknowledgement of their possible restriction in application?

(d) Interpretation

Taking the benefits and harms into consideration, as well as the limitations of the study, any multiple testing and subgroup analyses, and the results from other similar studies if relevant, is the authors' interpretation of the trial findings consistent with the results?

(6) Other information

Are sources of **funding** documented and is there a **conflict of interest** statement for each of the investigators?

18.4 Paper 1

Bille, C., Auvigne, V., Libermann, S., Bomassi, E., Durieux, P. & Rattez, E. (2012) Risk of anaesthetic mortality in dogs and cats: an observational cohort study of 3546 cases. *Veterinary Anaesthesia and Analgesia* **39**, 59–68. (Reproduced with permission from the publisher, Wiley-Blackwell.)

Veterinary
Anaesthesia and Analgesia
            Formerly the Journal of Veterinary Anaesthesia

Veterinary Anaesthesia and Analgesia, 2012, **39**, 59–68   doi:10.1111/j.1467-2995.2011.00686.x

RESEARCH PAPER

Risk of anaesthetic mortality in dogs and cats: an observational cohort study of 3546 cases.

Christophe Bille*, Vincent Auvignet†, Stéphane Libermann*, Eric Bomassi*, Philippe Durieux* & Elise Rattez*

*Centre Hospitalier Vétérinaire des Cordeliers, Meaux, France

†Ekipaj, Angers, France

Correspondence: Christophe Bille, Centre Hospitalier Vétérinaire des Cordeliers, 29 avenue du maréchal Joffre, 77100, Meaux, France. E-mail: cbille@chvcordeliers.com

Abstract

Objective To evaluate the anaesthetic death risk for dogs and cats in a French private practice.

Study design Observational cohort study.

Animal population All small animals anesthetized at the Centre Hospitalier Vétérinaire des Cordeliers between April 15th, 2008 and April 15th, 2010.

Methods General anaesthesia was defined as a drug-induced unconsciousness characterised by a controlled and reversible depression of the central nervous system and analgesia, sufficient to allow endotracheal intubation. Patient outcome (alive or dead) was assessed at the end of anaesthesia defined as the meeting point of the return of consciousness, rectal temperature >36 °C and ability to maintain sternal recumbency. Death occurring during anaesthesia was recorded. Relationship between anaesthetic death and ASA status, species, age, nature of the procedure, anaesthetic protocol and occurrence of epidural administration of a combination of morphine and bupivacaine were analysed.

Results During the study period 3546 animals underwent general anaesthesia. The overall death rate in the present study was 1.35% (48 in 3546, 95% CI 0.96–1.75). The death rate of healthy animals (ASA 1 and 2) was 0.12% (3 in 2602 95% CI 0.02–0.34). For sick animals (ASA status 3 and over), the overall death rate was 4.77% (45 in 944 95% CI 3.36–6.18). The death rates in the ASA 3, 4 and 5 categories were 2.90%, 7.58% and 17.33%, respectively. The main factor associated with increased odds of anaesthetic death in ASA categories 3 and over was poor health status (ASA physical status classification). The nature of the procedure the patient underwent and epidural administration of a combination of morphine and bupivacaine were not correlated with the occurrence of death during anaesthesia. Neither species nor age effects were detected.

Conclusion and clinical relevance Specific factors were associated with increased odds of anaesthetic death, especially poor health status. Efforts must be directed towards thorough preoperative patient evaluation and improvement of clinical conditions if possible. Identification of risk factors before anaesthesia should lead to increased surveillance by trained staff. This could result in better outcomes.

Keywords anaesthetic, cat, death, dog, mortality, risk, small animal.

Introduction

In the last 30 years, the risk of anaesthetic death has been studied in dogs and cats by teams in different countries (Clarke & Hall 1990; Dodman & Lamb 1992; Dyson et al. 1998; Hosgood & Scholl 1998, 2002; Gaynor et al. 1999; Joubert 2000; Nicholson & Watson 2001; Williams et al. 2002;

Redondo et al. 2007; Brodbelt et al. 2006, 2008a,b; Alef et al. 2008).

The most recent study of anaesthetic deaths (Brodbelt et al. 2008a) included 98,036 dogs and 79,178 cats and defined anaesthetic or sedation-related death as a perioperative death (including euthanasia) occurring after pre-medication and within 48 hours of termination of the procedure, except when death or euthanasia was due solely to inoperable surgical or pre-existing medical conditions. Considering animals of all American Society of Anesthesiologists (ASA) grades, cumulative incidences of anaesthetic and sedation-related death were reported to be 0.17% in dogs and 0.24% in cats. This is higher than the 0.01–0.02% reported in human anaesthesia (Biboulet et al. 2001; Newland et al. 2002).

There is no consensus on the definition of anaesthetic mortality (Arbous et al. 2001). Discrepancies between different reports may result from the studied population. Some authors have included animals that underwent general anaesthesia while others included patients undergoing either general anaesthesia or sedation. Variations may be seen regarding the cause of death, some authors including death of any origin whilst others only considering death that cannot be explained by pre-existing medical conditions or surgical complications. Variations also occur over the study period. Sometimes, this is not clearly defined. Others define the study period as the time of anaesthesia or the time of surgery or set an end point between a few hours (Williams et al. 2002) to 48 hours after termination of the procedure (Brodbelt et al. 2006, 2008a,b).

In small animal practice, the risk of death during anaesthesia has shown to be related to different factors. It was increased in cats compared to dogs (Brodbelt et al. 2008a), in some particular breeds (Clarke & Hall 1990; Brodbelt et al. 2008a), in patients older than 12 years (Hosgood & Scholl 1998; Brodbelt et al. 2006, 2008b), in patients weighing <5 kg (Brodbelt et al. 2008b), in patients with poor health status (Clarke & Hall 1990; Dyson et al. 1998; Hosgood & Scholl 1998, 2002; Brodbelt et al. 2006, 2008a,b), if anaesthesia took place in a referral centre (Gaynor et al. 1999; Brodbelt et al. 2006, 2008a), if a procedure was urgent (Brodbelt et al. 2008b), if a surgical procedure was considered as major (Brodbelt et al. 2008b), if specific agents were used (Dyson et al. 1998) and if an inhalant agent alone was used for induction (Brodbelt et al. 2008b).

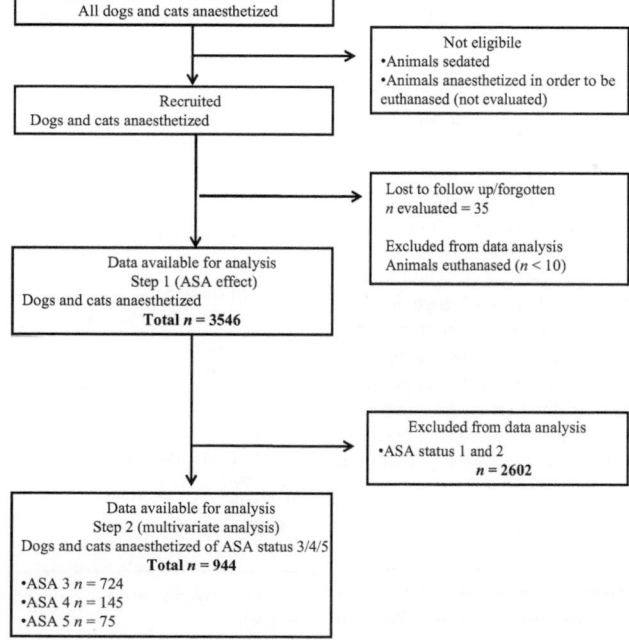

Figure 1 Flow diagram of the recruitment and follow-up of the anaesthetic cases.

© 2011 The Authors. Veterinary Anaesthesia and Analgesia

© 2011 Association of Veterinary Anaesthetists and the American College of Veterinary Anesthesiologists, **39**, 59–68

The aim of this study was to evaluate the anaesthetic death risk for dogs and cats in a French private practice. The authors hypothesised that cats would be at greater risk than dogs and that the anaesthetic death risk would be related to the patient's health status and age but not the nature of the drug used for induction of anaesthesia. To the author's knowledge, this is the first cohort study of small animal anaesthetic deaths undertaken in a single private practice in France.

Methods

We used an observational cohort study design. The observational character of the data collection implies that any decision made by an attending veterinarian on the anaesthetic procedure was not influenced in any way by the study design.

Patients' recruitment

This cohort study recruited all dogs and cats that underwent general anaesthesia at the Centre Hospitalier Vétérinaire des Cordeliers between April 15th 2008 and April 15th 2010 (Fig. 1). General anaesthesia was defined as a drug-induced unconsciousness characterised by a controlled and reversible depression of the central nervous system (CNS) and analgesia, sufficient to allow endotracheal intubation (Thurmon & Short 2007). Patients that were sedated or anaesthetized in order to be euthanased were not included. Sedation was defined as chemical restraint insufficient to allow endotracheal intubation.

The study period commenced when general anaesthesia was induced by administration of an injectable agent, whatever the route (intravenous (IV) or intramuscular (IM)), or with isoflurane and ended with the end of anaesthesia. This end was set at the last point at which anaesthetized patients could be systematically checked in a comparable manner. It was therefore defined as the meeting point of the return of consciousness, rectal temperature >36 °C and ability to maintain sternal recumbency.

Animals that were euthanased during anaesthesia because of medical reasons were excluded from the study.

Data collection

For all patients that were included, identification data, species and age were recorded. Prior to

anaesthetic induction, on the basis of history and clinical examination, the attending anaesthetist assessed the patient's ASA status and whether it would need laboratory tests or not. He then decided which of the anaesthetic protocols (see below) would be used. Any potential bias from such a decision was addressed by introducing the ASA status as a covariate in the final model

Epidural administration of a combination of morphine and bupivacaine by means of an injection or by placement of an epidural catheter was recorded.

The type of procedure the patient underwent was defined as: examination (chemical restraint was needed to perform a non-invasive procedure), orthopaedic or soft tissue surgery. Death occurring during anaesthesia was recorded.

Anaesthetic regimens

Premedication, induction and maintenance agents were recorded. For the data analysis, all premedication regimens were gathered in a 'premedication' category. As a consequence, the nature of the substance used and the route of administration were not taken into account. Any patient that did not receive premedication was included in a 'No' 'premedication' category.

Induction regimens were grouped into four categories: 'Ketamine', 'Thiopental', 'Propofol' and 'Other induction'. 'Other induction' included the use of fentanyl, isoflurane, etomidate, or their association with ketamine or thiopental (Table 1). Dogs given medetomidine or dexmedetomidine such

Table 1 Detail of induction regimens

Induction regimen	n
Medetomidine	12
Medetomidine + thiopental	3
Etomidate	1
Fentanyl	34
Isoflurane	64
Medetomidine + ketamine	34
Ketamine	204
Thiopental	302
Propofol	290
Total	944

n: number of dogs or cats, ASA grade 3–5, which received each regimen.

© 2011 Association of Veterinary Anaesthetists and the American College of Veterinary Anesthesiologists, **39**, 59–68

Risk of anaesthetic mortality in dogs and cats *C Bille et al.*

Table 2 Characteristics of the ASA 3, 4 and 5 study participants (*n* = 944)

	Total anaesthetized	Number of deaths	%	95% CI
Overall	944	45	4.77	3.36–6.18
ASA category				
ASA 3	724	21	2.90	1.61–4.19
ASA 4	145	11	7.59	2.93–12.24
ASA 5	75	13	17.33	8.10–26.57
Dog	683	33	4.83	3.15–6.51
Cat	261	12	4.60	1.87–7.33
Type of procedure				
Examination	272	9	3.31	1.00–5.62
Orthopaedic	151	7	4.64	0.95–8.32
Soft tissue	521	29	5.60	3.50–7.63
Induction agent				
Thiopental	302	20	6.62	3.66–9.59
Ketamine	204	9	4.41	1.35–7.47
Propofol	290	15	5.17	2.45–7.90
Other	148	1	0.68	0.02–3.70
Anaesthetic protocol				
Premedication + thiopental + isoflurane	271	19	7.01	3.79–10.23
Premedication + ketamine + isoflurane	166	9	5.42	1.67–9.17
Premedication + propofol + isoflurane	223	13	5.83	2.53–9.13
Other	284	4	1.41	0.39–3.57
Epidural				
No	872	38	4.36	2.95–5.77
Yes	72	7	9.72	2.19–17.26
Age				
<3 years old	263	14	5.32	2.42–8.23
>3 and ≤7 years old	246	13	5.29	2.29–8.28
>7 and ≤10 years old	207	8	3.86	1.00–6.73
>10 years old	228	10	4.37	1.51–7.26
Pre-anaesthetic blood tests				
Yes	325	15	4.61	2.18–7.05
No	619	30	4.85	3.07–6.62

that endotracheal intubation was carried out (*n* = 12) were also included in this group.

Two groups of maintenance regimes were defined: patients that received isoflurane and patients that did not. Patients that did not receive isoflurane were anaesthetized by means of total IV anaesthesia or IM injection of the induction agent with no further maintenance agent.

The overall anaesthetic regimen was then defined by the combination of the premedication, the induction and the maintenance regimens. Four groups were defined (Table 2):
• Use of premedication, induction of anaesthesia with ketamine, maintenance with isoflurane.
• Use of premedication, induction of anaesthesia with thiopental, maintenance with isoflurane.
• Use of premedication, induction of anaesthesia with propofol, maintenance with isoflurane.

• Use of any other anaesthetic regimen. This represented 66 different regimens.

For statistical means, animals were grouped according to their age. Groups were defined arbitrarily to obtain four categories of equal importance as shown in Table 2.

Data analysis

The data analysis was conducted following a two-step approach. As a first step, bivariate analysis was performed to analyse the relationship between ASA score and mortality (Mann–Whitney/Wilcoxon Two-Sample Test, EpiInfo 3.5.1; Centers for Disease Control and Prevention, GA, USA). 95% Confidence Intervals were calculated using the normal approximation when $n(1 - p) > 4$ and the binomial exact method in other cases (Epidat 3.1;

Table 3 Relation between peri-operative death, species and ASA status

		Peri-operative death			Dogs		Cats	
ASA	Total number of animals	n deaths	%	95% CI	Total number of dogs	n deaths	Total number of cats	n deaths
1	714	0	0.0	0.00–0.52	197	0	517	0
2	1888	3	0.12	0.003–0.46	1372	1	516	2
3	724	21	2.90	1.61–4.19	521	17	203	4
4	145	11	7.59	2.93–12.24	101	5	44	6
5	75	13	17.33	8.10–26.57	61	11	14	2
Total	3546	48	1.35	0.96–1.75	2252	34	1294	14

n: number of deaths.

Epidat : PanAmerican Health Organization, WA D.C., USA).

As a second step, because of the null to very low mortality in animals of ASA score 1 or 2 (see Results), only animals of ASA score of 3 or more were included. In other words, because the occurrence of the outcome is rare in the subpopulation of ASA score 1 or 2, the analysis of the relationship between death and other variables is of no benefit. In this second step, univariate and bivariate analyses were carried out, followed by a multivariate analysis of the data. The statistical unit was the animal and death the outcome variable. Logistic regression models were created using the GLM procedure of R software 2.9.0 (R Foundation for Statistical Computing, Austria). 'ASA category', 'Species', 'Type of procedure', 'Anaesthetic protocol', 'Epidural' and 'Age' were set as explanatory variables. The probability of wrongly rejecting the null hypothesis was set to 5%. A backward procedure was used. Variables were kept in the model if $p < 0.15$. Two-way interactions were tested and kept in the model if $p < 0.05$. For assessing the fit of the models receiver-operating characteristic (ROC) curves were constructed and the areas under curves (AUCs) were calculated.

Results

During the study period, 3546 animals underwent general anaesthesia. Animals lost to follow-up were estimated to be 35. The number of patients euthanased for medical reasons during general anaesthesia was evaluated at <10 (Fig. 1).

The first-step (univariate) analysis revealed that 48 animals out of 3546 (1.35%, 95% CI 0.96–1.75) died. No animal died in the ASA 1 category. The death rate increased with each grade of ASA status (Table 3). The second-step (multivariate) analysis was performed on the ASA 3, 4 and 5 categories. Nine hundred and forty-four patients of ASA status 3, 4 and 5 were included (Fig. 1). The characteristics of these 944 patients are shown in Table 2. Forty-five (4.77%, 95% CI 3.36–6.18) died during anaesthesia (Table 2).

When considering the multivariate model (Table 4), increasing ASA status was associated with increased odds of anaesthetic death. Also, when compared to the group 'other anaesthetic protocol', the group 'premedication + thiopental + isoflurane' was associated with increased odds of anaesthetic death. Increasing ASA category from 3 to 4 was associated with a 3.7-fold increase in the odds of death ($p = 0.001$, 95% confidence interval (CI) [1.7–8.1]). Increasing ASA category from 3 to 5 was associated with a 13.4-fold increase in the odds of death ($p < 0.001$, 95% CI [5.8–30.4]). Compared to the group 'premedication + thiopental + isoflurane', the group 'Other anaesthetic protocol' was associated with a 10-fold decrease in the odds of death ($p < 0.001$, 95% CI [0.0–0.3]). Compared to the group 'premedication + thiopental + isoflurane', the group 'premedication + propofol + isoflurane' showed a tendency for a decrease in the odds of death ($p = 0.08$, 95% CI [0.2–1.1]). Compared to the group 'premedication + thiopental + isoflurane', the group 'premedication + ketamine + isoflurane' showed a tendency for decrease

Risk of anaesthetic mortality in dogs and cats *C Bille et al.*

Table 4 Logistic regression modelling of the odds of anaesthetic death of animals undergoing anaesthesia

	OR	95% CI	p-value
ASA category*			
3	–	–	
4	3.7	1.7–8.1	0.001
5	13.4	5.8–30.4	<0.001
Species			
Dog	–	–	
Cat	1.9	0.9–3.9	0.11
Anaesthetic protocol†			
Premed + thiopental + isoflurane	–	–	
Other anaesthetic regimen	0.1	0.0–0.3	<0.001
Premed + ketamine + isoflurane	0.5	0.2–1.1	0.10
Premed + propofol + isoflurane	0.5	0.2–1.1	0.08
Epidural			
No	–	–	
Yes	2.2	0.9–5.3	0.09

Premed: premedication. *The OR represents a change from ASA 3 to ASA 4 or ASA 3 to ASA 5. †The OR represents a change from premedication + thiopental + isoflurane to either other anaesthetic regimen, premedication + ketamine + isoflurane or premedication + propofol + isoflurane.

in the odds of death ($p = 0.10$, 95% CI [0.2–1.1]). Although not statistically significant, there was a tendency for cats to be more at risk of dying during anaesthesia than dogs ($p = 0.11$, 95% CI [0.9–3.9]). There was a tendency for animals receiving an epidural combination of morphine and bupivacaine to be more at risk of anaesthetic death ($p = 0.09$, 95% CI [0.9–5.3]). After adjusting for other variables, the odds of death associated with the type of procedure were not significantly different. No age (data not shown) effect was detected. None of the interaction terms were significant and were therefore dropped out of the model. The AUC of the model was 0.74 indicating acceptable discrimination properties (Hosmer & Lemeshow 2000).

Discussion

The overall death rate in the present study was 1.35%. Results suggest that ASA status was significantly associated with increasing the odds of anaesthetic death in dogs and cats. When considering patients of ASA status 3 and over, the use of an anaesthetic protocol that included premedication, induction with thiopental and maintenance with isoflurane, was associated with increased odds

of anaesthetic death when compared to the group 'other anaesthetic regimen'. Results also suggest that, although not significant, there is a tendency for cats and animals receiving an epidural injection to be more at risk of anaesthetic death. Age was not found to be associated with an increase in the odds of death.

Many of the previously published studies have reported anaesthetic death rates of between 0.17% and 0.43% (Clarke & Hall 1990; Dodman & Lamb 1992; Dyson et al. 1998; Gaynor et al. 1999; Joubert 2000; Williams et al. 2002; Brodbelt et al. 2006, 2008a; Alef et al. 2008), which are lower than those reported here. However, there are two surveys (Hosgood & Scholl 1998, 2002) which have reported death rates similar to those seen in this current study.

As discussed earlier, it is difficult to compare different studies on anaesthetic death as case definitions and methods differ. It must also be remembered that in the earlier surveys, anaesthetic agents differed, and the computing power to calculate odds ratios was not always available.

This study was designed to provide a high rank of evidence when considering anaesthetic death risk factors. A cohort observational study was thought to be adequate (Holmes 2007). Major difficulties encountered when building this type of cohort observational study were thought to be: 1) including a representative group of the exposed population; and 2) limiting the loss related to poor follow-up. Therefore it was decided that all anaesthetized patients should be included.

Some animals were lost to follow up when data were not recorded by the administrator. Reasons included the administrator being unaware that anaesthesia had taken place, usually for a minor, short and uneventful procedure. Occasionally the administrator postponed filling out the data sheet and had forgotten a procedure that took place at the end of the day. It was estimated that one animal was lost to poor follow-up every 3 weeks; a total of 35 patients.

The end of the study period was defined as the meeting point of the return of consciousness, rectal temperature >36 °C and ability to maintain sternal recumbency. An end point of 48 hours after the procedure as set in veterinary (Brodbelt et al. 2006, 2008a,b) and human literature (Newland et al. 2002) or at the discharge of the patient (Wolters et al. 1996) would probably have increased the death rate, as animals that died in the immediate

© 2011 The Authors. Veterinary Anaesthesia and Analgesia
© 2011 Association of Veterinary Anaesthetists and the American College of Veterinary Anesthesiologists, **39**, 59–68

postoperative period would then have been taken into account. In the current study, from practice, this type of end point would have led to a selection bias by excluding many animals undergoing minor procedures that were not seen 48 hours after the procedure took place.

The major reason for euthanasia during anaesthesia was the diagnosis of an inoperable tumour. As these animals were to be excluded from the study, no data were prospectively recorded, and therefore, the number of euthanased patients was estimated retrospectively. The authors acknowledge it would have been preferable to record the number of such patients.

The study's objective was to evaluate anaesthetic death of any cause, so no attempt was made to classify the cause of death. Thus deaths from medical or surgical complications were included. This is different from other studies (Brodbelt et al. 2006, 2008a,b), where authors defined anaesthetic or sedation-related death as death that could not be explained totally by pre-existing medical or surgical complications.

A potential selection bias comes from the fact that the Centre Hospitalier Vétérinaire des Cordeliers is a referral centre. A difference in anaesthetic mortality has been observed when comparing practice-based studies (Clarke & Hall 1990; Dodman & Lamb 1992; Dyson et al. 1998; Joubert 2000; Williams et al. 2002), referral-studies (Hosgood & Scholl 1998, 2002; Gaynor et al. 1999; Brodbelt et al. 2006) or both (Brodbelt et al. 2008a,b). Referral practices usually anaesthetize a greater proportion of patients classified in the ASA 3, 4 and 5 categories. In our case, these categories represent 26.6% of the anaesthetized population. This is more than the 5–10% described in the practice-based studies (Clarke & Hall 1990; Dyson et al. 1998), and could explain the higher percentage of deaths in our study.

In this study, sick patients, as assessed by ASA score, had higher risk of anaesthetic death than did healthy animals. The ASA status is correlated to anaesthesia-related death in humans (Vancanti et al. 1970; Wolters et al. 1996; Jones & Cossart 1999; Biboulet et al. 2001; Newland et al. 2002) and in domestic animals (Clarke & Hall 1990; Dodman & Lamb 1992; Dyson et al. 1998; Hosgood & Scholl 1998, 2002; Brodbelt et al. 2006, 2008a,b). The death rate increases with each grade of ASA status (Table 3). This suggests that there is a causal relationship between these variables. The published absolute mortality rates of the ASA

classes has shown variations in veterinary studies, with 0.05–0.10% for ASA 1 and 2 categories and 1–2% for ASA 3, 4 and 5 categories (Dyson et al. 1998; Hosgood & Scholl 1998, 2002; Brodbelt et al. 2006, 2008a,b). Our data show a mortality rate of 0.12% for ASA 1 and 2 categories and 4.76% for ASA 3, 4 and 5 categories. These variations can be explained in part by differences in assessment of the patient's ASA physical status. In our case, we tried to limit this variability by having one attending veterinarian (CB) review and, if necessary, reassess the ASA status, on the basis of the patient charts.

The anaesthetic protocol was established by the veterinarian in charge, in light of his experience. Anaesthetist's experience is a subjective concept and is hard to analyse. It refers to numerous factors as patient condition, species, breed, body weight, nature of the illness, nature of the procedure, personal habits and preferences, personal perception and interpretation of an illness, owners' wishes, time of the day, work load, experience of co-workers (nurse and/or surgeon), and economic aspects. Many of these factors could not be tested as variables in the logistic regression models and this could have led to a selection bias.

The 'premedication + thiopental + isoflurane' group was statistically correlated to anaesthetic deaths when compared to the group 'other anaesthetic regimen'. Although not statistically significant, there was a tendency for animals in the group 'premedication + thiopental + isoflurane' to be more at risk of anaesthetic death when compared to those in groups 'premedication + propofol + isoflurane' and 'premedication + ketamine + isoflurane'. This was unexpected. There is no clear explanation for this finding. The Centre Hosptalier Vétérinaire des Cordeliers tends to use an anaesthetic protocol that includes premedication, an injectable induction agent and maintenance using inhalation anaesthesia with isoflurane in very critical patients, which could lead to a selection bias, as these protocols might therefore include a relatively larger number of anaesthetic deaths. This potential bias was addressed by introducing the ASA status as a covariate in the final model.

The authors have analysed the raw interactions between anaesthetic protocol and variables that were shown to increased the odds of anaesthetic death or to have tendency to increase the odds of anaesthetic death in the logistic regression model (e.g. ASA status, epidural and species). However, anaesthetic protocols were not randomly assigned.

Therefore, when considering raw associations, most variables are significantly associated. Moreover, ASA status and anaesthetic protocol, epidural injection and anaesthetic protocol, species and anaesthetic protocol were significantly correlated (data not shown). Because of these numerous correlations it was decided that raw interactions would not be interpreted and that only the logistic regression model would be satisfactory.

No satisfactory explanation was identified to explain why the 'premedication + thiopental + isoflurane' group was overrepresented in anaesthetic deaths. Using an 'other protocol' when compared to 'premedication + thiopental + isoflurane' was associated with a 10-fold decrease in the odds of anaesthetic death. This finding was expected. It is probable that, despite ASA classification, anaesthetist's experience leads to a subjective evaluation of the risk. This can lead to the establishment of 'another protocol'. This leads to a selection bias. The 'other protocol' category may then appear safer when in reality it is not and contains animals that where subjectively judged to be less at risk for anaesthetic death. As other protocol included many variations, numbers within any subcategory were too small for analysis.

The roles of premedication, induction and maintenance drugs in anaesthetic death have been studied (Clarke & Hall 1990; Dyson et al. 1998; Brodbelt et al. 2006, 2007, 2008a,b). The use of either acepromazine, atropine or medetomidine in premedication has been found to decrease the odds of anaesthetic death (Clarke & Hall 1990; Dyson et al. 1998; Brodbelt et al. 2006, 2008a). The use of xylazine in the anaesthetic protocol in dogs has been shown to be associated with an increase in the odds of anaesthetic death (Dyson et al. 1998). No correlation has been found previously between the use of either ketamine, thiopental of propofol and anaesthetic death (Dyson et al. 1998; Brodbelt et al. 2006, 2008a).

Dog owners might be more likely to seek medical attention than cat owners. A selection bias could therefore enhance the association between dogs and anaesthesia-related death, compared to cats. Also, cats' health status is, in general, less easily assessable than dogs', possibly resulting in poorer preoperative assessment of the feline patients. Finally, a type-II error could explain the tendency for cats to be more prone to anaesthetic death when compared to dogs. It could be induced by the small number of subjects (944) enrolled in our study. Therefore, the tendency for cats to be more prone to anaesthesia-related death

could have been significant if a greater number of patients had been included. In other studies there are conflicting results. Some authors concluded that cats were more prone to anaesthetic death when compared to dogs (Clarke & Hall 1990; Hosgood & Scholl 1998, 2002; Brodbelt et al. 2008a). Other teams found no correlation (Dyson et al.1998; Gaynor et al. 1999) or found dogs to be more at risk (Dodman & Lamb 1992), especially when considering the ASA 1 and 2 categories (Dyson et al.1998).

To the authors' knowledge, this is the first time that epidural injection of a combination of morphine and bupivacaine has been tested as a risk factor for anaesthetic death. In our study, animals that received an epidural injection showed a statistically not-significant tendency to be more at risk of anaesthetic death. This tendency was unexpected.

The epidural solution of morphine and bupivacaine was prepared as described by Valverde (2008). In this study epidural anaesthesia was performed only by one single veterinarian (CB), thus introducing a potential selection bias. Epidural injections were not equally distributed because they depend on which anaesthetist was on duty and a heavy workload could have led to the absence of epidural injections in patients that would have otherwise received one.

Animals were grouped arbitrarily according to their age in order to obtain four categories as shown in Table 2. It is unlikely that these categories are representative of the metabolic state of the patients. The <3 years old category contained neonates, paediatrics and young adult patients. However, number of subjects enrolled was too low to allow a more detailed classification and an age effect on anaesthetic mortality could have gone undetected. One team has shown that animals over 12 years old were 7.1 times more at risk of an anaesthetic death when compared to animals of 0.5–8 years old (Brodbelt et al. 2008a). Another study concluded that, in dogs, age was associated with anaesthetic death (Hosgood & Scholl 1998).

Our study did not permit identifying the nature of the procedure as a potential risk factor for anaesthetic death. We chose to classify the nature of the procedure on the basis of its technical description (e.g. examination, soft tissue, orthopaedics), in accordance to earlier publications (Dyson et al. 1998; Hosgood & Scholl 1998, 2002). Other authors have chosen to classify interventions into major or minor procedures (Brodbelt et al. 2007,

2008a). However, there is currently no universally agreed definition of what constitutes a major or a minor procedure. However, it has only been by this classification that procedure has been shown to be to be a risk factor for anaesthetic death in cats and dogs (Brodbelt et al. 2007, 2008a). This is in accordance with the human literature (Wolters et al. 1996; Newland et al. 2002). Studies that have found a significant effect of the nature of the procedure are mainly in large-scale studies including 72,959, 79,178 and 98,036 anaesthetized patients respectively (Newland et al. 2002; Brodbelt et al. 2007, 2008a). In our study, the small number of animals means that a type-II error may have prevented a significant correlation between procedures and death from being shown.

How applicable are our estimates to other veterinary practices? This is an important question because the Centre Hospitalier Vétérinaire des Cordeliers has a different caseload from most practitioners and many of the anaesthetized patients are presented because of the severity of their condition and the necessity for a complex surgical procedure. Patients of clinical status of ASA 3, 4 and 5 represented 26.6% of our anaesthetized population whereas practice-based studies have shown that 5–10% of the patients were in these categories. Also, anaesthesia might not be routinely monitored the same way in every practice. This includes the presence of trained staff and/or the use of monitoring devices (electrocardiogram, pulse oximetry, non-invasive or invasive blood pressure monitoring and capnography).

In conclusion, the risk of anaesthetic death appears to be comparable with risk reported internationally. Patients of ASA status 3 and over appear to be considerably more at risk than patients of ASA status 1 and 2. These animals should be thoroughly prepared for anaesthesia and closely monitored by well-trained staff.

References

Alef M, Von Praun F, Oechtering G (2008) Is routine preanaesthetic haematological and biochemical screening justified in dogs? Vet Anaesth Analg 35, 132–140.

Arbous MS, Grobbee DE, Kleef JWV et al. (2001) Mortality associated with anaesthesia: a qualitative analysis to identify risk factors. Anaesthesia 56, 1141–1153.

Biboulet P, Aubas P, Dubourdieu J et al. (2001) Fatal and non fatal cardiac arrests related to anesthesia. Can J Anaesth 48, 326–332.

Brodbelt DC, Hammond R, Tuminaro D et al. (2006) Risk factors for anaesthetic-related death in referred dogs. Vet Rec 158, 563–564.

Brodbelt DC, Pfeiffer DU, Young LE et al. (2007) Risk factors for anaesthetic-related death in cats: results from the confidential enquiry into perioperative small animal fatalities (CEPSAF). Br J Anaesth 99, 617–623. aem229.

Brodbelt DC, Blissitt KJ, Hammond RA et al. (2008a) The risk of death: the confidential enquiry into perioperative small animal fatalities. Vet Anaesth Analg 35, 365–373.

Brodbelt DC, Pfeiffer DU, Young LE et al. (2008b) Results of the confidential enquiry into perioperative small animal fatalities regarding risk factors for anesthetic-related death in dogs. J Am Vet Med Assoc 233, 1096–1104.

Clarke KW, Hall LW (1990) A survey of anaesthesia in small animal practice: AVA/BSAVA report. Vet Anaesth Analg 17, 4–10.

Dodman NH, Lamb LA (1992) Survey of small animal anesthetic practice in Vermont. J Am Anim Hosp Assoc 28, 439–444.

Dyson DH, Maxie MG, Schnurr D (1998) Morbidity and mortality associated with anesthetic management in small animal veterinary practice in Ontario. J Am Anim Hosp Assoc 34, 325–335.

Gaynor JS, Dunlop CI, Wagner AE, Wertz EM, Golden AE, Demme WC (1999) Complications and mortality associated with anesthesia in dogs and cats. J Am Anim Hosp Assoc. Jan–Feb;35 (1), 13–17.

Holmes MA (2007) Evaluation of the evidence. Vet Clin North Am Small Anim Pract 37, 447–462.

Hosgood G, Scholl DT (1998) Evalution of age as a risk factor for perianesthetic morbidity and mortality in the dog. J Vet Emerg Crit Care 8, 222–236.

Hosgood G, Scholl DT (2002) Evaluation of age and American Society of Anesthesiologists (ASA) physical status as risk factors for perianesthetic morbidity and mortality in the cat. J Vet Emerg Crit Care 12, 9–15.

Hosmer DW, Lemeshow S (2000) Applied Logistic Regression, Wiley Series in Probability and Mathematical Statistics, October 2000 (2nd edn). John Wiley, NY, USA. pp. 392. ISBN: 978-0-471-35632-5.

Jones HJ, Cossart L (1999) Risk scoring in surgical patients. Br J Surg 86, 149–157.

Joubert KE (2000) Routine veterinary anaesthetic management practices in South Africa. J S Afr Vet Assoc 71, 166–172.

Newland MC, Ellis SJ, Lydiatt CA et al. (2002) Anesthetic-related cardiac arrest and its mortality: a report covering 72,959 anesthetics over 10 years from a US teaching hospital. Anesthesiology 97, 108–115.

Nicholson A, Watson A (2001) Survey on small animal anaesthesia. Aust Vet J 79, 613–619.

Redondo JI, Rubio M, Soler G, Serra I, Soler C, Gomez-Villamandos RJ (2007) Normal values and incidence of cardiorespiratory complications in dogs during general

Risk of anaesthetic mortality in dogs and cats *C Bille et al.*

anaesthesia. A review of 1281 cases. J Vet Med. A 54, 470–477.

Thurmon JC, Short CE (2007) History and overview of veterinary anesthesia. In: Veterinary Anesthesia and Analgesia (4th edn) Lumb XX, Jones XX (eds). Blackwell publishing, Ames, USA. pp. 3–6.

Valverde A (2008) Epidural analgesia and anesthesia in dogs and cats. Vet Clin North Am Small Anim Pract 38, 1205–1230.

Vancanti CJ, Van Houton RJ, Hill RC (1970) A statistical analysis of the relationship of physical status to post-operative mortality in 63388 cases. Anesth Analg 49, 564–566.

Williams LS, Levy JK, Robertson SA et al. (2002) Use of the anesthetic combination of tiletamine, zolazepam, ketamine, and xylazine for neutering feral cats. J Am Vet Med Assoc 220, 1491–1495.

Wolters U, Wolf T, Stützer H et al. (1996) ASA classification and perioperative variables as predictors of postoperative outcome. Br J Anaesth 77, 217–222.

Received 29 October 2010; accepted 8 February 2011.

© 2011 The Authors. Veterinary Anaesthesia and Analgesia
© 2011 Association of Veterinary Anaesthetists and the American College of Veterinary Anesthesiologists, **39**, 59–68

18.5 Critical appraisal of paper 1

(1) Title and abstract

(a) The title states that the study is an observational cohort study.

(b) The abstract, which is structured, defines its primary objective as evaluating the anaesthetic death risk for dogs and cats in a French private practice. The design is described, as are the methods, results and conclusions. No limitations are listed in the abstract.

(2) Introduction

(a) The rationale for the study has been set out logically and clearly on pages 59–60. Necessary information from previous studies has been included.

(b) The primary aim of the study is indicated on page 61 (LHS). The outcome of interest is identified as the anaesthetic death risk for dogs and cats. The authors explicitly hypothesize that '*cats would be at greater risk than dogs*' and (as a secondary objective although not stated as such) '*that the anaesthetic death risk would be related to the patient's health status and age but not the nature of the drug used for induction of anaesthesia.*' Note that what the authors are hypothesizing is not, in either case, the null hypothesis that they are testing, but rather their views on the potential outcome. There was no publication of new evidence after the cohort study was initiated, and so it was not necessary to modify the original study protocol.

(3) Materials and methods

(a) Animals

(i) The number of animals anaesthetized is stated in the Results section (p. 63, LHS) as 3546; 944 of these animals were analysed in the second phase of the statistical analysis (Figure 1 and p. 61, RHS). The authors provide a flow chart (Figure 1) that shows the recruitment and follow-up of the anaesthetic cases. The choice of animals is clearly stated in the Patients' recruitment section (p. 61) as '*all dogs and cats that underwent general anaesthesia at the Centre Hospitalier Vétérinaire des Cordeliers between April 15th 2008 and April 15th 2010.*' The authors do not state where the hospital is in the text but all but one of the authors are listed as working in this hospital in Meaux, France. The end of follow-up is defined (p. 61, Patients' recruitment) as '*the meeting point of the return of consciousness, rectal temperature >36°C and ability to maintain sternal recumbency.*'

(ii) The study was conducted using an appropriately wide range of animals (Tables 2 and 3). Only dogs and cats were of interest, and all dogs and cats that underwent anaesthesia in the relevant period were included. Although the authors collected information on species, they do not report the results in the paper. Exclusions are documented on page 61 (Patients' recruitment); those patients sedated or anaesthetized in order to be euthanased or that were euthanased during anaesthesia because of medical reasons were excluded.

(b) General methodology

All methods are clearly presented in the Data collection section (p. 61) and in the Anaesthetic regimens section (pp. 61–2).

(c) Study design

The study is clearly stated as an observational cohort study (p. 61, Methods). The authors explain (p. 61, Patients' recruitment) that all the animals underwent general anaesthesia at the Centre Hospitalier Vétérinaire des Cordeliers, between 15 April 2008 and 15 April 2010. The authors were aware that a bias might arise from the decision to use a particular anaesthetic protocol, and this was addressed by introducing the American Society of Anesthesiologists (ASA) status as a covariate in the multivariable model (p. 61, Data collection). Potential selection biases are documented in the Discussion section (p. 65, LHS and p. 66, LHS). Randomization and blinding were not relevant in this observational study.

(d) Variables

(i) The only outcome of interest was whether or not there was an anaesthetic death (specifically stated on p. 63, LHS).

(ii) There were no secondary outcomes.

(iii) No changes to outcomes were made after the start of the study.

(iv) There is a clear description of explanatory variables: ASA status, species, type of procedure, anaesthetic protocol, epidural and age (p. 63, LHS).

(e) Sample size

There is no power statement to justify the overall sample size. Subgroup analysis was performed on the 944 animals that belonged to ASA categories 3, 4 and 5. The subgroup was defined because the authors found that there were no deaths in ASA category 1 and only three deaths in ASA category 2: the sample size of the subgroup was not based on power calculations but was, nevertheless, substantial at 944.

(f) Statistical methods

(i) The unit of investigation is clearly identified as the animal (p. 63, LHS).

(ii) All the statistical methods employed for all data analyses are clearly identified (pp. 62–3, Data analysis). To summarize: as a first step, the non-parametric Mann–Whitney test was performed to analyse the relationship between ASA score and mortality. Confidence intervals are provided for the percentage of deaths in each ASA category. As a second step, univariate and bivariate analyses, followed by multivariate (strictly 'multivariable') logistic regression, were performed on animals with an ASA score of 3 or more. ROC (receiver operating characteristic) curves were constructed to assess the fit of the models.

(iii) The statistical methods in the paper are appropriate. The authors explain that they grouped age into '*four categories of equal importance*' (p. 62, RHS and Table 2). 'Importance' is not explained: the authors probably mean groups of approximately equal size, as suggested by the group sizes in Table 2.

(iv) The only numerical variable was age in years. This was grouped arbitrarily (p. 62, RHS) into four categories, as shown in Table 2.

(v) There were no additional analyses other than the subgroup analysis explained in Part 3e.

(vi) There are no missing data other than the losses to follow-up (see Part 3f(vii)).

(vii) There were 35 animals that were lost to follow-up/forgotten (p. 63, Results, LHS and Figure 1). They were excluded from the analysis (Figure 1) and there was no attempt to estimate the missing data.

(viii) It was not necessary to perform a sensitivity analysis (no assumptions were violated and a very small proportion of animals were lost to follow-up).

(ix) Information about software and significance level is given on pages 62–3 (Data analysis). Mann–Whitney/Wilcoxon tests were analysed by EpiInfo 3.5.1 (Centers for Disease Control and Prevention, GA, USA). Confidence intervals were calculated using Epidat 3.1 (Epidat: PanAmerican Health Organization, WA, DC USA). Logistic regression models were created using R software 2.9.0 (R Foundation for Statistical Computing, Austria). The significance level was set to 5% (but it was 15% for variables kept in the backward stepwise logistic regression model).

(4) Results

(a) Animal numbers and dates

(i) There is a clear report of the number of subjects included at each stage of the study in the flow chart (Figure 1).

(ii) The numbers of and reasons for exclusions and the numbers of losses to follow-up are documented (p. 63, Results, LHS; p. 64, RHS paragraph 5; and Figure 1).

(iii) The authors explain that recruitment was between 15 April 2008 and 15 April 2010 (p. 61, Patients' recruitment).

(b) Baseline data

See Point 4c(i).

(c) Descriptive data

(i) The characteristics at baseline of study participants are not provided for the whole group of animals. However, some of this information is given in Tables 1 and 2 for the 944 animals who were in ASA categories 3, 4 and 5. Sex, species, developmental stage and weight distributions of the animals are not summarized. Numbers of dogs and cats in each ASA status group are shown in Table 3.

(ii) Housing of the animals is not relevant.

(iii) Covariate adjusted odds ratios are provided for group comparisons in Table 4.

(iv) There is no indication of the number of participants, if any, with missing data for each variable of interest.

(v) The follow-up time is defined as the meeting point of the return of consciousness, rectal temperature >36°C and ability to maintain sternal recumbency; it is not necessary to summarize this (e.g. as mean).

(d) Numbers analysed

The number of animals anaesthetized and analysed in the first phase is stated in the Results section (p. 63, LHS) as 3546; 944 of these animals were analysed in the second phase of the statistical analysis (Figure 1 and p. 63, RHS).

(e) Outcomes of interest

(i) **Main outcome of interest.** The outcome of interest was death. Information is provided on deaths in each ASA category for the whole sample of 3546 animals, and separately for these dogs and cats, in Table 3. Some additional information on deaths according to potential risk factors is provided in Table 2 for the subset of 944 animals that were in ASA categories 3, 4 and 5.

(ii) **Magnitude of the effect of interest.** The estimated risk of death for the whole group of 3546 animals, as well as in each ASA category, is provided in Table 3. The analysis revealed that 48 animals out of 3546 (1.35%) died. The estimated risk of death in ASA categories 1–5 were 0.0%, 0.12%, 2.90%, 7.59% and 17.33%, respectively. (Note: the proportion of perioperative deaths in ASA category 3 is actually 0.16% and not 0.12% as in the table.) The estimated odds ratio is provided in Table 4 for each of a number of potential risk factors for the subgroup of

944 animals in ASA categories 3–5. Significant risk factors were: (i) ASA categories 4 and 5 compared to ASA category 3 (estimated OR = 3.7 and 13.4, respectively); and (ii) 'other anaesthetic regimen' (i.e. a group comprising 66 different regimens that excluded the three regimens defined by the bullet points on p. 62, LHS) compared to premed + thiopental + isoflurane (estimated OR = 0.1), which was not what the authors expected at the start of the study. Although the authors hypothesized that cats would be at greater risk than dogs, this was not a significant effect in the logistic regression (OR = 1.9, $P = 0.11$). The authors have provided only covariate adjusted estimates in Table 4, obtained from the logistic regression analysis. It is assumed that they included these covariates after each was found to be significant in the univariable analyses that preceded the logistic regression analysis (p. 63, LHS), although this is not explicitly stated. Four times in the Results section, the authors report 'a tendency' for a decrease/increase in the odds/risk of dying for one group compared with another. This approach to reporting results that are not statistically significant is potentially misleading.

(iii) **Precision of the effect of interest.** The 95% confidence intervals for the risk of death for the whole group (0.96 to 1.75: p. 63, RHS), and according to ASA status, are provided in Table 3. Ninety-five per cent confidence intervals for the odds ratios of various risk factors for the subset of 944 animals are provided in the text and Table 4 (p. 63, RHS and p. 64, LHS).

(f) Additional analyses

Most of the results relate to the subgroup of 944 patients that were in ASA categories 3–5. The authors decided to do these *post hoc* analyses because only three deaths occurred in ASA categories 1 and 2.

(g) Harms

This is not relevant in an observational cohort study.

(5) Discussion

(a) Deciding whether the results are important

(i) The key findings summarized with reference to the study objectives are stated in the final paragraph of the paper (p. 67), '*the risk of anaesthetic death appears to be comparable with risk reported internationally. Patients of ASA status 3 and over appear to be considerably more at risk than patients of ASA status 1 and 2.*' The authors also state that '*When considering patients of ASA status 3 and over, the use of an anaesthetic protocol that included premedication, induction with thiopental and maintenance with isoflurane, was associated with increased odds of anaesthetic death when compared to the group "other anaesthetic regimen"*' (p. 64, Discussion, paragraph 1).

(ii) The results make biological sense, although we agree with the authors that the finding regarding the relatively better outcome from the 'other' group of anaesthetic regimens was unexpected.

(iii) The 95% confidence interval for the risk of death for animals in ASA category 1 is 0.0% to 0.52% rising to 8.10% to 26.57% for those in ASA category 5 (Table 3). The lower limit of the confidence interval for those in ASA category 5 is substantially greater than the upper limit of that for those in ASA category 1, suggesting that this is an important and unambiguous result. Furthermore, the upper limit of the confidence interval for those in ASA category 5 is high at 26.57%, further emphasizing the importance of the result and the implication for those animals in the highest ASA category. In addition, the 95% confidence interval for the odds ratio of death in ASA category 5 compared with category 3 in the subset of 944 animals is 5.8 to 30.4. Both of these limits are substantially greater than 1 and emphasize the importance of ASA status in evaluating the risk of anaesthetic death for dogs and cats.

(iv) The number needed to treat is not relevant in this observational study.

(v) Although the odds ratios are provided for the subset of 944 patients with ASA status 3, 4 and 5, the actual risk of anaesthetic death is also provided for each ASA category for the whole group of 3546 animals.

(vi) Herd immunity is not relevant in this study.

(b) Limitations

The authors discuss study limitations, including potential sources of bias, in the Discussion on pages 65 and 66. In particular, they say that '*A potential selection bias comes from the fact that the Centre Hospitalier Vétérinaire des Cordeliers is a referral centre*' and '*Referral practices usually anaesthetize a greater proportion of patients classified in the ASA 3, 4 and 5 categories*' (p. 65, LHS). They also say that '*The anaesthetic protocol was established by the veterinarian in charge, in light of his experience. Anaesthetist's experience is a subjective concept and is hard to analyse. It refers to numerous factors . . . . Many of these factors could not be tested as variables in the logistic regression models and this could have led to a selection bias*' (p. 65, RHS). In addition, in relation to the significant odds of anaesthetic death in those animals receiving 'premedication + thiopental + isoflurane' compared with those in the 'other protocol' group, '*It is probable that, despite ASA classification, anaesthetist's experience leads to a subjective evaluation of the risk. This can lead to the establishment of "another protocol". This leads to a selection bias*' (p. 66, LHS). The authors state that '*Dog owners might be more likely to seek medical attention than cat owners. A selection bias could therefore enhance the association between dogs and anaesthesia-related death, compared to cats. Also, cats' health status is, in general, less easily assessable than dogs*', possibly resulting in poorer preoperative assessment of the feline patients.' The authors believe that, because there was a '*small number of subjects (944) . . . the tendency for cats to be more prone to anaesthesia-related death could have been significant if a greater number of patients had been included*' (p. 66, last paragraph LHS and first paragraph RHS). Finally, the authors believe that the arbitrary age grouping was unlikely to be representative of the metabolic state of patients. '*However, number of subjects enrolled was too low to allow a more detailed classification and an age effect on anaesthetic mortality could have gone undetected'* (p. 66, RHS paragraph 4).

(c) Generalizability
The authors discuss the generalizability of their findings to other veterinary practices on page 67 (LHS). They note that the '*Centre Hospitalier Vétérinaire des Cordeliers has a different caseload from most practitioners and many of the anaesthetized patients are presented because of the severity of their condition and the necessity for a complex surgical procedure. Patients of clinical status of ASA 3, 4 and 5 represented 26.6% of our anaesthetized population whereas practice-based studies have shown that 5–10% of the patients were in these categories. Also, anaesthesia might not be routinely monitored the same way in every practice.'*

(d) Interpretation
Taking the limitations of the study, and subgroup analyses, and the results from other similar studies, we believe the authors' interpretation of the study findings is consistent with the results.

(6) Other information
No sources of funding are documented nor is there a conflict of interest statement for each of the investigators.

18.6 Paper 2

Lori, J.C., Stein, T.J. & Thamm, D.H. (2010) Doxorubicin and cyclophosphamide for the treatment of canine lymphoma: a randomized, placebo-controlled study. *Veterinary and Comparative Oncology* **8** (3) 188–95. (Reproduced with permission from the publisher, Wiley-Blackwell.)

Veterinary and
Comparative Oncology

Original Article   DOI: 10.1111/J.1476-5829.2010.00215.x

Doxorubicin and cyclophosphamide for the treatment of canine lymphoma: a randomized, placebo-controlled study*

J. C. Lori[1], T. J. Stein[2] and D. H. Thamm[1]

[1] Animal Cancer Center, Colorado State University College of Veterinary Medicine, Fort Collins, CO, USA
[2] School of Veterinary Medicine, University of Wisconsin-Madison, Madison, WI, USA

Abstract

Median survival times (STs) for doxorubicin-treated canine lymphoma range from 5.7 to 9 months. Because dogs treated with multi-agent protocols have longer STs, we sought to evaluate whether adding cyclophosphamide would improve outcome in canine lymphoma patients while maintaining an acceptable level of toxicity. Thirty-two dogs with stage III–V multicentric lymphoma were treated with doxorubicin every 3 weeks for five total cycles and prednisone at a tapering dose for the first 4 weeks. Dogs were randomized to receive either cyclophosphamide or placebo concurrently. Seventeen dogs received doxorubicin and placebo, while 15 dogs received doxorubicin and cyclophosphamide. Response, toxicity, progression-free interval (PFI) and ST were evaluated. The combination of doxorubicin and cyclophosphamide was well tolerated, causing no increase in adverse events over doxorubicin alone. Despite a numeric improvement in outcome in cyclophosphamide treated dogs, the addition of cyclophosphamide did not result in statistically improved response rate, PFI or ST.

Keywords
adriamycin, cancer, chemotherapy, cytoxan, dog

Introduction

Lymphoma is the most common haematopoietic neoplasm in dogs. Standard of care treatment involves multi-agent chemotherapy protocols that incorporate doxorubicin. Most combination protocols are so-called CHOP-based, which use cyclophosphamide, doxorubicin, vincristine and prednisone, with 80–90% complete response (CR) rates and median survival times (STs) of approximately 12 months reported[1,2]; however, the use of multi-agent protocols is not always possible because of cost or time constraints on the part of owners.

Doxorubicin is an anthracycline derived from the *Streptomyces* yeast. It has multiple mechanisms of action. These include intercalation of DNA, which leads to inhibition of protein synthesis and free radical formation, and inhibition of topoisomerase enzymes. Major toxicities associated with doxorubicin are bone marrow suppression, gastrointestinal upset, including nausea, vomiting and diarrhoea, and myocardial toxicity, which is cumulative and dose limiting.[3–6] Single-agent therapy with doxorubicin results in STs greater than those of prednisone alone for the treatment of canine lymphoma. Reported remission durations range from 4.3 to 6.8 months, STs from 5.7 to 9 months, and reported response rates of 59–85%.[7–11]

Cyclophosphamide is an alkylating agent that can be given orally in dogs, with relatively little toxicity, including bone marrow suppression and sterile haemorrhagic cystitis.[3,12–15] Although doxorubicin has been evaluated as a single agent for lymphoma

Correspondence address:
Dr D. H. Thamm
Animal Cancer Center
Colorado State University
College of Veterinary
Medicine
300 W. Drake Road
Fort Collins, CO 80523-1620
e-mail:
dthamm@colostate.edu

*This data was presented in part at the meeting of the Veterinary Cancer Society on October 17, 2009 in Austin, Texas.

in dogs, cyclophosphamide has not. The ability to administer cyclophosphamide and prednisone orally allows for these drugs to be given concurrently with doxorubicin with minimal time or effort on the part of the owner, and with little added expense. Previously, cyclophosphamide was evaluated in combination with doxorubicin as a maintenance protocol following induction with vincristine and L-asparaginase for 28 dogs with stage III–V lymphoma. In this study, the median remission duration was 173 days (5.7 months), which appeared similar to those in single-agent doxorubicin protocols.[16] Data regarding first-line use of doxorubicin/cyclophosphamide combination chemotherapy have not been reported to our knowledge.

The purpose of this prospective study was to evaluate whether the addition of oral cyclophosphamide to five doses of doxorubicin and oral prednisone would increase median progression-free interval (PFI), response rate, ST or toxicity in dogs with treatment-naïve multicentric lymphoma.

Materials and methods

Patient population

Thirty-two dogs with multicentric lymphoma that were presented to the Animal Cancer Center at Colorado State University or the University of Wisconsin-Madison School of Veterinary Medicine between September of 2007 and October of 2008 were included in the study. The study design was prospective in nature. Dogs were eligible for the study if they were stage II–V, substage a or b and the owners elected to treat with single-agent doxorubicin. Breed, sex and age at diagnosis were recorded for each dog. All dogs were naïve to chemotherapy including corticosteroids. The staging system of the World Health Organization for canine lymphoma was used to determine stage

and substage. A complete blood count (CBC), serum chemistry and urinalysis were required for entry into the study. Thoracic radiographs, abdominal ultrasound and bone marrow aspirate were documented when performed for staging. Immunophenotype, as assessed by Polymerase Chain Reaction for antigen receptor rearrangement, immunohistochemistry, immunocytochemistry or flow cytometry, was recorded when available.

Treatment

If owners chose single-agent doxorubicin as treatment, and elected to enroll in the study, dogs were randomized to receive either cyclophosphamide or placebo. The randomization scheme was generated by using the web site Randomization.com (http://www.randomization.com). Patients were treated with doxorubicin ($30 \, \mathrm{mg \, m^{-2}}$) IV every 3 weeks for a total of five cycles and prednisone at a tapering dose for the first 4 weeks (Table 1). Based on randomization to treatment or placebo group, patients received either cyclophosphamide (target dose $50 \, \mathrm{mg \, m^{-2}}$ daily for three days) or placebo concurrently, starting on the same day as the doxorubicin dosing.

Response and toxicity

CR (complete resolution of disease), partial response (at least 30% or greater reduction in sums of the longest diameters of measurable peripheral nodes), PFI, ST and number of grade 3/4 adverse events were compared between groups. Response was determined using the Response Evaluation Criteria in Solid Tumors (RECIST) criteria.[17] Stable disease was defined as neither a 30% decrease or 20% increase in the sums of the longest diameters of measurable peripheral lymph nodes, while progressive disease (PD) was defined as a greater than

Table 1. Chemotherapy protocol dogs were scheduled to receive

Drug and dosage	Weeks												
	1	2	3	4	5	6	7	8	9	10	11	12	13
Doxorubicin ($30 \, \mathrm{mg \, m^{-2}}$)	X			X			X			X			X
Cyclophosphamide ($50 \, \mathrm{mg \, m^{-2}}$ daily $\times$ 3 days) or Placebo	X			X			X			X			X
Prednisone ($\mathrm{mg \, kg^{-1} \, day^{-1}}$)	2	1.5	1	0.5									

20% increase in the sums of the longest diameters. The PFI was defined as the time from first treatment to the date of PD. The ST was calculated as the time from the date of the first treatment to the date of death. Toxicity was graded 1–4, and based on the Veterinary Co-operative Oncology Group common terminology criteria for adverse events.[18] Using this grading scheme, Grade 1 neutropenia was defined as 1500 cells μL^{-1} to the lower limit of normal, which was 2000 cells μL^{-1} for both institutions. Haematological toxicity was evaluated 7 days after the first treatment, and subsequently at the time of each treatment, if dosage adjustments were not made.

Upon completion of the five treatments, it was recommended that animals be seen once monthly for rechecks involving a physical examination. Blood work was performed at the discretion of the clinician. If lymph node enlargement was palpated, cytology was used to confirm relapse. Information regarding rescue therapy pursued following relapse was collected, and outcome information collected following relapse via recheck examinations and telephone conversations with owners and referring veterinarians.

Statistical analysis

Power analysis was performed prospectively and prior to enrollment of patients. With a planned total of 32 dogs to enroll, this study was powered to detect a 3.1-fold increase in PFI or ST with 80% power and a *P* value of 0.05. CR versus partial or no response and the presence of grade 3/4 adverse events were compared between groups for significance using a two-tailed Fisher's exact test. This test was also used to evaluate for differences between groups for substage, hypercalcaemia and T-cell immunophenotype, all of which have been associated with prognosis in previous studies. Stage was not evaluated as a result of inconsistencies in staging tests performed between patients. A Student's two-tailed unpaired *t*-test was used to compare age between groups. The PFI and ST curves were generated by the Kaplan–Meier product limit method. A log rank (Mantel–Cox) test was used to compare the curves. In all analyses, a *P* value of <0.05 was considered statistically significant. Statistical analyses were performed

using Prism 5 software (GraphPad, San Diego, CA, USA).

Results

Patients

Thirty-two dogs with lymphoma were included in the study. Patient characteristics by treatment group are listed in Table 2. All patients received full blood work as part of staging, while some patients received thoracic radiographs, abdominal ultrasound and/or bone marrow aspirates. There were no significant differences between the two groups with regard to age, weight, sex, substage, immunophenotype or the presence of hypercalcaemia.

Treatment and toxicity

The overall number of doses of doxorubicin and cyclophosphamide given ranged from 1 to 5 (median 5) for both groups. In the doxorubicin and placebo group, the mean starting dose of doxorubicin was 28.1 mg m^{-2} (range 19.7–30.3 mg m^{-2}). In the doxorubicin and cyclophosphamide group, the mean starting dose of doxorubicin was 27.7 mg m^{-2} (range 18.1–30.3 mg m^{-2}), while the mean starting dose of cyclophosphamide was 159 mg m^{-2}

Table 2. Patient characteristics by treatment group

	Doxorubicin + cyclophos- phamide (*n* = 15)	Doxorubicin + placebo (*n* = 17)	*P* value
Age (years)			0.83
Mean	8.25 ± 2.57	8.47 ± 3.07	
Median	8	9	
Range	5–13	2–14	
Body weight (mean in kg)	31.7 ± 4.1	33.3 ± 3.2	0.76
Sex			1.0
Male	10 (66.7%)	12 (64.7%)	
Female	5 (33.3%)	5 (35.2%)	
Substage			0.32
a	12 (80.0%)	16 (94.1%)	
b	3 (20.0%)	1 (5.9%)	
Immuno- phenotype			0.49
B	6 (40.0%)	5 (29.4%)	
T	2 (13.3%)		
Null		2 (11.8%)	
Hypercalcaemia	2 (13.3%)	1 (5.9%)	0.58

Table 3. Grade 3/4 adverse events by number of patients

	Cyclophosphamide	Placebo
Grade 3/4 toxicities[a]	6 (8 events)	5 (5 events)
Grade 3/4 haematological toxicities	6 (8 events)	3 (3 events)
Grade 3 anaemia	1	0
Grade 3 neutropenia	1	0
Grade 4 neutropenia	2	1
Grade 3 thrombocytopenia	2	2
Grade 4 thrombocytopenia	2	0
Grade 3/4 gastrointestinal toxicity	0	2
Grade 3 vomiting	0	2

[a]$P = 0.71$.

divided over 3 days (range 123–192 mg m^{-2}). The distribution of adverse events is outlined in Table 3. In the cyclophosphamide group, there were three animals that did not have a follow-up CBC 1 week after the first treatment. There were six animals in the cyclophosphamide group that had grade 3 or 4 haematological toxicity, and no animals with grade 3/4 gastrointestinal toxicity. Of these patients, there were two patients that had dose reductions, one in the patient that had grade 3 thrombocytopenia and grade 4 neutropenia, and the other in a patient with grade 4 neutropenia. When dose reductions were made, the doxorubicin was reduced, as it was unknown whether patients were receiving cyclophosphamide or placebo.

In the placebo group, there were also three animals that did not have a follow-up CBC 1 week after the first treatment. There were three patients in the placebo group that had grade 3 or 4 haematological toxicity, and two with grade 3/4 gastrointestinal toxicity. Two patients had dose reductions in the placebo group. There was no significant difference in the number of patients with grade 3/4 toxicities between groups ($P = 0.71$) or the number of dose reductions between groups ($P = 1.0$). There were two patients in the study that died or were euthanized as a result of presumed cardiac disease. Both of these patients were in the cyclophosphamide group. There was no significant difference in cardiac disease between the groups ($P = 0.21$). There were two patients that died 6 and 7 days after the first treatment in the placebo group of unknown

causes. Postmortem examinations were not performed on either patient. There were no other reported toxicities.

Outcome

Overall, there were 11/15 (73.3%) CRs in the cyclophosphamide group and 13/17 (76.4%) in the placebo group ($P = 0.65$). Most dogs experienced a CR by the time they were presented for their second treatment, although a few dogs did not achieve CR until after the second treatment. The median PFI for the cyclophosphamide group was 246 days (range of 7–337 days), while the PFI for the placebo group was 169 days (range 6–428; Fig. 1). This difference was not statistically significant ($P = 0.58$).

The median ST for the cyclophosphamide group was 423 days (range 7–564), while the median ST for the placebo group was 295 days (range 6–545; Fig. 2). This difference was also not statistically significant ($P = 0.11$). When evaluating rescue protocols received, 10 of the 10 dogs in the cyclophosphamide group eligible to receive rescue therapy were treated. Four dogs received CCNU, L-asparaginase and prednisone, three dogs received the investigational drug GS-9219 (Gilead Sciences, Foster City, CA, USA),[19,20] one dog received an additional dose of doxorubicin and cyclophosphamide, and two dogs received multiple rescue protocols consisting of idarubicin, vinblastine, L-asparaginase/vincristine/melphalan, Cyclophosphamide/vincristine/prednisone (COP), CCNU or bleomycin/DTIC. Of the eight dogs eligible to receive rescue therapy in the placebo group, five received rescue therapy. Two dogs received CCNU, L-asparaginase and prednisone, one dog

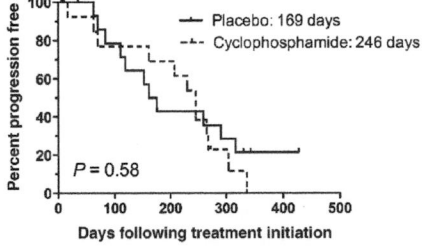

Figure 1. Kaplan Meier curve of progression free interval comparing cyclophosphamide and placebo groups.

© 2010 Blackwell Publishing Ltd, *Veterinary and Comparative Oncology*, **8**, 3, 188–195

192   J. C. Lori *et al.*

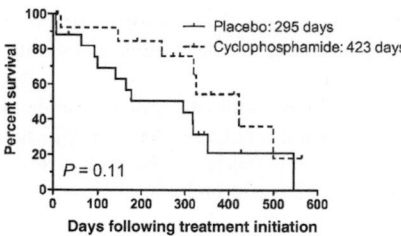

Figure 2. Kaplan Meier curve of survival time comparing cyclophosphamide and placebo groups.

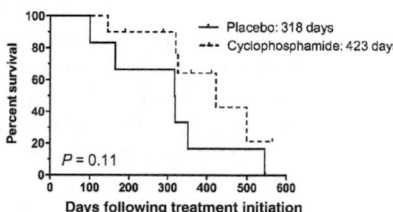

Figure 3. Kaplan Meier curve of survival time of dogs receiving rescue therapy comparing cyclophosphamide and placebo groups.

received cyclophosphamide and prednisone, and two dogs received multiple rescue protocols consisting of GS-9219, CCNU, L-asparaginase, vincristine or mitoxantrone. The difference in the percentage of dogs receiving rescue therapy at relapse between groups approached significance ($P = 0.06$). When only the dogs of each group that received rescue chemotherapy were compared for survival (Fig. 3), the median ST of cyclophosphamide dogs was 423 days, while that of placebo dogs was 318 days ($P = 0.11$). When the dogs receiving rescue therapy were separated from the eligible dogs who did not receive rescue, regardless of whether they received placebo or cyclophosphamide, dogs that received rescue therapy had a median ST of 352 days, which was significantly longer than those that did not receive rescue therapy (295 days; $P = 0.01$).

Discussion

This study compared outcome in dogs treated for multicentric lymphoma with doxorubicin, cyclophosphamide and prednisone to outcome in dogs treated with doxorubicin, placebo and prednisone. Results of the present study suggest that the combination of doxorubicin and cyclophosphamide for treatment of canine lymphoma was well tolerated, causing no significant increase in adverse events over doxorubicin alone. However, the addition of cyclophosphamide in this study did not result in significantly improved response, PFI or ST.

Although there was no statistical difference in the PFI or ST between the two groups, there was a longer median PFI and ST for the dogs treated with doxorubicin and cyclophosphamide. The most noticeable difference was in the ST between the two groups, with a ST of 423 days for the cyclophosphamide group versus 295 days for the placebo group. Given the differences in rescue therapy elected, we speculated that this difference could be explained in part by the difference in rescue protocols between groups. The cyclophosphamide group had a larger number of patients receiving rescue therapy than the placebo group, which statistically approached significance. When only patients that received rescue therapy were compared for survival between the two groups, the curves were similar to the initial survival curves (423 days versus 318 days for cyclophosphamide and placebo groups, respectively), with an equivalent P value, suggesting a minimal contribution of rescue therapy to patient outcome.

With a total of 32 dogs, this study was powered to detect a 3.1-fold increase in PFI or ST with 80% power and a P value of 0.05. In order to detect the 1.45-fold improvement in outcome observed in this study with 80% power, a total of 255 patients would have been required. Because of the minimal added expense, ease of administration, and lack of additional toxicity, it may be reasonable to add cyclophosphamide to doxorubicin and prednisone in this population. Given the limited power in this study, it may be dangerous to interpret that cyclophosphamide is not useful in addition to doxorubicin because of type II error, failing to accept the null hypothesis when it is in fact true.[21]

It has been previously shown that lymphoma dogs treated with single-agent doxorubicin are more responsive to rescue protocols than are dogs treated with COP.[8] It seems that the addition of cyclophosphamide does not negatively affect the ST of dogs receiving rescue therapy, given that the ST of cyclophosphamide treated dogs remained greater when patients not receiving rescue therapy were removed from the survival curve. Thus, the addition of cyclophosphamide remains more convenient and less expensive than CHOP-based protocols, and likely does not influence the response to rescue therapy negatively.

The two populations of dogs in this study were comparable in terms of age, sex, weight and potential prognostic factors. The randomization scheme avoided potential biases between groups. One limitation was that most of the dogs were not staged with a bone marrow aspirate and many were not immunophenotyped, owing to a lack of financial support for these aspects of the trial. This makes it difficult to compare the groups for these two important prognostic factors, and although statistical differences did not exist between the groups, this could have contributed to the differences in PFI and ST.

Ultimately, most dogs that achieve remission are likely to experience a relapse of disease, possibly representing the emergence of resistant tumour clones. It is somewhat intuitive that dogs receiving rescue therapy after relapsing following induction would have a longer ST than those receiving prednisone alone or no rescue therapy, although this has never been evaluated systematically in dogs with lymphoma. This study demonstrates that patients receiving some form of chemotherapy following relapse had a statistically longer ST than those that received palliative therapy (prednisone) or no treatment. This seems logical and again could have contributed to the longer numerical ST in the cyclophosphamide group, although the difference among the groups in those patients that received rescue therapy was not statistically significant.

Prednisone was administered in addition to the doxorubicin in this study, as the authors felt that it may improve quality of life during the induction period and could also increase response and survival. The results for the placebo group, with a median ST of 295 days (9.8 months) is similar to those reported historically for doxorubicin alone (median ST 5.7–9 months).[7–11] Similarly, there appears to be no difference in percentage of patients responding to treatment with the addition

of prednisone, although comparison with historical controls does not allow meaningful statistical evaluation.

Doxorubicin-associated cardiomyopathy did not seem to be a significant occurrence in this study. There were two patients in this study that died because of suspected cardiac disease, one euthanized because of heart failure and one that died of suspected heart failure. Neither of these patients' disease was confirmed to be a result of therapy with doxorubicin. Neither patient had a prescreening echocardiogram and one patient was a Doberman Pinscher, a breed known to be predisposed to dilated cardiomyopathy. Both of these patients were in the cyclophosphamide group, but there was no statistical difference in the incidence of cardiac disease between the two groups, although this study was not powered to detect such a small difference. It has been shown in people that cyclophosphamide given concurrently with doxorubicin may lower the cumulative dose necessary for the development of cardiac toxicity.[22] A cumulative dose of 180 mg m^{-2} was the maximum dose given in the cyclophosphamide group in one dog, the remainder receiving 150 mg m^{-2}. The addition of concurrent cyclophosphamide, although dosed over 3 days following the doxorubicin, did not seem to increase the development of cardiomyopathy.

In summary, we found no significant differences in the response rate, PFI, ST or prevalence of toxicity in dogs treated with doxorubicin, placebo and prednisone versus doxorubicin, cyclophosphamide and prednisone. This suggests that although well tolerated and given with little added expense, there was no statistical improvement in outcome with the addition of cyclophosphamide in the present population. The authors strongly feel that this question may be better answered in a larger population of dogs with lymphoma.

Acknowledgements

We would like to acknowledge Dr Jens Eickhoff for helpful discussions, as well as Drs Ruthanne Chun and David Vail for case management and helpful discussions. This study was funded in part by grant 1UL1RR025011 from the Clinical and Translational Science Award (CTSA) program of the National

194   J. C. Lori *et al.*

Center for Research Resources (NCRR) National Institutes of Health (NIH) to T. J. S.

References

1. Garrett LD, Thamm DH, Chun R, Dudley R and Vail DM. Evaluation of a 6-month chemotherapy protocol with no maintenance therapy for dogs with lymphoma. *Journal of Veterinary Internal Medicine* 2002; **16**: 704–709.
2. Keller E, MacEwen E and Rosenthal R. Evaluation of prognostic factors and sequential combination chemotherapy with doxorubicin for canine lymphoma. *Journal of Veterinary Internal Medicine* 1993; **7**: 289–295.
3. Chun R, Garrett LD and Vail DM. Cancer chemotherapy. In: *Withrow and MacEwen's Small Animal Clinical Oncology*, 4th edn, St Louis, Saunders, 2007: 163–191.
4. Langer S, Sehested M and Jensen P. Treatment of anthracycline extravasation with dexrazoxane. *Clinical Cancer Research* 2000; **6**: 3680–3686.
5. Cvetkovic R and Scott L. Dexrazoxane: a review of its use for cardioprotection during anthracycline chemotherapy. *Drugs* 2005; **65**: 1005–1024.
6. Mauldin GE, Fox PR, Patnaik AK, Bond BR, Mooney SC and Matus RE. Doxorubicin-induced cardiotoxicosis. *Journal of Veterinary Internal Medicine* 1992; **6**: 82–88.
7. Vail DM and Young KM. Canine lymphoma and lymphoid leukemia. In: *Withrow & MacEwen's Small Animal Clinical Oncology*, 4th edn, St Louis, Saunders, 2007: 699–733.
8. Carter R, Harris C and Withrow SJ. Chemotherapy of canine lymphoma with histopathological correlation: doxorubicin alone compared to COP as first treatment regimen. *Journal of the American Animal Hospital Association* 1987; **23**: 587–596.
9. Postorino NC, Susaneck SJ, Withrow SJ, Macy DW and Harris C. Single agent therapy with adriamycin for canine lymphosarcoma. *Journal of the American Animal Hospital Association* 1989; **25**: 221–225.
10. Mutsaers AJ, Glickman NW, DeNicola DB, Widmer WR, Bonney PL, Hahn KA and Knapp DW. Evaluation of treatment with doxorubicin and piroxicam or doxorubicin alone for multicentric lymphoma in dogs. *Journal of the American Veterinary Medical Association* 2002; **220**: 1813–1817.
11. Valerius K, Ogilvie G, Mallinckrodt C and Getzy D. Doxorubicin alone or in combination with asparaginase, followed by cyclophosphamide, vincristine, and prednisone for treatment of multicentric lymphoma in dogs: 121 cases (1987–1995). *Journal of the American Veterinary Medical Association* 1997; **210**: 512–516.
12. Charney S, Bergman P, Hohenhaus A, Mcknight J. Risk factors for sterile hemorrhagic cystits in dogs with lymphoma receiving cyclophosphamide with or without concurrent administration of furosemide: 216 cases (1990-1996). *Journal of the American Veterinary Medical Association* 2003; **222**: 1388–1393.
13. Crow S, Theilen G, Madewell B, Weller RE and Henness AM. Cyclophosphamide induced cystitis in the dog and cat. *Journal of the American Veterinary Medical Association* 1977; **171**: 259–262.
14. Stanton M and Legendre A. Effects of cyclophosphamide in dogs and cats. *Journal of the American Veterinary Medical Association* 1986; **188**: 1319–1322.
15. Peterson J, Couto C, Hammer A and Ayl AD. Acute sterile hemorrhagic cystitis after single intravenous administration of cyclophosphamide in three dogs. *Journal of the American Veterinary Medical Association* 1992; **201**: 1572–1573.
16. Price GS, Page RL, Fischer BM, Levine JF and Gerig TM. Efficacy and toxicity of doxorubicin/cyclophosphamide maintenance therapy in dogs with multicentric lymphosarcoma. *Journal of Veterinary Internal Medicine* 1991; **5**: 259–262.
17. Therasse P, Arbuck SG, Eisenhauer EA, Wanders J, Kaplan RS, Rubinstein L, Verweij J, Van Glabbeke M, van Oosterom AT, Christian MC and Gwyther SG. New guidelines to evaluate response to treatment in solid tumors. European Organization for Research and Treatment of Cancer, National Cancer Institute of the United States, National Cancer Institute of Canada. *Journal of the National Cancer Institute* 2000; **92**: 205–216.
18. Veterinary co-operative oncology group – common terminology criteria for adverse events (VCOG-CTCAE) following chemotherapy or biological antineoplastic therapy in dogs and cats. *Veterinary and Comparative Oncology* 2004; **2**: 195–213.
19. Reiser H, Wang J, Chong L, Watkins WJ, Ray AS, Shibata R, Birkus B, Cihlar T, Wu S, Li B, Liu X, Henne IN, Wolfgang GH, Desai M, Rhodes GR, Fridland A, Lee WA, Plunkett W, Vail D, Thamm DH, Jeraj R and Tumas DB. GS-9219 – a novel acyclic nucleotide analogue with potent antineoplastic activity in dogs with spontaneous non-Hodgkin's lymphoma. *Clinical Cancer Research* 2008; **14**: 2824–2832.
20. Vail DM, Thamm DH, Reiser H, Ray AS, Wolfgang GH, Watkins WJ, Babusis D, Henne IN, Hawkins MJ, Kurzman ID, Jeraj R, Vanderhoek M,

Plaza S, Anderson C, Wessel MA, Robat C, Lawrence J and Tumas DB. Assessment of GS-9219 in a pet dog model of non-Hodgkin's lymphoma. *Clinical Cancer Research* 2009; **15**: 3503–3510.

21. Baldi B and Moore DS. Inference in practice: the power of a statistical test. In: *The Practice of*

Statistics in the Life Sciences, C Bleyer, ed., New York City, W. H. Freeman and Company, 2009: 398–405.

22. Minow R, Benjamin R, Lee E and Gottlieb J. Adriamycin cardiomyopathy – risk factors. *Cancer* 1977; **39**: 1397–1402.

18.7 Critical appraisal of paper 2

(1) Title and abstract

(a) The title states that the study is a randomized, placebo-controlled trial and this is also mentioned in the abstract, albeit obliquely. The drugs used in the treated group are indicated in both the title and abstract.

(b) The abstract summarizes the primary objective as determining whether adding cyclophosphamide rather than a placebo to a regimen of doxorubicin every 3 weeks for five cycles and prednisone at a tapering dose for 4 weeks would improve the (unspecified) outcome in canine lymphoma dogs. The authors conclude in the abstract that there was a clinical but not statistical improvement with the addition of cyclophosphamide, and that the combination of drugs was well tolerated. The numbers of dogs in each treatment group are stated (17 in the placebo group and 15 in the cyclophosphamide group) but no effects of interest are provided and no limitations are mentioned in the abstract.

(2) Introduction

(a) The rationale is set out logically and clearly in the Introduction and references are provided for the details included (pp. 188–9). The authors provide information about toxicity associated with doxorubicin, as well as remission durations and survival times (STs) (p. 188, RHS). They explain that cyclophosphamide has relatively little toxicity (p. 188, RHS) and that the ability to administer cyclophosphamide and prednisone orally allows for these drugs to be given concurrently with doxorubicin with minimal time or effort on the part of the owner, and with little added expense (p. 189, LHS). However, first-line use of doxorubicin/cyclophosphamide combination chemotherapy has not been reported as far as the authors are aware.

(b) The purpose of the study was *'to evaluate whether the addition of oral cyclophosphamide to five doses of doxorubicin and oral prednisone would increase median progression-free interval (PFI), response rate,* *ST or toxicity in dogs with treatment-naïve multicentric lymphoma'* (p. 189, LHS, paragraph 2). No single primary outcome of interest is identified. Instead, there appear to be four outcomes of equal importance (PFI, response rate, ST and toxicity).

(3) Materials and methods

(a) Animals

(i) There were 32 dogs with multicentric lymphoma in the study, all presenting at two institutions in the USA between September 2007 and October 2008 (p. 189, Patient population, paragraph 1). Inclusion criteria are documented: dogs were eligible *'if they were stage II–V, substage a or b and the owners elected to treat with single-agent doxorubicin . . . dogs were naïve to chemotherapy including corticosteroids.'* In addition, *'A complete blood count (CBC), serum chemistry and urinalysis were required for entry into the study'* (p. 189, RHS, paragraph 1).

(ii) No indication is given of the breeds of the dogs included in the study. Hence we cannot assess if the study was conducted using an appropriately wide range of animals.

(b) General methodology

(i) The methods are clearly presented: all dogs had baseline information collected on breed, sex and age at diagnosis, stage using the World Health Organization (WHO) system for canine lymphoma, CBC (complete blood count), serum chemistry and urinalysis. Some dogs received thoracic radiographs, abdominal ultrasound and/or bone marrow aspirates for staging (p. 189, Patient population). Other information was recorded when available. The treatment regimen is detailed in Table 1 and described under 'Treatment' on page 189. Explanations are provided for the definitions of outcomes under 'Response and toxicity' on pages 189–90. The conditions for determining PFI and ST are clearly outlined (p. 190, LHS). Toxicity of the drugs was assessed rigorously based on defined criteria (p. 190, LHS), and dosage reduction of doxorubicin only (p. 191, LHS, paragraph 1) was made in the light of severe toxicity.

Physical examination at monthly intervals was continued during follow-up when lymph nodes were assessed quantitatively to assess whether the disease was stable or progressive (p. 189, Response and toxicity, RHS). '*If lymph node enlargement was palpated cytology was used to confirm relapse*' (p. 190, LHS, second paragraph). On relapse, rescue therapy was considered and details are given of various rescue protocols used (p. 191, RHS, last paragraph). Outcome information was '*collected following relapse via recheck examinations and telephone conversations with owners and referring veterinarians*' (p. 190, LHS, paragraph 2).

(ii) It would appear that the assessment methods were applied to all dogs, irrespective of group (pp. 189–90, Response and toxicity).

(c) Study design

The authors describe the design as prospective (p. 189, Patient population) and indicate that it was a randomized, placebo-controlled trial (p. 189, Treatment). They provide information about the setting and dates, explaining that dogs were presented to the Animal Cancer Center at Colorado State University or the University of Wisconsin-Madison School of Veterinary Medicine between September 2007 and October 2008 (p. 189, Patient population).

(i) The authors explain that dogs were randomized to the treatment groups and that the randomization scheme was generated by using the website http://www.randomization.com. No indication is given of the type of randomization, nor who enrolled the subjects and who assigned the participants to the treatments.

(ii) No information is provided about blinding apart from the statement in the Results section on page 191 (LHS, paragraph 1), which states that '*it was unknown whether patients were receiving cyclophosphamide or placebo.*'

(iii) No information is provided as to whether the allocation sequence was concealed from those assigning subjects to treatments and those responsible for care of the animals.

(iv) With the exception that they received different treatments, there is no indication that the groups were treated differently.

(d) Variables

(i) Consideration is given to all important outcomes, namely complete resolution of disease (CR), partial response (at least 30% or greater reduction in sums of the longest diameters of measurable peripheral nodes), progression-free interval (PFI), survival time (ST) and number of grade 3/4 adverse events.

(ii) There is no clear distinction between the primary and secondary outcomes. All outcomes listed in Part 3d(i) are treated with equal importance. These outcomes are precisely defined (pp. 189–90, Response and toxicity).

(iii) No changes were made to outcomes after the start of the study.

(iv) There is a clear description of treatments. All dogs were treated with intravenous doxorubicin (30 mg/m^2) every 3 weeks for a total of five cycles and prednisone at a tapering dose for the first 4 weeks. Dogs received either cyclophosphamide (target dose 50 mg/m^2 daily for 3 days) or placebo concurrently, starting on the same day as the doxorubicin dosing (p. 189, Treatment). Table 1 also defines the chemotherapy protocol over the time period of interest, with the dogs receiving five treatments of cyclophosphamide or placebo in this time. Dose reductions were made only in doxorubicin in dogs experiencing severe toxicity. No information is given about potential confounders and effect modifiers.

(e) Sample size

(i) There is a power statement to justify the overall sample size (p. 190, Statistical analysis): '*this study was powered to detect a 3.1-fold increase in PFI or ST with 80% power and a P value of 0.05*', although the authors do not state the form of the statistical analysis on which it is based. Furthermore, the PFI and ST data were compared between treatment groups using survival analysis, and there is no suggestion that this was used for the sample size determination nor any indication of what was the parameter of interest (e.g. the median survival time or the hazard ratio).

(ii) There is no reference to any pilot studies that informed the power analysis.

(iii) There were no interim analyses.

(iv) The authors performed subgroup analyses on the dogs receiving rescue therapy but no sample size calculations were performed in relation to this subgroup.

(f) Statistical methods

(i) It is clear throughout the study that the dog is the unit of investigation.

(ii) The authors explain (p. 190, Statistical analysis) that categorical data were compared between the groups using Fisher's exact test. An unpaired *t*-test was used to compare age. Kaplan–Meier curves were generated for PFI and ST, and a log-rank test used to compare them in the two treatment groups. Tests were two-tailed and a significance level of 0.05 used throughout.

(iii) The statistical methods described are appropriate, although there is no mention of checking the assumptions of Normality and homoscedasticity for the *t*-test, and the authors have not taken into account the potential clustering resulting from the dogs presenting to two institutions.

(iv) The numerical variables were not grouped and no transformations were taken of them.

(v) The authors performed subgroup analyses on those dogs receiving rescue therapy. These analyses were not specified *a priori* but are presented in the Results section (p. 192, LHS). The authors compared the survival experience between the two treatment groups considering only the dogs that received rescue therapy. They also disregarded treatment, and compared the survival experience in those receiving rescue therapy and those not receiving rescue therapy if eligible for it.

(vi) There do not appear to be any missing data other than three dogs in each treatment group with no follow-up CBC 1 week after the first treatment (p. 191, LHS), which is not an outcome of primary interest.

(vii) Two dogs in the cyclophosphamide group died or were euthanized because of presumed cardiac disease and two dogs died of unknown causes in the placebo group after the first treatment. No attempts were made to deal with these losses.

(viii) No sensitivity analyses were performed.

(ix) The authors specify a significance level of 0.05 and report that the data were analysed using Prism 5 software (p. 190, Statistical analysis).

(4) Results

(a) Animal numbers and dates

(i) The authors show clearly that 17 dogs were randomized to the placebo group and 15 dogs were randomized to the cyclophosphamide group (Table 2).

(ii) Information relating to an observational study is not relevant as the study is not observational.

(iii) The numbers of and reasons for losses to follow-up are documented (see Part 3f(vii)).

(iv) Dates are provided that define the periods of recruitment (see Part 3a(i)) but not of the follow-up period (see Part 4c(v)).

(b) Baseline data

(i) Table 2 shows the baseline data for each group.

(ii) The groups were comparable (see Part 4c(iii)).

(c) Descriptive data

(i) The baseline variables, including age, weight and substage, of each treatment group are summarized in Table 2.

(ii) Information on housing and husbandry conditions is not relevant to this study.

(iii) The groups are shown to be comparable with respect to the variables presented in Table 2: this is confirmed on page 190 under Patients. The authors performed hypothesis tests to confirm comparability and provide *P*-values. In fact, when using randomization for treatment allocation, hypothesis tests should not be employed. A hypothesis test is used to see if the difference between the two treatment groups is due to chance. Since the groups in this study have been created by randomization (i.e. a method based on chance), any difference between the baseline values cannot be due to treatment and must be due to chance.

(iv) There were no exclusions. The only losses to follow-up were those dogs that died (see Part 3f(vii)).

(v) The follow-up time for the survival analysis is shown in Figures 2 and 3 to be up to about 550 days or approximately 1.5 years. The total follow-up time is not provided in the text, although the authors state that 564 days was the maximum survival time for dogs in the cyclophosphamide group (p. 191, Outcome).

(d) Numbers analysed

(i) Since there were no protocol violations, intention-to-treat (ITT) analysis is not relevant.

(ii) A sensitivity analysis was not performed.

(e) Outcomes of interest

(i) **Main outcome of interest.** The authors provide summary measures for all the important outcomes. In particular, they indicate (p. 191, Outcome) that there were 11/15 (73.3%) complete remissions in the cyclophosphamide group and 13/17 (76.4%) in the placebo group. The median PFI was 246 days (range 7–337 days) in the cyclophosphamide group and 169 days (range 6–428 days) in the placebo group. The median ST was 423 days (range 7–564 days) in the cyclophosphamide group and 295 days (range 6–545 days) in the placebo group. The authors provide P-values to afford a comparison of the summary measures in the treatment groups. The authors report that $P = 0.65$ for the comparison of the proportions of CRs in the cyclophosphamide and placebo groups (p. 191, RHS, paragraph 2); however, Fisher's exact test actually shows

that $P > 0.99$. It should be noted, furthermore, that if they performed the log-rank test as part of the survival analysis for ST and PFI, as stated in the Statistical analysis section on page 190, the P-value for each treatment comparison compares the overall survival (or progression-free interval) experienced and not the median values.

Two additional outcomes are reported: the toxicity data (Table 3, which would be improved by including total number of dogs in each group), dose reductions and deaths (p. 191, LHS) and the ST of those dogs receiving rescue therapy following relapse (p. 191, RHS, last paragraph). As summarized in Table 3 and reported in the text, there were six animals in the cyclophosphamide group that had grade 3 or 4 haematological toxicity, no animals with grade 3/4 gastrointestinal toxicity (p. 191, LHS, paragraph 1) and there were three patients in the placebo group that had grade 3 or 4 haematological toxicity, and two with grade 3/4 gastrointestinal toxicity (p. 191, LHS, paragraph 2). There was no significant difference in the number of patients with grade 3/4 toxicities between groups ($P = 0.71$) or the number of dose reductions between groups ($P = 1.0$) (p. 191, LHS, paragraph 2).

Some confusion exists in the terminology used to indicate the condition of eligibility for rescue therapy; it would have been helpful to use the term 'relapse' in connection with the definitions of progressive disease (PD) and termination of PFI (p. 190, LHS, paragraph 1). The results of rescue therapy are discussed in Part 4f.

(ii) **Magnitude of the effect of interest.** The authors do not provide any effects of interest (e.g. the difference in proportions or hazard ratios).

(iii) **Precision of the effect of interest.** The precision of the effects of interest is not provided.

(f) Additional analyses

Post hoc comparisons were made between the two treatment groups of the proportions receiving rescue therapy. The authors state (p. 191, Outcome) that 10 out of the 10 dogs eligible to receive rescue therapy in the cyclophosphamide group received rescue therapy, and five of the eight dogs eligible to receive rescue therapy in the placebo group received rescue therapy. They also provide a *P*-value for the comparison of the proportions receiving rescue therapy at relapse on page 192 ($P = 0.06$), although it is not certain that these proportions correspond to 10/10 and 5/8 as a Fisher's exact test on these figures gives $P = 0.07$ when they are compared. In addition, the authors performed a *post hoc* subgroup analysis (p. 192, LHS, paragraph 1). They considered only the dogs that received rescue therapy, and compared the two treatment groups using survival analysis (Figure 3), noting that the median ST of cyclophosphamide dogs was 423 days, while that of placebo dogs was 318 days ($P=0.11$). We believe this was an ill-advised analysis since there were only 10 dogs in the cyclophosphamide group and five dogs in the placebo group on which to base this survival analysis.

Finally, the authors performed another *post hoc* comparison (p. 192, LHS) by separating the dogs receiving rescue therapy from the eligible dogs who did not receive rescue therapy, regardless of whether they received placebo or cyclophosphamide. The 15 (five in the cyclophosphamide group and 10 in the placebo group) dogs that received rescue therapy had a median ST of 352 days, which was significantly longer than that of the three (none in the cyclophosphamide group and three in the placebo group) dogs that did not receive rescue therapy but were eligible for it (295 days; $P = 0.01$). Again, numbers are small here and such an analysis is, in our view, ill-advised.

(g) Harms

The toxicities experienced by the dogs in the two treatment groups are documented on page 191 (LHS) and in Table 3. Although two dogs died of presumed cardiac disease in the cyclophosphamide group (p. 191, LHS, paragraph 2) and no dogs died of cardiac disease in the placebo group, there was no evidence of a difference in cardiac disease between the groups ($P = 0.21$). There were no other reported toxicities.

(5) Discussion

(a) Deciding whether the results are important

(i)   The key findings are summarized with reference to the study objectives (p. 193, last paragraph of Discussion). The authors state that they '*found no significant differences in the response rate, PFI, ST or prevalence of toxicity in dogs treated with doxorubicin, placebo and prednisone versus doxorubicin, cyclophosphamide and prednisone. This suggests that although well tolerated and given with little added expense, there was no statistical improvement in outcome with the addition of cyclophosphamide in the present population.*'

The authors write (p. 192, RHS, paragraph 3) that '*it may be dangerous to interpret that cyclophosphamide is not useful in addition to doxorubicin because of type II error, failing to accept the null hypothesis when it is in fact true.*' The latter part of this statement is incorrect – a Type II error occurs when we do not reject the null hypothesis when it is false. However, by referring to a Type II error (equal to one minus the power of the study), there is a suggestion that the lack of significance is due to low power. This is supported by the authors' final recommendation to investigate the treatment effect in a larger population of dogs with lymphoma.

(ii) Treatment with cyclophosphamide in addition to doxorubicin and prednisolone is a rational step to explore to prolong survival and quality of life. In this small prospective study (32 dogs) the authors anticipated a 3.1-fold improvement and achieved only a 1.45-fold response, which in this study was not statistically significant, which may, as indicated in Part 5a(i), be due to low power.

(iii) No confidence intervals for the effect of interest are provided so we cannot decide on that basis whether the results are clinically important or unambiguous.

(iv) There is no evaluation of the number of subjects needed to treat (NNT) with the cyclophosphamide rather than the placebo in order to prevent one dog developing the 'bad' outcome.

(v) It is not relevant to translate relative risks into absolute risks.

(vi) Herd immunity is not relevant in this study.

(b) Limitations

The authors list a number of limitations. They speculate that the differences in rescue therapy elected could explain the differences in ST between the two groups (p. 192, RHS, paragraph 2). They also note that the power of the study was limited, and suggest that with a greater sample size and consequently a greater power, the effect of cyclophosphamide might be more marked (p. 192, RHS, paragraph 3). Finally, the authors explain that a limitation of the study was that *'most of the dogs were not staged with a bone marrow aspirate and many were not immunophenotyped, owing to a lack of financial support for these aspects of the trial. This makes it difficult to compare the groups for these two important prognostic factors, and although statistical differences did not exist between the groups, this could have contributed to the differences in PFI and ST'* (p. 193, LHS, paragraph 2).

(c) Generalizability

There is no discussion about the generalizability of the results.

(d) Interpretation

The authors conclude that *'although well tolerated and given with little added expense, there was no statistical improvement in outcome with the addition of cyclophosphamide in the present pop-ulation'* (p. 193, last paragraph of Discussion). This statement is consistent with their results and highlights that they can only make inferences about the population from which their dogs were taken. They recognize that their study may be underpowered as they go on to suggest that the question would be better answered with a larger population of dogs with lymphoma.

(6) Other information

The authors state (p. 193, Acknowledgements) that the study was funded in part by grant 1UL1RR025011 from the Clinical and Translational Science Award (CTSA) program of the National Center for Research Resources (NCRR) National Institutes of Health (NIH) to T. J. Stein (pp. 193–4). There is no conflict of interest statement.

18.8 General conclusion

So we have now come to the end of this book. We hope we have guided you through the basic steps of statistics and its applications, and you have sufficient confidence to tackle your own study design, data collection and analysis. We trust you will continue to build your confidence in your own abilities. It may be worth remarking that it has been said that you can torture the data to confess to anything, but a good statistics training controls your choices and limits your excesses. As you go on learning, you should not be too proud to consult someone who has more experience than you of statistical procedures. We wish you every success in all your statistical adventures!

Solutions to exercises

Chapter 1

1.1 (a) **F**: there are several sources of variation between animals, the most important being genetic variation. Biological variation describes it; it does not cause it. (b) **T**. (c) **F**: statistics deals with the problems of biological variation, but offers other benefits as well. (d) **F**: since we can rarely sample whole populations, there will always be an element of uncertainty in the conclusions we draw about biological data. Statistics deals with the biological variation in such a way as to quantitate that uncertainty. (e) **F**: no, this is known as technical error or fatigue!

1.2 (a) **F**: to achieve this, a sample would not have to be random. (b) **F**: a sample cannot claim to represent the full range of the population. (c) **F**: a sample does not claim to be made up of only 'normal' animals. (d) **T**: yes, a random sample aims to be representative. (e) **T**: a random sample excludes biases imposed by the process of selection.

1.3 (a) **T**. (b) **F**: a nominal variable is a particular type of categorical variable. (c) **F**: a nominal scale relates to a categorical variable which is not directly measurable. (d) **F**: percentages are numerical. (e) **F**: ranked data are measured on an ordinal scale.

1.4 (a) **S**: enzyme activity is temperature dependent; if the temperature falls, the enzyme

activity will be reduced. All samples will be similarly affected. (b) **S**: the readings will be raised or lowered to the nearest 0.5 degree mark, which is not random. (c) **S**: a zero offset will be present affecting every reading equally. (d) **S**: the scales will have been calibrated by activation after the load is placed. Should the scales be activated before the load is placed, this will probably induce a systematic error due to hysteresis. (e) **R**: this is a random error caused by attempts to read beyond the sensitivity of the instrument.

1.5 (a) **H**: there is no existing population of treated cows. (b) **R**: the population includes all horses at livery. (c) **R**: all fleas on all dogs in Liverpool make up this population. (d) **H**: there is no existing population of treated dogs. (e) **R**: the population includes all blood glucose readings from diabetic dogs.

1.6 (a) **N**: nominal since the classes are descriptive. (b) **C**: the percentage scale is continuous between 0 and 100, delimited only by the accuracy of the values. (c) **C**: light absorbance is measured on a continuous but arbitrary scale. (d) **O**: this arbitrary scale has only integer values, and a particular interval on the scale does not necessarily represent the same change in performance as we move up the scale. So, for example, the difference between 2 and 4 does not necessarily indicate the same change in performance as that between 5 and 7. (e) **C**: progesterone values are continuous, limited only by the sensitivity of the

Statistics for Veterinary and Animal Science, Third Edition. Aviva Petrie and Paul Watson.
© 2013 John Wiley & Sons, Ltd. Published 2013 by John Wiley & Sons, Ltd.

assay. (f) **N**: two classes defined by appearance. (g) **C**: optical density is another light intensity assay – a continuous scale. (h) **D**: litter size is an integer scale $1 - n$. (i) **O**: body condition is a sliding scale with various classes given numerical values but without any expectation that the intervals between classes are identical. (j) **D**: this is another integer scale since we are concerned only with counts in a year. (k) **C**: this is a continuous scale because the total number of counts divided by the total time in minutes results in a value that is not an integer. (l) **D**: although time is a continuous scale, since it is divided into days (integers), it should be considered to be D.

Chapter 2

2.1 (a) **T**. (b) **F**: the pie chart is useful for categorical data. (c) **T**. (d) **F**: the bar chart is useful for categorical or discrete data. (e) **T**.

2.2 (a) **F**: the mean will be unduly influenced by the extreme values and will overestimate the central tendency. (b) **T**. (c) **T**: this is the geometric mean. (d) **T**. (e) **T**: this is the median.

2.3 (a) **T**. (b) **F**. (c) **F**: for symmetrically distributed data, the range is approximately equal to four times the standard deviation. (d) **T**. (e) **F**: the standard deviation is the square root of the variance.

2.4 (a) **F**: the reference range can be determined as the difference between the 2.5th and 97.5th percentiles if the data are skewed. (b) **T**. (c) **F**: the reference range is meant to be representative of the population of healthy animals. A small sample is inadequate. (d) **F**: it is determined as mean ± 1.96SD, often approximated by mean ± 2SD. (e) **F**: the difference between the largest and smallest observations is the range, which may be unduly influenced by outliers.

2.5 (a) Class intervals of 1.0 l/min give eight classes and the data are shown to display a unimodal distribution. (b) With a class interval of 0.2 l/min, there are 36 classes and only 25 data values, too many class intervals to be useful. (c)

With a class interval of 5.0 l/min, nearly all the observations are in one class and only two classes are represented. We get no sense of the distribution of the data. Clearly (a) is the most appropriate.

2.6 (a) Both axes have inadequate labelling; the tick marks have no scales. (b) This is a histogram, but it is drawn as a bar chart. The vertical bars should be attributed to represent the continuous variable on the axis. (c) Again, the x-axis is inadequately labelled; we are left to guess what are the units for the scale; they must be included. (d) The slices of the pie chart give details neither of the numbers involved, nor of the percentages represented by the slices. These figures should be added.

2.7 Arranged in ascending order, the rates (%) are: 29.2, 34.2, 44.4, 64.2, 64.7, 67.6, 75.0, 76.2 and 80.0. There are nine observations, so the median is the $(9 + 1)/2 = 5$th observation in the ordered set, i.e. the median is 64.7%.

2.8 Mean = 761.2/16 = 47.58 g, median = 51.95 g (the arithmetic mean of 51.9 and 52.0). The mean and the median do not coincide, indicating that the data are skewed. The mean is less than the median, indicating that the data are skewed to the left.

2.9 Range = 2.5 to 8.6 = 6.1 μmol/l; variance = 3.57 $(\mu$mol/l$)^2$; standard deviation = 1.89 μmol/l.

2.10 (a) When the data are arranged in order of magnitude, the percentiles are those values of the variable which divide the data set into 100 equal parts. The 1st percentile has 1% of the ordered observations below it and 99% above it. The 5th percentile has 5% of the ordered observations below it and 95% above it, etc. (b) The median is the value of an observation in a data set which has as many observations above it as below it when the observations are arranged in increasing order of magnitude. It is equal to the 50th percentile. If the number of observations, n, in the data set is odd, it is the $(n + 1)/2$th observation in the ordered set. If n is even, it is usually taken as the arithmetic mean of the middle two observations. (c) The interquartile range is the difference between the 1st and 3rd quartiles, i.e. the 25th and 75th percentiles. It contains the central 50% of the ordered observations, with 25% of them lower than the lower limit of the range, and 25% of them above the upper limit of the range. (d) The reference range is the range of values of a variable such that values of the variable are expected to lie on or between them if the individual is healthy with respect to that variable. It is generally defined as the range containing the central 95% of the observations for that variable in a population of healthy individuals. If the variable is Normally distributed, it is calculated as the mean ± 1.96SD. If the distribution is skewed, it is often taken as the range of values from the 2.5th to the 97.5th percentiles. It is also sometimes called the normal range or reference interval.

Chapter 3

3.1 (a) **F**: the Normal distribution is symmetrical. (b) **T**. (c) **F**: the limits that contain 95% of the distribution are mean ± 1.96SD. (d) **F**: this is a particular Normal distribution, i.e. the Standard Normal distribution. (e) **F**: the term 'Normal' in statistics describes the Gaussian distribution and not the 'normal' or healthy population.

3.2 (a) **F**: z is a continuous random variable because the Standard Normal distribution is a continuous distribution. (b) **F**: the mean equals 0 and the standard deviation equals 1. (c) **T**. (d) **F**: it is x which has a mean of μ and a standard deviation of σ if z has a Standard Normal distribution. (e) **T**.

3.3 (a) **T**. (b) **F**: it is the Normal distribution. (c) **F**: a Normal distribution is a theoretical probability distribution and should not be confused with 'normal' or healthy individuals. In this case, the variable simply follows a Normal distribution. (d) **F**: the Standard Normal distribution always has a mean of 0 and an SD of 1. (e) **F**: if data have a distribution which is skewed to the right, then a log transformation is likely to Normalize

it. The data are then said to follow the Lognormal distribution.

3.4 (a) The probability of a six when she rolls one die = 1/6; the probability of a six in the second die = 1/6. The probability of a double six, using the multiplication rule, is $(1/6) \times (1/6) = 0.028$. Similarly, the probability of a double of any other number is also 0.028. Hence, using the addition rule, the probability of either a double six, or a double five, . . . , or a double one is $6 \times 0.028 = 0.17$. There is, therefore, a very small chance that they will purchase a bitch using this approach, and he is right to have second thoughts. (b) The chance of a six in one roll of a single die is 1/6. The chance of not getting a six in one roll is 5/6. Using the multiplication rule, the chance of not getting a six in the three rolls of a single die is $(5/6)^3 = 0.58$. Hence, there is now a much better chance that they will get a bitch. These calculations are based on the model approach to probability.

3.5 (a) The data are approximately Normally distributed. (b) The data are skewed to the right, but the log data are approximately Normally distributed.

3.6 The Poisson distribution; the mean and variance of the counts should be equal.

3.7 (a) The Standardized Normal Deviate (SND) = $(0.40 - 0.37)/0.066 = 0.45$. Reference to Table A.1 gives a two-tailed probability of 0.6527. Hence the required percentage is half this, i.e. 32.7%. (b) SND = $(0.30 - 0.37)/0.066 = -1.061$. The two-tailed area in Table A.1 is 0.2891. Hence the required percentage is 14.5%. (c) The percentage of values below 0.40 l/l is $100 - 32.7 = 67.3\%$, the percentage of values below 0.30 l/l is 14.5%; hence the required percentage = $67.3 - 14.5 = 52.8\%$. (d) The lower limit is the value below which 5% of the observations fall; it is derived from the equality $-1.64 = (x_1 - 0.37)/0.066$, which gives $x_1 = 0.26$ l/l. The upper limit is the value above which 5% of the observations fall; it is derived from the equality $1.64 = (x_2 - 0.37)/0.066$, which gives

$x_2 = 0.48$ l/l. The required range is therefore 0.26 to 0.48 l/l.

3.8 (a) (i) From Table A.1, $0.0455 \times 1/2 = 0.0228$. (ii) From Table A.1, $0.3173 \times 1/2 = 0.1587$. (b) (i) From Table A.2, 1.64. (ii) From Table A.2, −1.96.

3.9 With an assumed Normal (symmetrical) distribution, we would expect 50% of cows to calve by the mean of 278 days, therefore the probability of not calving by 278 days is 0.5. For two cows each to calve before 278 days (independent events), the probability is given by $0.5 \times 0.5 = 0.25$ or 25%.

3.10 The conditional probability of Mollie choosing a female pup for Stephanie, having already chosen a male pup for Stephen (where the probability of a male pup on the first selection is $2/4 = 0.5$), is the probability of choosing a female pup out of the remaining three pups, two of whom are female, i.e. it is $2/3 = 0.66$. Hence the probability of Mollie achieving her aim is the product of these two probabilities, i.e. it is $0.5 \times 0.66 = 0.33$.

Chapter 4

4.1 (a) **F**: the SEM relates to the precision of the sample mean, and not the individual observations. (b) **F**: it is the standard deviation which measures the spread of the observations. (c) **T**. (d) **T**. (e) **T**.

4.2 (a) **F**: it contains the population mean with 95% certainty. (b) **T**. (c) **F**: it is the reference range that contains, usually, 95% of the observations in the population. (d) **F**: you should add and subtract 2 standard errors to the sample mean. (e) **T**.

4.3 (a) **F**: it is the population mean plasma potassium that lies between these values. (b) **T**. (c) **T**. (d) **F**: the confidence interval is for the population mean and does not relate to individual values. (e) **F**: there is a 5% chance that the population mean lies outside the interval.

4.4
(a) 95% CI $= 2.35 \pm 1.96 \times \sqrt{(0.16/100)} = 2.272$ to 2.428 mg/kg
    99% CI $= 2.35 \pm 2.58 \times \sqrt{(0.16/100)} = 2.247$ to 2.453 mg/kg
(b) 95% CI $= 34.8 \pm 2.064 \times 13.0/\sqrt{25} = 29.434$ to 40.166 ng/ml
    99% CI $= 34.8 \pm 2.797 \times 13.0/\sqrt{25} = 27.528$ to 42.072 ng/ml

4.5 (a) The estimated proportion of joint lameness is $5/60 = 0.0833$ (i.e. 8.33%) therefore the 95% CI $= 0.0833 \pm 1.96 \times \sqrt{(0.0833)(1 - 0.0833)/60}$ $= 0.013$ to 0.153. (b) Wider. (c) Narrower.

Chapter 5

5.1 (a) **F**: randomization is used so that biases associated with the allocation of animals to the different treatments are avoided. (b) **T**. (c) **F**: a control group can be incorporated into the design whether or not randomization is used. (d) **T**. (e) **F**: blinding is another issue, unrelated to random allocation.

5.2 (a) **F**: treatment is given to each chicken so that this is an experimental study. (b) **F**: the chickens are assessed both before and after they have received treatment, so the trial is longitudinal. (c) **F**: the chickens are followed forward in time, so the study is prospective. (d) **T**. (e) **F**: a sample survey is a particular type of observational study and this is an experimental study.

5.3 (a) **F**: the wash-out period eliminates the carry-over effect. (b) **F**: the randomization ensures that there is no allocation bias. A wash-out period should eliminate the carry-over effect. (c) **F**: a parallel group design is one in which each animal receives only one treatment and the treatment comparison is made between animals. (d) **T**. (e) **F**: a between-animal comparison provides less precise treatment effects than a within-animal comparison.

5.4 (a) Longitudinal study – it follows the bitches forward in time. (b) Experimental – there was an intervention in one of the groups. (c) Neither – cohort and case–control studies are only observational studies. (d) A case–control study in which incontinent bitches and matched controls are traced back in time to see whether they had been spayed.

5.5 The *laissez-faire* approach does not subject the cats to any stress comparable with the surgical intervention. Any differences, therefore, are not due solely to the surgical repair but to the stresses of anaesthesia, etc. The proper controls should be subjected to a sham operation although this would be ethically unacceptable with clinical cases.

5.6 (a) Dose levels in dogs should be investigated with stratified randomization allowing for the differences in body weight. Common strata are large, medium and toy dogs. It might be advisable to use restricted randomization within each of the strata, particularly if the number of dogs available for study is not great. (b) Grouped randomization (because it is a treatment for a worm infestation) with groups of, say, four to eight animals penned in small subplots of the two plots. In addition it would be sensible to have restricted randomization of the groups to treatment or control to ensure balance. (c) Each litter is a group. The litters are allocated at random to one of the two preparations. (d) Despite the word 'group' in the description, this is not a group investigation. Animals are allocated using restricted randomization to each of the treatments at each location (which can be regarded as a stratum); this should result in the required balance.

5.7 (a) Estimated risk of a large farm being positive = 33/57 = 0.579 (i.e. 57.9%). Estimated risk of a small farm being positive = 20/68 = 0.294 (i.e. 29.4%). Estimated prevalence of positive farms = 53/125 = 0.424 (i.e. 42.4%). (b) Estimated RR = 0.579/0.294 = 1.97. It is estimated that the risk of a farm being positive is nearly two times greater if the farm was large rather than small.

Estimated ARR = 0.579 − 0.294 = 0.285. It is estimated that for every 100 farms, approximately 29 of them were positive because they were large rather than small. (c) Estimated odds ratio = (33/24)/(20/48) = 3.3. The odds of a farm being positive is estimated to be over three times greater if the farm was large rather than small. The estimated RR = 1.97, which is smaller than the OR. The OR and RR are similar only if the prevalence of positive farms is low. In this case the prevalence is estimated to be 42.4%, which is not low.

Chapter 6

6.1 (a) **F**: the null hypothesis concerns the population means. (b) **T**. (c) **F**: it is only the result of the test which is or is not significant, not the null hypothesis. (d) **F**: the null hypothesis is a statement of fact that may or may not be true. (e) **F**: the null hypothesis is not expressed in terms of what is expected.

6.2 (a) **F**: it could also refer to the left-hand side, but not both sides. (b) **F**: the tails of the test influence the *P*-value which is the probability of rejecting the null hypothesis when it is true, whereas the power is the probability of rejecting the null hypothesis when it is false. (c) **F**: most tests are two-tailed because it is very unusual to be sure that any treatment difference can be in only one direction. (d) **T**. (e) **F**: the decision to use a one-tailed test does not relate to the sample size but rather to the biological certainty that, if a treatment difference exists, it can only be in one direction.

6.3 (a) **F**: the *P*-value is the probability of obtaining a result as or more extreme than the one observed if the null hypothesis is true. (b) **F**: the null hypothesis is a stated theory about the population parameter(s) that is either true or false. (c) **F**: the *P*-value relates what is observed in the sample to what is hypothesized about the population; the null hypothesis is either true or false, and no probability is attached to it in the hypothesis test. (d) **T**. (e) **T**.

6.4 (a) **F**: the null hypothesis is a statement about the population parameter(s) that is either true or false; there is no probability attached to it in the hypothesis test. (b) **F**: the alternative hypothesis is also a statement about the population parameter(s) that is true or false. (c) **T**. (d) **F**: the P-value must relate what is observed in the sample to what is hypothesized in the population. (e) **F**: see (a).

6.5 (a) **F**: the test statistic is a mathematical expression in which the sample values are substituted to determine a P-value. This is used to decide whether there is evidence to reject the null hypothesis about a population parameter (such as the mean). (b) **F**: see (a). (c) **T**. (d) **F**: it is the P-value that has to be lower than a stated value (typically 0.05) in order for the result of the test to be significant. (e) **F**: significance tests can be performed using small and large samples. The test is more powerful if the sample size is large.

6.6 (a) **F**: if the null hypothesis is not rejected, all we can say is that there is no evidence to show that the two means are different. This is not the same as establishing equivalence. (b) **T**. (c) **F**: if the two treatments are equivalent, the relevant confidence interval for the effect of interest must lie wholly within the equivalence interval, whereas if one treatment is not inferior, only the lower limit of the confidence interval has to lie above the lower limit of the equivalence interval. (d) **F**: the equivalence interval is an interval relating to the effect of interest which is considered by experts to be of no clinical importance. (e) **T**.

6.7 The null hypothesis is that the mean muscle tension in the populations is the same when using the novel drug and when using the control. The alternative hypothesis is that the two population means are different. This is a two-sided alternative; there is no biological reason for presuming that any difference, should it exist, can be in only one direction. The null hypothesis is essentially the same when using an existing drug – it is that the mean muscle tension in the populations is the same on the novel drug as on the existing treat-

ment. Again, the alternative hypothesis is that the two population means are different (direction unspecified).

6.8 The null hypothesis is that the proportions of ponies who fail the test are the same in the population of ponies who are trained by the new system and in the population of ponies who are trained in the traditional manner. The alternative hypothesis is that these two proportions are not equal (direction unspecified).

6.9 The 95% confidence interval for the true mean temperature is $37.3 \pm 2.06(0.7/\sqrt{26}) = 37.0$ to $37.6°C$. Since $37.5°C$, the optimum mean temperature for hatching, lies within this confidence interval, this incubator can be used in the hatchery.

Chapter 7

7.1 (a) **F**: the sample sizes do not have to be equal but, if they are, the assumption of Normality is less important. (b) **F**: it is used on independent groups of observations. Performing a two-sample t-test on paired or dependent data will lead to a loss of power. (c) **F**: the null hypothesis assumes that the two population means are equal. (d) **T**. (e) **F**: the paired t-test should be used on dependent data rather than the two-sample t-test, irrespective of sample size.

7.2 (a) **T**. (b) **T**. (c) **F**: the paired t-test should be used on paired or related data, irrespective of sample size. However, if the sample size is very small, a non-parametric alternative may be preferred. (d) **F**: the two-sample t-test should be used for comparing the means of independent groups of observations. (e) **F**: the paired t-test makes the assumption that the differences between the pairs are Normally distributed.

7.3 (a) Paired comparison. (b) H_0: the population mean difference in plasma lactate concentration when the horse is cantering and when it is on a treadmill is zero. (c) The differences are approximately Normally distributed. Paired t-test test statistic = 2.51, df = 9, P = 0.033. (d)

Reject the null hypothesis that the mean difference in the population is zero. We cannot consider the exercise exerted by the horses to be of similar metabolic demand in both situations. The 95% confidence interval for the mean difference is 0.077 to 1.503 mmol/l.

7.4 (a) Two independent groups. (b) H_0: the population mean sperm numbers are the same using the two methods. (c) The observations in each sample are approximately Normally distributed. The mean (SEM) sperm numbers ($\times 10^6$) using the AV and EE methods are 63.46 (6.72) and 43.90 (6.07), respectively: the two variances (587.63 and 368.76) are not significantly different (Levene's test gives $P = 0.471$). The two-sample t-test statistic = 2.09, $df = 21$, $P = 0.049$. (d) The 95% confidence interval for the difference in means is 0.12 to 39.00×10^6. The result of the test is just significant at the 5% level indicating that the AV method is likely to be able to obtain more sperm, and the difference in means could be as great as 39×10^6 sperm.

7.5 This is a one-sample t-test of the null hypothesis that there is no difference between the mean urea value from this laboratory in January and 7.5 mmol/l. The test statistic is $(9.7 - 7.5)/0.22 = 10.00$ on 139 degrees of freedom. Hence $P < 0.001$, and there is evidence to reject the null hypothesis. It would seem that the laboratory overestimated plasma urea in cats in January.

7.6 The design is inappropriate because there is no control group, i.e. horses who do not go through the breaking programme, but are followed for the same length of time in otherwise identical circumstances. In the given design, the increase in cardiopulmonary function could be a consequence of time alone, unrelated to the effect of the breaking programme. An appropriate design should include a control group; then the change in cardiopulmonary function after 8 weeks should be evaluated for each horse, and the changes in the two groups compared using a two-sample test, such as the two-sample t-test.

7.7 (a) The 95% confidence interval for the difference in the mean percentage of protein binding in the two species is -12.7% to 32.3%, with an estimated difference in means of 9.8%. Since this CI spans zero, there is no evidence to reject the null hypothesis that the two population means are equal. Wasfi *et al.* inferred that the two means are the same. However, lack of evidence to find a significant difference does not imply that the means are the same. (b) The statistical test used by the second set of investigators was the two-sample t-test. The null hypothesis is that the mean percentage of protein binding in the population of horses and camels is equal. (c) The two assumptions of the two-sample t-test are that the distribution of the percentages in each group is approximately Normal and that the two groups have the same variances. In addition, it is assumed that the observations in each group are independent. (d) The Normality assumption is a reasonable assumption as the box plot shows that the median is approximately in the middle of the box, which is approximately in the middle of the whiskers in each group. Levene's F-test in the output has $P = 0.007$, so the null hypothesis that the two variances are the same should be rejected, i.e. this implies that the constant variance assumption is not satisfied. Instead, a P-value using a modified t-test, shown in the bottom line of the table in the output, should be used. (e) $P = 0.006$ so there is evidence to reject the null hypothesis that the two means are equal in the population, i.e. the mean percentage of protein binding is significantly greater in camels than in horses. (f) Wasfi *et al.* had a non-significant result and so there was no evidence to reject the null hypothesis, but this is not the same as concluding that the means are equal. The different results are probably due to the fact that the power of the Wasfi *et al.* study would have been very low to detect the difference as significant, since the sample size was very small in their study (only six horses and five camels). (g) The 95% CI is broadly interpreted to mean that we can say with 95% confidence that the true difference in means lies within these values (where the mean percentage of protein binding in camels is subtracted from that of horses).

7.8 (a) The two tests are the paired t-test and Wilcoxon signed rank test. (b) The assumption underlying the paired t-test is that the differences (between secondary and tail) are Normally distributed. There are no distributional assumptions underlying the Wilcoxon signed rank test, which is a non-parametric test. (c) Using the confidence interval for the mean difference in feather Hg in tail and secondary feathers for each type of eagle, there is significantly more mean feather Hg in the tail than in the secondary feathers of (i) tawny and (ii) eagle owls. This can be established because the confidence interval in each case excludes zero. Because both are 95% confidence intervals, we can say that $P < 0.05$ in each case. We can therefore conclude that there is evidence to reject the null hypothesis that the true mean difference is zero. (d) The mean of the difference between the tail and secondary feather Hg is significantly greater in eagle owls than in tawny owls, $P < 0.05$. This can be established because the upper limit of the mean of the difference between tail and secondary feather Hg in tawny owls is lower than the lower limit of the mean of the difference between tail and secondary feather Hg in eagle owls, i.e. there is no overlap between the 95% confidence intervals for the two mean differences. (e) Two tests are the two-sample t-test and the Mann–Whitney test (almost identical to the Wilcoxon rank sum test).

Chapter 8

8.1 (a) **T**. (b) **F**. (c) **T**. (d) **F**: the data should be analysed as a repeated measures ANOVA if the data are matched. (e) **F**: the null hypothesis states that the population means are all the same.

8.2 (a) **F**: the test makes no assumptions about the means, only that the data are Normally distributed. (b) **T**. (c) **T**. (d) **F**: the F-test compares variances and not means. (e) **F**: the F-test compares variances. Equal variances is an assumption of the two-sample t-test, so the F-test may precede the t-test to validate this assumption, but will be followed by the t-test only if the intention is to compare two means.

8.3 The data are approximately Normally distributed in each sample. The estimated variances of Group 1 and Group 2 are 0.671 and 2.313 kg^2, respectively. The sample sizes are 15 and 13, respectively. The ratio of these two variances, the larger over the smaller, is 3.345; this follows the F-distribution with 12 df in the numerator, and 14 df in the denominator. The percentage points in Table A.5b, which correspond to two-sided P-values of 0.05 and 0.01 (i.e. we look at $P = 0.025$ and $P = 0.005$ in the table), are 3.05 and 4.43, respectively. Since 3.345 lies between these two values, $0.01 < P < 0.05$; we reject the null hypothesis that the two variances are equal, and would have to perform a modified t-test or a non-parametric test to compare the average liver weights in the two groups.

8.4 The null hypothesis is that there is no difference between the true mean intensities in the three diluent solutions. The data are approximately Normally distributed in each group. Levene's test (performed on the computer, but you could do a series of F-tests by hand, adjusting the P-values using Bonferroni's correction) shows that the three variances are not significantly different (test statistic = 3.27, $P = 0.06$). A one-way ANOVA (see Display 8.2) gives an F-ratio of 13.66, $df = 2, 18, P = 0.0002$ (Sig. = 0.000 in the output, indicating that $P < 0.001$). Hence there is a significant difference between at least two of the means, suggesting that egg yolk dilution affects the binding of the fluorophore to the sperm membrane. The sample means (SEM) of the 1%, 5% and 25% egg yolk solutions are 0.999 (0.017), 0.950 (0.078) and 0.846 (0.040), respectively. *Post hoc* Bonferroni's tests show that the 25% egg yolk solution has a mean intensity that is significantly less than that of either of the other two solutions ($P < 0.05$), but that no other two means are significantly different from each other ($P > 0.05$). The mean square of the within-groups source of variation is 0.0029, and this is used as the combined estimate of variance in the calculation of confidence intervals (i.e. this is the s^2 in the formula for the confidence interval given in Section 7.4.3). The 95% confidence intervals for the difference in means between the 25% and each of the 1% and 5% egg yolk solutions are (0.087, 0.219) and (0.085, 0.125), respectively.

8.5 (a) The diagram is a box-and-whisker plot, sometimes just called a box plot. For a given treatment group, the heavy line in the middle of the box is the median, the box shows the upper and lower quartiles of the distribution (i.e. it contains the central 50% of the ordered observations) and the whiskers contain the central 95% of the ordered observations. Sometimes outliers are shown at the extremes. (b) The test is the two-sample *t*-test (devised by Student). (c) The null hypothesis is that the mean MRT values are the same in the moxidectin and doramectin groups in the population. (d) The assumptions are that the data are approximately Normally distributed in each group and that the variances of the observations are the same (i.e. same spread). (e) Yes, it would appear that the assumptions are reasonable. From the box plot, we can see that MRT is approximately Normally (symmetrically) distributed in each group as the median is approximately in the middle of the box, which is more or less in the middle of the whiskers. Also, the spread of the observations appears similar in the two groups. In addition, Levene's test examines the null hypothesis that the variances of the two groups are equal. $P = 0.091$ from this test so there is insufficient evidence to reject the null hypothesis. Hence we may take the variances to be equal in the *t*-test. (f) The table of results gives $P = 0.000$ (using the first line of results since we can assume equal variances). This indicates that $P < 0.001$ and there is strong evidence to reject H_0. This suggests that the mean MRT is significantly greater in the moxidectin group of goats than in the doramectin group. (g) The estimated effect of interest is the difference in mean MRT between the two groups. This is estimated as 7.77 days with a 95% confidence interval of 7.06 to 8.47 days.

Chapter 9

9.1 (a) **F**: the *t*-test is for comparing two means from numerical data. (b) **F**: the *F*-test is for comparing variances. (c) **T**. (d) **F**: McNemar's test is for paired categorical responses, and these data are not paired. (e) **F**: the null hypothesis is not about a theoretical distribution.

9.2 (a) **F**: it is the expected frequencies that have to be greater than 5. (b) **F**: the degrees of freedom are $(2 - 1)(2 - 1) = 1$. (c) **T**. (d) **F**: the null hypothesis is that there is no difference between these proportions. (e) **F**: the data are binary categorical, and cannot be Normally distributed.

9.3 This is a test of a single proportion; the null hypothesis is that the proportion of dairy cattle in the local area does not differ from the national proportion. The estimated proportion of dairy cows in the local area = $359/1375$ = 0.261. Thus $Test_6 = \dfrac{|0.261 - 0.29| - 1/2750}{\sqrt{0.29(1 - 0.29)/1375}} = 2.34$.
Referring this value to Table A.1, we find that $P = 0.0193$. Hence we reject the null hypothesis $(P = 0.02)$ – it seems that the committee was right and this area has a lower percentage of dairy cows in the cattle population.

9.4 This is a test of two proportions; we can use the Chi-squared test to test the null hypothesis that the true proportions of bitches that have mammary nodules are equal in those bitches that had MPA and in those without MPA. The table shows the observed frequencies; the expected frequencies are in brackets:

	MPA +ve	MPA −ve	Total
With nodules	21 (15.6)	13 (18.4)	34
Without nodules	12 (17.4)	26 (20.6)	38
Total	33	39	72

Hence $Test_7 = 5.4$ (with the continuity correction), and $P = 0.020$. There is evidence to reject the null hypothesis. From this prospective cohort study, we would conclude that MPA administration does appear to increase the risk of subsequent mammary nodules. Note that the estimated proportions which had nodules are $21/33 = 0.636$ and $13/39 = 0.333$ in the groups with and without MPA, respectively. The estimated difference in the two proportions is 0.303. The 95% CI for the difference in the true proportions is $(0.636 - 0.333) \pm 1.96 \times 0.113 = (0.082, 0.524)$.

9.5 We show the observed frequencies of sheep with and without liver fluke infestation and with a positive or negative response to a diagnostic ELISA test in the following contingency table:

	ELISA +ve	ELISA −ve	Total
Egg shedding +ve	39	14	53
Egg shedding −ve	16	74	90
Total	55	74	143

We use McNemar's test: $Test_9 = (|16 - 14| - 1)^2 \div (16 + 14) = 1/30 = 0.03$. This has a Chi-squared distribution on 1 degree of freedom. Referring to Table A.4, we find that $P > 0.05$. Hence we do not have evidence to reject the null hypothesis. The two sample proportions with positive results are $53/143 = 0.37$ by the egg-shedding approach, and $55/143 = 0.38$ by the ELISA test. The 95% confidence interval for the difference in the true proportions is

$$(0.38 - 0.37) \pm 1.96 \frac{1}{143} \sqrt{16 + 14 - \frac{(16 - 14)^2}{143}}$$
$$= 0.01 \pm 1.96 \times 0.038$$
$$= (-0.07, 0.09).$$

9.6 (a) There was no randomization of dogs to treatment groups. (b) The observed frequencies are displayed in the table:

	Pu	Control	Total
Tumour	67	45	112
No tumour	53	18	71
Total	120	63	183

(c) Chi-squared test with continuity correction. (d) The expected values in the four cells of the table are each greater than 5. (e) We are 95% certain that the true/population percentage of adult beagles without any intervention developing mammary tumours lies between 60.2% and 82.6%. (f) The confidence intervals provided give the range of values within which we expect the true percentage developing mammary tumours to lie in each treatment group. If there is no overlap between the two 95% confidence intervals, then there is a significant difference ($P<0.05$) between the two percentages. However, if there is overlap, then the percentages may or may not be significantly different. In this study, there was overlap between the two confidence intervals, so we cannot say whether or not there is a significant difference between the percentages using this approach. (g) The authors seem to have taken the lower limit of the confidence interval for the percentage of mammary tumours in the plutonium group of dogs and the upper limit of the confidence interval for the control dogs. (h) A useful confidence interval is that which relates to the difference in the percentages developing mammary tumours of any kind in the two groups. (The estimated difference in these percentages is $71.4\% - 55.8\% = 15.6\%$.) If the 95% confidence interval excludes zero, then this is an indication that the two percentages are significantly different with $P < 0.05$.

9.7 In order to calculate the Chi-squared goodness-of-fit statistic, we must combine some of the categories since there are expected frequencies which are less than 5. Combining the frequencies for 0–3 pregnant ewes, and for 7 and 8 pregnant ewes, we find that $Test_8 = 3.9553 + 0.0127 + 0.0302 + 0.2582 + 0.9732 = 5.23$ with 3 *df*. Referring to Table A.4 we obtain $0.10 < P < 0.25$ (in fact, a computer analysis gives $P = 0.16$). Hence we can assume that the observed distribution of the number of pregnant ewes conforms with the Binomial distribution with $\pi = 0.64$.

9.8 (a) Frequency table for the data in Exercise 9.8:

Standard collar	New collar		Total
	Lost	Retained	
Lost	6	2	8
Retained	19	8	27
Total	25	10	35

(b) Percentage lost new collar $= 100 \times 25/35 = 71.4\%$, percentage lost standard collar $= 100 \times 8/35 = 22.9\%$. (c) McNemar's test. (d) The percentage of cats losing either type of cat collar is the same in both populations. (e) The percentage of cats losing the different types of collar is not the same in both populations. (f) The significance level of the test is the cut-off for the P-value which determines significance, i.e. if the P-value is less than the significance level, then the null hypothesis is rejected in favour of the alternative hypothesis. The usual significance level is 0.05. (g) The Type I error of a test is the error that is made when the null hypothesis is rejected when it is true. The probability of making a Type I error is the chance of making this mistake by incorrectly rejecting the null hypothesis. The significance level of the test is the maximum chance of making a Type I error. (h) There is a 0.05% chance of getting the observed sample values/frequencies, or values more extreme, if the null hypothesis is true. (i) The pet-shop owner would have rejected the null hypothesis and concluded that the percentage of cats losing the new type of collar is significantly greater than that losing the standard collar.

Chapter 10

10.1 (a) **F**: it lies between −1 and +1. (b) **F**: the assumption of Normality of at least one of the variables is important only for hypothesis testing; both variables should be Normally distributed if the confidence interval is to be calculated. (c) **T**. (d) **F**: it is zero if there is no linear relationship between the two variables; there could be a non-linear relationship. (e) **F**: this is the interpretation of the regression coefficient, β.

10.2 (a) **F**: this is the function of the correlation coefficient. (b) **T**. (c) **T**. (d) **F**: it assumes that the residuals are Normally distributed, and that y is Normally distributed for each value of x. (e) **F**: the x variable is assumed capable of measurement without error and is used to predict the y variable. There is no distinction between the two variables in correlation analysis.

10.3 (a) There appears to be an approximately linear relationship between CFT and ELISA (see Figure 10.10a), with ELISA values increasing as the CFT values increase. (b) The Model summary table (see Display 10.2) shows that the estimated correlation coefficient is 0.737. (c) From the Coefficients table, we find that the estimated regression line is ELISA = 1.21 + 0.020CFT. (d) From the Model summary table, $R^2 = 0.54$; this is derived from (137.467)/(253.269) obtained from the ANOVA table. Thus, 54% of the varia-

tion in ELISA values is explained by its linear relationship with CFT; 46% is unexplained. Since only just over half the variation is explained, we might conclude that the model does not fit very well. (e) From the box-plot (Figure 10.10b) we see that, although there is a suggestion that the residuals are slightly skewed to the right, they may be regarded as being approximately Normally distributed. The residuals in the scatter diagram (Figure 10.10d) appear to be randomly scattered around a mean of about zero, indicating that a linear relationship between CFT and ELISA is reasonable. The residuals in the scatter diagram (Figure 10.10c) have constant variability for increasing predicted values of ELISA. There is only one pair of readings of ELISA and CFT for each donkey. Hence, we can conclude that all the assumptions underlying the linear regression are satisfied. (f) The ANOVA table is testing the null hypothesis that the true slope of the line is zero. The P-value of 0.000 given in the output (indicating $P < 0.001$) shows that there is evidence to reject this null hypothesis in favour of the alternative hypothesis that the true slope is not zero. (g) The slope of the line (from the Coefficients table) is 0.0198 (i.e. 1.98E-02) with an estimated standard error of 0.002 and 95% CI = (0.017, 0.023). Thus, as we increase CFT by 1 unit, we increase the ELISA by 0.0198 units on average (although, we believe with 95% confidence, that this average increase could be as low as 0.017 or as great as 0.023). (h) The t-test in the Coefficients table (test statistic = 12.03) and the F-test in the ANOVA table (test statistic = 144.82) both indicate $P < 0.001$ (i.e. Sig. = 0.000). Hence there is strong evidence to reject the null hypothesis that the true slope is equal to zero.

10.4 (a) The correlation coefficient measures the linear association between rugal fold thickness and body weight. A coefficient of zero indicates there is no linear association. A coefficient of one indicates that there is perfect positive association. This coefficient is positive and, judged subjectively, quite large, suggesting that there is a strong positive linear association between the two variables. (b) The P-value results from the hypothesis test that the true correlation coefficient is zero. Since $P < 0.001$ is very small, there is strong evidence to reject the null hypothesis. (c) The slope of the line represents the average change in y per unit change in x; thus we estimate that as the dog's body weight increases by 1 kg, its rugal thickness increases, on average, by 0.069 mm. (d) The fraction is the square of the correlation coefficient $= 0.71 \times 0.71 = 0.50$; thus 50% of the variance in y is explained by the regression, and 50% is unexplained. (e) The regression line is a questionable fit as it explains only half the variance in y, in spite of the correlation coefficient being highly significant.

10.5 (a) $r = 0.158$ obtained from the Model summary table (it is R in this table in Display 10.3). (b) The outcome or dependent variable is the number of cases of lameness and the explanatory or independent variable is the amount of rainfall. They were chosen in this way for the regression analysis as it would be of interest to predict the number of cases of lameness from the amount of rainfall and not the other way round. (c) $Y = 31.235 + 0.081x$ where Y is the predicted value of the number of cases of lameness and x is the amount of rainfall. This equation is obtained from the first column of the Coefficients table. (d) The estimated slope of the line is 0.081 cases per millimetre of rainfall. This means that we estimated the number of cases of lameness to increase on average by 0.081 for each millimetre increase in the amount of rainfall in a fortnight (or equivalently, the number of cases of lameness will increase on average by eight for each 100 mm increase in the amount of rainfall). The 95% confidence interval for the slope is from -0.133 to 0.294 cases per millimetre rainfall. This means that these figures contain the true slope with 95% certainty. (e) H_0: the true slope in the population of the regression line of cases of lameness on amount of rainfall is zero. The t-test statistic for this hypothesis is 0.782 and $P = 0.442$. Since the P-value is greater than the significance level of 0.05, there is no evidence to reject the null hypothesis that the true slope is zero. Hence there is no evidence that there is a linear relationship between rainfall and lameness. (f) The square of the correlation coefficient is 0.025. This can be interpreted to mean that only 2.5% of the

variation in cases of lameness is explained by its linear relationship with amount of rainfall. The remaining 97.5% is unexplained by the relationship. Hence the line is a very poor fit.

10.6 (a) The correlation coefficient is dimensionless, and has no units of measurement. (b) The estimated correlation coefficient is positive and so, in general, the penguin's rate of oxygen consumption increases as its heart rate increases. (c) The null hypothesis is that the Pearson correlation coefficient is zero in the population of Macaroni penguins. (d) The 95% confidence interval for the correlation coefficient can be interpreted broadly as indicating that the interval from 0.703 to 0.971 contains the true correlation coefficient with 95% certainty. More strictly, on repeated sampling the true correlation coefficient would be contained in this interval on 95% of occasions. (e) 82% of the variation in oxygen consumption can be attributed to its linear relationship with heart rate. This value is obtained by squaring 0.904 and multiplying by 100. (f) The assumptions made in testing the null hypothesis about the Pearson correlation coefficient are that both of the variables are numerical, and that at least one of them is Normally distributed. Both of them should be Normally distributed if the confidence interval for the correlation coefficient is to be determined. (g) The value of the correlation coefficient would be expected to increase if the range of values of the heart beat was greater than 125–225 beats/min.

10.7 (a) There are various deficiencies. In particular, at what level is significance achieved? What are the values given: are they means? What is the figure after the ±: is it the SD? What differences were found significant: are they the difference in means? How many male horses were there? (b) A regression analysis has been performed in which the dependent variable is month of age and the explanatory variable is BGP. This implies that it would be of interest to predict the month of age from the BGP, whereas the opposite is true. The outcome and explanatory variables should be interchanged. (c) -1.68 is the estimated regression coefficient, which is an estimate of the gradient or slope of the line. It represents the average change in the age of the horse in months for a unit change in BGP. (d) Apart from the fact that the regression equation should be used to predict the BGP from the age of the horse, and not *vice versa*, an estimated equation should never be used beyond the range of values in the sample. No horse in the sample would have had a zero value for BGP, and so the equation should not be used in this instance.

Chapter 11

11.1 (a) **F**: the residuals should be Normally distributed. (b) **T**. (c) **T**: this is a particular application of multiple regression, the analysis of covariance, when the means can be compared whilst adjusting for other variables. (d) **F**: the sample size should be about 10 times greater than the number of independent variables. (e) **F**: the reverse is true.

11.2 (a) **F**: the correlation coefficient lies between these limits. (b) **F**: again, confusion with the correlation coefficient. (c) **T**. (d) **F**: this is R^2. (e) **F**: it is the correlation coefficient which is independent of the units of measurement.

11.3 (a) **F**: we use logistic regression analysis when the dependent variable is binary. The explanatory variables may be binary or numerical. (b) **F**: the exponential of a logistic regression coefficient is interpreted as an estimated odds ratio. (c) **T**. (d) **T**. (e) **F**: we use conditional logistic regression analysis when we have matched data and a binary outcome variable.

11.4 (a) **F**: Poisson regression analysis can be used on data that relate to any species or circumstance, provided the event of interest follows a Poisson distribution. (b) **T**. (c) **T**. (d) **F**: the exponential of the coefficients of a Poisson regression model represents the ratio of the rates of the event as the relevant explanatory variable increases by 1 unit. (e) **F**: maximum likelihood is used to estimate the coefficients in a Poisson regression model.

11.5 (a) **T**. (b) **F**: the level 2 unit represents the cluster which contains a number of level 1 units. (c) **F**: the use of generalized estimating equations does not require any distributional assumptions about the between-cluster residuals. (d) **T**. (e) **F**: the random intercepts model with a single explanatory variable for clustered data assumes that the regression lines for each cluster have the *same* slope and different intercepts which vary randomly about the mean intercept.

11.6 (a) Clearly, the authors felt that a single variable with three levels (none, early and late) is strictly a nominal variable. It would be inappropriate to include a nominal explanatory variable, unless it is binary, in a multivariable regression analysis as its coefficient cannot be interpreted in a meaningful way. Instead, the authors used two dummy variables. For example, they chose never cat ownership as the reference category for investigating the risk of cat sensitization and created two dummies, one for the early and one for the late cat ownership categories, each comparing their associated category with never cat ownership. (b) The adjusted OR of 0.32 implies that the odds of sensitization in an early cat owner was 0.32 of that in a never cat owner, after adjusting for the other variables in the logistic model, i.e. the odds were reduced by 68% if the child was an early cat owner. The adjusted OR of 0.51 implies that the odds of an early cat ownership child having allergic rhinitis were 0.51 of that in a never cat owner (for these comparisons, early cat ownership was taken as the reference category), after adjusting for the other variables in the logistic model; i.e. the odds were reduced by 49% if the child was an early cat owner compared to a never cat owner. (c) The odds ratio is an adjusted odds ratio because its derivation takes into account the effect of the other variables in the logistic regression model. It is looking at the independent effect of that particular variable on the outcome of interest. (d) The *P*-value for each OR is $P < 0.05$. We can assume this because the 95% confidence intervals for both of the odds ratios exclude one. (e) A Chi-squared test.

Chapter 12

12.1 (a) **T**. (b) **F**: the reverse is true. (c) **F**: non-parametric tests tend to be less powerful than their parametric counterparts if all the assumptions underlying the parametric test are satisfied. (d) **T**. (e) **F**: the tests do not generally incorporate parameter estimates in their calculation.

12.2 (a) **T**. (b) **T**. (c) **F**. (d) **F**: the data on each variable are converted to ranks but they do not have to be initially measured on a ranking scale. (e) **T**: then it is difficult to establish the distribution of the data.

12.3 The correct way to analyse these data is to consider the set of differences in each group. These differences are not related, so that any test which relies on paired data is inappropriate. (a) **F**. (b) **F**. (c) **T**. (d) **F**. (e) **F**: the sample size is probably too small to perform a two-sample t-test because it is difficult, if not impossible, to establish whether the data are Normally distributed in each group and whether there is constant variance.

12.4 (a) There is a strong positive relationship between the scores which appears to be approximately linear. (b) The subjective method assigns arbitrary scores to measure the degree of fluorescence, i.e. they are on an ordinal scale and, therefore, Pearson's correlation coefficient is inappropriate. (c) $r_s = 0.90$, $P < 0.002$, from Table A.7 since $0.90 > 0.8182$, the tabulated percentage point for significance at the 0.2% level with a sample size of 12. Hence we reject the null hypothesis that the true correlation coefficient is zero, and conclude that there is a significant relationship between the two scoring systems. Note that the 95% confidence limits for the correlation coefficient are 0.67 to 0.97, which is quite wide (to be expected since the sample size is small). Although a significant association exists, the lower confidence limit indicates that ρ_s may be as low as 0.67.

12.5 A Wilcoxon rank sum test computer analysis gives $P = 0.035$ (although when corrected for ties, $P = 0.030$). If performing the test by hand, we rank the two groups together and find the sum of the ranks of the bitches from the large litters $= 3.5 + 7.5 + 12 + 12 + 12 + 16 + 16 + 18 + 19 = 116$. (Note, the sum of the ranks of the bitches from the small litters $= 1 + 3.5 + 3.5 + 3.5 + 7.5 + 7.5 + 7.5 + 12 + 12 + 16 = 74$.) Referring to Table A.10 with sample sizes of 9 and 10, we find that 116 exceeds the tabulated 5% significance level limits of 65–115 (or alternatively, with sample sizes of 10 and 9, 74 is less than the tabulated limits of 75–125). However, 116 lies within the 1% significance level limits of 58–122. Hence we reject the null hypothesis that the median litter sizes are the same in the populations, $0.01 < P < 0.05$ (computer analysis gives $P = 0.035$). There is evidence to indicate that litter size is inherited. The median litter sizes for the bitches from the large litters is 5 (range 3–7), and from the small litters is 4 (range 2–5).

12.6 We find the differences in weight (before – after). The differences are (kg): +2.2, +0.4, +4.3, +1.0, +2.1, −1.4, −1.2, +0.7, 0.0, +0.4, −0.3, +0.7, +0.2, −0.3, +0.6, +1.8, +0.5, +0.2. These differences are skewed to the right, so that a non-parametric test, the Wilcoxon signed rank test, is advocated. The null hypothesis is that the samples come from populations with identical distributions and the same median, or from the same population, which would indicate that the dogs' weight is unaffected by the diet. The alternative hypothesis is that they do not come from populations with identical distributions or the same median. The ranks of the differences are 16, 5.5, 17, 11, 15, 13, 12, 9.5 (we ignore the zero difference), 5.5, 3.5, 9.5, 1.5, 3.5, 8, 14, 7 and 1.5, respectively. There are only four negative differences, and there are 13 positive differences. The sum of the ranks of the negative differences $= 12 + 13 + 3.5 + 3.5 = 32$. We refer this sum to Table A.9, and find that $P < 0.05$ (since 32 lies outside 34–119) but >0.02 (since 32 lies within 28–125). Hence we reject the null hypothesis $0.02 < P < 0.05$. In fact, a computer analysis gives $P = 0.04$. The median weight loss (with 25th and 75th percentiles) is 0.45 (−0.08, 1.20) kg. On the basis of this analysis, we would conclude that the novel diet is effective in promoting weight loss. However, this is a poorly designed trial since there is no control group of dogs that do not receive the novel diet. Hence, we cannot be sure that the observed loss in weight can be attributed to the novel diet: perhaps the dogs would have lost weight without it. Question 12.7 shows the results in a control group of dogs without the diet.

12.7 We find the differences between the dogs' weights before and after (B − A) the standard diet. They are +3.1, +0.6, +2.9, −1.0, +2.9, −1.8, −3.0, −0.9, −0.6, +0.6, −1.2, +1.6, +0.7, −0.2, −0.9, +1.7, +0.7 and +0.2 kg, respectively. They are not Normally distributed. The differences in weights for the dogs on the novel diet (Exercise 12.6) are: +2.2, +0.4, +4.3, +1.0, +2.1, −1.4, −1.2, +0.7, 0.0, +0.4, −0.3, +0.7, +0.2, −0.3, +0.6, +1.8, +0.5 and +0.2 kg. These differences are skewed to the right. The null hypothesis is that the distributions of the differences in weight loss between the dogs in the population on the novel diet and those on the standard diet are the same. This is a two-sample test of the differences; we can use the Wilcoxon rank sum test to test the null hypothesis. We rank the two groups together and find the sum of the ranks of one of the two groups, say the novel diet group. The sum of these ranks is 3 + 4.5 + 10 + 11 + 13 + 15 + 15 + 17 + 18 + 19 + 21 + 24.5 + 24.5 + 27 + 30 + 31 + 32 + 36 = 351.5. We cannot refer this sum to Table A.10 because the sample sizes are too great. Instead, we find

$$Test_{14} = \frac{351.5 - 18(18+18+1)/2}{\sqrt{18(18)(18+18+1)/12}} = 0.59$$

which we refer to Table A.1 which gives $P = 0.56$. Hence we have insufficient evidence to reject the null hypothesis. Note, a computer analysis also gives $P = 0.56$. Thus there is no evidence to indicate that the novel diet promotes weight loss in obese dogs. The median weight loss (25th, 75th percentiles) in the novel diet group of dogs is 0.45 kg (−0.08, 1.2 kg), and in the standard diet group it is 0.40 kg (−0.93, 1.63 kg).

12.8 (a) The Friedman two-way ANOVA is the appropriate analysis because the data are dependent – there is a response for each dog for each of the three conditions. The null hypothesis is that the percentage aminopeptidase responses in the three different conditions come from the same population or from populations with the same median. Because the data are not homoscedastic (i.e. the variances are not constant), and recognizing that both the numerator and the denominator of the variable of interest (the percentages) are random variables (leading to some theoretical difficulties), we suggest analysing the data using a non-parametric approach. (b) The result of the Friedman ANOVA is significant ($P = 0.006$) so that we have evidence to reject the null hypothesis. We can infer that the aminopeptidase responses do not come from populations with the same median. We are particularly interested to know whether the response in the presence of gluten is different from that of either the negative or positive controls. Wilcoxon signed rank tests comparing the results of the gluten responses with the negative and the positive controls give $P = 0.027$ for each comparison (if we employ the Bonferroni correction – see Section 8.6.3 – in each case (i.e. multiply the P-value by 2), we would only obtain borderline significance). It would seem that the aminopeptidase response in the presence of gluten is suppressed, a surprising result and one which certainly deserves to be explored further.

12.9 (a) It was sensible to perform non-parametric tests in this study because the sample sizes in the two groups were very small (five and six) so that it is impossible to establish the distribution of the data in each group. (b) Apart from small sample sizes, other reasons for using a non-parametric test would be if the assumptions (e.g. Normality, constant variance) of the proposed parametric test are not satisfied, or if the data are measured on a categorical scale rather than a numerical scale. (c) The Wilcoxon rank sum test is an appropriate non-parametric test to use when it is of interest to compare the observations in two independent groups, as was the case when the aqueous VEGF level was compared in the ischaemic and control groups. The Wilcoxon signed rank test is an appropriate non-parametric test to use when it is of interest to compare related, i.e. paired, observations within a group, as was the case when the VEGF level was compared in the same rabbit on different days, and then averaged over all the rabbits. (d) The null hypothesis relating to $P = 0.03$ is that the VEGF levels on day 1 from the ischaemic and control groups of rabbits were obtained from populations which have similar distributions and the same median, and the null hypothesis relating to $P = 0.06$ is that the VEGF levels of rabbits with anterior segment ischaemia on day 1 and day 14 come from populations with identical distributions and the same median, or from the same population. (e) $P = 0.03$ and $P = 0.04$ for the comparison of VEGF levels in the two groups on days 1 and 14, respectively, imply that the VEGF level is significantly greater in the ischaemic group than in the controls on both of these days. $P = 0.06$ implies that there is no significant decrease in VEGF level in the group of ischaemic rabbits at day 14 compared with day 1. (f) The appropriate summary measures for the rank sum test would be the median in each group with a range, CI or percentiles together with the difference in medians with a CI. For the signed rank test the median at each day could be reported (with CI, range or percentiles) but, more importantly, the median difference between day 1 and day 14 should be reported with a CI, range or percentiles.

Chapter 13

13.1 (a) **F**: it Normalizes data that are skewed to the right. (b) **T**. (c) **T**: in particular when the standard deviation is proportional to the mean. (d) **F**: it is not used for proportions. The logistic transformation is appropriate. (e) **F**: non-parametric tests are often applied when the sample size is small.

13.2 (a) **T**: if you increase the power, you have a greater chance of detecting a real difference. (b) **T**. (c) **F**: it is easier to detect, as significant, a large treatment difference than a small one, so that you will need fewer animals if the treatment effect is greater. (d) **T**: if you have underestimated the standard deviation, then the treatment effect relative to the standard deviation will be smaller, and therefore harder to detect. Also, if there is more variability in the data, it will be

harder to detect a treatment difference unless you increase the sample size. (e) **F**: if the standardized difference is increased, this means that the treatment effect relative to the standard deviation is greater. As it is easier to detect a large difference, you can decrease the sample size.

13.3 (a) **F**: a long time-lag precludes an early decision and wastes information from further subjects. (b) **T**. (c) **F**: selection and allocation are two different processes, and one does not imply the other. (d) **T**. (e) **F**: a cluster sample is less precise than a simple random sample. The greatest precision is achieved if it is designed so that the units within a cluster are as different as possible, and the cluster means are as alike as possible.

13.4 (a) **F**: a meta-analysis is a quantitative systematic review that combines the results of relevant studies to produce and investigate an estimate of the overall effect of interest. (b) **T**. (c) **T**. (d) **T**. (e) **F**: the forest plot is used to display the different estimates of the effect of interest together with the overall estimate of the effect and relevant confidence intervals.

13.5 This is a two-tailed test. Even though we are interested in the decline in Hb content, we cannot exclude the possibility that the Hb content of the blood might rise in the course of the investigation. (a) The standardized difference = $1/(0.96) = 1.04$; hence we need about 30 animals (15 per group). (b) About 40 animals would be required to raise the power to 90%, i.e. 20 per group. (c) About 44 animals would be required, i.e. 22 per group. (d) The standardized difference is now $1/(1.3) = 0.77$; hence about 55 animals would be required, i.e. 28 per group. (e) Instead of 20 animals in each group, we require $40(1 + 2)^2/(4 \times 2) = 45$ animals in total, i.e. $45/3 = 15$ with the infestation and 30 controls.

13.6 (a) The standardized difference = $2 \times (1.0)/(1.7) = 1.18$, so we require about 36 horses for this trial. (b) Only 55%, i.e. too low to be of any real use. (c) For a sample size of 20, the power of the test increases to just over 75%.

13.7 The standardized difference is $(90-50) \div \sqrt{70(100-70)} = 0.8$. This trial will require about 55 animals in total, with 28 in each group.

13.8 (a) The significance level is the cut-off for the *P*-value which leads to rejection of the null hypothesis. Typically the significance level is 0.05. Then, if the *P*-value from the test is less than 0.05, the null hypothesis is rejected. If the *P*-value is equal to or greater than 0.05, there is no evidence to reject the null hypothesis. (b) The power of the test is the probability (often expressed as a percentage) of rejecting the null hypothesis when it is false. It is the probability of correctly detecting an effect of a given magnitude as significant. Thus in the study quoted, a power of 80% means there is an 80% chance of finding a significant difference of at least 5 days in the mean days to slaughter weight if there really is a difference. (c) The significance level is the cut-off for the probability of a Type I error. The power of the test is 1 minus the probability of a Type II error. (d) Decrease – it is easier to find a difference if the significance level is increased. (e) Increase – it is harder to be more sure of detecting a difference. (f) Decrease – it is easier to detect a larger difference.

Chapter 14

14.1 (a) T. (b) F: this is the positive predictive value. (c) F: although the sensitivity and the specificity of a test are related, so that as one is increased, the other decreases, one is not the complement of the other. (d) T. (e) F: the sensitivity and specificity of a test are not affected by the prevalence of the disease.

14.2 (a) F: this is for a categorical variable. (b) F: this only determines whether a systematic difference or bias is present. (c) F: the correlation coefficient does not assess how close the points are to the line of equality. (d) T: this measure gives an indication of the maximum likely difference between two measurements. We can use this measure to determine the limits of agreement. (e) F: we are interested in the differences if we are investigating agreement, so s_w should not be

used as the actual measure of agreement. Note that it is possible to calculate the appropriate measure of agreement from this quantity.

14.3 (a) F: there are too few points in the series. (b) T. (c) F: the information on the changes that a given animal undergoes is lost. Multiple comparisons may lead to spurious *P*-values. (d) F: multiple comparisons may lead to spurious *P*-values. The results of successive tests are not independent. (e) T: the use of summary measures is a correct approach. The difference between the initial and final response in an animal may be the correct summary measure in a particular circumstance.

14.4 (a) T. (b) F: a Cox regression analysis may be used when there are censored data but it can also be used when there are no censored data. (c) T. (d) F: two survival curves are compared in a Cox regression by assessing the significance of the relative hazard associated with the variable whose categories distinguish the two survival curves. The logrank test is commonly used when a Kaplan–Meier survival analysis is performed when there is only one explanatory variable of interest, that which distinguishes the two curves. (e) F: this is not an assumption underlying a Cox regression analysis.

14.5 (a) F: a Pearson correlation coefficient of 0.95 indicates that the points in the scatter diagram were close to or on the line of best fit. For there to be almost perfect agreement, the points should be close to or on the 45° line through the origin. (b) F: the kappa measure of agreement can only be evaluated for categorical data. HU values are, as indicated, numerical. (c) T: if the Pearson correlation coefficient is close to one, the only reason for Lin's concordance correlation coefficient to be low is because there is a systematic effect, i.e. poor accuracy. (d) F: poor precision would imply that the points in the scatter diagram were not close to the line of best fit. Since the Pearson correlation coefficient was close to one, this would not have been true. (e) F: the difference between these correlation coefficients could arise if there was poor accuracy.

Since the Pearson correlation coefficient was close to one, there was good precision.

14.6 (a) **F**: a ROC curve is a plot of the sensitivity against 1 minus the specificity when each is expressed as a proportion. (b) **T**. (c) **F**: it is a plot of the true-positive rate against the false-positive rate. (d) **F**: if the AUROC is 0.5 then the diagnostic test is no better than chance at discriminating between those with and without the disease. (e) **T**.

14.7 (a) For a cut-off value of >90 U/l, sensitivity = $100 \times (43/46) = 93.5\%$, specificity = $100 \times (80/92) = 87.0\%$. (b) This cut-off value produces a test with both a high sensitivity and a high specificity, and is a worthwhile diagnostic test. (c) With a cut-off value of >500 U/l, sensitivity = $100 \times (37/46) = 80.4\%$, specificity = $100 \times (88/92) = 95.7\%$. Hence, when the cut-off value is raised, the sensitivity is compromised so that the test has a lesser ability to detect HAC, although the specificity of the test is substantially the same. (d) The PPV is very low, indicating that it is unlikely that a dog with a positive test result actually has HAC. Thus, the test is unreliable for establishing whether the dog has HAC. However, because the NPV = 100%, then we would expect all dogs with CAP ≤90 U/l not to have HAC. It would seem that the CAP test should not be used as a screening tool but is a useful diagnostic device for dogs in which HAC is indicated. (e) Using the data in the table, we find that PPV = $100 \times (43/45) = 95.6\%$ and NPV = $100 \times (80/83) = 96.4\%$. The PPV is very different from what was obtained from the serum samples submitted to the laboratory in the 3-month period because the prevalence of HAC is very different in the two data sets. In the original investigations, the results of which are shown in the table, the observed prevalence is $100 \times (46/138) = 33.3\%$. In the wider population, the prevalence is very much lower, so that the PPV is also lower.

14.8 The likelihood ratio of a positive test result (LR_+) is equal to the sensitivity divided by (100 − specificity) when the sensitivity and spe-

cificity are each expressed in percentage terms. Hence $LR_+ = 61/(100 - 99.9) = 610$. Using Fagan's nomogram, we connect the pre-test probability (i.e. the prevalence) of 34% to the likelihood ratio of 610 and extend the line so formed to the post-test probability axis. This suggests that the chance that a mithun has brucellosis if it tests positive using the standard tube agglutination test is greater than 99%.

14.9 The frequencies that we would expect if there were chance agreement along the diagonal (starting from the top) are 17.69 (i.e. this is $35 \times 143/283$), 23.32, 19.26 and 1.22. Observed agreement along the diagonal = $(34 + 16 + 14 + 3)/283 = 67/283 = 0.267$; chance agreement = $(17.69 + 23.32 + 19.26 + 1.22)/283 = 61.49/283 = 0.217$; so kappa = $(0.267 - 0.217)/(1 - 0.217) = 0.025$. This represents poor agreement. Poor agreement implies that the scores before and after treatment are dissimilar. We can see from the table of results that the scores tend to improve after treatment, suggesting that treatment has improved the condition of foot rot in this flock.

14.10 We find the differences between the duplicate readings (these are, corrected to two decimal places, −0.09, 0.00, 0.09, −0.02, −0.01, 0.03, −0.04, 0.11, −0.01, −0.05 and 0.09 mmol/l, respectively). We also find the means of the duplicate readings (these are, corrected to two decimal places, 3.71, 4.30, 3.59, 3.16, 3.34, 3.04, 3.11, 3.25, 2.99, 2.79 and 2.93 mmol/l, respectively). When we plot the difference against the mean, we obtain a random scatter of points approximately evenly scattered around the zero difference line. In fact, the mean of these differences is 0.010 mmol/l and the estimated standard deviation of the differences is 0.064 mmol/l. A paired *t*-test investigating the differences between the readings gives a test statistic of 0.49 and $P = 0.63$, indicating that there is no systematic difference. The limits of agreement are approximately $0.010 \pm 2 \times 0.064 = -0.118$ mmol/l to 0.138 mmol/l. We expect 95% of the differences to lie between these limits; the maximum likely difference between two readings (equal to the British Standards repeatability coefficient) is approximately $2 \times 0.064 = 0.128$ mmol/l. In addition, using the formula provided in Section 14.4.2(a), we estimate Lin's concordance correlation coefficient to be 0.99. Since there is no evidence of a systematic effect, we also estimate the intraclass correlation coefficient to be 0.99 by determining the Pearson correlation coefficient between 22 pairs of readings (i.e. the 11 pairs in Table 14.7 and the 11 pairs obtained by switching the members of each pair in the table). Thus, we can see that this assay is highly repeatable, with both good precision and accuracy.

Chapter 15

15.1 (a) **F**: the investigator cannot ignore the consequences of his/her actions. (b) **F**: ethics committees are of course primarily concerned with these matters but that does not absolve the investigator from responsibility in this area. (c) **T**. (d) **F**: research involving animals cannot focus exclusively on the welfare of the experimental animals since this would rule out most procedures. (e) **T**.

15.2 (a) **F**: data from different locations can be included in other statistical approaches. (b) **F**: it is the GIS that provides the mapping facility. (c) **F**: although time can be included this is not the purpose of spatial statistics. (d) **T**. (e) **T**.

15.3 (a) **F**: veterinary surveillance may record events, but it is not its purpose to provide a clinical veterinary examination. (b) **T**. (c) **F**: this is the responsibility of professional veterinary organizations. (d) **F**: veterinary surveillance may record animal movements but does not control them. (e) **F**: veterinary surveillance is not involved in licensing slaughter houses.

15.4 (a) **T**. (b) **F**: this is the preserve of molecular genetics. (c) **T**. (d) **F**: quantitative genetics employs both parametric and non-parametric methods. (e) **F**: this is the preserve of molecular genetics.

15.5 (a) The goat population is not uniformly distributed, with a concentration of goats within the southern provinces. The preponderance of

positive herds are located within the 2009 vaccination area. (b) The majority of areas with higher goat density are located within the 2009 vaccination area. (c) (i) The goat density is evenly distributed throughout the 12 regions of the Netherlands. (ii) The occurrence of Q fever is unrelated to the herd distribution. (iii) The numbers of serology-only positive-testing herds are no different from the numbers of both serology- and bulk milk-positive herds. (iv) The occurrence of Q fever is unrelated to the goat density.

Chapter 16

16.1 (a) **F**: although EBVM draws heavily on the peer-reviewed published scientific literature, it also considers any other communicated information on its merits. Of concern is reliability and this depends partly on study design and veracity. (b) **F**: while EBVM may help to justify clinical decisions, its prime intention is to improve practice. (c) **T**. (d) **F**: EBVM brings a systematic and scientific formality to the process of using the evidence available in contrast to the older practice of 'clinical judgement' alone. (e) **T**.

16.2 (a) **F**: the NNT is the number of animals we need to treat with the novel treatment instead of the control treatment to prevent one adverse outcome. (b) **F**. (c) **T**. (d) **T**. (e) **F**: the ratio of the risks is the relative risk.

16.3 (a) **F**: it is hoped that you will keep up to date with your field, but EBVM requires you to be far more focused about seeking answers to specific clinical problems, working from the question to the answer, rather than hoping that you will come across a relevant article in your general reading. (b) **F**: this is a secondary result of EBVM. It is not its primary intention. (c) **T**. (d) **T**: what you gather in evidence from afar is then integrated with your local knowledge and experience to arrive at the most appropriate clinical decision, so EBVM does not eliminate your experience. (e) **F**: you are responsible for your own clinical decisions – EBVM provides the evidence to guide your decision-making.

16.4 Only (a) is not a component of PICO. The 'P' stands for patient or problem and not *P*-value.

16.5 (a), (b), (d) and (e) are each one of the steps of EBVM but (d) is not.

16.6 (a) There was investigator blinding (but no mention of whether the owner of the dog was blind to the treatments), a placebo control, randomization of limbs to treatments and an intention-to-treat analysis. (b) The authors do not say which kind of Wilcoxon test they used. Since the limbs in a dog were randomized to the treatments and thus each animal acted as its own control, a paired analysis would be appropriate, in which case the Wilcoxon signed rank test would be appropriate. As the authors found that baseline scores were not significantly different, the authors could have performed this Wilcoxon test on the actual scores rather than on the percentage change from baseline. Since they have used the percentage reduction from baseline for each limb for the analysis, and have provided the median percentage reduction from baseline in each group (rather than the median of the set of differences in the percentage reduction for each dog), there is a suggestion that they performed a two-sample Wilcoxon rank sum test; this would be inappropriate as the within-dog differences are ignored. Furthermore, the authors say that they performed a Fisher's (exact) test to compare the percentage of lesions that decreased by 50% or greater. Fisher's exact test is a two-sample test that ignores the paired nature of the data. McNemar's test is a test that compares proportions in paired samples, and this would be more appropriate for this study. (c) Both *P*-values indicate that the results were highly significant, with the percentage reduction from baseline scores being higher for tacrolimus-treated sites ($P = 0.0003$) and a greater percentage of tacrolimus-treated feet having lesions that decreased by at least 50% ($P < 0.0001$). (d) The main effects of interest are not provided. They would be: (i) the difference in the percentage reduction from baseline of lesional scores in the treatment and placebo groups; and (ii) the difference in the percentage with scores decreased by 50% or more at the study end in the two groups. (e) Although the CI is wide, the tacrolimus-treated sites showed a major reduction in clinical scores over the 6-week period, with the lower limit indicating a minimum median reduction of 39%. Vaseline showed what appears to be no effect of clinical importance, with the upper limit of the confidence interval being 13%, well below the lower limit of confidence interval for tacrolimus. The way the CIs are expressed is potentially confusing because of difficulty in distinguishing the minus sign from the dash. (f) Yes, there is evidence that tacrolimus was more effective than placebo in reducing the severity of localized skin lesions in dogs.

Appendix A
Statistical tables

Acknowledgements

Table A.1 Modified from Altman (1991) *Practical Statistics for Medical Research*, with permission. Copyright CRC Press, Boca Raton.

Table A.3 Modified from *Geigy Scientific Tables*, Vol. 2 (1990), 8th edn, Ciba-Geigy Ltd, with copyright permission from the Company Archives of Novartis Ltd, Basel.

Table A.4 Condensed from Table 8 of Pearson, E.S. and Hartley, H.O. (1966) *Biometrika Tables for Statisticians*, 3rd edn, by permission of Oxford University Press on behalf of the Biometrika Trust.

Table A.5 Condensed from *Geigy Scientific Tables*, Vol. 2 (1990), 8th edn, Ciba-Geigy Ltd, with copyright permission from the Company Archives of Novartis Ltd, Basel.

Table A.6 Modified from *Geigy Scientific Tables*, Vol. 2 (1990), 8th edn, Ciba-Geigy Ltd, with copyright permission from the Company Archives of Novartis Ltd, Basel.

Table A.7 Modified from Altman, D.G. (1991) *Practical Statistics for Medical Research*, with permission. Copyright CRC Press, Boca Raton.

Table A.8 Condensed from Siegel, S. and Castellan, N.J. (1988) *Nonparametric Statistics for the Behavioral Sciences*, 2nd edn, McGraw-Hill, New York, and used with permission of the McGraw-Hill Companies Inc.

Table A.9 Reproduced from Altman, D.G. (1991) *Practical Statistics for Medical Research*, with permission. Copyright CRC Press, Boca Raton.

Table A.10 Extracted from *Geigy Scientific Tables*, Vol. 2 (1990), 8th edn, Ciba-Geigy Ltd, with copyright permission from the Company Archives of Novartis Ltd, Basel.

Statistics for Veterinary and Animal Science, Third Edition. Aviva Petrie and Paul Watson.
© 2013 John Wiley & Sons, Ltd. Published 2013 by John Wiley & Sons, Ltd.

Table A.1 The Standard Normal distribution (two-tailed *P*-values from values of *z*, the SND)

The tabulated value is the *P*-value in the two tails of the Standard Normal distribution corresponding to a specified value (critical value or percentage point) of the Standardized Normal Deviate

$$z = \frac{x - \mu}{\sigma}$$

where *x* is a Normally distributed variable with mean = μ and standard deviation = σ (see Section 3.5.3(c)).

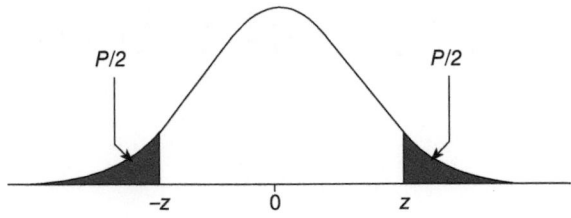

Example: if $z = 1.96$, then the two-tailed *P*-value = 0.05 ($P = 0.025$ in each tail).

Table A.1 The Standard Normal distribution (two-tailed P-values from values of z, the SND).

z	P	z	P	z	P	z	P	z	P	z	P
0.00	1.0000	0.53	0.5961	1.04	0.2983	1.56	0.1188	2.08	0.0375	2.59	0.0096
0.01	0.9920	0.54	0.5892	1.05	0.2937	1.57	0.1164	2.09	0.0366	2.60	0.0093
0.02	0.9840	0.55	0.5823	1.06	0.2891	1.58	0.1141	2.10	0.0357	2.61	0.0091
0.03	0.9761	0.56	0.5755	1.07	0.2846	1.59	0.1118	2.11	0.0349	2.62	0.0088
0.04	0.9681	0.57	0.5687	1.08	0.2801	1.60	0.1096	2.12	0.0340	2.63	0.0085
0.05	0.9601	0.58	0.5619	1.09	0.2757	1.61	0.1074	2.13	0.0332	2.64	0.0083
0.06	0.9522	0.59	0.5552	1.10	0.2713	1.62	0.1052	2.14	0.0324	2.65	0.0080
0.07	0.9442	0.60	0.5485	1.11	0.2670	1.63	0.1031	2.15	0.0316	2.66	0.0078
0.08	0.9362	0.61	0.5419	1.12	0.2627	1.64	0.1010	2.16	0.0308	2.67	0.0076
0.09	0.9283	0.62	0.5353	1.13	0.2585	1.65	0.0989	2.17	0.0300	2.68	0.0074
0.10	0.9203	0.63	0.5287	1.14	0.2543	1.66	0.0969	2.18	0.0293	2.69	0.0071
0.11	0.9124	0.64	0.5222	1.15	0.2501	1.67	0.0949	2.19	0.0285	2.70	0.0069
0.12	0.9045	0.65	0.5157	1.16	0.2460	1.68	0.0930	2.20	0.0278	2.71	0.0067
0.13	0.8966	0.66	0.5093	1.17	0.2420	1.69	0.0910	2.21	0.0271	2.72	0.0065
0.14	0.8887	0.67	0.5029	1.18	0.2380	1.70	0.0891	2.22	0.0264	2.73	0.0063
0.15	0.8808	0.68	0.4965	1.19	0.2340	1.71	0.0873	2.23	0.0257	2.74	0.0061
0.16	0.8729	0.69	0.4902	1.20	0.2301	1.72	0.0854	2.24	0.0251	2.75	0.0060
0.17	0.8650	0.70	0.4839	1.21	0.2263	1.73	0.0836	2.25	0.0244	2.76	0.0058
0.18	0.8572	0.71	0.4777	1.22	0.2225	1.74	0.0819	2.26	0.0238	2.77	0.0056
0.19	0.8493	0.72	0.4715	1.23	0.2187	1.75	0.0801	2.27	0.0232	2.78	0.0054
0.20	0.8415	0.73	0.4654	1.24	0.2150	1.76	0.0784	2.28	0.0226	2.79	0.0053
0.21	0.8337	0.74	0.4593	1.25	0.2113	1.77	0.0767	2.29	0.0220	2.80	0.0051
0.22	0.8259	0.75	0.4533	1.26	0.2077	1.78	0.0751	2.30	0.0214	2.81	0.0050
0.23	0.8181	0.76	0.4473	1.27	0.2041	1.79	0.0735	2.31	0.0209	2.82	0.0048
0.24	0.8103	0.77	0.4413	1.28	0.2005	1.80	0.0719	2.32	0.0203	2.83	0.0047
0.25	0.8026	0.78	0.4354	1.29	0.1971	1.81	0.0703	2.33	0.0198	2.84	0.0045
0.26	0.7949	0.79	0.4295	1.30	0.1936	1.82	0.0688	2.34	0.0193	2.85	0.0044
0.27	0.7872	0.80	0.4237	1.31	0.1902	1.83	0.0672	2.35	0.0188	2.86	0.0042
0.28	0.7795	0.81	0.4179	1.32	0.1868	1.84	0.0658	2.36	0.0183	2.87	0.0041
0.29	0.7718	0.82	0.4122	1.33	0.1835	1.85	0.0643	2.37	0.0178	2.88	0.0040
0.30	0.7642	0.83	0.4065	1.34	0.1802	1.86	0.0629	2.38	0.0173	2.89	0.0039
0.31	0.7566	0.84	0.4009	1.35	0.1770	1.87	0.0615	2.39	0.0168	2.90	0.0037
0.32	0.7490	0.85	0.3953	1.36	0.1738	1.88	0.0601	2.40	0.0164	2.91	0.0036
0.33	0.7414	0.86	0.3898	1.37	0.1707	1.89	0.0588	2.41	0.0160	2.92	0.0035
0.34	0.7339	0.87	0.3843	1.38	0.1676	1.90	0.0574	2.42	0.0155	2.93	0.0034
0.35	0.7263	0.88	0.3789	1.39	0.1645	1.91	0.0561	2.43	0.0151	2.94	0.0033
0.36	0.7188	0.89	0.3735	1.40	0.1615	1.92	0.0549	2.44	0.0147	2.95	0.0032
0.37	0.7114	0.90	0.3681	1.41	0.1585	1.93	0.0536	2.45	0.0143	2.96	0.0031
0.38	0.7039	0.91	0.3628	1.42	0.1556	1.94	0.0524	2.46	0.0139	2.97	0.0030
0.39	0.6965	0.92	0.3576	1.43	0.1527	1.95	0.0512	2.47	0.0135	2.98	0.0029
0.40	0.6892	0.93	0.3524	1.44	0.1499	1.96	0.0500	2.48	0.0131	2.99	0.0028
0.41	0.6818	0.94	0.3472	1.45	0.1471	1.97	0.0488	2.49	0.0128	3.00	0.0027
0.42	0.6745	0.95	0.3421	1.46	0.1443	1.98	0.0477	2.50	0.0124	3.10	0.00194
0.43	0.6672	0.96	0.3371	1.47	0.1416	1.99	0.0466	2.51	0.0121	3.20	0.00137
0.44	0.6599	0.97	0.3320	1.48	0.1389	2.00	0.0455	2.52	0.0117	3.30	0.00097
0.45	0.6527	0.98	0.3271	1.49	0.1362	2.01	0.0444	2.53	0.0114	3.40	0.00067
0.46	0.6455	0.99	0.3222	1.50	0.1336	2.02	0.0434	2.54	0.0111	3.50	0.00047
0.47	0.6384	1.00	0.3173	1.51	0.1310	2.03	0.0424	2.55	0.0108	3.60	0.00032
0.48	0.6312	1.01	0.3125	1.52	0.1285	2.04	0.0414	2.56	0.0105	3.70	0.00022
0.49	0.6241	1.02	0.3077	1.53	0.1260	2.05	0.0404	2.57	0.0102	3.80	0.00014
0.50	0.6171	1.03	0.3030	1.54	0.1236	2.06	0.0394	2.58	0.0099	3.90	0.00010
0.51	0.6101			1.55	0.1211	2.07	0.0385			4.00	0.00006
0.52	0.6031										

Table A.2 The Standard Normal distribution (values of *z*, the SND, from *P*-values)

The one-tailed *P*-value is that in which the total probability is contained in the tail area to the right of the Standardized Normal Deviate

$$z = \frac{x - \mu}{\sigma}$$

where *x* is a Normally distributed variable with mean = μ and standard deviation = σ. The two-tailed *P*-value is that in which half of the total probability is contained in the tail area to the right of *z*, the SND, and the other half is contained in the tail area to the left of $-z$ (see Section 3.5.3(d)).

Table A.2 Tail area probabilites and corresponding values of the SND, *z*.

Two-tailed probability	SND, *z*	One-tailed probability
1.00	0.00	0.50
0.90	0.13	0.45
0.50	0.67	0.25
0.25	1.15	0.125
0.20	1.28	0.10
0.15	1.44	0.075
0.10	1.64	0.05
0.05	1.96	0.025
0.02	2.33	0.01
0.01	2.58	0.005
0.005	2.81	0.0025
0.001	3.29	0.0005

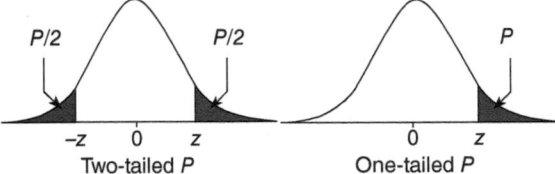

Two-tailed *P*   One-tailed *P*

Table A.3 The *t*-distribution

This table contains the critical value (percentage point), t_p, of the *t*-distribution which corresponds to a particular two-tailed *P*-value for specified degrees of freedom. If the test statistic follows the *t*-distribution with known degrees of freedom, then the *P*-value for the two-tailed hypothesis test is calculated by determining where the absolute value (i.e. ignoring its sign) of the observed test statistic lies in relation to the critical values in the table. If its value is greater than the tabulated critical value, then the *P*-value for the test is less than the relevant tabulated *P*-value. If its value lies between two adjacent critical values, then the *P*-value for the test lies between the corresponding tabulated *P*-values.

Example: if the observed test statistic = 2.72 on 15 degrees of freedom, then since 2.72 > 2.602, $P < 0.02$. Furthermore, since 2.72 lies between 2.602 and 2.947, $0.01 < P < 0.02$.

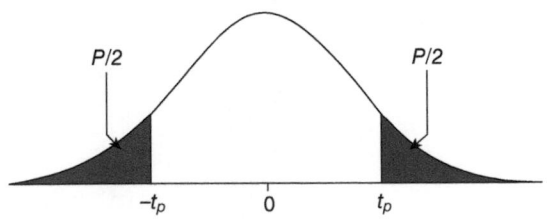

Table A.3 Percentage points of the *t*-distribution.

df	\multicolumn{13}{c}{Two-tailed *P*-values}
	0.9	0.8	0.7	0.6	0.5	0.4	0.3	0.2	0.1	0.05	0.02	0.01	0.001
1	0.158	0.325	0.510	0.727	1.000	1.376	1.963	3.078	6.314	12.706	31.821	63.657	636.619
2	0.142	0.289	0.445	0.617	0.816	1.061	1.386	1.886	2.920	4.303	6.965	9.925	31.598
3	0.137	0.277	0.424	0.584	0.765	0.978	1.250	1.638	2.353	3.182	4.541	5.841	12.924
4	0.134	0.271	0.414	0.569	0.741	0.941	1.190	1.533	2.132	2.776	3.747	4.604	8.610
5	0.132	0.267	0.408	0.559	0.727	0.920	1.156	1.476	2.015	2.571	3.365	4.032	6.869
6	0.131	0.265	0.404	0.553	0.718	0.906	1.134	1.440	1.943	2.447	3.143	3.707	5.959
7	0.130	0.263	0.402	0.549	0.711	0.896	1.119	1.415	1.895	2.365	2.998	3.499	5.408
8	0.130	0.262	0.399	0.546	0.706	0.889	1.108	1.397	1.86	2.306	2.896	3.355	5.041
9	0.129	0.261	0.398	0.543	0.703	0.883	1.100	1.383	1.833	2.262	2.821	3.250	4.781
10	0.129	0.260	0.397	0.542	0.700	0.879	1.093	1.372	1.812	2.228	2.764	3.169	4.587
11	0.129	0.260	0.396	0.540	0.697	0.876	1.088	1.363	1.796	2.201	2.718	3.106	4.437
12	0.128	0.259	0.395	0.539	0.695	0.873	1.083	1.356	1.782	2.179	2.681	3.055	4.318
13	0.128	0.259	0.394	0.538	0.694	0.870	1.079	1.350	1.771	2.160	2.650	3.012	4.221
14	0.128	0.258	0.393	0.537	0.692	0.868	1.076	1.345	1.761	2.145	2.624	2.977	4.140
15	0.128	0.258	0.393	0.536	0.691	0.866	1.074	1.341	1.753	2.131	2.602	2.947	4.073
16	0.128	0.258	0.392	0.535	0.690	0.865	1.071	1.337	1.746	2.120	2.583	2.921	4.015
17	0.128	0.257	0.392	0.534	0.689	0.863	1.069	1.333	1.741	2.110	2.567	2.898	3.965
18	0.127	0.257	0.392	0.534	0.688	0.862	1.067	1.330	1.734	2.101	2.552	2.878	3.922
19	0.127	0.257	0.391	0.533	0.688	0.861	1.066	1.328	1.729	2.093	2.539	2.861	3.883
20	0.127	0.257	0.391	0.533	0.687	0.860	1.064	1.325	1.725	2.086	2.528	2.845	3.850
21	0.127	0.257	0.391	0.532	0.686	0.859	1.063	1.323	1.721	2.080	2.518	2.831	3.819
22	0.127	0.256	0.390	0.532	0.686	0.858	1.061	1.321	1.717	2.074	2.508	2.819	3.792
23	0.127	0.256	0.390	0.532	0.685	0.858	1.060	1.319	1.714	2.069	2.500	2.807	3.767
24	0.127	0.256	0.390	0.531	0.685	0.857	1.059	1.318	1.711	2.064	2.492	2.797	3.745
25	0.127	0.256	0.390	0.531	0.684	0.856	1.058	1.316	1.708	2.060	2.485	2.787	3.725
26	0.127	0.256	0.390	0.531	0.684	0.856	1.058	1.315	1.706	2.056	2.479	2.779	3.707
27	0.127	0.256	0.389	0.531	0.684	0.855	1.057	1.314	1.703	2.052	2.473	2.771	3.690
28	0.127	0.256	0.389	0.530	0.683	0.855	1.056	1.313	1.701	2.048	2.467	2.763	3.674
29	0.127	0.256	0.389	0.530	0.683	0.854	1.055	1.311	1.699	2.045	2.462	2.756	3.659
30	0.127	0.256	0.389	0.530	0.683	0.854	1.055	1.310	1.697	2.042	2.457	2.750	3.646
40	0.126	0.255	0.388	0.529	0.681	0.851	1.050	1.303	1.684	2.021	2.423	2.704	3.551
50	0.126	0.255	0.388	0.528	0.679	0.849	1.047	1.299	1.676	2.009	2.403	2.678	3.497
100	0.126	0.254	0.386	0.526	0.677	0.845	1.042	1.291	1.661	1.984	2.364	2.626	3.391
200	0.126	0.254	0.386	0.525	0.676	0.843	1.039	1.286	1.653	1.972	2.345	2.601	3.340
∞	0.126	0.253	0.385	0.524	0.674	0.842	1.036	1.282	1.645	1.960	2.326	2.576	3.291

Table A.4 The Chi-squared (χ^2) distribution

This table contains the critical value (percentage point), χ^2_p, of the χ^2-distribution which corresponds to a particular P-value for specified degrees of freedom. Note that the P-value relates to the upper tail of the χ^2-distribution. If the test statistic follows the χ^2-distribution with known degrees of freedom, then the P-value for the hypothesis test is calculated by determining where the observed test statistic lies in relation to the critical values in the table. If the observed test statistic is greater than the critical value, then the P-value for the test is less than the tabulated P-value. If the observed test statistic lies between two adjacent critical values, then the P-value for the test lies between the corresponding tabulated P-values.

Example: if the observed test statistic = 20.3 on 10 degrees of freedom, then since $20.3 > 18.307$, $P < 0.05$. Furthermore, since 20.3 lies between 18.307 and 20.48, $0.025 < P < 0.05$.

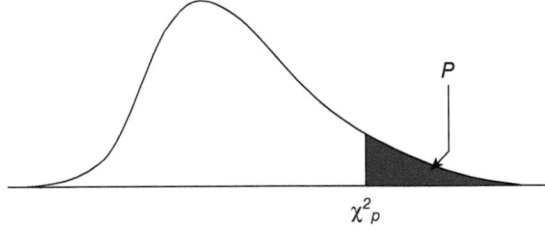

Table A.4 The Chi-squared (χ^2) distribution.

| df | \multicolumn{7}{c}{One-tailed P-value} |
	0.500	0.250	0.100	0.050	0.025	0.010	0.001
1	0.45	1.32	2.71	3.84	5.02	6.63	10.83
2	1.39	2.77	4.61	5.99	7.38	9.21	13.82
3	2.37	4.11	6.25	7.81	9.35	11.34	16.27
4	3.36	5.39	7.78	9.49	11.14	13.28	18.47
5	4.35	6.63	9.24	11.07	12.83	15.09	20.52
6	5.35	7.84	10.64	12.59	14.45	16.81	22.46
7	6.35	9.04	12.02	14.07	16.01	18.48	24.32
8	7.34	10.22	13.36	15.51	17.53	20.09	26.12
9	8.34	11.39	14.68	16.92	19.02	21.67	27.88
10	9.34	12.55	15.99	18.31	20.48	23.21	29.59
11	10.34	13.70	17.28	19.68	21.92	24.72	31.26
12	11.34	14.85	18.55	21.03	23.34	26.22	32.91
13	12.34	15.98	19.81	22.36	24.74	27.69	34.53
14	13.34	17.12	21.06	23.68	26.12	29.14	36.12
15	14.34	18.25	22.31	25.00	27.49	30.58	37.70
16	15.34	19.37	23.54	26.30	28.85	32.00	39.25
17	16.34	20.49	24.77	27.59	30.19	33.41	40.79
18	17.34	21.60	25.99	28.87	31.53	34.81	42.31
19	18.34	22.72	27.20	30.14	32.85	36.19	43.82
20	19.34	23.83	28.41	31.41	34.17	37.57	45.32
21	20.34	24.93	29.62	32.67	35.48	38.93	46.80
22	21.34	26.04	30.81	33.92	36.78	40.29	48.27
23	22.34	27.14	32.01	35.17	38.08	41.64	49.73
24	23.34	28.24	33.20	36.42	39.36	42.98	51.18
25	24.34	29.34	34.38	37.65	40.65	44.31	32.62
26	25.34	30.43	35.56	38.89	41.92	45.64	54.05
27	26.34	31.53	36.74	40.11	43.19	46.96	55.48
28	27.34	32.62	37.92	41.34	44.46	48.28	56.89
29	28.34	33.71	39.09	42.56	45.72	49.59	58.30
30	29.34	34.80	40.26	43.77	46.98	50.89	59.70
40	39.34	45.62	51.80	55.76	59.34	63.69	73.40
50	49.33	56.33	63.17	67.50	71.42	76.15	86.66
60	59.33	66.98	74.40	79.08	83.30	88.38	99.61
70	69.33	77.58	85.53	90.53	95.02	100.42	112.32
80	79.33	88.13	96.58	101.88	106.63	112.33	124.84
90	89.33	98.64	107.56	113.14	118.14	124.12	137.21
100	99.33	109.14	118.50	124.34	129.56	135.81	149.45

Table A.5 The *F*-distribution

Tables A.5a and A.5b contain the critical values (percentage points) of the *F*-distribution, F_p, which correspond to a specified *P*-value for v_1 degrees of freedom in the numerator and v_2 degrees of freedom in the denominator of the test statistic. If the test statistic follows the *F*-distribution with known degrees of freedom, then we can calculate the *P*-value by determining where the observed test statistic lies in relation to the critical values in the table. Note that the tabulated *P*-value relates to the *upper* tail of the *F*-distribution.

For a *one-sided* hypothesis test (as in the ANOVA; see Section 8.5), if the observed test statistic is greater than the critical value, then the *P*-value for the one-sided test is less than the tabulated *P*-value. If the observed test statistic lies between two adjacent critical values, then the *P*-value lies between the corresponding tabulated *P*-values. We are more likely to use Table A.5a if the test is one-sided.

Example: for a *one-sided* test, if the observed test statistic = 4.41 on 5 (numerator) and 6 (denominator) degrees of freedom, then since 4.41 > 4.39, $P < 0.05$. Furthermore, since 4.41 lies between 4.39 and 8.75, $0.01 < P < 0.05$.

Occasionally, we have a *two-sided* hypothesis test (e.g. when comparing two variances from independent groups: see Section 8.3). To determine significance at a given level, we have to compare our observed test statistic with the critical value in the table that corresponds to the tabulated *P*/2. Thus, a two-sided *P*-value of 0.05 corresponds to the tabulated $P = 0.025$; a two-sided *P*-value of 0.01 corresponds to the tabulated $P = 0.005$. We are more likely in this situation to use Table A.5b.

Example: for a *two-sided* test, if the observed test statistic = 6.0 on 2 (numerator) and 9 (denominator) degrees of freedom, then since 6.0 lies between 5.71 (the critical value for $P = 0.025$) and 10.11 (the critical value for $P = 0.005$), $0.01 < P < 0.05$.

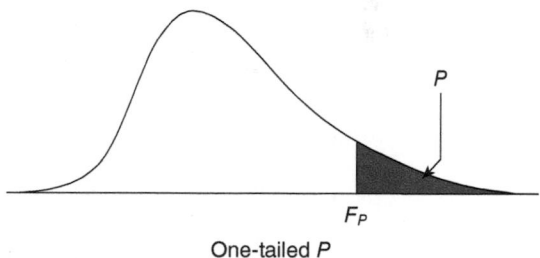

One-tailed *P*

Table A.5a   Percentage points of the F-distribution ($P = 0.05$ and $P = 0.01$).

df denominator, v_2	P	1	2	3	4	5	6	7	8	12	24	∞
1	0.05	161.4	199.5	215.7	224.6	230.2	234.0	236.8	238.9	243.9	249.1	254.3
	0.01	**4052**	**5000**	**5403**	**5625**	**5764**	**5859**	**5928**	**5981**	**6106**	**6235**	**6366**
2	0.05	18.51	19.00	19.16	19.25	19.30	19.33	19.35	19.37	19.41	19.45	19.50
	0.01	**98.50**	**99.00**	**99.17**	**99.25**	**99.30**	**99.33**	**99.36**	**99.37**	**99.42**	**99.46**	**99.50**
3	0.05	10.13	9.55	9.28	9.12	9.01	8.94	8.89	8.85	8.74	8.64	8.53
	0.01	**34.12**	**30.82**	**29.46**	**28.71**	**28.24**	**27.91**	**27.67**	**27.49**	**27.05**	**26.60**	**26.13**
4	0.05	7.71	6.94	6.59	6.39	6.26	6.16	6.09	6.04	5.91	5.77	5.63
	0.01	**21.20**	**18.00**	**16.69**	**15.98**	**15.52**	**15.21**	**14.98**	**14.80**	**14.37**	**13.93**	**3.46**
5	0.05	6.61	5.79	5.41	5.19	5.05	4.95	4.88	4.82	4.68	4.53	4.36
	0.01	**16.26**	**13.27**	**12.06**	**11.39**	**10.97**	**10.67**	**10.46**	**10.29**	**9.89**	**9.47**	**9.02**
6	0.05	5.99	5.14	4.76	4.53	4.39	4.28	4.21	4.15	4.00	3.84	3.67
	0.01	**13.75**	**10.92**	**9.78**	**9.15**	**8.75**	**8.47**	**8.26**	**8.10**	**7.72**	**7.31**	**6.88**
7	0.05	5.59	4.74	4.35	4.12	3.97	3.87	3.79	3.73	3.57	3.41	3.23
	0.01	**12.25**	**9.55**	**8.45**	**7.85**	**7.46**	**7.19**	**6.99**	**6.84**	**6.47**	**6.07**	**5.65**
8	0.05	5.32	4.46	4.07	3.84	3.69	3.58	3.50	3.44	3.28	3.12	2.93
	0.01	**11.26**	**8.65**	**7.59**	**7.01**	**6.63**	**6.37**	**6.18**	**6.03**	**5.67**	**5.28**	**4.86**
9	0.05	5.12	4.26	3.86	3.63	3.48	3.37	3.29	3.23	3.07	2.90	2.71
	0.01	**10.56**	**8.02**	**6.99**	**6.42**	**6.06**	**5.80**	**5.61**	**5.47**	**5.11**	**4.73**	**4.31**
10	0.05	4.96	4.10	3.71	3.48	3.33	3.22	3.14	3.07	2.91	2.74	2.54
	0.01	**10.04**	**7.56**	**6.55**	**5.99**	**5.64**	**5.39**	**5.20**	**5.06**	**4.71**	**4.33**	**3.91**
12	0.05	4.75	3.89	3.49	3.26	3.11	3.00	2.91	2.85	2.69	2.51	2.30
	0.01	**9.33**	**6.93**	**5.95**	**5.41**	**5.06**	**4.82**	**4.64**	**4.50**	**4.16**	**3.78**	**3.36**
14	0.05	4.60	3.74	3.34	3.11	2.96	2.85	2.76	2.70	2.53	2.35	2.13
	0.01	**8.86**	**6.51**	**5.56**	**5.04**	**4.69**	**4.46**	**4.28**	**4.14**	**3.80**	**3.43**	**3.00**
16	0.05	4.49	3.63	3.24	3.01	2.85	2.74	2.66	2.59	2.42	2.24	2.01
	0.01	**8.53**	**6.23**	**5.29**	**4.77**	**4.44**	**4.20**	**4.03**	**3.89**	**3.55**	**3.18**	**2.75**
18	0.05	4.41	3.55	3.16	2.93	2.77	2.66	2.58	2.51	2.34	2.15	1.92
	0.01	**8.29**	**6.01**	**5.09**	**4.58**	**4.25**	**4.01**	**3.84**	**3.71**	**3.37**	**3.00**	**2.57**
20	0.05	4.35	3.49	3.10	2.87	2.71	2.60	2.51	2.45	2.28	2.08	1.84
	0.01	**8.10**	**5.85**	**4.94**	**4.43**	**4.10**	**3.87**	**3.70**	**3.56**	**3.23**	**2.86**	**2.42**
30	0.05	4.17	3.32	2.92	2.69	2.53	2.42	2.33	2.27	2.09	1.89	1.62
	0.01	**7.56**	**5.39**	**4.51**	**4.02**	**3.70**	**3.47**	**3.30**	**3.17**	**2.84**	**2.47**	**2.01**
40	0.05	4.08	3.23	2.84	2.61	2.45	2.34	2.25	2.18	2.00	1.79	1.51
	0.01	**7.31**	**5.18**	**4.31**	**3.83**	**3.51**	**3.29**	**3.12**	**2.99**	**2.66**	**2.29**	**1.80**
60	0.05	4.00	3.15	2.76	2.53	2.37	2.25	2.17	2.10	1.92	1.70	1.39
	0.01	**7.08**	**4.98**	**4.13**	**3.65**	**3.34**	**3.12**	**2.95**	**2.82**	**2.50**	**2.12**	**1.60**
120	0.05	3.92	3.07	2.68	2.45	2.29	2.17	2.09	2.02	1.83	1.61	1.25
	0.01	**6.85**	**4.79**	**3.95**	**3.48**	**3.17**	**2.96**	**2.79**	**2.66**	**2.34**	**1.95**	**1.38**
∞	0.05	3.84	3.00	2.60	2.37	2.21	2.10	2.01	1.94	1.75	1.52	1.00
	0.01	**6.63**	**4.61**	**3.78**	**3.32**	**3.02**	**2.80**	**2.64**	**2.51**	**2.18**	**1.79**	**1.00**

Table A.5b Percentage points of the F-distribution ($P = 0.025$ and $P = 0.005$).

df denominator, ν_2	P	df numerator, ν_1										
		1	2	3	4	5	6	7	8	12	24	∞
1	0.025	647.8	799.5	864.2	899.6	921.8	937.1	948.2	956.7	976.7	997.2	1018
	0.005	**16211**	**20000**	**21615**	**22500**	**23056**	**23437**	**23715**	**23925**	**24426**	**24940**	**25465**
2	0.025	38.51	39.00	39.17	39.25	39.30	39.33	39.36	39.37	39.41	39.46	39.50
	0.005	**198.5**	**199.0**	**199.2**	**199.2**	**199.3**	**199.3**	**199.4**	**199.4**	**199.4**	**199.5**	**199.5**
3	0.025	17.44	16.04	15.44	15.10	14.88	14.73	14.62	14.54	14.34	14.12	13.90
	0.005	**55.55**	**49.80**	**47.47**	**46.19**	**45.39**	**44.84**	**44.43**	**44.13**	**43.39**	**42.62**	**41.83**
4	0.025	12.22	10.65	9.98	9.60	9.36	9.20	9.07	8.98	8.75	8.51	8.26
	0.005	**31.33**	**26.28**	**24.26**	**23.15**	**22.46**	**21.97**	**21.62**	**21.35**	**20.70**	**20.03**	**19.32**
5	0.025	10.01	8.43	7.76	7.39	7.15	6.98	6.85	6.76	6.52	6.28	6.02
	0.005	**22.78**	**18.31**	**16.53**	**15.56**	**14.94**	**14.51**	**14.20**	**13.96**	**13.38**	**12.78**	**12.14**
6	0.025	8.81	7.26	6.60	6.23	5.99	5.82	5.70	5.60	5.37	5.12	4.85
	0.005	**18.63**	**14.54**	**12.92**	**12.03**	**11.46**	**11.07**	**10.79**	**10.57**	**10.03**	**9.47**	**8.88**
7	0.025	8.07	6.54	5.89	5.52	5.29	5.12	4.99	4.90	4.67	4.42	4.14
	0.005	**16.24**	**12.40**	**10.88**	**10.05**	**9.52**	**9.16**	**8.89**	**8.68**	**8.18**	**7.65**	**7.08**
8	0.025	7.57	6.06	5.42	5.05	4.82	4.65	4.53	4.43	4.20	3.95	3.67
	0.005	**14.69**	**11.04**	**9.60**	**8.81**	**8.30**	**7.95**	**7.69**	**7.50**	**7.01**	**6.50**	**5.95**
9	0.025	7.21	5.71	5.08	4.72	4.48	4.32	4.20	4.10	3.87	3.61	3.33
	0.005	**13.61**	**10.11**	**8.72**	**7.96**	**7.47**	**7.13**	**6.88**	**6.69**	**6.23**	**5.73**	**5.19**
10	0.025	6.94	5.46	4.83	4.47	4.24	4.07	3.95	3.85	3.62	3.37	3.08
	0.005	**12.83**	**9.43**	**8.08**	**7.34**	**6.87**	**6.54**	**6.30**	**6.12**	**5.66**	**5.17**	**4.64**
12	0.025	6.55	5.10	4.47	4.12	3.89	3.73	3.61	3.51	3.28	3.02	2.72
	0.005	**11.75**	**8.51**	**7.23**	**6.52**	**6.07**	**5.76**	**5.52**	**5.35**	**4.91**	**4.43**	**3.90**
14	0.025	6.30	4.86	4.24	3.89	3.66	3.50	3.38	3.29	3.05	2.79	2.49
	0.005	**11.06**	**7.92**	**6.68**	**6.00**	**5.56**	**5.26**	**5.03**	**4.86**	**4.43**	**3.96**	**3.44**
16	0.025	6.12	4.69	4.08	3.73	3.50	3.34	3.22	3.12	2.89	2.63	2.32
	0.005	**10.58**	**7.51**	**6.30**	**5.64**	**5.21**	**4.91**	**4.69**	**4.52**	**4.10**	**3.64**	**3.11**
18	0.025	5.98	4.56	3.95	3.61	3.38	3.22	3.10	3.01	2.77	2.50	2.19
	0.005	**10.22**	**7.21**	**6.03**	**5.37**	**4.96**	**4.66**	**4.44**	**4.28**	**3.86**	**3.40**	**2.87**
20	0.025	5.87	4.46	3.86	3.51	3.29	3.13	3.01	2.91	2.68	2.41	2.09
	0.005	**9.94**	**6.99**	**5.82**	**5.17**	**4.76**	**4.47**	**4.26**	**4.09**	**3.68**	**3.22**	**2.69**
30	0.025	5.57	4.18	3.59	3.25	3.03	2.87	2.75	2.65	2.41	2.14	1.79
	0.005	**9.18**	**6.35**	**5.24**	**4.62**	**4.23**	**3.95**	**3.74**	**3.58**	**3.18**	**2.73**	**2.18**
40	0.025	5.42	4.05	3.46	3.13	2.90	2.74	2.62	2.53	2.29	2.01	1.64
	0.005	**8.83**	**6.07**	**4.98**	**4.37**	**3.99**	**3.71**	**3.51**	**3.35**	**2.95**	**2.50**	**1.93**
60	0.025	5.29	3.93	3.34	3.01	2.79	2.63	2.51	2.41	2.17	1.88	1.48
	0.005	**8.49**	**5.79**	**4.73**	**4.14**	**3.76**	**3.49**	**3.29**	**3.13**	**2.74**	**2.29**	**1.69**
120	0.025	5.15	3.80	3.23	2.89	2.67	2.52	2.39	2.30	2.05	1.76	1.31
	0.005	**8.18**	**5.54**	**4.50**	**3.92**	**3.55**	**3.28**	**3.09**	**2.93**	**2.54**	**2.09**	**1.43**
∞	0.025	5.02	3.69	3.12	2.79	2.57	2.41	2.29	2.19	1.94	1.64	1.00
	0.005	**7.88**	**5.30**	**4.28**	**3.72**	**3.35**	**3.09**	**2.90**	**2.74**	**2.36**	**1.90**	**1.00**

Table A.6 Pearson's correlation coefficient (*r*)

This table contains critical values of the sample correlation coefficient, *r*; it is used to test the null hypothesis that the true correlation coefficient (*ρ*) is equal to zero. For a given sample size (number of pairs), if the absolute value (i.e. ignoring its sign) of the sample correlation coefficient, *r*, is greater than the critical value, then the two-tailed *P*-value of the test is less than the tabulated *P*-value. If the sample correlation coefficient lies between two adjacent critical values, then the *P*-value for the test lies between the corresponding tabulated *P*-values. See Section 10.3.2(b) if the sample size is greater than 150.

Note: this table can also be used to test the significance of Spearman's rank correlation coefficient (see Section 12.7.4), provided the sample size is greater than 10 pairs. If the sample size is 10 or less, refer to Table A.7.

Example: if the sample size is 14 and *r* = 0.70, then since 0.70 > 0.6614, *P* < 0.01. Furthermore, since 0.70 lies between 0.6614 and 0.7800, 0.001 < *P* < 0.01.

Table A.6 Critical values of Pearson's correlation coefficient (*r*).

Sample size	Two-tailed *P*-value			Sample size	Two-tailed *P*-value		
	0.05	0.01	0.001		0.05	0.01	0.001
3	0.9969	0.9999	1.0000	23	0.4132	0.5256	0.6402
4	0.9500	0.9900	0.9990	24	0.4044	0.5151	0.6287
5	0.8783	0.9587	0.9911	25	0.3961	0.5052	0.6177
6	0.8114	0.9172	0.9741	26	0.3882	0.4958	0.6073
7	0.7545	0.8745	0.9509	27	0.3809	0.4869	0.5974
8	0.7067	0.8343	0.9249	28	0.3739	0.4785	0.5880
9	0.6664	0.7977	0.8983	29	0.3673	0.4705	0.5790
10	0.6319	0.7646	0.8721	30	0.3610	0.4629	0.5703
11	0.6021	0.7348	0.8471	35	0.3338	0.4296	0.5322
12	0.5760	0.7079	0.8233	40	0.3120	0.4026	0.5007
13	0.5529	0.6835	0.8010	45	0.2940	0.3801	0.4742
14	0.5324	0.6614	0.7800	50	0.2787	0.3610	0.4514
15	0.5139	0.6411	0.7604	55	0.2656	0.3445	0.4317
16	0.4973	0.6226	0.7419	60	0.2542	0.3301	0.4143
17	0.4821	0.6055	0.7247	70	0.2352	0.3060	0.3850
18	0.4683	0.5897	0.7084	80	0.2199	0.2864	0.3611
19	0.4555	0.5751	0.6932	90	0.2072	0.2702	0.3412
20	0.4438	0.5614	0.6788	100	0.2172	0.2830	0.3569
21	0.4329	0.5487	0.6652	150	0.1603	0.2097	0.2660
22	0.4227	0.5368	0.6524				

Table A.7 Spearman's rank correlation coefficient (r_s)

This table contains critical values for Spearman's rank correlation coefficient, r_s, for small samples; it is used to test the null hypothesis that the true correlation coefficient (ρ_s) is equal to zero. If the sample size (number of pairs) is greater than 15, you can refer to Table A.6, which provides a good approximation. For a given sample size, if the absolute value (i.e. ignoring its sign) of the sample rank correlation coefficient, r_s, is greater than the critical value, then the two-tailed P-value of the test is less than the tabulated P-value. If the sample rank correlation coefficient lies between two adjacent critical values, then the two-tailed P-value for the test lies between the corresponding tabulated P-values.

Example: if the sample size is 6 and $r_s = 0.85$, since $0.85 > 0.8286$, $P < 0.05$. Furthermore, since $0.8286 < 0.85 < 0.8857$, $0.02 < P < 0.05$.

Table A.7 Critical values of Spearman's rank correlation coefficient.

Sample size	Two-tailed P-value				
	0.1	0.05	0.02	0.01	0.002
4	0.8000	–	–	–	–
5	0.8000	0.9000	0.9000	–	–
6	0.7714	0.8286	0.8857	0.9429	–
7	0.6786	0.7450	0.8571	0.8929	0.9643
8	0.6190	0.7143	0.8095	0.8571	0.9286
9	0.5833	0.6833	0.7667	0.8167	0.9000
10	0.5515	0.6364	0.7333	0.7818	0.8667
11	0.5273	0.6091	0.7000	0.7455	0.8364
12	0.4965	0.5804	0.6713	0.7273	0.8182
13	0.4780	0.5549	0.6429	0.6978	0.7912
14	0.4593	0.5341	0.6220	0.6747	0.7670
15	0.4429	0.5179	0.6000	0.6536	0.7464

Table A.8 The sign test

This table contains two-tailed P-values for the sign test of the null hypothesis that the proportion of positive (or negative, whichever is the smaller) differences is equal to one half (see Section 12.3). k is the number of positive differences; n is the number of non-zero differences. Note that probabilities less than 0.001 are omitted.

Example: if $k = 3$ and $n = 10$, $P = 0.344$.

Table A.8 Two-tailed P-values for the sign test.

						k				
n	0	1	2	3	4	5	6	7	8	9
4	1.00	0.624	1.00	–	–	–	–	–	–	–
5	0.062	0.376	1.00	–	–	–	–	–	–	–
6	0.032	0.218	0.688	1.00	–	–	–	–	–	–
7	0.016	0.124	0.454	1.00	–	–	–	–	–	–
8	0.008	0.070	0.290	0.726	1.00	–	–	–	–	–
9	0.004	0.040	0.180	0.508	1.00	–	–	–	–	–
10	0.002	0.022	0.110	0.344	0.754	1.00	–	–	–	–
11	0.001	0.012	0.066	0.226	0.548	1.00	–	–	–	–
12	–	0.006	0.038	0.146	0.388	0.774	1.00	–	–	–
13	–	0.004	0.022	0.092	0.266	0.582	1.00	–	–	–
14	–	0.002	0.012	0.058	0.180	0.424	0.790	1.00	–	–
15	–	–	0.008	0.036	0.118	0.302	0.608	1.00	–	–
16	–	–	0.004	0.022	0.076	0.210	0.554	0.804	1.00	–
17	–	–	0.002	0.012	0.050	0.144	0.332	0.630	1.00	–
18	–	–	0.002	0.004	0.030	0.096	0.238	0.480	0.814	1.00
19	–	–	–	0.004	0.020	0.064	0.168	0.360	0.648	1.00
20	–	–	–	0.002	0.012	0.042	0.116	0.264	0.504	0.824

Table A.9 The Wilcoxon signed rank test

This table contains the critical values for a two-tailed Wilcoxon signed rank test of n non-zero differences (see Section 12.4). It uses the sum of the positive ranks, T_+, or the negative ranks, T_-, of the differences. Then if T_+ (or T_-) is equal to or lies outside the tabulated critical values, the P-value for the two-sided test is less than the tabulated P-value.

Example: if the number of non-zero differences is 10, and $T_+ = 4$, then since 4 is less than the lower limit of the interval 5–50, $P < 0.02$. However, since 4 lies in the interval 3–52, $P > 0.01$. Hence $0.01 < P < 0.02$.

	Two-tailed P-value				
n	0.1	0.05	0.02	0.01	0.001
4	–	–	–	–	–
5	0–15	–	–	–	–
6	2–19	0–21	–	–	–
7	3–25	2–26	0–28	–	–
8	5–31	3–33	1–35	0–36	–
9	8–37	5–40	3–42	1–44	–
10	10–45	8–47	5–50	3–52	–
11	13–53	10–56	7–59	5–61	0–66
12	17–61	13–65	9–69	7–71	1–77
13	21–70	17–74	12–79	9–82	2–89
14	25–80	21–84	15–90	12–93	4–101
15	30–90	25–95	19–101	15–105	6–114
16	35–101	29–107	23–113	19–117	9–127
17	41–112	34–119	28–125	23–130	11–142
18	47–124	40–131	32–139	27–144	14–157
19	53–137	46–144	37–153	32–158	18–172
20	60–150	52–158	43–167	37–173	21–189
21	67–164	58–173	49–182	42–189	26–205
22	75–178	66–187	55–198	48–205	30–223
23	83–193	73–203	62–214	54–222	35–241
24	91–209	81–219	69–231	61–239	40–260
25	100–225	89–236	76–249	68–257	45–280

Table A.9 Critical values for the Wilcoxon signed rank test.

Table A.10 The Wilcoxon rank sum test

This table contains the critical values for a two-tailed Wilcoxon rank sum test comparing two samples of size n_1 and n_2, with $n_1 < n_2$ (see Section 12.5). Suppose T_1 is the sum of the ranks of the smaller sample. If $T_1 \leq$ the lower critical value in the table, or if $T_1 \geq$ the upper critical value, then the two-tailed P-value of the test is less than the relevant tabulated P-value.

Example: if $n_1 = 10$, $n_2 = 14$ and $T_1 = 83$, then since 83 lies outside the limits 91–159 in Table A.10a, then $P < 0.05$; since 83 lies within the limits 81–169 in Table A.10b, then $P > 0.01$. Hence $0.01 < P < 0.05$.

Table A.10a Critical values for the Wilcoxon rank sum test. Two-tailed $P = 0.05$.

n_1	4	5	6	7	8	9	10	11	12	13	14	15
n_2												
4	10–26	16–34	23–43	31–53	40–64	49–77	60–90	72–104	85–119	99–135	114–152	130–170
5	11–29	17–38	24–48	33–58	42–70	52–83	63–97	75–112	89–127	103–144	118–162	134–181
6	12–32	18–42	26–52	34–64	44–76	55–89	66–104	79–119	92–136	107–153	122–172	139–191
7	13–35	20–45	27–57	36–69	46–82	57–96	69–111	82–127	96–144	111–162	127–181	144–201
8	14–38	21–49	29–61	38–74	49–87	60–102	72–118	85–135	100–152	115–171	131–191	149–211
9	14–42	22–53	31–65	40–79	51–93	62–109	75–125	89–142	104–160	119–180	136–200	154–221
10	15–45	23–57	32–70	42–84	53–99	65–115	78–132	92–150	107–169	124–188	141–209	159–231
11	16–48	24–61	34–74	44–89	55–105	68–121	81–139	96–157	111–177	128–197	145–219	164–241
12	17–51	26–64	35–79	46–94	58–110	71–127	84–146	99–165	115–185	132–206	150–228	169–251
13	18–54	27–68	37–83	48–99	60–116	73–134	88–152	103–172	119–193	136–215	155–237	174–261
14	19–57	28–72	38–88	50–104	62–122	76–140	91–159	106–180	123–201	141–223	160–246	179–271
15	20–60	29–76	40–92	52–109	65–127	79–146	94–166	110–187	127–209	145–232	164–256	184–281
16	21–63	30–80	42–96	54–114	67–133	82–152	97–173	113–195	131–217	150–240	169–265	190–290
17	21–67	32–83	43–101	56–119	70–138	84–159	100–180	117–202	135–225	154–249	174–274	195–300
18	22–70	33–87	45–105	58–124	72–144	87–165	103–187	121–209	139–233	159–257	179–283	200–310
19	23–73	34–91	46–110	60–129	74–150	90–171	107–193	124–217	143–241	163–266	184–292	205–320
20	24–76	35–95	48–114	62–134	77–155	93–177	110–200	128–224	147–249	167–275	188–302	211–329

Table A.10b Critical values for the Wilcoxon rank sum test. Two-tailed $P = 0.01$.

n_1	4	5	6	7	8	9	10	11	12	13	14	15
n_2												
4	–	–	21–45	28–56	37–67	46–80	57–93	68–108	81–123	94–140	109–157	125–175
5	–	15–40	22–50	29–62	38–74	48–87	59–101	71–116	84–132	98–149	112–168	128–187
6	10–34	16–44	23–55	31–67	40–80	50–94	61–109	73–125	87–141	101–159	116–178	132–198
7	10–38	16–49	24–60	32–73	42–86	52–101	64–116	76–133	90–150	104–169	120–188	136–209
8	11–41	17–53	25–65	34–78	43–93	54–108	66–124	79–141	93–159	108–178	123–199	140–220
9	11–45	18–57	26–70	35–84	45–99	56–115	68–132	82–149	96–168	111–188	127–209	144–231
10	12–48	19–61	27–75	37–89	47–105	58–122	71–139	84–158	99–177	115–197	131–219	149–241
11	12–52	20–65	28–80	38–95	49–111	61–128	73–147	87–166	102–186	118–207	135–229	153–252
12	13–55	21–69	30–84	40–100	51–117	63–135	76–154	90–174	105–195	122–216	139–239	157–263
13	13–59	22–73	31–89	41–106	53–123	65–142	79–161	93–182	109–203	125–226	143–249	162–273
14	14–62	22–78	32–94	43–111	54–130	67–149	81–169	96–190	112–212	129–235	147–259	166–284
15	15–65	23–82	33–99	44–117	56–136	69–156	84–176	99–198	115–221	133–244	151–269	171–294
16	15–69	24–86	34–104	46–122	58–142	72–162	86–184	102–206	119–229	136–254	155–279	175–305
17	16–72	25–90	36–108	47–128	60–148	74–169	89–191	105–214	122–238	140–263	160–288	180–315
18	16–76	26–94	37–113	49–133	62–154	76–176	92–198	108–222	125–247	144–272	164–298	184–326
19	17–79	27–98	38–118	50–139	64–160	78–183	94–206	111–230	129–255	148–281	168–308	189–336
20	18–82	28–102	39–123	52–144	66–166	81–189	97–213	114–238	132–264	152–290	172–318	193–347

Table A.11 The table of random numbers

Table A.11   Table of random numbers (derived using Microsoft Excel Version 5.0).

77267	67258	38499	94709	46989	44360	46788	62666	67551	79212
72309	70484	25843	72251	82013	70561	14058	38073	53571	91594
54395	89438	92622	45780	29108	53340	85537	50232	28477	93512
98270	62867	44084	98370	59635	25367	30528	58516	78666	83753
66032	31218	29309	26890	34700	43168	09914	47240	51526	51115
57277	70054	60345	84988	24257	19358	39083	63075	67491	55733
85981	87059	50122	80180	98114	64749	75696	59666	43806	52538
75254	50278	61364	84524	18067	94064	42011	21085	79258	44419
71820	17948	38074	48411	63605	34244	96320	36384	80985	79176
55759	77728	41765	61731	27045	81464	44584	11390	85593	69342
92725	91260	25468	94632	44972	96413	93134	29630	70497	71787
18169	44658	95643	71214	61018	90640	59106	76377	90625	15455
55710	88227	84684	33948	29576	57306	96961	90832	52720	38631
49556	24412	93967	63006	69252	52089	29551	62555	54033	39961
87891	87778	61646	24558	16210	81147	16734	24214	45062	64957
18699	87766	21808	40788	77612	97617	34199	86693	51631	17475
96353	24916	71714	97492	42680	14894	87091	51667	10183	28272
58932	54779	81765	17127	76773	52970	52430	56064	62116	48515
60376	97508	91787	84684	39870	12608	11299	30277	87317	61131
71521	34632	82603	56428	71537	10548	10765	51679	45875	12404
17760	37556	52225	68445	18626	67414	62242	51329	80427	11747
36901	23375	21348	32148	47612	60511	24558	91901	50626	65405
17488	34113	69144	24953	13842	90301	38518	59852	96747	96478
16435	63514	78929	62326	89294	48853	35503	43729	89186	36601
79145	37322	17054	61899	74394	58695	77454	81735	98688	91397
96388	61117	31714	58107	85666	47675	33123	08943	75625	06598
38147	23339	32981	80989	96940	44860	39707	84883	26243	59861
95893	06491	95520	91538	35285	17192	80784	32664	49226	25919
53544	31391	23798	36857	16786	19639	93659	66776	34108	74268
03513	34015	78337	46158	92198	99481	70804	73939	39152	44116
92737	89927	81721	33548	78029	62464	53482	54191	95898	66099
10688	61502	73817	63841	87058	23377	24045	99470	17509	26636
51658	59565	61280	48120	38438	57832	25639	84632	38523	89459
53916	57066	46906	18657	79932	93039	62470	22405	78427	92145
40912	63211	63856	61644	18635	02946	30842	24031	36992	37917
75159	14888	59932	74222	39075	33201	33747	53800	79883	26609
25224	72513	58746	52366	73436	74699	80799	56699	16557	58671
82703	53196	34797	28093	97105	56797	39992	67944	00310	49311
51627	41127	86363	48078	27726	37269	21629	21785	25822	95264
02574	68647	82762	80442	70966	95743	56140	58213	78202	60038

Appendix B
Tables of confidence intervals

Table B.1   95%* confidence intervals from a single sample: summary of results (see relevant sections for assumptions and explanation of notation).

Parameter	95% confidence interval	Section
Mean (μ)	$\bar{x} \pm t_{0.05}\text{SEM} = \bar{x} \pm t_{0.05}\dfrac{s}{\sqrt{n}}$ where degrees of freedom $= n - 1$	4.5
Proportion (π) (Sensitivity, Specificity, PPV, NPV)	$p \pm 1.96\sqrt{\dfrac{p(1-p)}{n}}$ where $p = \dfrac{r}{n}$	4.7, 14.2.2, 14.2.7
Pearson correlation coefficient (ρ)	$\dfrac{e^{2z_1}-1}{e^{2z_1}+1}$ to $\dfrac{e^{2z_2}-1}{e^{2z_2}+1}$ where $z = \dfrac{1}{2}\log_e \dfrac{1+r}{1-r}$ $z_1 = z - \dfrac{1.96}{\sqrt{(n-3)}}$, $z_2 = z + \dfrac{1.96}{\sqrt{(n-3)}}$	10.3.2(b)
Regression coefficient (β)	$b \pm t_{0.05}\text{SE}(b)$ where degrees of freedom $= n - 2$	10.4.6
Relative risk (RR)	$\exp\left(\log_e \text{RR} \pm 1.96\sqrt{\dfrac{1}{r_1}+\dfrac{1}{r_2}-\dfrac{1}{n_1}-\dfrac{1}{n_2}}\right)$ where $\text{RR} = p_1/p_2$ and $p_1 = r_1/n_1$ and $p_2 = r_2/n_2$	5.2.3(a)
Odds ratio (OR)	$\exp\left(\log_e \text{OR} \pm 1.96\sqrt{\dfrac{1}{r_1}+\dfrac{1}{r_2}+\dfrac{1}{n_1-r_1}+\dfrac{1}{n_2-r_2}}\right)$ where $\text{OR} = \dfrac{r_1(n_2-r_2)}{r_2(n_1-r_1)}$	5.2.3(b)
Absolute risk reduction (ARR)	$(p_1 - p_2) \pm 1.96\sqrt{\dfrac{p_1(1-p_1)}{n_1}+\dfrac{p_2(1-p_2)}{n_2}}$ where $p_1 = r_1/n_1$ and $p_2 = r_2/n_2$ are the two risks Call these limits ARR_L and ARR_U	5.2.3, 9.4.3(c), 16.5.3
Number needed to treat (NNT)	$100/\text{ARR}_U$ to $100/\text{ARR}_L$	16.5.3
Kappa measure of agreement (κ)	$\kappa \pm 1.96\sqrt{\dfrac{p_0(1-p_0)}{n(1-p_c)^2}}$	14.4.3

*Replace 1.96 by appropriate percentage point of the Standard Normal distribution (see Table A.2) if a different CI is required, e.g. replace 1.96 by 2.58 for a 99% CI. Similarly, replace $t_{0.05}$ by $t_{0.01}$ for a 99% confidence interval.

Statistics for Veterinary and Animal Science, Third Edition. Aviva Petrie and Paul Watson.
© 2013 John Wiley & Sons, Ltd. Published 2013 by John Wiley & Sons, Ltd.

Table B.2 95%* confidence intervals from two samples: summary of results (see relevant sections for assumptions and explanation of notation).

Parameter	95% confidence interval	Section
Difference in means $(\mu_1 - \mu_2)$: (a) Independent samples (equal variances)	$(\bar{x}_1 - \bar{x}_2) \pm t_{0.05} \mathrm{SE}(\bar{x}_1 - \bar{x}_2)$ where degrees of freedom $= n_1 + n_2 - 2$ $\mathrm{SE}(\bar{x}_1 - \bar{x}_2) = \sqrt{s^2\left(\dfrac{1}{n_1} + \dfrac{1}{n_2}\right)}$ $s^2 = \dfrac{(n_1 - 1)s_1^2 + (n_2 - 1)s_2^2}{n_1 + n_2 - 2}$	7.4.3
(b) Paired samples	$\bar{d} \pm t_{0.05}\dfrac{s_d}{\sqrt{n}}$ where degrees of freedom $= n - 1$ and s_d is the SD of the differences	7.5.3
Difference in proportions $(\pi_1 - \pi_2)$: (a) Independent samples	$(p_1 - p_2) \pm 1.96\sqrt{\dfrac{p_1(1 - p_1)}{n_1} + \dfrac{p_2(1 - p_2)}{n_2}}$	9.4.3(c)
(b) Paired samples	$(p_1 - p_2) \pm 1.96\dfrac{1}{m}\sqrt{(f + g) - \dfrac{(f - g)^2}{m}}$ where e, f, g and h are defined in Table 9.4 and $p_1 = \dfrac{e + f}{m}$ and $p_2 = \dfrac{e + g}{m}$ so $p_1 - p_2 = \dfrac{f - g}{m}$	9.6.3

*The above are 95% CIs. For a different CI, replace the 1.96 in the formula by the appropriate percentage point in the table of the Standard Normal distribution (see Table A.2), e.g. for a 90% CI, replace 1.96 by 1.64. Similarly, replace $t_{0.05}$ by $t_{0.10}$ for a 90% CI.

Appendix C
Glossary of notation

We have used algebraic and mathematical notation throughout this book. The following glossary may help you understand some of that notation.

Mathematical symbols and transformations

∞ Infinity.

$\pm$ This means that, in turn, we add and subtract the quantity following the sign to the quantity preceding it, to obtain two separate quantities. Hence, $x \pm y$ gives $(x + y)$ and $(x - y)$.

$\geq$ The value preceding the sign is greater than or equal to the value after it.

$\leq$ The value preceding the sign is less than or equal to the value after it.

$\log x$ This is the logarithm (log) of the number x. Sometimes we put brackets around the x if it aids clarification. See Section 13.2 for the uses of the logarithmic transformation. Logarithms can take different bases, the most usual ones being 10 and e (see below). In general terms, if $\log_y(x) = z$, then $x = y^z$, where the base of the logarithm is the number y. As long as we are consistent in using a particular base of a logarithm, and specify which base we are using, we can use the logarithm to any base. *Remember that the log of zero is infinity, and that we can only take logs of positive numbers.* We can obtain the values of logarithms from special tables or more usually from hand calculators. If we have two numbers a and b, say, then
(i) the log of their product is equal to the sum of the logs,
$$\log(ab) = \log(a) + \log(b)$$
(ii) the log of their quotient is equal to the difference in their logs,
$$\log(a/b) = \log(a) - \log(b).$$

$\log_e x$ This is the Napierian or natural logarithm of x to base e, often written as $\ln x$, where e is the constant 2.71828. The logarithm to base e of a quantity x is the value z such that $x = e^z$. These logs are used most often in statistics and are generally used in computer packages.

$\log_{10} x$ This is the common logarithm to base 10 of x. If $\log_{10}(x) = z$, then $x = 10^z$. So, for example, $\log_{10}(10) = 1$ and $\log_{10}(100) = 2$. Logs to base 10 were used to simplify multiplication and division, relying on addition and subtraction instead, but are rarely used for this purpose now because of the advent of calculators and computers.

e^x This is the exponential function, sometimes written $\exp(x)$. If $x = \log_e(y)$, then $y = e^x$ is the antilogarithm of x. Thus, if we have taken a logarithmic transformation of a variable, we can transform back to the original scale by taking the antilog, using the exponential function of a calculator. Note that if we have taken logs to base 10 as a transformation, we can transform back to the original scale by using the antilog function 10^x.

$\text{logit}(p)$ The logistic (logit) transformation of a proportion, p, such that $\text{logit}(p) = \log_e\{p/(1 - p)\}$.

$|x|$ The vertical lines to the left and right of the x indicate that we should ignore the sign of x, i.e. we should consider its 'absolute value'. So, for example, $|-15.5| = |15.5| = 15.5$.

$\displaystyle\sum_{i=1}^{n} x_i$ Commonly abbreviated to Σx. The Greek letter 'sigma', Σ, indicates that we are summing the values of the variable, x, for all the n individuals in the sample, i.e. from $i = 1$ to $i = n$. The abbreviation (Σx) which omits the values of i both above and below the summation sign, and as the subscript of x, is used when no confusion can result. Clearly,
$$\sum_{i=1}^{n} x_i = x_1 + x_2 + x_3 + \ldots + x_n$$

$\displaystyle\sum_{i=1}^{n}(x_i - \bar{x})^2$ Commonly abbreviated to $\Sigma(x - \bar{x})^2$. It is called the sum of squared deviations, the corrected sum of squares or simply the sum of squares. We take the sample mean, $\bar{x}$, from each value of x in the sample, and then square this difference; repeating this procedure for all n values of x in the sample, we obtain a set of n squared differences which we then add up.

Statistics for Veterinary and Animal Science, Third Edition. Aviva Petrie and Paul Watson.
© 2013 John Wiley & Sons, Ltd. Published 2013 by John Wiley & Sons, Ltd.

Common notation

x_i If x denotes the value of a variable, such as age or systolic blood pressure, then the subscript, i, indicates that we are referring to the value of that variable for the ith individual in the sample or the population. If there are n individuals in the sample, then the sample values for that variable are $(x_1, x_2, x_3, \ldots, x_n)$.

$\bar{x}$ The sample mean of the variable, x. It is pronounced 'x bar', and is equal to the sum of all the values of x in the sample divided by the number of observations, n, in the sample (see Section 2.6.1). Hence

$$\bar{x} = \frac{x_1 + x_2 + x_3 + \ldots + x_n}{n} = \frac{1}{n}\sum_{i=1}^{n} x_i, \text{ often written as } \frac{1}{n}\sum x$$

b Often used to refer to an estimated regression coefficient.

F A particular continuous probability distribution.

H_0 The null hypothesis (H nought).

p The proportion of 'successes' in a sample, i.e. the proportion of individuals in the sample possessing some characteristic.

P The P-value; the probability of obtaining the observed results (or more extreme results) if the null hypothesis is true.

r The sample estimate of Pearson's product moment correlation coefficient, expressed as

$$r = \frac{\sum (x - \bar{x})(y - \bar{y})}{\sqrt{\sum (x - \bar{x})^2 \sum (y - \bar{y})^2}}$$

r^2 The square of the correlation coefficient, the proportion of the variance of one variable explained by its linear relationship with another variable. It is sometimes called the coefficient of determination.

R The multiple correlation coefficient equal to the square root of the coefficient of determination.

R^2 The coefficient of determination. It is the proportion of the variance of the response variable, y, explained by its relationship with the explanatory variables in a multiple regression analysis.

r_s The sample estimate of Spearman's rank correlation coefficient. It is equal to the Pearson product moment correlation coefficient between the ranks of the observations in the sample.

s The estimated population standard deviation obtained from a sample of n observations, thus

$$s = \sqrt{\frac{\sum_{i=1}^{n}(x_i - \bar{x})^2}{n - 1}}$$

     Its square, s^2, is the estimated population variance.

t A particular continuous probability distribution.

$t_{0.05}$ This is the percentage point or critical value of the t-distribution (see Table A.3) that gives a total tail area probability of 0.05, i.e. 2.5% of the total area under the curve is contained in the tail to the left of $-t_{0.05}$, and 2.5% is contained in the tail to the right of $t_{0.05}$.

$Test_i$ The test statistic used to test a particular null hypothesis ($i = 1, 2, \ldots, 14$).

α The Greek letter 'alpha'. It may refer to the constant term in a regression equation; alternatively, it sometimes refers to the significance level of a hypothesis test (the cut-off value for the P-value leading to rejection of the null hypothesis).

β The Greek letter 'beta'. It usually refers to the true value of a regression coefficient representing the gradient of the line in simple linear regression.

χ^2 The Greek letter 'chi' which is squared; a particular continuous probability distribution.

δ The Greek letter 'delta'. Sometimes used to refer to a difference of interest in the population.

κ The Greek letter 'kappa'. A measure of agreement for categorical variables.

μ The lower case Greek letter 'mu'. It represents the population mean. If there are N observations on the variable, x, in the population, then

$$\mu = \frac{1}{N}\sum_{i=1}^{N} x_i$$

π The Greek letter 'pi'. The proportion of individuals in the population possessing some characteristic.

ρ The Greek letter 'rho'. The population value of the Pearson's product moment correlation coefficient.

ρ_s The Greek letter 'rho' with subscript 's'. The population value of Spearman's rank correlation coefficient.

σ The Greek letter 'sigma'. The population standard deviation. If there are N observations on the variable, x, in the population, then

$$\sigma = \sqrt{\frac{\sum_{i=1}^{N}(x_i - \mu)^2}{N}}$$

     Its square, σ^2, is the population variance.

Abbreviations

AF	Attributable fraction.
ANCOVA	Analysis of covariance.
ANOVA	Analysis of variance.
AR	Attributable risk.
ARR	Absolute risk reduction; the difference in two risks.
ARRIVE	Guidelines, consisting of a 20-point checklist based on CONSORT, of the essential information that should be included in publications reporting animal research.
AUROC	Area under the receiver operating characteristic curve.
CI	Confidence interval; it contains the parameter of interest with a prescribed probability.
CONSORT	A statement which provides, in the form of a checklist and flowchart, guidance to authors on how they should report a randomized controlled trial.
CV	Coefficient of variation: the standard deviation expressed as a percentage of the mean.
df	The degrees of freedom of a statistic, i.e. the number of independent observations contributing to the value of the statistic.
DNA	Deoxyribonucleic acid.
EBM	Evidence-based medicine.
EBVM	Evidence-based veterinary medicine.
EQUATOR	International network that seeks to improve the reliability and value of medical research literature by promoting transparent and accurate reporting of research studies.
GEE	Generalized estimating equation.
GIS	Geographical or geospatial information system.
GLM	Generalized linear model.
ICC	Intraclass correlation coefficient; if individual units are contained within a cluster, it expresses the variation between clusters as a proportion of the total variation.
IRR	Incidence rate ratio; the ratio of two incidence rates, often the incidence rate of disease in the treated group divided by that in the control group.
IU	International unit.
LR	Likelihood ratio; the ratio of two likelihoods. For example, in the context of a diagnostic test, it may be the ratio of the likelihoods of a positive test result in animals with and without the disease.
LRS	Likelihood ratio statistic which uses the ratio of two likelihoods to compare two regression models.
LSD	Least significant difference: a multiple comparison tests of means.
MANOVA	Multivariate analysis of variance.
MAR	Missing at random.
MAUP	Modifiable area unit problem.
MCAR	Missing completely at random.
MLE	Maximum likelihood estimation; a process which obtains estimates of the parameters in a model by maximizing the likelihood.
MLM	Multilevel model.
mRNA	Messenger ribonucleic acid.
NMAR	Not missing at random.
NNT	Number needed to treat with a novel treatment instead of a control treatment to prevent one adverse outcome.
NPV	Negative predictive value of a diagnostic or screening test – the proportion of those testing negative who really are disease-free.
OR	Odds ratio; the ratio of two odds, usually the odds of the disease in those exposed to the factor, divided by the odds of disease in those not exposed to the factor.
PAF	Population attributable fraction.
PAR	Population attributable risk.
PPV	Positive predictive value of a diagnostic or screening test – the proportion of those testing positive who actually have the disease.
PRISMA	A statement to guide the reporting of systematic reviews and meta-analyses to assess the benefits and harms of a healthcare intervention.
RCT	Randomized controlled trial.
RD	Risk difference.
REFLECT	A statement providing an evidence-based minimum set of items for reporting livestock trials with production, health and food-safety outcomes.
RNA	Ribonucleic acid.

ROC	Receiver operating characteristic curve.
RR	Relative risk; the ratio of two risks, usually the risk of disease in those with the factor divided by the risk in those without the factor.
RRR	Relative risk reduction equal to 1 – RR.
SD	Standard deviation of a set of observations.
SE(*b*)	Standard error of a statistic, *b*.
SEM	Standard error of the sample mean. Sometimes abbreviated to SE.
SND	Standardized Normal Deviate given by

$$z = \frac{x - \mu}{\sigma}$$

where the variable, x, is Normally distributed with mean = μ and SD = σ. The SND has a Normal distribution with mean = 0 and SD = 1.

STARD	Guidelines for reporting diagnostic accuracy studies.
STROBE	Guidelines for reporting cohort, case–control and cross-sectional studies.
VIF	Variance inflation factor: a measure which can provide evidence of collinearity between variables.

Appendix D
Glossary of terms

a priori **probability**   a way of evaluating the probability of an outcome solely on the basis of a theoretical model. Hence it may be called the model definition of probability.

absolute risk reduction (ARR)   the difference in two risks. *See also* attributable risk.

accuracy   refers to how well the observed value of a quantity agrees with the true value.

addition rule   the probability of either of two mutually exclusive events occurring is the sum of the probability of each event.

adjusted R^2 a corrected value of R^2 (*see* coefficient of determination) which allows multiple regression models with differing numbers of explanatory variables to be compared when assessing goodness-of-fit.

administrative censoring   occurs in survival analysis when animals may be observed for varying lengths of time because they have been recruited into the study at different times and there is a single time point at which the study period ends.

all subsets selection   the process of determining an optimal regression model which examines all the possible models for the various combinations of the explanatory variables of interest.

alternative hypothesis   the proposition (statement) which disagrees with the hypothesis under test (the null hypothesis).

Altman's nomogram   a graphic representation showing the relationship between sample size, power and standardized difference; it can be used to determine any one with knowledge of the other two. The standardized difference is a reflection of the variability of the observations and the minimum magnitude of the effect of interest considered important.

analysis of covariance (ANCOVA)   an extension to the analysis of variance which takes account of the values of one or more subsidiary variables (the covariates).

analysis of variance (ANOVA)   a powerful collection of parametric statistical procedures for the analysis of data, essentially comparing the means of various groups of data. It relies on separating the total variation of a variable into its component parts which are associated with defined sources of variation.

ANCOVA   *see* analysis of covariance.

angular transformation   *see* arcsine transformation.

ANOVA   *see* analysis of variance.

arcsine transformation   a transformation for a proportion, p, to $\sin^{-1}\sqrt{p}$. It linearizes a sigmoid curve and stabilizes variance. Also called the angular transformation or inverse sine transformation.

area under the ROC curve (AUROC)   describes the overall ability of a diagnostic test to distinguish between animals with and without disease. This area represents the probability that a randomly chosen diseased animal has a higher predicted probability of having the disease than a randomly chosen disease-free animal. Also called c statistic.

arithmetic mean usually abbreviated to the mean; a measure of location. It is the sum of the observations divided by the number of observations in the set.

ARRIVE guidelines a framework produced with the intention of improving the reporting of research using laboratory animals.

artificial pairing two different animals which have been matched with respect to any variables that may be thought to influence response.

attributable fraction (AF) the attributable risk expressed as a proportion of those exposed.

attributable risk (AR) the risk of a particular outcome in those exposed to a factor of interest minus the risk in those unexposed. Also called the absolute risk reduction (ARR) or the risk difference (RD).

AUROC *see* area under the ROC curve.

autoregressive series a time series in which the value of an observation is dependent on the preceding observation(s).

average a measure of location of a set of observations which describes central tendency, e.g. mean, median, mode.

backward step-down selection the process of selecting an optimal regression model in which, starting with all the explanatory variables in the model, we remove them sequentially (beginning with the variable which contributes the least) until the deletion of a variable significantly increases the residual variance.

bar chart a diagram in which every category of a variable is represented by the length of a bar depicting the number or percentage of individuals belonging to that category.

Bayes' theorem underlies Bayesian inference which uses the current evidence from a study to update the prior probability of a particular outcome (e.g. disease) to produce the posterior probability of the outcome.

Berkson–Gage analysis an approach used in survival analysis when survival times are grouped into intervals; it bases the calculations on the methods involved in actuarial life tables.

Berkson–Gage survival curve a survival curve based on actuarial life tables; its calculations require knowledge of the time intervals within which the critical events (e.g. death) occur.

bias systematic distortion of the data.

bimodal a distribution which has two modes or modal groups.

binary variable a discrete random variable with only two possible values. Also called a dichotomous variable.

Binomial distribution a discrete probability distribution of a variable representing the number of successes in trials in which there are only two outcomes – success (with a fixed probability) and failure.

bio-equivalence study used to show that two formulations of a drug have similar bioavailability (when the same amount of drug gets into the body for each formulation).

bioinformatics the application of computer science and information technology to the field of biology and medicine. Also called computational biology.

biological (clinical) importance the considered judgement of what is relevant in the particular circumstances of the investigation; it should be contrasted with statistical significance.

biological variation an inherent variability in biological material such that measurements taken from different individuals or from one time to another will rarely be identical.

biometry a broad numerical approach to biology including study design, data collection, analysis, display and the drawing of appropriate conclusions. *See also* statistics.

Bland and Altman plot a scatter diagram used to assess the agreement between two sets of numerical results measured on the same scale and on the same individuals. The difference between each pair is plotted against their mean.

blind either the carer of the animals in a clinical trial or the investigator, or both, have no knowledge of the specific treatments the animals receive. Also called masked.

block a group of individuals in an experimental design which are observed in particular circumstances (e.g. after individuals are allocated a treatment). Blocks are usually created to isolate sources of variability, so that the individuals within a block exhibit less variability than in the general population.

blocked randomization a method of randomly allocating individuals to treatments with the aim of achieving approximately equal numbers of individuals in each treatment group. Also called restricted randomization.

Bonferroni's correction a method of reducing the risk of a Type I error when using multiple comparisons; it involves multiplying the *P*-value obtained from any one test by the number of multiple comparisons.

bootstrapping a computer-intensive iterative method of estimating parameters of interest based on resampling. A sample of size *n* is taken, with replacement, from the original sample of size *n*. This process is repeated multiple times and the distribution of the estimates of the parameter of interest obtained from the multiple samples is used to provide an overall estimate of the parameter, together with its associated confidence interval.

box-and-whisker plot a diagram that shows the distribution of numerical or ordinal data. It usually comprises a box whose horizontal limits are defined by the upper and lower quartiles enclosing the central 50% of the observations, with the median marked by a horizontal line within the box. The whiskers are vertical lines extending from the box as low as the 2.5th percentile and as high as the 97.5th percentile. Also known as a box plot.

British Standards Institution repeatability coefficient a measure of the repeatability of a method; it gives an indication of the maximum difference likely to occur between two measurements.

c **statistic** *see* area under the ROC curve.

capture–tag–recapture method a method of estimating the size of a wildlife population.

cartogram a diagrammatic presentation, commonly of geographically-bound statistical data, on a map base or distorted map base.

case–control study a form of observational study. At the start of the investigation, we identify animals as being either diseased (cases) or healthy (controls). Then we assess whether the animals in the two groups have differences in past exposure to various risk factors.

categorical (qualitative) variable each individual belongs to one of two or more mutually exclusive categories of the variable.

censored data animals in survival analysis who are alive (or the event of interest has not occurred, if the event is not death) at the end of the study or who are lost to follow-up.

central tendency indicates a position which represents the middle of a group of observations.

centring the process of subtracting a mean or some other value from each observed value of an explanatory variable to ensure a meaningful interpretation of the intercept and regression coefficient(s) in a regression model.

Chi-squared (χ^2) distribution a continuous probability distribution which is often used in hypothesis testing of proportions.

Chi-squared (χ^2) test a non-parametric test, based on the Chi-squared distribution, which is often used to compare proportions.

Chi-squared (χ^2) test for trend a specific Chi-squared test used to determine whether there is a trend in proportions classified by an ordinal variable.

clinical field trial a comparative study involving new treatments or preventive measures applied under natural, field or semi-field conditions.

clinical heterogeneity exists when studies in a meta-analysis are not comparable because of differences in the populations, definition of variables, etc.

clinical prior in a Bayesian analysis, it expresses the opinions of well-informed specialists or is derived from reputable published material.

clinical trial a form of experimental study in controlled conditions which is designed to assess the effectiveness of one or more treatments or preventive measures when these are applied to humans or animals.

cluster randomization *see* group randomization.

cluster sampling a form of random sampling in which subdivisions or clusters of the population are identified; a simple random sample of clusters is selected and all the units within the selected clusters studied.

clustered design   *see* repeated measures design.

Cochrane Collaboration   an international network of experts and consumers who continually update systematic reviews and make them available.

Cochran's Q test   an extension of McNemar's test for related samples that provides a method for testing for differences between three or more matched sets of data when the variable of interest has two categories (e.g. success/failure). Also used in meta-analysis as a test for homogeneity.

coefficient of determination (R^2)   the proportion of the total variance of the dependent variable, y, in a regression model which is explained by the regression.

coefficient of variation (CV)   the standard deviation expressed as a percentage of the mean.

Cohen's kappa coefficient (κ)   a measure of the agreement, corrected for chance agreement, between pairs of results measured on the same categorical scale.

cohort study   a form of observational study. We start by defining groups (cohorts) of animals by the exposure of the animals in the groups to the factors of interest; we usually follow these animals forward in time and observe the outcome (e.g. disease).

collinearity (multicollinearity)   when two or more of the explanatory variables in a multiple regression model exhibit a linear relationship and are very highly correlated.

competing risks   occur in survival analysis when, in a particular individual, one event precludes the occurrence of the event of interest that defines a failure.

complete randomized block design   each block in the experimental design contains a complete set of treatments.

computational biology   *see* bioinformatics.

conditional logistic regression   a form of logistic regression analysis used when the study involves matched individuals.

conditional probability   the conditional probability of an event B occurring is the probability of B occurring, given that the event A has already occurred.

confidence band, region or interval for the line   the region around a linear regression line within which we believe the true line lies with a prescribed degree of certainty.

confidence interval   the range of values which contains a population parameter (e.g. the mean) with a given probability. Strictly, 95% of the 95% confidence intervals obtained by repeatedly taking samples of the same size from the population would contain the parameter.

confidence limits   the upper and lower values of the confidence interval.

confounder   an explanatory variable which is related both to the response of interest and to another (or more than one) explanatory variable so that it is impossible to separate the effects of the two explanatory variables on the response.

CONSORT statement   provides, in the form of a checklist and flowchart, guidance to authors on how they should report a randomized clinical trial on human subjects.

contemporary control   animals are assigned to control or test treatment at similar times within the study period.

contingency table   a table of frequencies which shows how individuals are classified into the different categories of two or more factors.

continuity correction   a correction applied to a test statistic to facilitate the approximation of a discrete distribution (of the test statistic) to a continuous distribution (such as the Chi-squared distribution).

continuous scale   all values are theoretically possible (perhaps limited by an upper and/or lower boundary), e.g. height, weight.

continuous variable   one which can take an infinite set of possible values in a range.

control group   a group of individuals (i) in an experimental study who receive either the standard treatment or no active treatment, or (ii) in an observational study who are not subjected to the risk factor under investigation. It is used as a basis for comparison with the group of individuals (i) receiving the active treatment(s) or (ii) who are exposed to the risk factor.

controlled clinical trial a clinical trial that includes a control group.

Cook's distance an overall measure of influence, used in regression analysis, which incorporates both leverage and residual values.

correlation changes in one variable tend to be accompanied by changes in the other variable, either in the same (or opposite) directions.

correlation coefficient Pearson's correlation coefficient measures the degree of linear association between two variables. *See also* Spearman's rank correlation coefficient.

covariate one of a number of factors that may influence the response. Also called an explanatory or independent variable or prognostic factor.

Cox proportional hazards regression model an advanced regression approach to survival analysis, used when we desire to investigate the effect of several variables on survival and also to take censored data into account. The ratio of the hazards is assumed constant over time.

critical value the value of a test statistic, determined from a theoretical probability distribution, which corresponds to a given tail area probability (say, 0.05). Also called a percentage point.

cross-over trial two or more treatments are applied in random order to each individual animal. The aim is to examine the effects of the treatments within the animals, rather than between animals, thereby enhancing the precision of the estimate of the difference between treatments.

cross-sectional study one in which we take all our measurements on the individuals included in the study concurrently.

cross-sectional time series *see* random effects model.

cumulative relative frequency distribution shows the accumulated proportions of individuals which are contained in a category (class) and in all lower categories.

cumulative relative frequency polygon a diagram showing a cumulative relative frequency distribution. It is formed by joining cumulative relative frequencies which correspond to the class midpoints.

Declaration of Helsinki a statement of ethical principles for medical research involving human subjects, developed in 1964 in Helsinki, Finland.

degrees of freedom (*df*) the number of independent observations contributing to the value of a statistic, i.e. the number of observations available to evaluate that statistic minus the number of restrictions on those observations.

dependent variable the variable in a regression model which can be predicted by the explanatory (independent) variable(s). Also called the response or outcome variable.

descriptive statistics that branch of statistics concerned with describing and characterizing the data distribution and summarizing and displaying the findings.

design the plan of the study or experiment which should take into account any factors which may affect the response of interest.

diagnostic service analyses animal samples for the benefit of health monitoring and diagnosis of disease.

diagnostic test a procedure that is able to distinguish between diseased and healthy animals.

diagram a means of displaying data pictorially.

diffuse prior *see* vague prior.

digit preference when there is an element of judgement involved in making readings from instruments, certain digits between 0 and 9 are more commonly chosen than others; it varies from individual to individual.

discrete (discontinuous) scale data can take only integer values, typically counts, e.g. litter size, clutch size, parity.

discrete variable taking only a finite set of possible values.

distance sampling a method of estimating parameters of interest using a sampling procedure which obtains estimates by recording the number and frequency of species from a transect line. The method is based on the proposition that the detection of randomly distributed subjects declines with distance from the transect line.

distribution *see* empirical frequency distribution; probability distribution.

distribution-free tests *see* non-parametric tests.

DNA (deoxyribonucleic acid) a nucleic acid that carries the genetic information in a cell.

dot diagram/plot used to show the distribution of a data set. Each observation is marked as a dot on a line calibrated in the units of measurement of the variable.

double-blind neither the carer(s) of the animals in a clinical trial nor the assessor of response to treatment (test or control) is aware of which treatment each animal is receiving.

dummy *see* placebo.

dummy variable the variable which has codes (typically 0 and 1) to represent the outcomes of a binary nominal or ordinal variable. By choosing one category of a nominal categorical variable with k categories to be the reference category in a regression analysis, a series of $(k - 1)$ dummy variables can be created, each allowing one of the categories to be compared with the reference category. Also called an indicator variable.

Duncan's multiple range test a multiple comparison test of means that adjusts the P-values to avoid spuriously significant results arising from multiple testing.

effect a measure of the comparison of interest. *See also* treatment effect.

effect modification *see* interaction.

element a single object or individual or unit of investigation.

empirical Bayes a modified Bayesian analysis in which the observed data are used to estimate the prior.

empirical frequency distribution shows the frequency of occurrence of the observations in a data set.

enthusiastic prior optimistic in nature, reflecting the best plausible outcome in a Bayesian analysis before the sample data are available.

epidemiological study concerned with investigating the aetiology of a disease by determining whether various factors (termed risk factors) are associated with the occurrence and distribution of the disease in the population.

EQUATOR Network an international initiative that seeks to improve the reliability and value of medical research literature by promoting transparent and accurate reporting of research studies.

equivalence interval the range of values for the effect of interest in a clinical trial which is considered of no clinical importance.

equivalence study used to show that the clinical effectiveness of one treatment is similar to that of the existing treatment.

estimation the process of generating an approximation of a population parameter using sample data.

evidence-based veterinary medicine (EBVM) the conscientious, explicit and judicious use of the current best evidence in making decisions about the care of individual animals.

experimental study we intervene in the study; we then observe the effect of our intervention on the response of interest, usually with a view to establishing whether a change in response may be directly attributable to our action.

experimental unit the basic subject for experimentation; it is usually the individual animal, but may, for example, be a group of animals. The entire assembly of the experimental units is the population from which a sample may be taken.

explanatory variable *see* independent variable.

extra-Binomial variation occurs when the residual variation is greater than would be expected from Binomial sampling variation when fitting a logistic model.

extra-Poisson variation occurs when the residual variation is greater than would be expected from a Poisson model.

F-distribution a continuous probability distribution; it is used to compare variances.

F-test *see* variance ratio test.

factor a variable with one or more categories (levels) into which individuals can be classified.

Fagan's nomogram a diagram which is used in the context of diagnostic tests to convert the pre-test probability into the post-test probability via the likelihood.

Fisher's exact test a test for which the exact *P*-value is calculated in a hypothesis test of data presented in a contingency table; this approach is preferable to using the Chi-squared approximation to the Chi-squared test statistic when the expected frequencies in the table are very small.

fixed effect the levels or categories of the factor of interest comprise the entire population (e.g. treatments in a clinical trial).

fixed sample size plans study designs in which the sample size is predetermined before the data are collected.

forest plot a diagram used in a meta-analysis which shows the estimated effect in each study as well as their average and associated confidence intervals.

forward step-up selection the process of selecting an optimal regression model; we start with the explanatory variable which contributes the most to the explained variation in *y*, and include more variables in the equation, progressively, until the addition of an extra variable does not significantly improve the situation.

fourfold table a contingency table with two rows (representing the two categories of a binary variable) and two columns (representing the two categories of a second binary variable). Also called a two-by-two table.

frailty model a random effects proportional hazards model, used when analysing survival in clustered data where failure times are not independent.

frame a complete list of sampling units.

frequency the number of times a particular value (or range of values) of a variable occurs.

frequency definition of probability relies on counting the frequency of occurrence of the event in a large number of repetitions of similar trials.

frequency distribution *see* empirical frequency distribution; probability distribution.

frequency matching the groups of cases and controls are chosen so they have the same average value of a potential risk factor. Also called group matching.

frequentist inference uses only the current evidence provided by the sample data to draw conclusions about the population, in contrast to Bayesian inference which uses prior beliefs as well. It relies on the frequency approach to probability (this defines the probability of an event as the proportion of times the event occurs if the experiment is repeated many times). Also called classical inference.

frequentist theory associated with the frequency definition of probability, i.e. the proportion of times that the event of interest would occur if the experiment were repeated many times.

Friedman two-way ANOVA a non-parametric equivalent to the two-way ANOVA.

funnel plot a scatter diagram used in meta-analysis in which the sample size of a study, or some measure related to it, is plotted against the effect of interest to produce a funnel of points. An absence of points where the sample size is small and where there is no positive effect may indicate the presence of publication bias.

Gaussian distribution *see* Normal distribution.

gene a unit of inheritance in Mendelian terms and, in molecular terms, a region of DNA which is transcribed into mRNA, and this is then used to synthesize protein.

generalized estimating equation (GEE) used to estimate parameters and their standard errors in a regression model which represents a two-level hierarchical structure; it does not assume a particular probability distribution for the random effects. Also called marginal or population-averaged models.

generalized linear model (GLM) a general form for a regression model in which the mean value of the response variable which has a known probability distribution is related, via a link function, to a linear combination of the explanatory variables.

genome the complete set of genes in an organism, tissue or cell.

genomics the branch of molecular biology concerned with the structure, function, evolution and mapping of genomes.

geographical or geospatial information system (GIS) a data-handling system that merges statistical analysis, database technology and cartography.

geometric mean   a measure of location. It is the antilog of the arithmetic mean of the log-transformed values of a variable.

geospacial analysis   an approach to applying statistical analysis and other informational techniques to geographically based data.

goodness-of-fit   examines the agreement between an observed set of values and another set of values which are derived under some particular theory or hypothesis.

group   a collection of animals or experimental units.

group matching   *see* frequency matching.

group randomization   the randomization process is applied to the whole group of units rather than to the individual units within a group. Also called cluster randomization.

group sequential design   involves interim analyses of the data.

hazard   used in survival analysis to describe the instantaneous probability of experiencing the event of interest (e.g. death) at a particular time.

hazard ratio   the ratio of two hazards.

herd immunity   if the experimental unit is the animal rather than the group, the protection afforded the vaccinated animals leads to a reduced prevalence of disease in the group environment, resulting in a reduced incidence of disease in the control animals.

heterogeneity   an effect of interest (typically a variance) is not equal in all of a number of groups.

heteroscedasticity   the variances (or some other measure of variability) are not equal in different groups.

hierarchical model   *see* random effects model.

histogram   a two-dimensional diagram illustrating a frequency distribution of a continuous variable. Usually, the horizontal axis represents the units of measurement of the variable; rectangles above each class interval indicate the frequency for that class by their area.

historical control   animals are not assigned to control or test treatment(s) contemporaneously; information from historical controls is obtained from past records.

homogeneity   an effect of interest (typically a variance) is equal in all relevant groups.

homoscedasticity   the variances (or some other measure of variability) are equal in different groups.

human error   variability in the measurements due to human mistakes.

hypothesis testing   the process of formulating and testing a proposition about the population using the sample data.

hypothetical (or infinite) population   the population does not exist but can be conceptualized (e.g. the population of animals who might receive a novel treatment).

hysteresis   the phenomenon whereby a series of values recorded as they are increasing in magnitude are different from those when they are decreasing in magnitude; seen in some instruments.

I^2 a statistic providing a measure of heterogeneity in a meta-analysis. It takes a value from 0% (no heterogeneity) to 100%.

identity link   the link function used in simple and multiple regression; the mean value of the response variable in this form of generalized linear model is not transformed when it is related to a linear function of the covariates.

imputation   a procedure that replaces each missing observation in a data set by an estimated value.

incidence (of a condition)   the number (percentage) of new cases of the condition (e.g. disease) that develop in a defined time period.

incidence rate ratio (IRR)   the ratio of two incidence rates. Also called a relative rate.

incomplete block designs   each block in an experiment does not contain the entire set of treatments.

independent   two events are independent if the probability of one occurring is not affected by the occurrence of the other event.

independent variable   the variable in a regression analysis which is used to predict the value of the dependent or response variable. It is also called the regressor, the explanatory or predictor variable or, if there is more than one, the covariate.

indicator variable *see* dummy variable.

inferential statistics that branch of statistics concerned with drawing conclusions about a population using sample information.

inferiority study used to show that the clinical effectiveness of one treatment is no worse than that of the existing treatment.

influential point an observation which alters the values of one or more parameter estimates if omitted from a regression analysis.

informative censoring occurs in survival analysis when the probability that an animal is censored is related to the probability that the animal will experience the failure.

informative prior in a Bayesian analysis provides strong information so that the likelihood has little influence on the posterior.

instability or drift a form of instrumental error in which the calibration varies.

instrumental error inaccuracies introduced by the mechanical or electronic devices used to make the measurements.

intention-to-treat the process of statistical analysis of data from an experiment in which animals which deviate from the protocol (e.g. by stopping treatment) are analysed as if they are still in the treatment groups to which they were originally assigned.

interaction exists between two variables if the variables do not act independently on the response of interest. In the context of analysis of variance, there is an interaction between two variables when the difference in the response between any two levels of one variable is not constant for the different levels of the other variable. Also called effect modification.

interim analysis a decision is made, before the fixed sample size investigation starts, to perform an analysis of the data at a predetermined time before the end of the investigation. Hence the term 'repeated significance test'.

internal pilot study incorporates its results into the main study.

interquartile range the range of values which encloses the central 50% of the observations if the observations are arranged in rank order.

intraclass correlation coefficient (ICC) the ratio of the between-cluster variance to the total variance; it describes the proportion of the total variance in a set of clustered measurements which is attributed to the difference between clusters.

inverse sine *see* arcsine transformation.

isodemographic map a diagram of an area that has a demographic base distorting its geographic base.

jackknifing a computer-intensive process of estimating parameters and their associated confidence intervals. Each of the n individuals in the study is removed in turn and the parameter(s) of interest estimated from the sample comprising the remaining $n - 1$ individuals. The distribution of these n estimates is used to provide an overall estimate and confidence interval for the parameter.

Kaplan–Meier survival curve a survival curve based on known survival times and which incorporates censored data.

kappa coefficient *see* Cohen's kappa coefficient.

Kendall's tau a non-parametric correlation coefficient.

Kolmogorov–Smirnov test a goodness-of-fit test to test whether data come from a particular distribution (e.g. the Normal) or whether two groups of data come from the same distribution.

Kruskal–Wallis one-way ANOVA a non-parametric equivalent to the one-way ANOVA, used to compare independent groups of observations.

kurtosis a term used to describe the peakedness of a unimodal frequency curve.

laboratory experiment a particular form of experimental study in the laboratory in which the experimental intervention is highly regulated and controlled.

learning objectives task-oriented terms indicating what you should be able to 'do' when you have mastered the concepts to test your growing understanding; if you are able to perform the tasks specified in the learning objectives, you have understood the concepts.

least significant difference (LSD) test   a multiple comparisons test of means that adjusts the *P*-values to avoid spuriously significant results arising from multiple testing.

level   a particular category of a qualitative variable or factor, e.g. dose levels of a drug, different treatments.

level 1 unit   the individual at the lowest level of a multilevel structure; a group of level 1 units (e.g. piglets) is nested within a level 2 unit (e.g. sow).

level 2 unit   the individual at the second lowest level of a multilevel structure; in a two-level structure, each two-level unit (e.g. sow) gives rise to a number of level 1 units (the piglets).

level of significance   *see* significance level.

Levene's test   a parametric test used to investigate the equality of variance in two or more groups.

leverage   the extent to which an individual's value(s) of the explanatory variable(s) in a regression analysis differs from the mean value of the explanatory variable(s).

likelihood   the probability of getting the observed results, given the model.

likelihood ratio statistic (LRS)   uses the ratio of two likelihoods to compare two regression models.

limits of agreement   in the Bland and Altman diagram it is the range of values between which most (usually 95%) of the differences between pairs of observations lie.

linear   a straight line.

linear correlation coefficient   a measure of the linear association between two variables.

linear regression analysis   a formal process of estimating the coefficients of the linear regression equation and making inferences from it.

linear regression equation   describes the linear relationship between two variables when one variable is dependent on the other.

link function   a particular transformation (e.g. the logistic transformation in logistic regression or the log transformation in Poisson regression) of the mean value of the response variable in a generalized linear model; it is modelled as a linear combination of the explanatory variables.

Lin's concordance correlation coefficient   a measure of agreement between pairs of measurements evaluated on the same numerical scale. It encompasses both precision (the closeness of points to the line of best fit when one member of the pair is plotted against the other) and accuracy (the closeness of the best fitting line to the 45° line through the origin). Its value is 1 when there is perfect agreement and 0 when there is no agreement.

listwise deletion   all individuals with any missing data are omitted from the analysis.

logistic (logit) transformation   the transformation, $\log_e\{p/(1-p)\}$, of the proportion, p, used to linearize a sigmoid curve.

logistic regression   *see* multiple linear logistic regression.

Lognormal distribution   a continuous probability distribution. If data which are skewed to the right are log transformed, and the resulting distribution is Normal, the data are said to approximate a Lognormal distribution.

logrank test   a non-parametric test that compares survival curves.

longitudinal study   one in which we investigate changes in the same individuals over time.

lower quartile   the 25th percentile. Also called the first quartile.

Mann–Whitney *U* test   a non-parametric test used to compare two groups of independent observations. It produces the same *P*-value as the Wilcoxon rank sum test.

Mantel–Haenszel method   the correct approach to combining the results contained in contingency tables which relate to different strata of the population.

marginal model   *see* generalized estimating equation.

mask   *see* blind.

matching   the process of making groups of interest comparable with respect to relevant characteristics.

maximum likelihood estimation (MLE)   a process which obtains estimates of the parameters in a model by maximizing the likelihood.

McNemar–Bowker test   an extension of McNemar's test for related samples that provides a method for comparing two paired data sets (e.g. when an animal is assessed by each of two observers) when the ordinal variable of interest has more than two categories.

McNemar's test a test, based on the Chi-squared test, which compares two proportions in paired data.

mean *see* arithmetic mean.

mean square the sum of squares divided by the degrees of freedom; an estimate of variance.

measure of agreement describes how well pairs of observations conform to one another; it may be calculated as twice the SD of the differences between pairs of observations measured on a numerical scale.

measure of dispersion provides an indication of the degree of scatter shown by observations; it is usually a measure of how widely scattered the observations are in either direction from their average.

measure of location some form of average which measures the central tendency of the data set.

median a measure of location. It is the central value in the set of observations which have been arranged in rank order.

median survival time the time which corresponds to a survival probability of 0.5 in survival analysis.

meta-analysis (overview) a systematic approach to combining the quantitative information from several independent studies of a given condition in order to produce, if appropriate, an overall estimate of the effect of interest.

metabolites the intermediates and products of metabolism.

metabolomics the scientific study of all the metabolites, small molecules generated in the process of metabolism in cells, tissues and organs.

method agreement also called reproducibility – concerned with gauging the similarity of different methods of measurement, e.g. different observers using the same technique, or a single observer using different techniques.

method of least squares a mathematical technique for finding the best-fitting line through a series of points. It relies on minimizing the sum of the squared residuals.

missing at random (MAR) the probability that the value of a variable for an individual is missing does not depend on that variable, but depends on the known values of the other variables.

missing completely at random (MVAR) the probability that the value of a variable for a given individual is missing does not depend on any variable.

mixed model *see* random effects model.

modal group or modal class the group or class of a frequency distribution which contains more observations than any other class.

mode the most commonly occurring observation in a set of observations.

model an algebraic description of the relationship between two or more variables.

model definition of probability *see a priori* probability.

model sensitivity indicates the extent to which parameter estimates in a regression model are affected by the data from one or more individuals.

modifiable area unit problem (MAUP) arises when data collected in relation to specific geographical point locations are amalgamated into areas for comparison: the choice of area boundaries can precipitate potentially misleading conclusions.

molecular genetics the study of the structure and functions of DNA at a molecular level.

mRNA (messenger ribonucleic acid) RNA molecules formed by transcription of DNA which carry the instruction for the synthesis of protein in a cell.

multicollinearity *see* collinearity.

multilevel model (MLM) *see* random effects model.

multinomial logistic regression a modification of logistic regression analysis used when the outcome variable is nominal with more than two categories. Also called polycotomous logistic regression.

multiple comparisons the process of performing many hypothesis tests in a data set; it results in increasing the risk of a Type I error unless adjustments are made.

multiple correlation coefficient (R) the square root of the coefficient of determination. R

measures the association between the observed values of the dependent variable and the values of it obtained from the equation.

multiple imputation a process of imputation which relies on creating a number of imputed data sets which are each analysed, and then the results combined to obtain overall estimates of parameters and their standard errors.

multiple linear logistic regression a particular form of a generalized linear model used when the outcome of interest is binary, indicating whether or not an individual possesses a characteristic. The logistic regression equation describes the linear relationship between the explanatory variables and the logit transformation of the proportion of individuals with the characteristic. Often simply called logistic regression.

multiple linear regression equation a multivariable model, often called multiple regression, which provides a mathematical expression to describe the linear relationship between two or more explanatory variables and a dependent variable.

multiplication rule the probability of two independent events occurring is the product of the probability of each event.

multi-stage sampling a simple random sample of clusters is selected from a population of clusters. In two-stage sampling, a simple random sample of units is selected for observation from the selected clusters. This process can be extended to encompass more stages.

multivariable regression model a mathematical model which comprises one dependent variable and two or more explanatory variables. Often called a multiple regression model.

multivariate analysis a general term traditionally used to describe a number of techniques which examine several response or dependent variables simultaneously, when every individual takes a value for each of the variables.

natural pairing litter mates, or some other biological association, provide the experimental material.

negative control the animal receives no active treatment. A negative control group is a group of such animals.

negative predictive value (NPV) the proportion of animals with a negative test result (i.e. shown by the test not to have the disease) which are disease-free.

Newman–Keuls test a multiple comparisons test of means that adjusts the P-values to avoid spuriously significant results arising from multiple testing.

nominal scale the distinct categories which define the variable are unordered and each can be assigned a name, e.g. coat colour.

non-inferiority study used to show that the clinical effectiveness of one treatment is not substantially worse than that of the existing treatment.

non-informative censoring *see* uninformative censoring.

non-parametric tests often called distribution-free tests – methods which make no assumptions about the underlying data distributions.

Normal or Gaussian distribution a continuous probability distribution. It is a bell-shaped distribution and is approximated by many biological variables.

Normal plot a diagram scaled in such a way that Normally distributed data are exhibited as a straight line. Deviations from the straight line suggest that the data are not Normally distributed.

normal range *see* reference range or reference interval.

not missing at random (NMAR) the missingness of data depends not only on the observed data but also on the unobserved (missing) data.

null hypothesis (H_0) the term given to the proposition (about the population) that is under test in a hypothesis testing procedure. In general, it is expressed in terms of no effect, e.g. no difference in population means.

number needed to treat (NNT) the number of animals the clinician needs to treat with a novel treatment instead of a control treatment in order to prevent the occurrence of one adverse outcome. A simple way to express the benefit of a novel treatment.

numerical measure a characteristic which takes a quantitative value.

numerical (quantitative) variable numerical values on a well-defined scale.

observational study we merely observe the animals in the study and record the relevant measurements on those animals; we make no attempt to intervene, for example, by administering treatments or withholding factors which we feel may affect the course of the condition.

odds of exposure the ratio of the probability of being exposed to the probability of being unexposed.

odds ratio (OR) the ratio of two odds, usually the odds of disease in the group exposed to a factor divided by the odds of disease in the unexposed group; an estimate of the relative risk when the disease is rare.

one-sample *t*-test a parametric test based on the *t*-distribution used to test H_0 that the true mean takes a particular value.

one-sided test a hypothesis test in which the *P*-value is determined by referring the test statistic to only a single tail of a theoretical probability distribution. The *a priori* decision to make a test one-sided relies on the specification of the alternative hypothesis which must indicate the direction of the effect of interest based on the impossibility of the effect occurring in the other direction.

one-tailed probability the *P*-value resulting from a one-sided test such that all the probability of interest is contained in only a single tail area of the theoretical distribution.

one-tailed test *see* one-sided test.

one-way ANOVA an extension of the two-sample *t*-test used when we wish to compare the means of more than two independent groups of observations.

one-way repeated measures ANOVA may be regarded as an extension of the paired *t*-test when means are to be compared in three or more groups of related observations.

ordered variable a categorical variable which has some basis of order or ranking in the various categories, e.g. body condition scores, age categories.

ordinal logistic regression a modification of logistic regression analysis used when the outcome variable is ordinal with more than two categories.

ordinal scale the categories which constitute the variable have some intrinsic order but the intervals between the various categories cannot be interpreted in a consistent manner.

outcome variable *see* dependent variable.

outlier an observation whose value is highly inconsistent with the main body of the data.

overview *see* meta-analysis.

P-value in a hypothesis test this is the probability of obtaining the observed results (or more extreme results) if the null hypothesis is true.

paired observations each observation in one group is paired or individually matched with an observation in the other group.

paired *t*-test a parametric test, whose test statistic follows Student's *t*-distribution, which compares the means in two populations using matched pairs of observations.

parallel group design each individual animal receives only one treatment, and treatment comparisons are made between groups of animals rather than within animals.

parallel testing when using two (or more) diagnostic tests, both tests are administered to all animals and an animal is regarded as testing positive if at least one test has a positive result.

parameter a characteristic in the population, such as the mean or SD, which describes a particular feature of a distribution.

parametric test this investigates a hypothesis about the parameter(s) of a distribution and makes assumptions about the underlying form of the distribution of the observations, e.g. that it is Normal.

partial regression coefficient the coefficient in the multiple regression equation which corresponds to a particular explanatory variable. It is generally different from the regression coefficient which would be obtained by regressing the dependent variable on that explanatory variable alone, omitting the other explanatory variables from the equation altogether. It is sometimes called the regression coefficient.

Pearson's product moment correlation coefficient *see* correlation coefficient.

percentage point the upper percentage point (percentile) is the value of the variable which has $p\%$ of the distribution of the variable to the right of it. The lower percentage point has $p\%$ to the left of it. For a two-tailed test, we consider the percentage of the distribution in both tails, i.e. to the right and left of the relevant percentage points.

percentiles the values of the variable which divide the total frequency into 100 equal parts.

performance indicator in a surveillance context this is a specifically designed key measure of quality, sensitivity and quantity of a surveillance system, used to evaluate whether the achievements of a disease surveillance programme are fulfilling the purposes for which they were established.

pharmaceutical and agrichemical industries industrial and commercial companies whose products may raise issues concerned with risks to human health derived from farming, e.g. drug residues in carcasses at slaughter, pesticides and fertilizer residues in plants.

pictogram a diagram, often used to display the frequency distribution of a categorical data set, in which the frequency in a category is indicated by some measure (e.g. the height, number of repeated images) of a pictorial representation of a relevant object.

pie chart a diagram used to display the frequency distribution of a categorical data set. It is a circle divided into segments with each segment portraying a different category of the qualitative variable. The area of a segment is proportional to the percentage of individuals in that category.

pilot study a small-scale preliminary investigation.

placebo a pharmacologically inert substance identical in appearance to the test treatment, which dissociates the pharmacological effect of treatment from any suggestive element (the placebo effect) imposed by the receipt of treatment.

placebo effect the response induced by suggestion on the part of the animal attendants or investigators when the animal receives a placebo (dummy) treatment.

Poisson distribution a discrete probability distribution of the count of the number of events occurring randomly in time or space at a constant rate on average.

Poisson regression analysis a particular form of a generalized linear model (with a log link function) used when the outcome of interest is a rate which is assumed to be constant over the period of interest; the individuals in the study may have different follow-up times.

polycotomous logistic regression *see* multinomial logistic regression.

polynomial a non-linear or curvilinear relationship described by a regression equation in which the degree of the polynomial is determined by the power of the explanatory variable(s), e.g. for the explanatory variable, x, the quadratic equation includes the term x^2, the cubic equation includes the term x^3, etc.

population the complete finite (real) or infinite (hypothetical) collection of observational units.

population attributable fraction (PAF) the difference between the risk of a particular outcome in the whole population and the risk in the group unexposed to some factor of interest (i.e. the PAR) expressed as a proportion of the risk in the whole population.

population attributable risk (PAR) the difference between the risk of a particular outcome in the whole population and the risk in the group unexposed to some factor of interest.

population-averaged model *see* generalized estimating equation.

population survey an observational study of the entire population, e.g. a census.

positive control in clinical trials, a standard therapy against which a novel therapy is compared. In laboratory studies, it is a treatment inducing the maximum response.

positive predictive value (PPV) the proportion of animals with a positive test result (i.e. shown by the test to have the disease) which have the disease.

posterior probability an individual's belief relating to a particular outcome (e.g. that an animal has a certain disease); it is quantified after performing an experiment or conducting a trial by using the current evidence from that study to update the prior probability. The term is integral to Bayesian inference.

post-test probability the posterior probability of an event (e.g. a disease outcome) obtained by using the current best evidence (the diagnostic test result) to update the pre-test or prior probability.

power-efficiency a way of comparing the power of a parametric test and that of its non-parametric equivalent. It is the extent to which the sample size of the non-parametric test needs to be increased to make it as powerful as its parametric equivalent.

power (of a test) the probability that a test will reject the null hypothesis when the null hypothesis is false; it is the chance of detecting as statistically significant an effect of a given magnitude.

precision refers to how well repeated observations agree with one another.

predictive value *see* negative predictive value; positive predictive value.

predictor variable *see* independent variable.

pre-test probability in the context of a disease outcome, it is the prior probability of the disease (e.g. its prevalence in the population) which is updated using the current best evidence (e.g. a diagnostic test result) to obtain the post-test or posterior probability of the disease.

prevalence (of a condition) the number (percentage) of cases of the condition (e.g. disease) that exist at a specific instant in time (point prevalence) or in a defined interval of time (period prevalence).

prior probability an individual's belief relating to a particular outcome (e.g. that an animal has a certain disease); its value is assumed before performing an experiment or conducting a trial. The term is integral to Bayesian inference.

PRISMA guidelines a framework to help authors report systematic reviews and meta-analyses to assess the benefits and harms of a healthcare intervention.

probability the chance of a particular event occurring.

probability density function the curve, defined by a mathematical formula, which describes the relative frequency distribution of the pop-ulation. The total area under the curve is unity, and the proportion of observations between any two limits is the area under the curve between these limits.

probability distribution a theoretical distribution which we specify mathematically, and use to calculate the theoretical probability of an event occurring.

probability sampling any method of selection of a sample that is based on the theory of probability, for example, random sampling.

prognostic factor *see* covariate.

propensity score a score (usually generated by logistic regression) that describes the chance of an animal falling into one of the categories of the (usually binary) explanatory variable that is of the greatest interest (e.g. 'treatment' in a non-randomized study). Used as a basis for matching, stratification or as a covariate in a regression model to overcome problem of confounding.

proportion the ratio of the number of events of interest to the total number of events.

proportional hazards the ratio of the hazards is constant over time.

proportional hazards regression model *see* Cox proportional hazards regression model.

proportional or scale error a technical error in which the magnitude of the inaccuracy in measurement increases (or decreases) with the magnitude of the value.

prospective longitudinal study the study is conducted forwards in time from a defined starting point.

proteome the complete set of proteins expressed by an organism, tissue or cell.

proteomics the scientific study of the entire protein complement of a cell, tissue or organism.

publication bias the tendency for authors to submit only papers with positive findings to journals and for journals to accept only significant results for publication, thereby giving undue weight to positive treatment effects in meta-analyses.

published scientific literature information available to the student and professional from the work of others and published in scientific journals, textbooks and magazines and electronically (e.g. on the internet).

qualitative variable an individual belongs to any one of two or more distinct categories of the variable. Also called a categorical variable.

quality control ensuring that processes and procedures are carried out in a consistently satisfactory manner so that the results are trustworthy.

quantitative genetics the study of genetic variation of complex traits using probabilistic (statistical) models.

quantitative variable *see* numerical (quantitative) variable.

random allocation assigning of animals to groups (e.g. treatments) in a randomized manner (i.e. the process is based on chance). Also referred to as randomization.

random effect the levels of the factor of interest represent individual members of a sample from the population of interest (e.g. individual pigs sampled from a population of Gloucester Old Spot pigs).

random effects model a regression model for a hierarchical data structure in which the random effect for a two-level model is the source of error attributable to the level 2 units. Also called a multilevel model, cross-sectional time series model, hierarchical model or a mixed model.

random error the recorded values are evenly distributed above and below the true value; it is due to unexplained sources.

random intercepts model a particular form of random effects model in which, for a two-level structure (i.e. level 1 units within clusters), the linear regression equations for the clusters have the same slope but intercepts that vary randomly about the mean intercept.

random sample a selection made from the population such that every individual in the sample has an equal chance of selection, and the selection of one individual has no influence on the selection of subsequent individuals.

random selection the process, using a method based on chance, whereby individuals are chosen to be included in a random sample.

random variable a variable which can take various values with given probabilities. All the values that the random variable can take, with their associated probabilities, comprise the probability distribution of the random variable.

randomization this is the same as random allocation. In addition, a set of objects is said to be randomized if they are arranged in random order.

randomized block a particular ANOVA design in which each of the treatments in the investigation is randomly allocated to the units within a 'block', the complete design comprising a number of such blocks.

randomized controlled trial (RCT) a clinical trial which incorporates at least one control group, and which uses randomization to allocate the animals to the different treatment and control groups.

range the difference between the largest and smallest observations in a data set.

rank order a systematized arrangement of the data values in ascending or descending order.

ranks the successive numbers, starting at 1, assigned to the values of the observations in a data set which have been arranged in ascending (or descending) order. Thus, the rank of the smallest observation is 1, of the next smallest is 2, etc.

rate number of new events per unit of investigation per unit time.

raw data *see* readings.

readings primary measurements taken from individual animals or biological samples; also called values or raw data.

real (or finite) population the individuals in the population that actually exist (cf. hypothetical population).

receiver operator characteristic (ROC) curve a plot of the sensitivity against 1 minus the specificity for different cut-off values of the variable that is to be used to discriminate between two disease outcomes (present/absent). The ROC curve may be used to assess the discriminatory ability of a test, define the optimal cut-off (often corresponding to the point in the curve closest to the top left-hand corner of the diagram) or compare two or more diagnostic tests.

reference interval *see* reference range or reference interval.

reference prior in a Bayesian analysis it represents minimal prior information and is usually used as a baseline against which other priors can be compared.

reference range or reference interval the range of values of a variable that defines the healthy population, usually calculated as the interval which encompasses the central 95% of the observations from this population; if the data are Normally distributed, it is defined by the mean ± 1.96 SD. Sometimes called the normal range.

REFLECT statement an evidence-based minimum set of items for reporting livestock trials with production, health and food-safety outcomes. It focuses on field trials and challenge studies with either therapeutic or preventive interventions.

regression coefficient the coefficient which corresponds to a particular explanatory variable in a regression equation. Sometimes, the constant term (the intercept) in simple linear regression is also referred to as a regression coefficient, as is a partial regression coefficient in a multivariable regression equation.

regression diagnostics the processes used to check the assumptions underlying a regression model and to determine outliers and influential cases.

regression model an algebraic description of the relationship between a response variable and one or more explanatory variables.

regression of y on x the equation (usually a linear model) which describes the relationship between a dependent variable, y, and an explanatory variable, x.

regression to the mean a phenomenon whereby animals which may have been selected for study because they had extreme measurements on the variable of interest, are likely to have measurements which are closer to the average if the measurement is repeated on a second occasion.

regressor variable *see* independent variable.

relative frequency distribution shows the proportion or percentage of observations in each class or category of the distribution.

relative rate *see* incidence rate ratio.

relative risk (RR) the ratio of two risks, usually the ratio of the risk of disease in the 'exposed' group to the risk of disease in the 'unexposed' group. It provides a measure of the strength of the association between the disease and the exposure to the factor. If the relative risk is unity, then exposure to the factor does not affect the animal's chance of developing the disease; if it is greater than unity it indicates the increased risk associated with 'exposure'.

relative risk reduction (RRR) the difference in the risks of the event of interest between the treated and control groups (i.e. the ARR), expressed as a proportion of the risk in the control group.

reliability reflects the amount of error, both random and systematic, inherent in any measurement. It encompasses repeatability, reproducibility, validity and stability.

repeatability the extent to which replicate measurements in identical circumstances of a particular technique or instrument or observer are the same.

repeated measures design an experimental design where each animal is investigated at every level of a factor, so the effects of interest are examined on a within-animal basis; e.g. when each animal receives all treatments or is investigated at a number of time points. Also called clustered design. *See also* one-way repeated measures ANOVA.

repeated significance tests hypothesis tests performed at intermediate stages of a trial. *See also* interim analysis.

replication we take more than one measurement on the variable of interest on each individual.

reproducibility *see* method agreement.

residual in general, the residual is the difference between two quantities; in regression, it is the difference between the observed value of the response variable and its value predicted by the model.

residual mean square *see* residual variance.

residual variance that part of the total variance of a variable which remains after the effects of certain factors have been removed; it measures the variability which cannot be explained by the model. The residual variance is the residual mean square in an ANOVA.

response variable   *see* dependent variable.

restricted   randomization   *see*   blocked randomization.

retrospective longitudinal study   the study is conducted by looking backwards in time from a defined starting point.

risk difference (RD)   *see* attributable risk.

risk of disease   number of new cases expressed as a proportion of those initially at risk.

RNA (ribonucleic acid)   a nucleotide used in key metabolic processes for all steps of protein synthesis in all living cells.

robust procedure   a hypothesis test is robust if the probabilities of the Type I and Type II errors are hardly affected when the assumptions underlying the test are not fulfilled.

robust standard error   estimation of standard error based on the variability in the data set rather than on that assumed by the regression model and is therefore robust to violations of the assumptions of the regression model.

rounding error   inaccuracy introduced due to rounding off the number string to a lesser number of decimal places or significant figures.

runs test   a non-parametric test used to investigate randomness of a binary variable in a single group.

sample   a subgroup drawn from the population.

sample size   the number of individuals included in an investigation when a subgroup of the population is studied.

sample survey   an observational study which uses sample data to provide information about the population from which the sample was taken.

sampling distribution of the mean   the distribution of the sample means; it is a hypothetical distribution obtained by taking all possible repeated samples (without replacement) of a given size from a population, and calculating the sample mean in each sample. These sample means can be plotted to show the distribution in diagrammatic form.

sampling distribution of the proportion   the distribution of the sample proportions; it is a hypothetical distribution obtained by taking all possible repeated samples (without replacement) of a given size from a population, and calculating the sample proportion in each sample.

sampling error   the difference between the sample statistic and the population parameter that it is estimating, present because we have taken only a sample of observations from the population, and are not looking at it in its entirety.

sampling units   the population is divided into non-overlapping parts called units (e.g. individual animals, different herds); the sampling process involves selecting a subgroup of these units from the population. The units may then be called sampling units.

sampling variation   describes the fact that the values of a statistic (e.g. the sample mean which estimates the population mean) will not be identical in different samples of a given size drawn from the same population. The variance and the SD of the sampling distribution of the statistic describe this sampling variation (the SD of the sampling distribution is called the standard error of the statistic).

saturated model   a model that has at least as many variables as individuals in the sample.

scaling   the process of dividing or multiplying the value of an explanatory variable by a suitable constant to provide a more meaningful interpretation of the parameter in a regression model.

scatter diagram   a two-dimensional plot in which each axis represents the scale of measurement of one of two variables; each point corresponds to the relevant co-ordinate values on the two scales.

sceptical prior   reflects the pessimistic or worst possible outcome in a Bayesian analysis before the sample data are available.

Scheffe's test   a multiple comparisons test of means that adjusts the P-values to avoid spuriously significant results arising from multiple testing.

screening   a process of identifying asymptomatic animals which are at risk of a particular disease.

self-pairing the animal acts as its own control in a clinical trial, and so receives both treatments, preferably in random order.

sensitivity the effectiveness of a diagnostic or screening test to identify animals with the disease. It is the proportion of true positives identified by the test as positive.

sensitivity analysis performed to assess how robust or sensitive the results of a statistical analysis are to the methods and assumptions of that analysis and/or to the data values included in the analysis.

sequential testing when using two (or more) diagnostic tests, one test is administered to all animals but only animals positive from the first test receive the second test.

sequential trial the sample size is not fixed in advance but depends on the results as they become available. A formal approach to the analysis has to be devised; it takes into account considerations such as the significance level and precision, and depends on stopping rules which allow the trial to terminate in favour of a particular treatment if certain conditions are met.

serial correlation a measurement of serial dependence in a sequence of observations, such as a time series. Its presence implies that the deviations about any long-term trends are associated.

series testing when using two (or more) diagnostic tests, both tests are administered to all animals and the animal is regarded as testing positive only if it has positive results from both tests.

Shapiro–Wilk W test investigates whether a data set follows a specific probability distribution, typically the Normal distribution.

sign test a non-parametric test used to investigate data in a single group, or from related pairs of subjects.

significance level a cut-off for the *P*-value such that the null hypothesis will be rejected if the *P*-value from a hypothesis test falls below this cut-off value; the cut-off is decided upon before the test is conducted and is often chosen as 0.05. Then if $P < 0.05$, we say that the test is significant at the 5% level. The significance level is the maximum chance of making a Type I error.

simple linear regression a regression equation with only one explanatory variable. Also called univariable linear regression.

simple random sampling a method of sampling in which every unit in the population has an equal chance of being selected.

simple randomization we randomly allocate animals to the different treatment groups without using any refinements or restrictions.

single-blind only one of these two parties – the carer or the assessor – is blind to the treatment that an animal receives in a clinical trial. Also called single-masked.

single-masked *see* single-blind.

skewed to the left (negatively skewed) the frequency distribution is not symmetrical but has an extended left-hand tail.

skewed to the right (positively skewed) the frequency distribution is not symmetrical but has an extended right-hand tail.

skewness a term used to describe the asymmetry of a frequency distribution.

spatial autocorrelation occurs when there is a relationship between the values of a single variable that is due to the geographical areas in which these values occur; this implies that there is a dependency between the values of the variable in one location and in neighbouring areas.

spatial statistics modifications, extensions and additions to statistical techniques that focus on the importance of locations or spatial arrangement.

Spearman's rank correlation coefficient a non-parametric equivalent to Pearson's product moment correlation coefficient; it measures the association (not necessarily linear) between two variables which may be ordinal.

specificity the effectiveness of a diagnostic or screening test to identify non-diseased animals. It is the proportion of true negatives identified by the test as negative.

square of the correlation coefficient (r^2) the proportion of the variance of one variable explained by its linear relationship with another variable. It is sometimes called the coefficient of determination.

stability concerns the long-term repeatability of measurements.

standard deviation (SD) a measure of spread which may be regarded, approximately, as an average of the deviations of the observations from the arithmetic mean. It is equal to the square root of the variance.

standard deviation of the proportion the standard deviation of the sampling distribution of a proportion; usually called the standard error of the proportion. It is a measure of the precision of p as an estimate of π.

standard error of measurement an estimate of the variability of the individual measurements in a repeatability study. It is equal to the square root of half the variance of the differences between the observations within pairs of measurements.

standard error of the estimate a measure of the precision of the sample statistic as an estimate of the population parameter. It is equal to the standard deviation of the sampling distribution of the statistic.

standard error of the mean (SEM) the standard deviation of the sampling distribution of the mean; it is a measure of the dispersion of the sample means and of the precision of the sample mean as an estimate of the population mean.

Standard Normal distribution a Normal distribution with a mean of zero and a standard deviation of 1 (unity).

standardized difference used in the calculations of sample size required for a hypothesis test; it is based on the meaningful treatment effect (one which we should not like to overlook) divided by the relevant standard deviation.

Standardized Normal Deviate (SND), z a variable which follows the Normal distribution with a mean of zero and a standard deviation of unity.

STARD guidelines a framework created with a view to improving the accuracy and completeness of reporting of studies of diagnostic accuracy.

statistic a sample estimate of a population parameter. Sometimes called a sample statistic, although since a statistic always relates to the sample, strictly, the word 'sample' is redundant.

statistical heterogeneity exists when there is a statistically significant difference between the effects of interest in a meta-analysis.

statistical inference the process of generalizing to the population from the sample; it enables us to draw conclusions about certain features of a population when only a subgroup of that population – the sample – is available for investigation.

statistical significance the result of a hypothesis test is statistically significant if the decision is made to reject the null hypothesis; statistical significance should be contrasted with biological importance.

statistics defined narrowly, this is the skills of data manipulation and analysis, but generally in biological science it is taken to mean a wider numerical approach to the science. *See also* biometry.

stem-and-leaf diagram a diagram, generally computer generated, which shows the distribution of a data set; the stem is the core value of the observations (e.g. the unit value before the decimal place) and each leaf is a sequence of ordered single digits, one for each observation, which follow the core value (e.g. the first decimal place).

stepwise selection the process of determining an optimal regression equation; it is essentially a step-up procedure which starts with one variable and adds more variables successively, but it allows the variables in the equation to be dropped according to defined statistical criteria specified by the computer package.

stratified randomization we divide the population into different strata according to the categorization of the key potentially confounding variables; then, within each stratum, we randomly allocate animals to each of the treatment groups.

stratified sampling the population is divided into strata and a simple random sample of units is selected from each stratum.

stratum one of a number of groups, each comprising different individuals that collectively make up the population (or sample).

STROBE statement provides guidelines for reporting cohort, case–control, and cross-sectional studies

Student's *t*-distribution *see t*-distribution.

subjective probability personal view of probability which is to regard it as a measure of the strength of belief an individual has that a particular event will occur.

substantial prior in a Bayesian analysis, it provides considerable empirical or theoretical relevant information about the unknown parameter with the consequence that the posterior departs substantially from the likelihood.

sum of squares the sum of the squared deviations of each observation from the mean; it is used in the calculations of mean squares in the analysis of variance.

summary measure a quantity which reduces a set of measurements to a single value which represents an important feature of that data set; for example, the maximum response in a series of measurements over time for an individual. Use of a summary measure considerably simplifies the analysis of repeated measures data by reducing a series of values for each individual to a single quantity.

superiority trial used to determine whether two or more treatments are statistically significantly different.

survey we examine an aggregate of animals or other such units in an observational study in order to derive values for estimates of various parameters in the population.

survival analysis the analysis of the time to a critical event, e.g. death, in a group of animals in which there may be censored data.

symmetrical distribution the shape of the distribution to the right of a central value is a mirror image of that to the left of the central value.

systematic error one in which the recorded value is systematically above (or below) its true value.

systematic review a qualitative, clearly defined examination of published and unpublished results which collates the information to answer questions, often about the effectiveness of a treatment.

systematic sampling a method of selecting a sample of elements from the population. A random start point in the frame is chosen (the *k*th element) and then a selection is made of every *k*th element thereafter; apart from the choice of the initial element, this is not random sampling.

***t*-distribution** discovered by 'Student', a pseudonym for W. S. Gosset, it is a continuous probability distribution; the distribution is symmetrical about the mean, and is characterized by the degrees of freedom. As the degrees of freedom increase, it becomes more like the Normal distribution.

***t*-test** these are significance tests based on Student's *t*-distribution. *See* one-sample *t*-test; paired *t*-test; unpaired *t*-test.

table an orderly arrangement, usually of numbers or words in rows and columns, which exhibits a set of facts in a distinct and comprehensive way.

tails tails of a frequency distribution represent the frequencies at the extremes of the distribution.

technical variations or errors variability in the measurements due to a variety of instrumental causes and to human error.

test statistic a quantity which follows a theoretical probability distribution and which forms the basis for performing a hypothesis test. By referring the value of the test statistic computed from the sample data to the appropriate probability distribution, we can determine the P-value and decide whether we have enough evidence to reject the null hypothesis.

theoretical probability distribution a mathematical formula from which the probability of each value of a discrete random variable can be determined, and which, if the random variable is continuous, defines the curve such that the probability that the variable falls in an interval is determined by the area under the curve within this interval.

time series a long series of measurements made at many successive points in time. Usually, the successive observations are dependent so that the magnitude of one value influences the magnitude of the next, i.e. we have an auto-regressive series.

time-dependent variable changes over time during the course of the study.

trait genetically determined phenotype or characteristic of an organism.

transcriptomics the scientific study of the expression profile of mRNA in a cell, tissue or organism.

transformation a mathematical manipulation (e.g. taking the log) of each value in the entire data set in an attempt to produce a new data set which conforms to the particular requirements of the analysis, e.g. Normality, a linear relationship or constant variance.

treatment effect a parameter specification of the treatment comparison of interest, e.g. the difference in means between the treatment and control groups.

Tukey's test a multiple comparisons test of means that adjusts the *P*-values to avoid spuriously significant results arising from multiple testing.

two-by-two table *see* fourfold table.

two-sample *t*-test *see* unpaired *t*-test.

two-sided test a hypothesis test in which the *P*-value is determined by relating the test statistic to both tails of a theoretical distribution. The *a priori* decision to make a test two-sided relies on the specification of the alternative hypothesis which does not indicate the direction of the treatment effect.

two-tailed probability the *P*-value resulting from a two-sided test in which all the probability of interest is contained in both tails (i.e. the sum of the right- and left-hand tail areas) of the probability distribution.

two-tailed test *see* two-sided test.

two-way ANOVA an analysis of data which examines the effect of two factors on a response variable, when each of these factors possesses two or more levels.

Type I error we reject the null hypothesis when it should not be rejected, i.e. when it is true. The maximum probability of making a Type I error is the significance level of the test.

Type II error we fail to reject the null hypothesis when it should be rejected, i.e. when it is false.

unbiased free from bias or systematic error.

unbiased estimate (of the population parameter) the mean of the sampling distribution of the sample statistic coincides with the population parameter which the statistic is estimating.

unimodal a distribution which has a single mode or modal group.

uninformative censoring occurs in survival analysis when the probability that an animal is censored is not related to the probability that the animal will experience the failure. Also called non-informative censoring.

uninformative prior in a Bayesian analysis does not influence the posterior probability as it provides no relevant information.

univariable regression model a mathematical model which comprises one outcome or dependent variable and one explanatory variable. Also called simple regression.

univariate analysis the analysis of data which comprises a single dependent or response variable.

unpaired *t*-test a parametric test, whose test statistic follows Student's *t*-distribution, used to compare the means in two independent populations. It is also called the two-sample *t*-test.

upper quartile the 75th percentile. Also called the third quartile.

vague prior in a Bayesian analysis, the sample data swamps the prior information so that the posterior and likelihood are virtually equal. Also called a diffuse prior.

validity concerned with determining whether the measurement is actually measuring what it purports to be measuring.

values *see* readings.

variable a characteristic which can take values which vary from individual to individual or group to group, e.g. height, weight, sex (male or female).

variance a measure of dispersion. It is the square of the standard deviation.

variance inflation factor (VIF) a measure which can provide evidence of collinearity between variables. If R_i^2 is equal to the proportion of variance explained by the regression of the variable x_i on the remaining explanatory variables in a regression model, the $\text{VIF}_i = 1/(1 - R_i^2)$. A value greater than 10 may suggest collinearity.

variance ratio test (*F*-test) a parametric test, based on the *F*-distribution, used to compare two variances.

verification bias arises in the evaluation of diagnostic tests when the gold standard test is not a true reflection of the disease state of the animal.

veterinary surveillance the process of collecting, collating and analysing information on animal diseases and infections in order to provide early indication of changing patterns of animal health which may affect productivity or pose a threat to human health.

Wald test statistic used to test the significance from zero of a regression coefficient whose estimate is obtained by maximum likelihood; it follows the Normal distribution.

weighted kappa coefficient a modification of Cohen's kappa coefficient that takes into account the extent to which paired ordinal measurements agree.

weighted mean the arithmetic mean of a set of observations where a particular weight is attached to each observation so that the observation assumes the required degree of importance.

Wilcoxon rank sum test a non-parametric test used to compare the distributions of data in two independent populations. It produces the same *P*-value as the Mann–Whitney *U* test, and may be used as the non-parametric alternative to the two-sample *t*-test.

Wilcoxon signed rank test a non-parametric test used to compare the distributions of data in two populations of matched pairs of observations. It may be used as the non-parametric alternative to the paired *t*-test.

withdrawal withdrawals from a study are animals which are lost to follow-up during the course of the study, perhaps because their owners move out of the area, so that information is not available for these animals from the time that they withdrew: their data are not accessible and cannot be analysed. Withdrawals from treatment (animals with protocol violations, such as stopping treatment because of side effects) which are not lost to follow-up should have their responses included in the statistical analysis.

Yates' correction an adjustment applied to the Chi-squared test statistic when it is used to test a hypothesis in a 2×2 contingency table. It makes the discrete distribution of the test statistic a better approximation to the continuous Chi-squared distribution.

zero error a technical error whereby the instrument fails to register a true zero reading.

zoonosis any infectious disease that can be transmitted naturally between animals, both wild and domestic, and humans.

Appendix E
Flowcharts for selection of appropriate tests

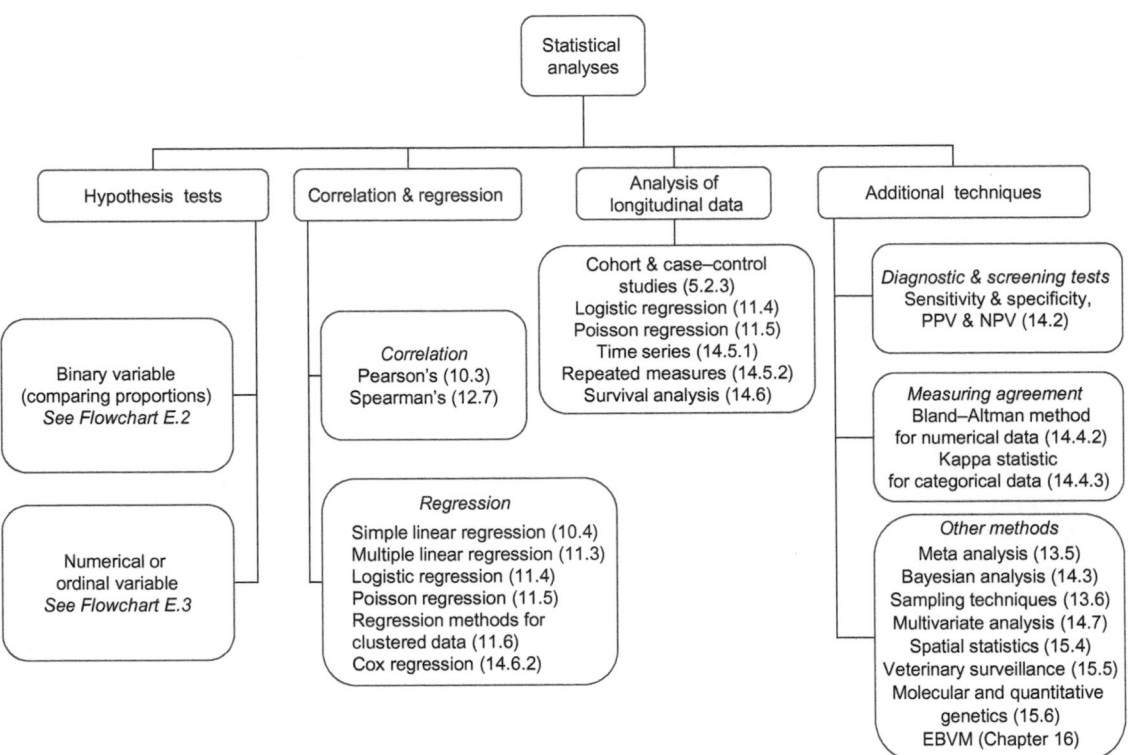

Figure E.1 Statistical analyses (section numbers in brackets).

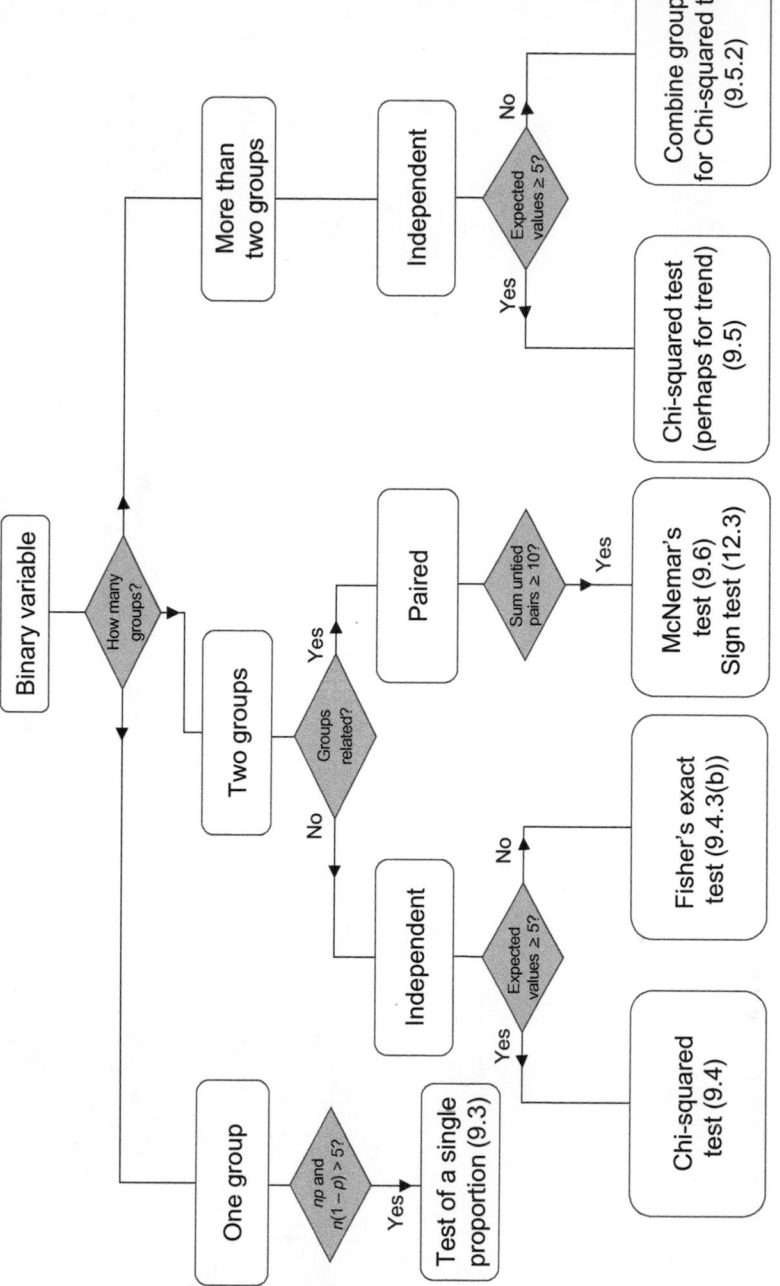

Figure E.2 Flowchart for choosing appropriate tests for proportions derived from a binary variable.

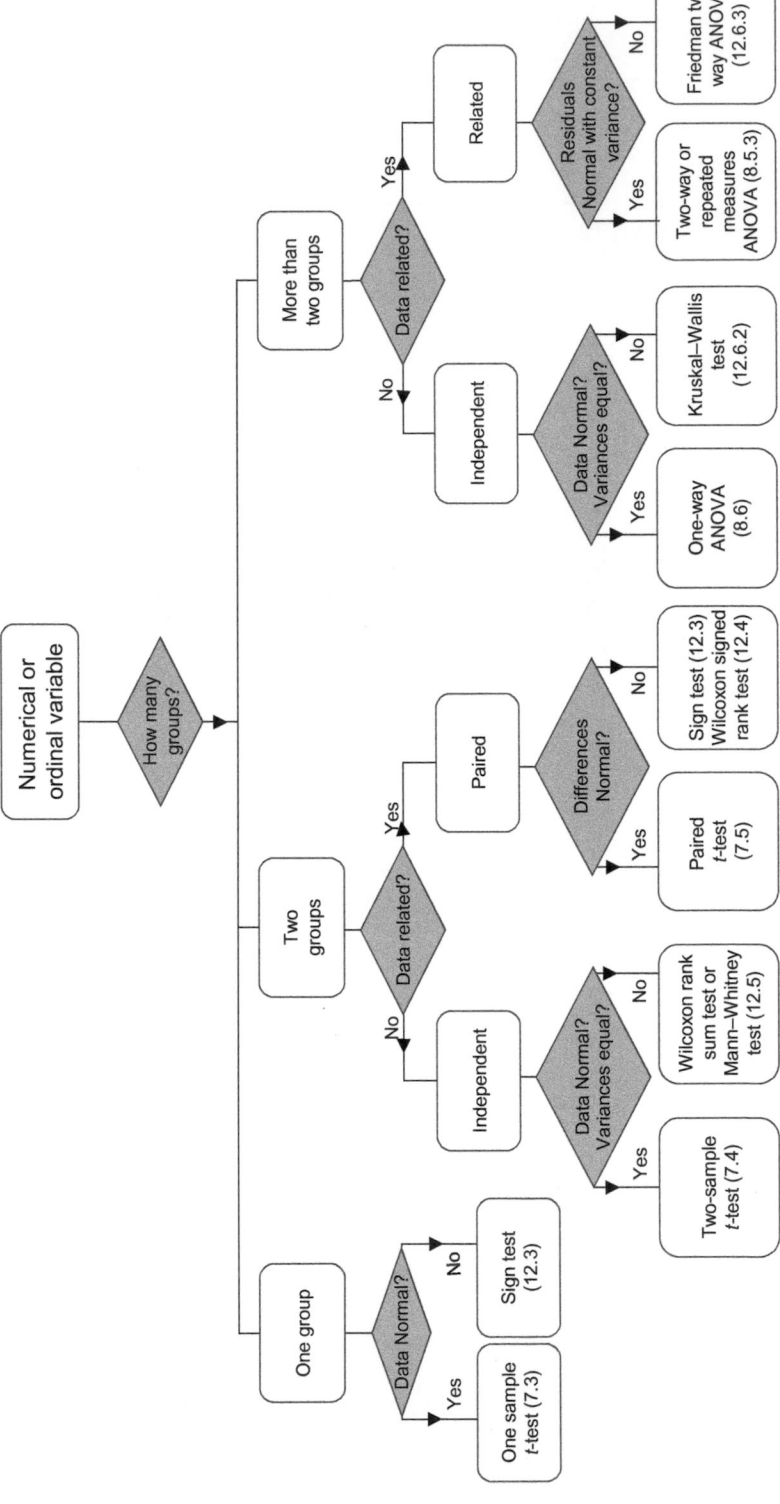

Figure E.3 Flowchart for choosing appropriate test for numerical or ordinal variables.

References

Agresti, A. (1996) *An Introduction to Categorical Data Analysis*. Wiley-Interscience, New York.

Agresti, A. (2010) *Analysis of Ordinal Categorical Data*, 2nd edn. John Wiley & Sons, Hoboken, NJ.

Alexander, F.E. & Boyle, P. (1996) *Methods for Investigating Localized Clustering of Disease*. International Agency for Research on Cancer Scientific Publications No. 135. IARC, Lyon, France.

Allen, M.P. (1997) *Understanding Regression Analysis*. Plenum Press, New York.

Allison, P.D. (2001) *Missing Data*. Sage Publications, Thousand Oaks, CA.

Altman, D.G. (1980) Statistics and ethics in medical research: III. How large a sample? *British Medical Journal* **281**, 1336–8.

Altman, D.G. (1991) *Practical Statistics for Medical Research*. Chapman & Hall/CRC Press, London.

Altman, D.G. & Bland, J.M. (1995) Absence of evidence in not evidence of absence. *British Medical Journal* **311**, 485.

Altman, D.G. & Bland, J.M. (1997) Units of analysis. *British Medical Journal* **314**, 1874.

Altman, D.G., Machin, D., Bryant, T.N. & Gardner, M.J. (eds) (2000) *Statistics with Confidence*, 2nd edn. BMJ Books/Blackwell Publishing, Oxford.

Altman, D.G., Schulz, K.F., Moher, D. *et al.*; CONSORT GROUP (Consolidated Standards of Reporting Trials) (2001) The revised CONSORT statement for reporting randomized trials: explanation and elaboration. *Annals of Internal Medicine* **134**, 663–94.

Armitage, P. (1975) *Sequential Medical Trials*, 2nd edn. Blackwell Scientific Publications, Oxford.

Armitage, P., Berry, G. & Matthews, J.N.S. (2002) *Statistical Methods in Medical Research*, 4th edn. Blackwell Science, Oxford.

Bajer, A., Behnke, J.M., Pawelczyk, A., Kulis, K., Sereda, M.J. & Sinski, E. (2005) Medium-term temporal stability of the helminth component community structure in bank voles (*Clethrionomys glareolus*) from the Mazury Lake District region of Poland. *Parasitology* **130**, 213–28.

Balding, D.J., Bishop, M. & Cannings, C. (2007) *Handbook of Statistical Genetics*. John Wiley & Sons, Chichester, UK.

Barber, P.J. & Elliott, J. (1998) Feline chronic renal failure: calcium homeostasis in 80 cases diagnosed between 1992 and 1995. *Journal of Small Animal Practice* **39**, 108–16.

Bensignor, E. & Olivry, T. (2005) Treatment of localized lesions of canine atopic dermatitis with tacrolimus ointment: a blinded randomized controlled trial. *Veterinary Dermatology* **16**, 52–60.

Bernardo, J.M. & Smith, A.F. (2000) *Bayesian Theory*. John Wiley & Sons, Chichester, UK.

Bessell, P.R., Shaw D.J., Savill, N.J. & Woolhouse, M.E. (2010) Estimating risk factors for farm-level transmission of disease: foot and mouth disease during the 2001 epidemic in Great Britain. *Epidemics* **2**, 109–15.

Bibby, C.J., Burgess, N.D. & Hill, D.A. (1992) *Bird Census Techniques*. Academic Press, London.

Bille, C., Auvigne, V., Libermann, S., Bomassi, E., Durieux, P. & Rattez, E. (2012) Risk of anaesthetic mortality in dogs and cats: an observational cohort study of 3546 cases. *Veterinary Anaesthesia and Analgesia* **39**, 59–68.

Birkett, M.A. & Day, S.J. (1994) Internal pilot studies for estimating sample size. *Statistics in Medicine* **13**, 2455–63.

Bland, J.M. & Altman, D.G. (1986) Statistical methods for assessing agreement between two methods of clinical measurement. *Lancet* **i**, 307–10.

Bland, J.M. & Altman, D.G. (1994) Matching. *British Medical Journal* **309**, 1128.

Bland, J.M. & Altman, D.G. (1998) Bayesians and frequentists. *British Medical Journal* **317**, 1151–60.

Bland, J.M. & Altman, D.G. (2007) Agreement between methods of measurement with multiple observations per individual. *Journal of Biopharmaceutical Statistics* **17**, 571–82.

Bland, J.M. & Kerry, S.M. (1997) Statistics notes: trials randomised in clusters. *British Medical Journal* **315**, 600.

Boden, L.A. & Parkin, T.D.H. (2008) Current guidelines on good reporting of analytical observational studies in epidemiology. *Equine Veterinary Journal* **40**, 84–6.

Borenstein, M., Hedges, L.V., Higgins, J.T.P. & Rothstein, H.R. (2009) *Introduction to Meta-Analysis*. Statistics in Practice. John Wiley & Sons, Chichester, UK.

Bossuyt, P.M., Reitsma, J.B., Bruns, D.E. *et al.* (2003a) Standards for reporting of diagnostic accuracy. Toward complete and accurate reporting of studies of diagnostic accuracy: the STARD initiative. Standards for Reporting of Diagnostic Accuracy. *British Medical Journal* **326**, 41–4.

Bossuyt, P.M., Reitsma, J.B., Bruns, D.E. *et al.* (2003b) Standards for reporting of diagnostic accuracy. The STARD statement for reporting of diagnostic accuracy: explanation and elaboration. *Clinical Chemistry* **49**, 7–18.

Bowker, A.H. (1948) A test for symmetry in contingency tables, *Journal of the American Statistical Association* **43**, 572–4.

British Standards Institution (BSI) (1975) *Precision of Test Methods 1: Guide for the determination and reproducibility for a standard test method (BS 597, Part 1)*. BSI, London.

Brookmeyer, R. & Stroup, D.F. (eds) (2003) *Statistical Principles and Methods for Public Health Surveillance*. Oxford University Press, New York.

Buckland, S.T., Anderson, D.R., Burnham, K.P. & Laake, J.L. (1993) *Distance Sampling: Estimating abundance of biological populations*. Chapman & Hall, London.

Burton, P., Gurrin, L. & Sly, P. (1998) Extending the simple linear regression model to account for correlated responses: an introduction to generalized estimating equations and multi-level mixed modelling. *Statistics in Medicine* **17**, 1261–91.

Burton, S.A., Lemke, K.A., Ihle, S.L. & MacKenzie, A.L. (1997) Effects of medetomidine on serum insulin and plasma glucose concentrations in clinically normal dogs. *American Journal of Veterinary Research* **58**, 1440–2.

Câmara, G., Monteiro, A.M., Druck Fucks, S. & Carvalho, M.S. (2008) *Spatial Analysis and GIS: A primer*. http://faculty.ksu.edu.sa/adosari/Documents/spatial_analysis_primer.pdf.

Carpenter, T.E. (2001) Methods to investigate spatial and temporal clustering in veterinary epidemiology. *Preventive Veterinary Medicine* **48**, 303–20.

Chang, J., Jung, J., Lee, H., Chang, D., Yoon, J. & Choi, M. (2011) Computed tomographic evaluation of abdominal fat in minipigs. *Journal of Veterinary Science* **12**, 91–4.

Chatfield, C. (2003) *The Analysis of Time Series: An introduction*, 6th edn. Chapman & Hall/CRC Press, Boca Raton, FL.

Chatterjee, S. & Hadi, A.S. (2006) *Regression Analysis by Example*, 4th edn. John Wiley & Sons, Hoboken, NJ.

Chhetri, B.K., Perez, A.M. & Thurmond, M.C. (2010) Factors associated with spatial clustering of foot-and-mouth disease in Nepal. *Tropical Animal Health and Production* **42**, 1441–9.

Chiappe, A., Gonzalez, G., Fradinger, E., Iorio, G., Ferretti, J.L., Zanchetta, J. (1999) The influence of age and sex in serum osteocalcin levels in thoroughbred horses. *Archives of Physiology and Biochemistry* **107**, 50–4.

Childs, J.E., Robinson, L.E., Sadek, R., Madden, A., Miranda, M.E. & Miranda, N.L. (1998) Density estimates of rural dog populations and an assessment of marking methods during a rabies vaccination campaign in the Philippines. *Preventative Veterinary Medicine* **33**, 207–18.

Ciba-Geigy Ltd (1990) *Geigy Scientific Tables*, Vol. 2, 8th edn. Ciba-Geigy Ltd, Basel.

Clark, C.R., Petrie, L., Waldner, C. & Wendell, A. (2004) Characteristics of the bovine claw associated with the presence of vertical fissures (sandcracks). *Canadian Veterinary Journal* **45**, 585–93.

Clegg, S.M., Kelly, J.F., Kimura, M. & Smith, T.B. (2003) Combining genetic markers and stable isotopes to reveal population connectivity and migration patterns in a neotropical migrant, Wilson's warbler (*Wilsonia pusilla*). *Molecular Ecology* **12**, 819–30.

Cochran, W.G. & Cox, G.M. (1957) *Experimental Designs*, 2nd edn. Wiley, New York.

Cockcroft, P. & Holmes, M. (2003) *Handbook of Evidence-based Veterinary Medicine*. Blackwell Publishing, Oxford.

Cohen, J. (1960) A coefficient of agreement for nominal scales. *Educational and Psychological Measurement* **20**, 37–46.

Cohen, J. (1968) Weighted kappa: nominal scale agreement with provision for scale disagreement or partial credit. *Psychological Bulletin* **70**, 213–20.

Cohen, J. (1988) *Statistical Power Analysis for the Behavioral Sciences*, 2nd edn. Laurence Erlbaum Associates, Hillsdale, NJ.

Collet, D. (2003) *Modelling Survival Data in Medical Research*, 2nd edn. Chapman & Hall/CRC Press, Boca Raton, FL.

Corveleyn, S., Deprez, P., van der Weken, G., Baeyens, W. & Remon, J.P. (1996) Bioavailability of ketoprofen in horses after rectal administration. *Journal of Veterinary Pharmacology and Therapeutics* **19**, 359–63.

Coughlin, S.S., Trock, B., Criqui, M.H., Pickle, L.W., Browner, D. & Tefft, M.C. (1992) The logistic modeling of sensitivity, specificity, and predictive value of a diagnostic test. *Journal of Clinical Epidemiology* **45**, 1–7.

Coyne, R., Hiney, M. & Smith, P. (1996) Transient presence of oxytetracycline in blue mussels (*Mytilus edulis*) following its therapeutic use at a marine Atlantic salmon farm. *Aquaculture* **149**, 175–81.

Dahlberg, G. (1926) *Twin Births and Twins from a Hereditary Point of View*. University Press, Stockholm.

Diggle, P.J. (1990) *Time Series – A biostatistical introduction*. Clarendon Press, Oxford.

Diggle, P.J., Heagerty, P., Liang, K.L. & Zeger, S. (2002) *Analysis of Longitudinal Data*, 2nd edn. Oxford University Press, Oxford.

Dohoo, I., Martin, W. & Stryhn, H. (2010) *Veterinary Epidemiologic Research*, 2nd edn. AVC Inc., Charlottetown, Prince Edward Island, Canada.

Dolan, K. (1999) *Ethics, Animals and Science*. Blackwell Science, Oxford.

Dolan, K. (2000) *Laboratory Animal Law*. Blackwell Science, Oxford.

Donald, P.F. & Evans, A.D. (1995) Habitat selection and population size of Corn Buntings *Milaria calandra* breeding in Britain in 1993. *Bird Study* **42**, 190–204.

Doncaster, C.P. & Davey, A.J.H. (1997) *Analysis of Variance and Covariance: How to choose and construct models for the life sciences*. Cambridge University Press, Cambridge.

Donner, A. (1987) Statistical methodology for paired cluster designs. *American Journal of Epidemiology* **126**, 972–9.

Donner, A., Birkett, N. & Buck, C. (1981) Randomisation by cluster: samples size requirements and analysis. *American Journal of Epidemiology* **114**, 906–14.

Draper, N.R. & Smith, H. (1998) *Applied Regression Analysis*, 3rd edn. Wiley Series in Probability and Statistics. John Wiley & Sons, New York.

Drew, S.B. & Peters, A.R. (1994) Effect of buserelin on pregnancy rates in dairy cows. *Veterinary Record* **134**, 267–9.

Duchateau, L. & Janssen, P. (2010) *The Frailty Model*. Statistics for Biology and Health. Springer, New York.

Dufour, B. & Hendrikx, P. (2009) *Epidemiological Surveillance in Animal Health*, 2nd edn. CIRAD, FAO, OIE and AEEMA.

Dugard, P., Todman, J. & Staines, H. (2010) *Approaching Multivariate Analysis: A practical introduction*. Routledge, Hove, UK and New York.

Egger, M., Davey Smith, G. & Altman, D.G. (eds) (2001) *Systematic Reviews in Health Care: Meta-analysis in context*, 2nd edn. BMJ Publishing Group, London.

Eizaguirre, I., Urkia, N.G., Asensio, A.B., Zubillaga, I., Zubillaga, D., Vidales, C., Garcia-Arenzana, J.M. & Aldazabal, P. (2002) Probiotic supplementation reduces the risk of bacterial translocation in experimental short bowel syndrome. *Journal of Paediatric Surgery* **37**, 699–702.

Elliott, J., Rawlings, J.M., Markwell, P.J. & Barber, P.J. (2000) Survival of cats with naturally occurring chronic renal failure: effect of dietary management. *Journal of Small Animal Practice* **41**, 235–42.

Engels, J.M. & Diehr, P. (2003) Imputation of missing longitudinal data: a comparison of methods. *Journal of Clinical Epidemiology* **56**, 968–76.

England, G.C.W. (1992) *The cryopreservation of dog semen*. Fellowship thesis, Royal College of Veterinary Surgeons, London.

Enoe, C., Georgiadis, M.P. & Johnson, W.O. (2000) Estimation of sensitivity and specificity of diagnostic tests and disease prevalence when the true disease state is unknown *Preventive Veterinary Medicine* **45**, 61–81.

Escudero, E., Carceles, M.S., Diaz, M.S., Sutra, J.F., Galtier, P. & Alvinerie, M. (1999) Pharmacokinetics of moxidectin and doramectin in goats. *Research in Veterinary Science* **67**, 177–81.

Everitt, B.S. (1995) The analysis of repeated measures: a practical review with examples. *The Statistician* **44**, 113–35.

Everitt, B.S. & Dunn, G. (2001) *Applied Multivariate Data Analysis*, 2nd edn. Arnold Publishers, London.

Fagan, T.J. (1975) Nomogram for Bayes theorem [Letter]. *New England Journal of Medicine* **293**, 257.

Falconer, D.S. & Mackay, T.F.C. (1995) *Introduction to Quantitative Genetics*, 4th edn. Longman, Edinburgh.

Fasce, L., Tosca, M.A., Silvestri, M., Olcese, R., Pistorio, A. & Rossi, G.A. (2005) 'Early' cat ownership and the risk of sensitization and allergic rhinitis in Ligurian children with respiratory symptoms. *Annals of Allergy, Asthma and Immunology* **94**, 561–5.

Fisher, L.D. & Lin, D.Y. (1999) Time-dependent covariates in the Cox proportional-hazards regression model. *Annual Review of Public Health* **20**, 145–57.

Fisher, R.A. (1925) *Statistical Methods for Research Workers*. Oliver & Boyd, Edinburgh.

Fleiss, J.L. (1986) *The Design and Analysis of Clinical Experiments*. John Wiley & Sons, Hoboken, NJ (published online 2011).

Fleiss, J.L., Levin, B. & Paik, M.C. (2003) *Statistical Methods for Rates and Proportions*, 3rd edn. John Wiley & Sons, Hoboken, NJ.

Food and Drug Administration (1992) *Statistical Procedures for Bioequivalence Studies using Standard Two-treatment Crossover Design*. US Department of Health and Human Services, Public Health Service, US Food and Drug Administration, Rockville, MD.

Freemantle, N., Mason, J. & Eccles, M. (1999) Deriving treatment recommendations from evidence from randomized trials. The role and limitation of meta-analysis. *International Journal of Technology Assessment in Health Care* **15**, 304–15.

Gardiner, W.P. & Gettinby, G. (1998) *Experimental Design Techniques in Statistical Practice*. Horwood Publishing, Chichester, UK.

Gart, J.J. & Buck, A.A. (1996) Comparison of a screening test and a reference test in epidemiological studies II. A probabilistic model for the comparison of diagnostic tests *American Journal of Epidemiology* **83**, 593–602.

Geffré, A., Concordet, D., Braun, J. & Trumel, C. (2011) Reference Value Advisor: a new freeware set of macroinstructions to calculate reference intervals with Microsoft Excel. *Veterinary Clinical Pathology* **40**, 107–12. www.biostat.envt.fr/spip/spip.php?article63.

Gelman, A., Carlin, J.B., Stern, H.S., Rubin, D.B. & Dunson, D.B. (2013) *Bayesian Data Analysis*, 3rd edn. CRC Texts in Statistical Science. Chapman & Hall, London.

Gloster, J., Champion, H.J., Mansley, L.M., Romero, P., Brough, T. & Ramirez, A. (2005) The 2001 epidemic of foot-and-mouth disease in the United Kingdom: epidemiological and meteorological case studies. *Veterinary Record* **156**, 793–803.

Gloster, J., Jones, A., Redington, A., Burgin, L., Sørensen, J.H., Turner, R., Dillon, M., Hullinger, P., Simpson, M., Astrup, P., Garner, G., Stewart, P., D'Amours, R., Sellers, R. & Paton, D. (2010) Airborne spread of foot-and-mouth disease-model inter-comparison. *Veterinary Journal* **183**, 278–86.

Gomez-Puerta, L.A., Gavidia, C., Lopez-Urbina, M.T., Garcia, H.H. & Gonzalez, A.E. (2012) Efficacy of a oxfendazole against *Fasciola hepatica* in naturally infected sheep. *American Journal of Tropical Medicine and Hygiene* **86**, 486–8.

Graubard, B.I. & Korn, E.L. (1994) Regression analysis with clustered data. *Statistics in Medicine* **13**, 509–22.

Green, J.A., Butler, P.J., Woakes, A.J., Boyd, I.L. & Holder, R.L. (2001). Heart rate and rate of oxygen consumption of exercising Macaroni penguins. *Journal of Experimental Biology* **204**, 673–84.

Greenwood, J.J.D. & Robinson, R.A. (2006) General census methods. In: *Ecological Census Techniques. A handbook*, 2nd edn (ed. W.J. Sutherland), pp. 89–185. Cambridge University Press, Cambridge.

Greiner, M., Pfeiffer, D. & Smith, R.D. (2000) Principles and practical application of the receiver-operating characteristic analysis for diagnostic tests. *Preventive Veterinary Medicine* **45**, 43–59.

Gunning, R.F. & Walters, R.J.W. (1994) 'Flying scapulas', a post turnout myopathy in cattle. *Veterinary Record* **135**, 433–4.

Guo, S.Y. & Fraser, M.W. (2010) *Propensity Score Analysis: Statistical methods and applications*. Advanced Quantitative Techniques in the Social Sciences. Sage Publications, Thousand Oaks, CA.

Haber, M., Logini, I.M. & Halloran, M.E. (1991) Measures of the effects of vaccination in a randomly mixing population. *International Journal of Epidemiology* **20**, 300–10.

Hackshaw, A. (2009) *A Concise Guide to Clinical Trials*. Wiley-Blackwell, Chichester, UK.

Halloran, M.E. & Struchiner, C.J. (1991) Study designs for dependent happenings. *Epidemiology* **2**, 331–8.

Hawkins, T., Gala, R.R. & Dunbar, J.C. (1993) The effect of neonatal sex hormone manipulation on the incidence of diabetes in non-obese diabetic mice. *Proceedings of the Society for Experimental Biology and Medicine* **202**, 201–5.

Higgins, J.P.T., Thompson, S.G., Deeks, J.J & Altman, D.G. (2003) Measuring inconsistency in meta-analysis. *British Medical Journal* **327**, 556–60.

Hilbe, J.M. (2009) *Logistic Regression Models*. Chapman & Hall/CRC Press, Boca Raton, FL.

Hiraga, A., Kai, A., Kubo, K. & Sugano, S. (1997) Effects of low intensity exercise during the breaking period on cardiopulmonary function in Thoroughbred yearlings. *Journal of Equine Science* **8**, 21–4.

Hirsch, A.C., Philipp, H. & Kleemann, R. (2003) Investigation on the efficacy of meloxicam in sows with mastitis–metritis–agalactia syndrome. *Journal of Veterinary Pharmacology and Therapeutics* **26**, 355–60.

Hoeben, D., Mitjen, P. & de Kruif, A. (1997) Factors influencing complications during Caesarean section on the standing cow. *Veterinary Quarterly* **19**, 88–92.

Holdo, R.M., Holt, R.D. & Fryxell, J.M. (2009) Opposing rainfall and plant nutritional gradients best explain the wildebeest migration in the Serengeti. *American Naturalist* **173**, 431–45.

Hseih, F.Y. (1988) Sample size formulae for intervention studies with the cluster as unit of randomisation. *Statistics in Medicine* **8**, 1195–201.

Jackson, B., Eastell, R., Russell, R.G.G., Lanyon, L.E. & Price, J.S. (1996) Measurement of bone specific alkaline phosphatase in the horse: a comparison of two techniques. *Research in Veterinary Science* **61**, 160–4.

Jain, N.C., Vegad, J.L., Jain, N.K. & Shrivastava, A.B. (1982) Haematological studies on normal lactating Indian buffaloes. *Research in Veterinary Science* **32**, 52–6.

Jakovljevic, S. & Gibbs, C. (1993) Radiographic assessment of gastric mucosal fold thickness in dogs. *American Journal of Veterinary Research* **54**, 1827–30.

Jekel, J.F., Elmore, J.G. & Katz, D.L. (1996) *Epidemiology, Biostatistics and Preventive Medicine*. Saunders, Philadelphia.

Jones, B., Jarvis, J.A. & Ebbutt, A.F. (1966) Trials to assess equivalence: the importance of rigorous methods. *British Medical Journal* **313**, 36–9.

Julius, S.A. (2003) Tutorial in biostatistics: sample sizes for clinical trials with Normal data. *Statistics in Medicine* **23**, 1921–86.

Kalton, G. (1983) *Introduction to Survey Sampling*. Quantitative Applications in the Social Sciences. Sage Publications, Newbury Park, CA.

Kerry, S.M. & Bland, J.M. (1998) Sample size in cluster randomisation. *British Medical Journal* **316**, 549.

Kilkenny, C., Browne, W.J., Cuthill, I.C., Emerson, M. & Altman, D.G. (2010) Improving bioscience research reporting: the ARRIVE guidelines for reporting animal research. *PLoS Biology* **8** (6), e1000412.

Kilkenny, C., Parsons, N., Kadyszewski, E. *et al.* (2009) Survey of the quality of experimental design, statistical analysis and reporting of research using animals. *PLoS ONE* **4** (11), e7824. doi:10.1371/journal.pone.0007824.

Kirkwood, B.R. & Sterne, J.A.C. (2003) *Essential Medical Statistics*, 2nd edn. Blackwell Science, Oxford.

Klaas, I.C., Enevoldsen, C., Ersbøll, A.K. & Tölle, U. (2005) Cow-related risk factors for milk leakage. *Journal of Dairy Science* **88**, 128–36.

Kleinbaum, D.G. & Klein, M. (2005) *Survival Analysis: A self-learning text*. Statistics for Biology and Health. Springer, New York.

Kleinbaum, D.G. & Klein, M. (2010) *Logistic Regression: A self-learning text*, 3rd edn. Statistics for Biology and Health. Springer, New York.

Kleinbaum, D.G., Kupper, L.L., Nizam, A. & Muller, K.E. (2008) *Applied Regression Analysis and Multivariable Methods*, 4th edn. Duxbury, Pacific Grove, CA.

Ko, J.C., Nicklin, C.F., Heaton-Jones, T.G. & Kuo, W.C. (1998) Comparison of sedative and cardiorespiratory effects of diazepam, acepromazine, and xylazine in ferrets. *Journal of the American Animal Hospital Association* **34**, 234–41.

Krampe, A. and Kuhnt, S. (2007) Bowker's test for symmetry and modifications within the algebraic framework. *Computational Statistics and Data Analysis* **51**, 4124–42.

Krzanowski, W. (2000) *Principles of Multivariate Analysis: A user's perspective*. Oxford University Press, Oxford.

Kulkarni, D.D., Bhikane, A.U., Shaila, M.S., Varalakshmi, P., Apte, M.P. & Narladkar, B.W. (1996) Peste des petits ruminants in goats in India. *Veterinary Record* **138**, 187–8.

Laird, N.M. & Lange, C. (2011) *The Fundamentals of Modern Statistical Genetics*. Statistics for Biology and Health. Springer, New York.

Lajili, H., Humblot, P. & Thibier, M. (1991) Effect of PGF2 alpha treatment on conception rates of dairy cows treated with a GnRH agonist 12 to 14 days after artificial insemination. *Theriogenology* **36**, 335–47.

Landis, J.R. & Koch, G.C. (1977) The measurement of observer agreement for categorical data. *Biometrics* **33**, 159–74.

Lesaffre, E. (2008) Superiority, equivalence, and non-inferiority trials. *Bulletin of the New York University Hospital for Joint Disease* **66**, 150–4.

Levy, P.S. & Lemeshow, S. (2011) *Sampling of Populations: Methods and applications*, 4th edn. John Wiley & Sons, Hoboken, NJ.

Ley, S.J., Waterman, A.E. & Livingston, A. (1995) A field study of the effect of lameness on mechanical nociceptive thresholds in sheep. *Veterinary Record* **137**, 85–7.

Liberati, A., Altman, D.G., Tetzlaff, J. *et al.* and the PRISMA Group (2009) The PRISMA statement for reporting systematic reviews and meta-analyses of studies that evaluate health care interventions: explanation and elaboration. *PLoS Medicine* **6**, e1000100. doi:10.1371/journal.pmed. 1000100.

Lin, L.I-K. (1989) A concordance correlation coefficient to evaluate reproducibility, *Biometrics* **45**, 255–68.

Lin, L.I-K. (2000) A note on the concordance correlation coefficient. *Biometrics* **56**, 324–5.

Lin, L., Hedayat, A.S. & Wu, W. (2012) *Statistical Tools for Measuring Agreement*. Springer, Berlin.

Little, R.J.A. & Rubin, D.B. (2002) *Statistical Analysis with Missing Data*. John Wiley & Sons, Chichester, UK.

Little, T.W.A., Richards, M.S., Hussaini, S.N. & Jones, T.D. (1980) The significance of Leptospiral antibodies in calving and aborting cattle in south west England. *Veterinary Record* **106**, 221–4.

Lloyd, R.D., Bruenger, F.W., Angus, W., Taylor, G.N. & Miller, S.C. (1995) Mammary tumor occurrence in beagles given 239PU. *Health Physics* **69**, 385–90.

Lori, J.C., Stein, T.J. & Thamm, D.H. (2010) Doxorubicin and cyclophosphamide for the treatment of canine lymphoma: a randomized, placebo-controlled study. *Veterinary Comparative Oncology* **8** (3), 188–95.

Louis, T.A. (1991) Using empirical Bayes methods in biopharmaceutical research. *Statistics in Medicine* **10**, 811–29.

Lukacs, N.W., McCorkle, F.M. & Taylor, R.L. (1987) Monoamines suppress the phytohemagglutinin wattle response in chickens. *Developmental and Comparative Immunology* **11**, 759–68.

Lunn, D.J., Thomas, A., Best, N. & Spiegelhalter, D. (2000) WinBUGS – a Bayesian modelling framework: concepts, structure, and extensibility. *Statistics and Computing* **10**, 325–37.

Machin, D. & Campbell, M.J. (2005) *The Design of Studies for Medical Research*. John Wiley & Sons, Chichester, UK.

Machin, D., Campbell, M.J., Tan, S.B. & Tan, S.H. (2009) *Sample Size Tables for Clinical Studies*, 3rd edn. John Wiley & Sons, Chichester, UK.

Machin, D. & Cheung, Y.B. (2006) *Survival Analysis: A practical approach*. John Wiley & Sons, Chichester, UK.

Machin, D., Day, S. & Green, S.B. (eds) (2006) *Textbook of Clinical Trials*, 2nd edn. John Wiley & Sons, Chichester, UK.

Machin, D. & Fayers, P.M. (2010) *Randomized Clinical Trials: Design, practice and reporting*. Wiley-Blackwell, Chichester, UK.

Mandelbrot, B.B. (1967) How long is the coast of Britain? Statistical self-similarity and fractional dimension. *Science* **156**, 636–8.

Manly, B.F.J. (2007) *Randomisation, Bootstrap and Monte Carlo Methods in Biology*, 3rd edn. Chapman & Hall/CRC Press, Boca Raton, FL.

Marr, C.M. (2003) Defining the clinically relevant questions that lead to the best evidence: what is evidence-based medicine? *Equine Veterinary Journal* **35**, 333–6.

Martin, G.S., Strand, E. & Kearney, M.T. (1996) Use of statistical models to evaluate racing performance in Thoroughbreds. *Journal of the American Veterinary Medical Association* **209**, 1900–6.

Matthews, J.N.S. (2006) *An Introduction to Randomized Controlled Clinical Trials*, 2nd edn. Chapman & Hall/CRC Press, Boca Raton, FL.

McBride, G.B. (2005) A proposal for strength-of-agreement criteria for Lin's concordance correlation coefficient. *NIWA Client Report* HAM2005-062. http://www.medcalc. org/download/pdf/McBride2005.pdf.

McCoy, M.A., Goodall, E.A. & Kennedy, D.G. (1996) Incidence of bovine hypomagnesaemia in Northern Ireland and methods of magnesium supplementation. *Veterinary Record* **138**, 41–3.

Menard, S. (2001) *Applied Logistic Regression Analysis*, 2nd edn. Sage University Paper Series on Quantitative Applications in the Social Sciences No. 07-106. Sage University Press, Thousand Oaks, CA.

Mendenhall, W., Ott, L. & Scheaffer, R.L. (1971) *Elementary Survey Sampling*. Wadsworth, Belmont, PA.

Merrell, B. (1998) Improving lamb survival on hill and upland farms. *SVS Congress Veterinary Times* (Peterborough), pp. 6–7.

Mirowsky, J. & Ross, C.E. (2002) Depression, parenthood, and age at first birth. *Social Science and Medicine* **54**, 1281–98.

Moher, D., Cook, D.J., Eastwood, S. *et al.* for the QUOROM group (1999) Improving the quality of reporting of meta-analysis of randomized controlled trials: the QUOROM Statement. *Lancet* **354**, 1896–900.

Moher, D., Liberati, A., Tetzlaff, J., Altman, D.G. and the PRISMA Group (2009) Preferred reporting items for systematic reviews and meta-analyses: the PRISMA Statement. *PLoS Medicine* **6** (6), e1000097. doi:10.1371/journal. pmed1000097.

Montgomery, D.C., Jennings, C.L. & Kulahci, M. (2008) *Introduction to Time Series Analysis and Forecasting*, John Wiley & Sons, New York.

More, S.J. (2010) Improving the quality of reporting in veterinary journals: how far do we need to go with reporting guidelines? *Veterinary Journal* **184**, 249–50.

Muir, M., Stannett, A., Offer, J.E., Ball, P.J.H., Taylor, C. & Logue, D.N. (1998) Oestrus synchronisation combined with buserelin administration in beef cattle. *Veterinary Record* **143**, 143–4.

Muma, J.B., Samui, K.L., Oloya, J., Munyeme, M. & Skjerve, E. (2007) Risk factors for brucellosis in indigenous cattle reared in livestock-wildlife interface areas of Zambia. *Preventive Veterinary Medicine* **80**, 306–17.

Myers, W.L., Chang W.Y., Germaine, S.S., Van der Haegen, W.M. & Owens, T.E.. (2008) *An Analysis of Deer and Elk–Vehicle Collision Sites along State Highways in Washington State*. Completion Report. Washington Department of Fish and Wildlife, Olympia, WA.

Nanda, A.S., Dodson, H. & Ward, W.R. (1990) Relationship between an increase in plasma cortisol during transport-induced stress and failure of oestradiol to induce a luteinising hormone surge in dairy cows. *Research in Veterinary Science* **49**, 25–8.

Nelson, R.W., Duesberg, C.A., Ford, S.L., Feldman, E.C., Davenport, D.J., Kiernan, C. & Neal, L. (1998) Effect of dietary insoluble fibre on control of glycemia in dogs with naturally acquired diabetes mellitus. *Journal of the American Veterinary Medical Association* **212**, 380–6.

Newton, J.R., Hedderson, E.J., Adams, V.J., McGorum, B.C., Proudman, C.J. & Wood, J.L.N. (2004) An epidemiological study of risk factors associated with the recurrence of equine grass sickness (dysautonomia) on previously affected premises. *Equine Veterinary Journal* **36**, 105–12.

Nicholas, F.W. (2010) *Introduction to Veterinary Genetics*, 3rd edn. Wiley-Blackwell, Oxford.

O'Connor, A.M., Sargeant, J.M., Gardner, I.A. *et al.* (2010) The REFLECT Statement: methods and processes of creating reporting guidelines for randomized controlled trials for livestock and food safety. *Preventive Veterinary Medicine* **93**, 11–18.

Olsen, S.F., Martuzzi, M. & Elliott, P. (1996) Cluster analysis and disease mapping – why, when, and how? A step by step guide. *British Medical Journal* **313**, 863–6.

Overton, M.W., Sischo, W.M. & Reynolds, J.P. (2003) Evaluation of effect of estradiol cypionate administered prophylactically to post-parturient dairy cows at high risk for metritis. *Journal of the American Veterinary Medical Association* **223**, 846–51.

Parker, B.N.J., Foulkes, J.A., Jones, P.C., Dexter, I. & Stephens, H. (1988) Prediction of calving times from plasma progesterone concentration. *Veterinary Record* **122**, 88–9.

Pearson, E.S. & Hartley, H.O. (1966) *Biometrika Tables for Statisticians*, 3rd edn. Cambridge University Press, Cambridge.

Pearson, R.A. & Ouassat, M. (1996) Estimation of the liveweight and body condition of working donkeys in Morocco. *Veterinary Record* **138**, 229–33.

Peres, C.A. (1999) General guidelines for standardizing line-transect surveys of tropical forest primates. *Neotropical Primates* **7**, 11–16.

Peters, A.R., Martinez, T.A. & Cook, A.J. (2000) A meta-analysis of studies of the effect of GnRH 11–14 days after insemination on pregnancy rates in cattle. *Theriogenology* **54**, 1317–26.

Petrie, A. & Sabin, C. (2009) *Medical Statistics at a Glance*, 3rd edn. Wiley-Blackwell, Oxford.

Petrie, A. & Sabin, C. (2013) *Medical Statistics at a Glance Workbook*. Wiley-Blackwell, Oxford.

Pfeiffer, D.U. (2009) Analysis of spatial data. In: *Veterinary Epidemiological Research*, 2nd edn (eds I.R. Dohoo, W. Martin & H. Stryhn), pp. 679–713. AVC Inc., Charlottetown, Prince Edward Island, Canada.

Pfeiffer, D.U., Robinson, T.P., Stevenson, M., Stevens, K.M., Rogers, D.J. & Clements, A.C.A. (2008) *Spatial Analysis in Epidemiology*. Oxford University Press, Oxford.

Pocock, S.J. (1983) *Clinical Trials: A practical approach*. John Wiley & Sons, Chichester, UK.

Putter, H., Fiocco, M., Geskus, R.B. (2007) Tutorial in biostatistics: competing risks and multi-state models. *Statistics in Medicine* **26**, 2389–430.

Rabe-Hesketh, S. & Skrondal, A. (2012) *Multilevel and Longitudinal Modeling using Stata*, 3rd edn. Stata Press, College Station, TX.

Rajkhowa, S., Rahman, H., Rajkhowa, C. & Bujarbaruah, K.M. (2005) Seroprevalence of brucellosis in mithuns (*Bos frontalis*) in India. *Preventive Veterinary Medicine* **69**, 145–51.

Ramirez-Barrios, R.A., Barboza-Mena, G., Munoz, J., Angulo-Cubillan, F., Hernandez E., Gonzales, F. & Escalona, F. (2004) Prevalence of intestinal parasites in dogs under veterinary care in Maracaibo, Venezuela. *Veterinary Parasitology* **121**, 11–20.

Raudenbush, S.W. & Bryk, A.S. (2002) *Hierarchical Linear Models: Applications and data analysis Methods*, 2nd edn. Sage Publications: Thousand Oaks, CA.

Rettmer, I., Stevenson, J.S. & Corah, L.R. (1992) Pregnancy rates in beef cattle after administering a GnRH agonist 11 to 14 days after insemination. *Journal of Animal Science* **70**, 7–12.

Rinaldi, L., Musella, V., Biggeri, A. & Cringoli, G. (2006) New insights into the application of geographical information systems and remote sensing in veterinary parasitology. *Geospatial Health* **1**, 33–47.

Ripley, B.D. (2004) *Spatial Statistics*. Wiley Series in Probability and Statistics. John Wiley & Sons, Hoboken, NJ.

Russell, W. & Birch, R. (1959) *The Principles of Humane Experimental Technique*. Methuen, London.

Sackett, D. (1996) *Evidence-based Medicine – What It Is and What It Isn't*. www.cebm.net/ebm_is_isnt.asp.

Sainsbury, D. (1998) *Animal Health*, 2nd edn. Wiley-Blackwell, Oxford.

Salman, M.D. (ed.) (2003) *Animal Disease Surveillance and Survey Systems: Methods and applications*. Iowa State Press, Ames, IA.

Saratsis, Ph., Schmidt-Adamopoulou, B., Ypsilantis, P., Brozos, Ch. & Demertzis, A. (1998) Effect of buserelin on corpus luteum activity and the fertility of dairy cows. *Bulletin of the Hellenic Veterinary Medical Society* **49**, 34–8.

Sargeant, J.M., O'Connor, A.M., Gardner, I.A. *et al.* (2010) The REFLECT Statement: reporting guidelines for randomized controlled trials in livestock and food safety: explanation and elaboration. *Journal of Food Protection* **73**, 579–603.

Saxton, A. (2004) *Genetic Analysis of Complex Traits using SAS*. SAS Institute Inc., Cary, NC.

Schimmer, B., Luttikholt, S., Hautvast, J.L.A., Graat, E.A.M., Vellema, P. & van Duynhoven, Y.T.H.P. (2011) Seroprevalence and risk factors of Q fever in goats on commercial dairy goat farms in the Netherlands, 2009–2010. *BMC Veterinary Research* **7**, 81. http://www.biomedcentral.com/1746-6148/7/81.

Schönmann, N.J., BonDurant, R.H., Gardner, I.A., Van Hoosear, K., Baltzer, W. & Kachulis, C. (1994) Comparison of sampling and culture methods for the diagnosis of *Tritrichomonas foetus* infection in bulls. *Veterinary Record* **134**, 620–2.

Schulz, K.F., Altman, D.G. & Moher, D. for the CONSORT Group (2010) CONSORT 2010 Statement: updated guidelines for reporting parallel group randomised trials. *PLoS Medicine* **7** (3), e1000251. doi:10.1371/journal.pmed.1000251.

Schwartz, D., Flamant, R. & Lellouch, J. (1980) *Clinical Trials.* Academic Press, London.

Senn, S. (2002) *Cross-over Trials in Clinical Research*, 2nd edn. Wiley, Chichester, UK.

Siegel, S. & Castellan, N.J. (1988) *Nonparametric Statistics for the Behavioral Sciences*, 2nd edn. McGraw-Hill, New York.

Simm, G. (2002) *Genetic Improvement of Cattle and Sheep*, 2nd edn. CABI Publishing, Wallingford, UK.

Singer, P. (2005) *Animal Liberation*, 2nd edn. Pimlico Books/Random House. London.

Sloet van Oldruitenborgh-Oosterbaan, M.M. & Barneveld, A. (1995) Comparison of the workload of Dutch warmblood horses ridden normally and on a treadmill. *Veterinary Record* **137**, 136–9.

Smith, P.J. (2002) *Analysis of Failure and Survival Data.* Chapman & Hall/CRC Press, Boca Raton, FL.

Smith, P.J., French, A.T., Van Israel, N. *et al.* (2005) Efficacy and safety of pimobendan in canine heart failure caused by myxomatous mitral valve disease. *Journal of Small Animal Practice* **46**, 121–30.

Snijders, T.A.B. & Bosker, R.J. (2012) *Multilevel Analysis: An introduction to basic and advanced multilevel modeling*, 2nd edn. Sage Publications, London.

Solter, P.F., Hoffman, W.E., Hungerford, L.L., Peterson, M.E. & Dorner, J.L. (1993) Assessment of corticosteroid-induced alkaline phosphatase isoenzyme as a screening test for hyperadrenocorticism in dogs. *Journal of the American Veterinary Medical Association* **203**, 534–8.

Sorensen, D. & Gianola, D. (2002) *Likelihood, Bayesian and MCMC Methods in Quantitative Genetics.* Springer, New York.

Southey, B.R., Rodriguez-Zas, S.L. & Leymaster, K.A. (2004) Competing risks analysis of lamb mortality in a terminal sire composite population. *Journal of Animal Science* **82**, 2892–9.

Southwood, T.R.E. (1966) *Ecological Methods.* Methuen, London.

Spiegelhalter, D., Abrams, K.R. & Myles, J.P. (2004) *Bayesian Approaches to Clinical Trials and Health-Care Evaluation.* John Wiley & Sons, Chichester, UK.

Sprent, P. & Smeeton, N.C. (2007) *Applied Nonparametric Statistical Methods*, 4th edn. Chapman & Hall/CRC Press, Boca Raton, FL.

Stevenson, J.S., Phatak, A.P., Rettmer, I. & Stewart, R.E. (1993) Postinsemination administration of Receptal: follicular dynamics, duration of cycle, hormonal responses, and pregnancy rates. *Journal of Dairy Science* **76**, 2536–47.

Stookey, G.K., Warrick, J.M. & Miller, L.L. (1995) Effects of sodium hexametaphosphate on dental calculus formation in dogs. *American Journal of Veterinary Research* **56**, 913–18.

Støvring, M., Moe, L. & Glattre, E. (1997) A population-based case–control study of canine mammary tumours and clinical use of medroxyprogesterone acetate. *APMIS* **105**, 590–6.

Straus, S., Richardson, W.S., Glasziou, P. & Haynes, R.B. (2011) *Evidence-based Medicine: How to practice and teach EBM*, 4th edn. Churchill Livingstone, London.

Stroup, D.F., Berlin, J.A., Morton, S.C. *et al.* (2000) Meta-analysis of observational studies in epidemiology: a proposal for reporting. *Journal of the American Medical Association* **283**, 2008–12.

Stürmer, T., Joshi, M., Glynn, R.J., Avorn, J., Rothman, K.J. & Schneeweiss, S. (2006) A review of the application of propensity score methods yielded increasing use, advantages in specific settings, but not substantially different estimates compared with conventional multivariable methods. *Journal of Clinical Epidemiology* **59**, 437–47.

Sutton, A., Abrams, K., Sheldon, T.A. & Song, F. (2000) *Methods for Meta-Analysis in Medical Research*. Wiley, New York.

Tamuli, M.K. & Watson, P.F. (1994) Cold resistance in the live acrosome-intact subpopulation of boar spermatozoa acquired during incubation after ejaculation. *Veterinary Record* **135**, 160–2.

Tanaka, T., Matsuo, T. & Ohtsuki, H. (1998) Aqueous vascular endothelial growth factor increases in anterior segment ischemia in rabbits. *Japanese Journal of Ophthalmology* **42**, 85–9.

Themudo, G.E., Østergaard, J. & Ersbøll, A.K. (2011) Persistent spatial clusters of plasmacytosis among Danish mink farms. *Preventive Veterinary Medicine* **102**, 75–82.

Thompson, W.L., White, G.C. & Gowan, C. (1998) *Monitoring Vertebrate Populations.* Academic Press, New York.

Thrusfield, M. (2005) *Veterinary Epidemiology*, 3rd edn. Blackwell Publishing, Oxford.

Unwin, D.J. (1996) GIS, spatial analysis and spatial statistics. *Progress in Human Geography* **20**, 540–51.

Vandenbroucke, J.P., von Elm, E., Altman, D.G. *et al.* (2007) STROBE Initiative. Strengthening the Reporting of Observational Studies in Epidemiology (STROBE): explanation and elaboration. *PLoS Medicine* **4** (10), e297. PMID 17941715.

von Elm, E., Altman, D.G., Egger, M., Pocock, S.J., Gøtzsche, P.C. & Vandenbroucke, J.P. (2008) STROBE Initiative. The strengthening the Reporting of Observational Studies in Epidemiology (STROBE) Statement: guidelines for reporting observational studies. *Journal of Clinical Epidemiology* **61**, 344–9. PMID: 18313558.

Warriss, P.D. & Edwards, J.E. (1995) Estimating the live weight of sheep from chest girth measurements. *Veterinary Record* **137**, 123–4.

Wasfi, I.A., Abdel Hadi, A.A., Elghazali, M. *et al.* (2000) Comparative disposition of tripelennamine in horses and camels after intravenous administration. *Journal of Veterinary Pharmacology and Therapeutics* **23**, 145–52.

Watson, P.F. (1979) An objective method for measuring fluorescence of individual sperm cells labelled with 1-anilinonaphthalene-8-sulphonate (ANS) by means of photomicrography and densitometry. *Journal of Microscopy* **117**, 425–9.

Watson, P.F. & Petrie, A. (2010) Method agreement analysis – a review of correct methodology. *Theriogenology* **73**, 1167–79.

Welch, R.D., Smith, P.H., Malone, J.B., Holmes, R.A. & Geaghan, J.P. (1987) Herd evaluation of *Fasciola hepatica* infection levels in Louisiana cattle by an enzyme-linked immunosorbent assay. *American Journal of Veterinary Research* **48**, 345–7.

Whitehead, A. (2002) *Meta-Analysis of Controlled Clinical Trials*. Wiley, Chichester, UK.

Whiting, P., Rutjes, A.W., Reitsma, J.B., Bossuyt, P.M. & Kleijnen, J. (2003) The development of QUADAS: a tool for the quality assessment of studies of diagnostic accuracy included in systematic reviews. *BMC Medical Research Methodology* **10**, 3–25.

WHO (World Health Organization) (2005) *International Health Regulations*, 2nd edn. WHO Press, Geneva.

Wilesmith, J.W., Ryan, J.B., Hueston, W.D. & Hoinville, L.J. (1992) Bovine spongiform encephalopathy: epidemiological features 1985 to 1990. *Veterinary Record* **130**, 90–4.

Wilesmith, J.W., Wells, G.A.H., Ryan, J.B.M., Gavier-Widen, D. & Simmons, M.M. (1997) A cohort study to examine maternally associated risk factors for bovine spongiform encephalopathy. *Veterinary Record* **141**, 239–43.

Wilson, E.B. (1927) Probable inference, the law of succession, and statistical inference. *Journal of the American Statistical Association* **22**, 209–12.

Witmer, G.W. (2005) Wildlife population monitoring: some practical considerations. *Wildlife Research* **32**, 259–63.

Xu, S., Yonash, N., Vallejo, R.L. & Cheng, H.H. (1998) Mapping quantitative trait loci for binary traits using a heterogeneous residual variance model: an application to Marek's disease susceptibility in chickens *Genetica* **104**, 171–8.

Yi, N. & Xu, S. (2000) Bayesian mapping of quantitative trait loci for complex binary traits. *Genetics* **155**, 1391–403.

Yousey-Hindes, K., Newman, A., Eidson, M., Rudd, R., Trimarchi, C. & Cherry, B. (2011) Rabid foxes, rabid raccoons, and the odds of a human bite exposure, New York State, 1999–2007. *Journal of Wildlife Diseases* **47**, 228–32.

Zolfaghari, G., Esmaili-Sari, A., Ghasempouri, S.M. & Kiabi, B.H. (2007) Examination of mercury concentration in the feathers of 18 species of birds in southwest Iran. *Environmental Research* **104**, 258–65.

Zweig, M.H. & Campbell G. (1993) Receiver-operating characteristic (ROC) plots: a fundamental evaluation tool in clinical medicine *Clinical Chemistry* **39**, 561–77.

Index

Statistics for Veterinary and Animal Science, Third Edition. Aviva Petrie and Paul Watson.
© 2013 John Wiley & Sons, Ltd. Published 2013 by John Wiley & Sons, Ltd.

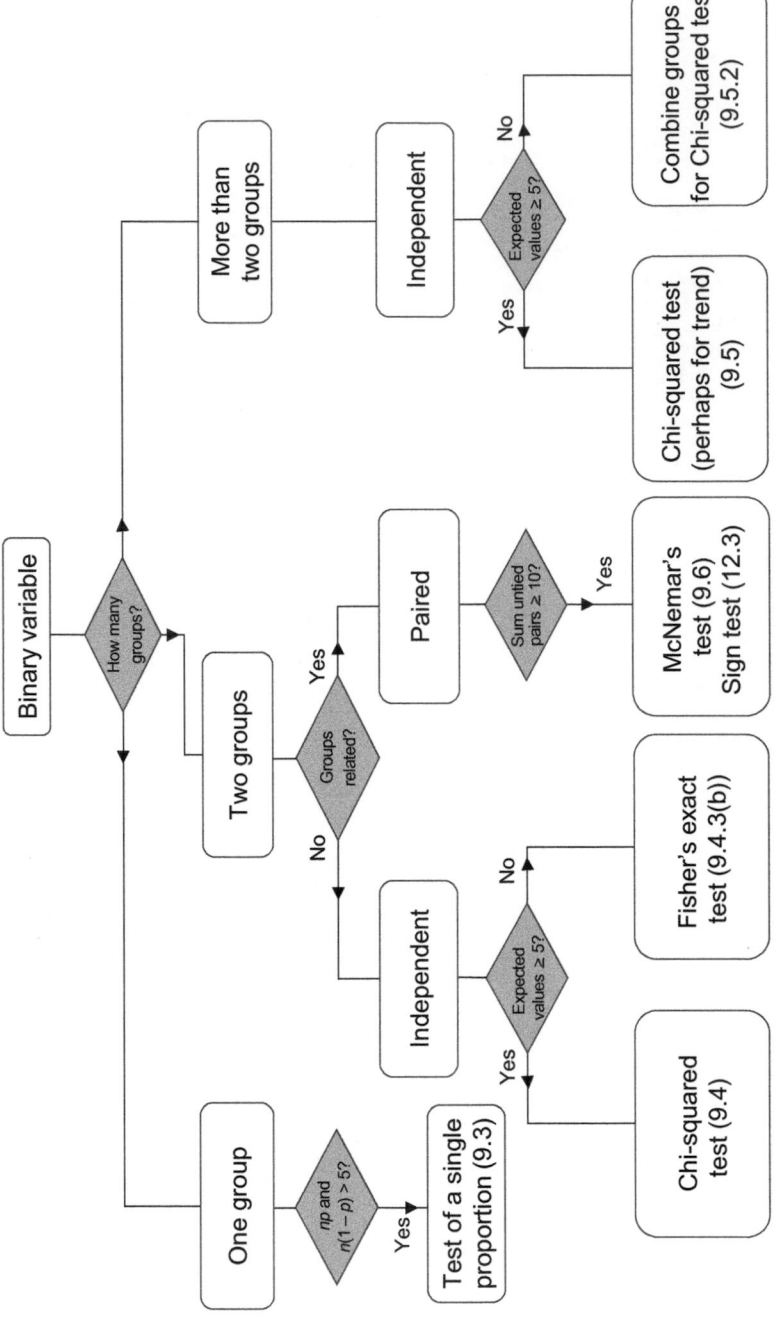

Figure E.2 Flowchart for choosing appropriate tests for proportions derived from a binary variable.

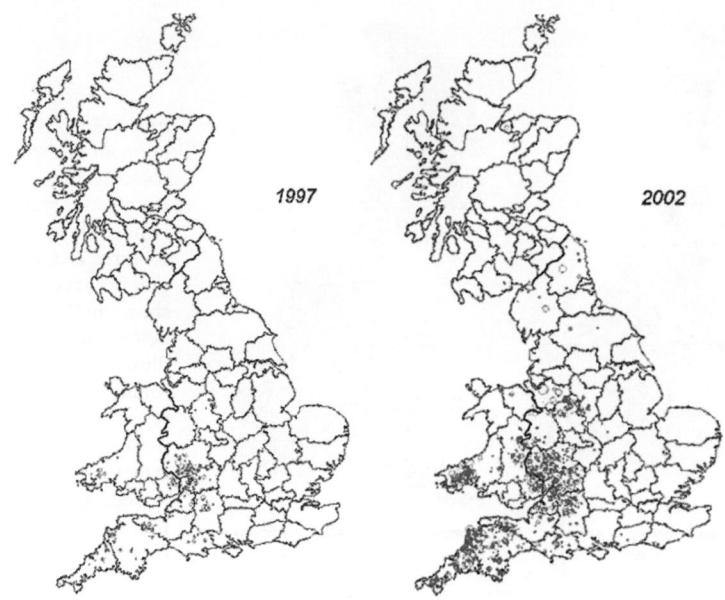

Plate 15.1 The change in bovine tuberculosis incidence in Great Britain between 1997 and 2002 (from http://www.scotland.gov.uk/Publications/2004/02/18855/32759, accessed 17 October 2012). Each map shows *confirmed* breakdown incidents commencing during a 12-month period. (A breakdown is defined as a herd with at least one animal with a positive TB skin test reaction.) The area enclosed by the circle is proportional to the number of skin test reactors in each breakdown. (Crown copyright. Contains public sector information licensed under the Open Government Licence v1.0.)

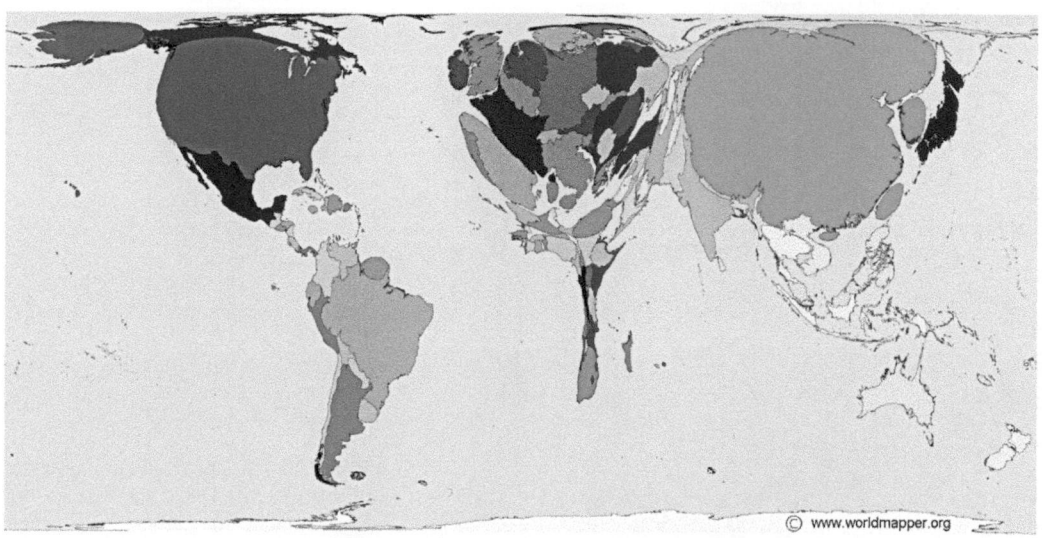

Plate 15.2 Cartogram of territory size showing the proportion of worldwide meat production per country (from http://www.worldmapper.org, accessed 17 October 2012, with permission. © SASI Group (University of Sheffield) and Mark Newman (University of Michigan)).

Statistics for Veterinary and Animal Science, Third Edition. Aviva Petrie and Paul Watson.
© 2013 John Wiley & Sons, Ltd. Published 2013 by John Wiley & Sons, Ltd.

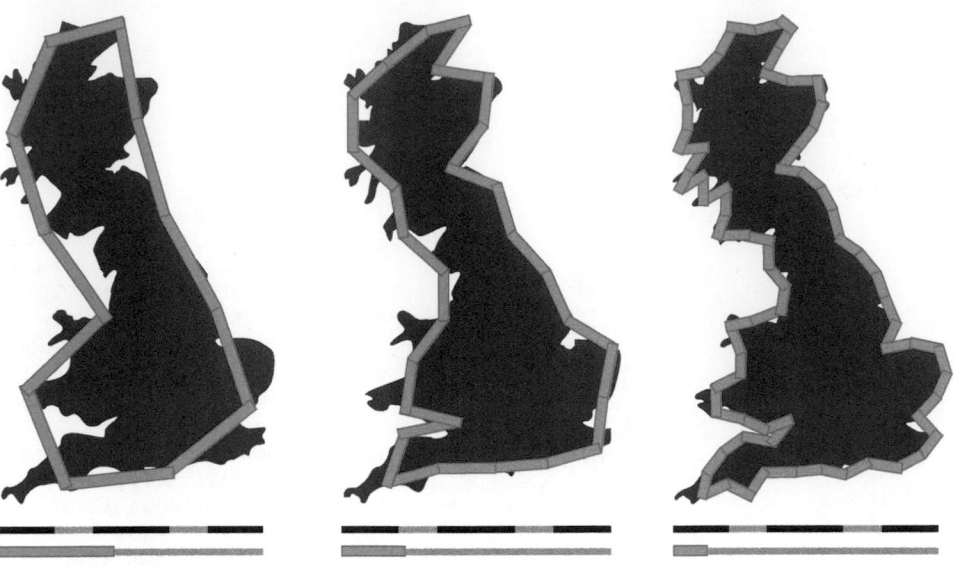

Plate 15.3 Measurement of the coastline of mainland Great Britain depending on three different unit distances shown in the bars below each illustration (from Mandelbrot, 1967, reprinted with permission from American Association for the Advancement of Science).

(a)

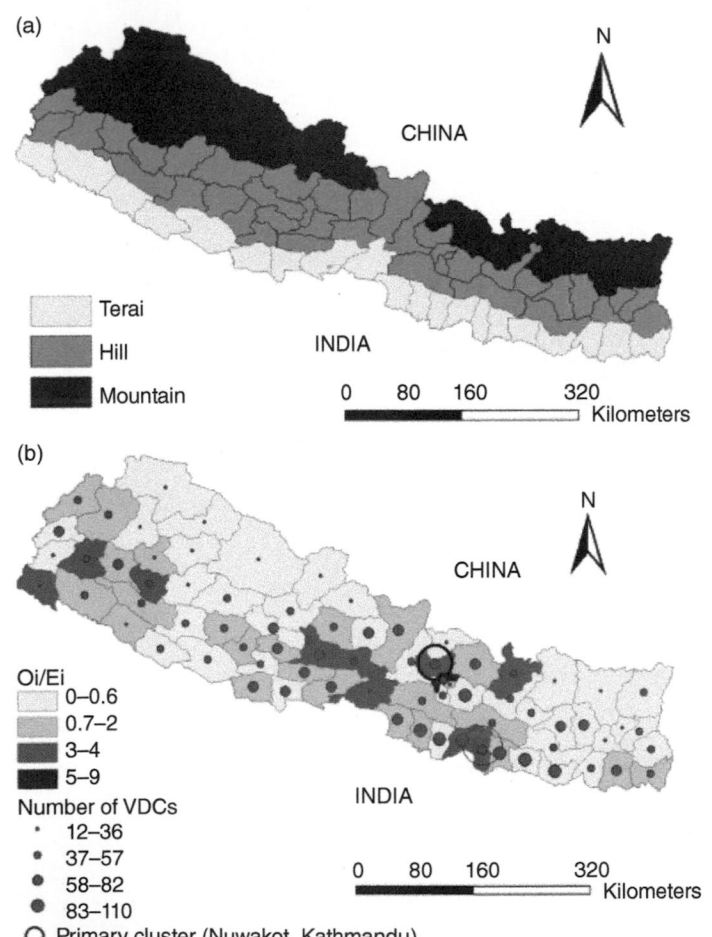

N

CHINA

Terai

Hill

Mountain

INDIA

0   80   160   320
                    Kilometers

(b)

N

CHINA

Oi/Ei
0–0.6
0.7–2
3–4
5–9

Number of VDCs
· 12–36
• 37–57
● 58–82
● 83–110
○ Primary cluster (Nuwakot, Kathmandu)
○ Secondary cluster (Mahottari, Saralahi)

INDIA

0   80   160   320
                    Kilometers

Plate 15.4 (a) The three ecogeographic regions of Nepal. (b) The total number of Village Development Committees (VDCs), and district-specific ratio of observed-to-expected foot-and-mouth-positive VDCs (Oi/Ei) for Nepal in 2004. The dark circle represents a primary spatial cluster (RR = 7.6) and the thin circle represents a secondary spatial cluster (RR = 2.7) of foot-and-mouth-positive VDCs identified using the spatial scan statistic (published under the Creative Commons Attribution License and reproduced with permission of the authors and the publisher, Springer).

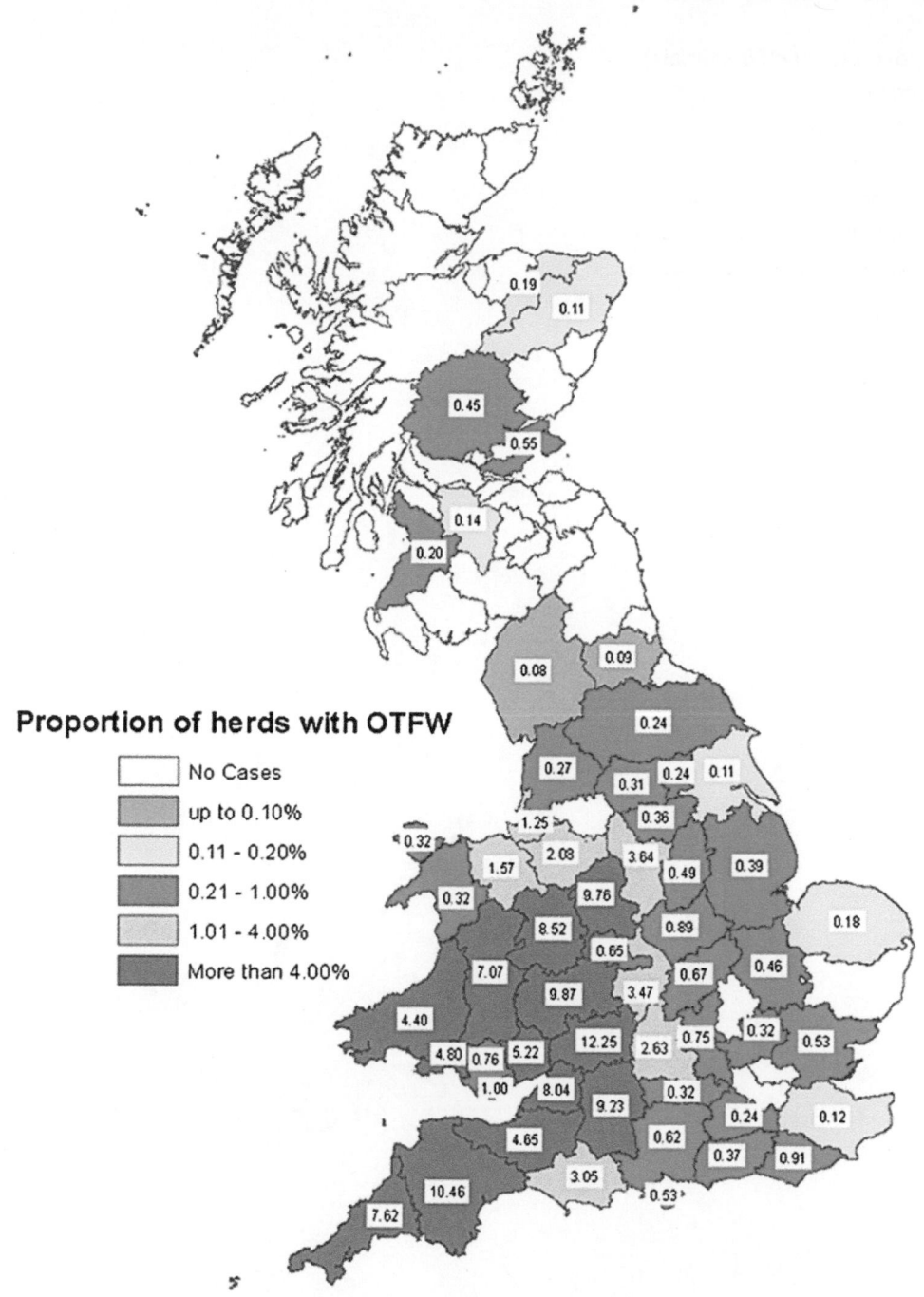

Plate 15.5 The proportions of herds (expressed as percentages) with official tuberculosis-free status withdrawn (OTFW) incidents by county between July 2009 and June 2010 (from http://archive.defra.gov.uk/foodfarm/farmanimal/diseases/atoz/tb/ documents/btb-surv-report.pdf, accessed 17 October 2012. Crown copyright. Contains public sector information licensed under the Open Government Licence v1.0).

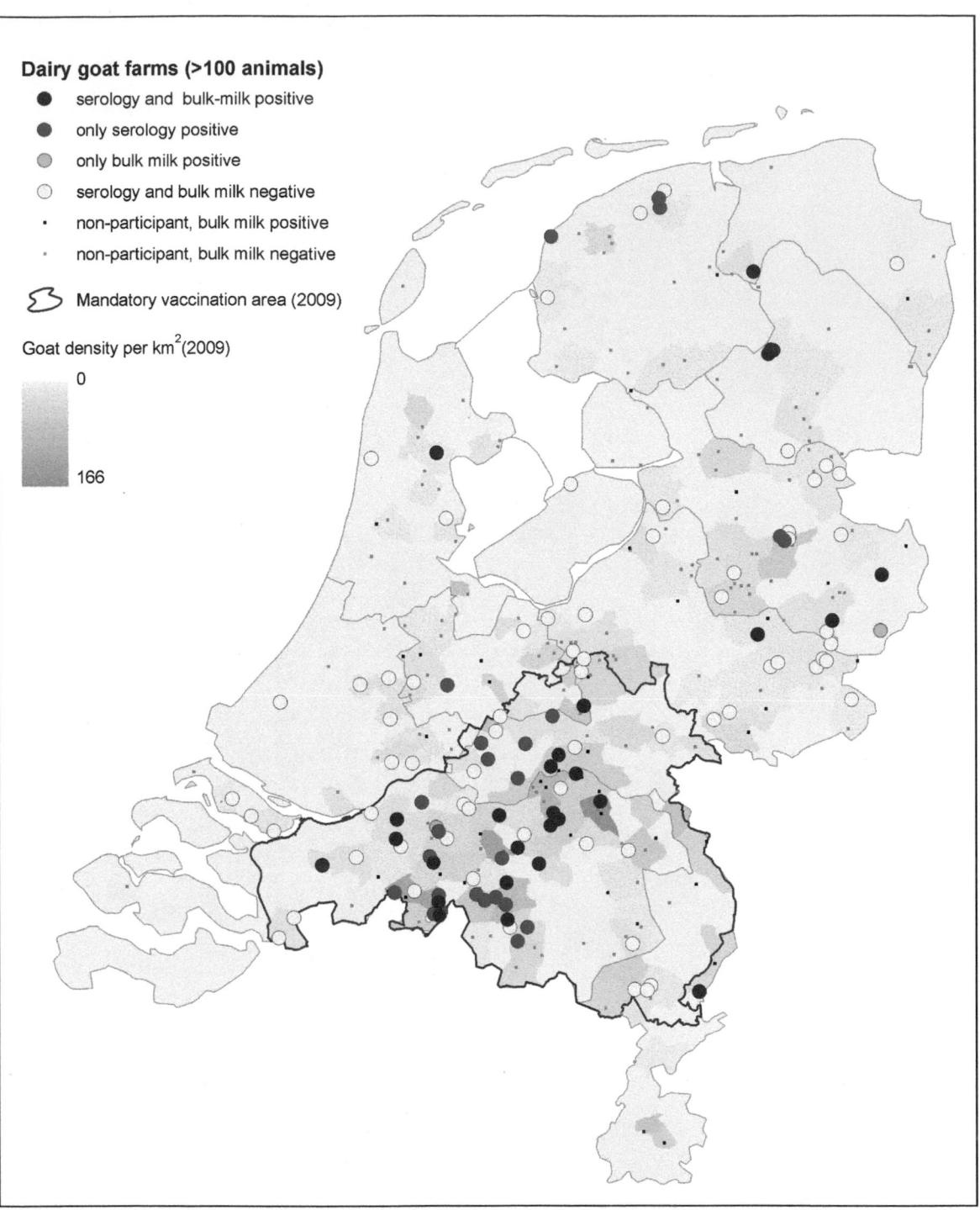

Plate 15.6 Map of the Netherlands showing the 12 provinces, the mandatory vaccination area (2009) and the geographic locations of 123 participating dairy goat farms (median 782 goats, range 120–4146) and 211 non-participating farms (median 689 goats, range 105–4733), the serological and bulk milk PCR (polymerase chain reaction) status of participating farms and bulk milk PCR status only of non-participating farms (from Schimmer *et al.*, 2011, reproduced with permission of the authors and Biomed Central).